AF719574

Malaria: Immune Response to Infection and Vaccination

Malaria: Immune Response to Infection and Vaccination

Editor: Jamie Spooner

FOSTER ACADEMICS
www.fosteracademics.com

www.fosteracademics.com

FOSTER ACADEMICS

Cataloging-in-Publication Data

Malaria : immune response to infection and vaccination / edited by Jamie Spooner.
p. cm.
Includes bibliographical references and index.
ISBN 978-1-64646-607-8
1. Malaria. 2. Malaria--Immunological aspects. 3. Malaria--Etiology. 4. Malaria--Vaccination.
5. Fever. 6. Protozoan diseases. I. Spooner, Jamie.
RA644.M2 M353 2023
614.532--dc23

© Foster Academics, 2023

Foster Academics,
118-35 Queens Blvd., Suite 400,
Forest Hills, NY 11375, USA

ISBN 978-1-64646-607-8 (Hardback)

This book contains information obtained from authentic and highly regarded sources. Copyright for all individual chapters remain with the respective authors as indicated. All chapters are published with permission under the Creative Commons Attribution License or equivalent. A wide variety of references are listed. Permission and sources are indicated; for detailed attributions, please refer to the permissions page and list of contributors. Reasonable efforts have been made to publish reliable data and information, but the authors, editors and publisher cannot assume any responsibility for the validity of all materials or the consequences of their use.

Trademark Notice: Registered trademark of products or corporate names are used only for explanation and identification without intent to infringe.

Contents

Preface

This book has been a concerted effort by a group of academicians, researchers and scientists, who have contributed their research works for the realization of the book. This book has materialized in the wake of emerging advancements and innovations in this field. Therefore, the need of the hour was to compile all the required researches and disseminate the knowledge to a broad spectrum of people comprising of students, researchers and specialists of the field.

Malaria refers to a type of mosquito-borne infectious disease that affects human beings and other animals. The symptoms of malaria typically include vomiting, fever, headaches and tiredness. It can result in major health issues including permanent organ damage and death, if not treated properly. It is caused by a single-celled parasite of the genus plasmodium. Malaria is diagnosed through antigen-based rapid diagnostic tests or microscopic examination of blood. Antimalarial medications such as atovaquone, mefloquine, primaquine, artemisinin drugs and doxycycline are used in the treatment of malaria. The use of vaccine considerably lowers the risk of malaria in young children. This book aims to understand the immune response to infection and vaccination in malaria. It includes some of the vital pieces of work being conducted across the world, on various topics related to this disease. The book is appropriate for students seeking detailed information on this medical condition as well as for experts.

At the end of the preface, I would like to thank the authors for their brilliant chapters and the publisher for guiding us all-through the making of the book till its final stage. Also, I would like to thank my family for providing the support and encouragement throughout my academic career and research projects.

Editor

1

A Synthetic Nanoparticle Based Vaccine Approach Targeting MSP4/5 is Immunogenic and Induces Moderate Protection Against Murine Blood-Stage Malaria

Kirsty L. Wilson[1,2], *Dodie Pouniotis*[2], *Jennifer Hanley*[1], *Sue D. Xiang*[1], *Charles Ma*[3], *Ross L. Coppel*[3] *and Magdalena Plebanski*[1,2*]

[1] *Department of Immunology and Pathology, Faculty of Medicine, Nursing and Health Sciences, Central Clinical School, Monash University, Melbourne, VIC, Australia,* [2] *School of Health and Biomedical Sciences, RMIT University, Bundoora, VIC, Australia,* [3] *Department of Microbiology, Monash University, Clayton, VIC, Australia*

***Correspondence:**
Magdalena Plebanski
magdalena.plebanski@rmit.edu.au

Malaria remains a significant health problem in many tropical and sub-tropical regions. The development of vaccines against the clinically active blood-stage of infection needs to consider variability and polymorphism in target antigens, and an adjuvant system able to induce broad spectrum immunity comprising both antibodies and helper T cells. Moreover, recent studies have shown some conventional pro-inflammatory adjuvants can also promote expansion of immunosuppressive regulatory T cells (Treg) and myeloid derived suppressor cells (MDSC), both of which could negatively impact malaria disease progression. Herein, we explore the ability of a model nanoparticle delivery system (polystyrene nanoparticles; PSNPs), previously proven to not induce conventional inflammation, Treg or MDSC, to induce immunity to MSP4/5 from *Plasmodium yoelii*, a member of the MSP4 and MSP5 family of proteins which are highly conserved across diverse malaria species including *P. falciparum*. The results show PSNPs-MSP4/5 conjugates are highly immunogenic, inducing immune responses comprising both T helper 1 (Th1) and Th2 cellular immunity, and a spectrum of antibody subclasses including IgG1, IgG2a, and IgG2b. Benchmarked against Alum and Complete Freund's Adjuvant (CFA), the immune responses that were induced were of comparable or higher magnitude, for both T cell frequencies by ELISpot and antibody responses in terms of ELISA end titer. Importantly, immunization with PSNPs-MSP4/5 induced partial protection against malaria blood-stage infection (50–80%) shown to be mechanistically dependent on interferon gamma (IFN-γ) production. These results expand the scope of adjuvants considered for malaria blood-stage vaccine development to those that do not use conventional adjuvant pathways and emphasizes the critical role of cellular immunity and specifically IFN-γ producing cells in providing moderate protection against blood-stage malaria comparable to Freunds adjuvant.

Keywords: blood-stage, malaria, nanoparticles, adjuvant, immunogenicity, protection

INTRODUCTION

Malaria remains a global health problem, affecting over 200 million people annually with ~40,000 deaths (1). It is caused by the plasmodium parasite, of which *Plasmodium falciparum* (*P. falciparum*) and *Plasmodium vivax (P. vivax)* are the most widespread. There is an urgent need for the development of an effective and long-lasting malaria vaccine. The most advanced pre-erythrocytic stage vaccine RTS, S provides <40% protection against disease in African populations (1, 2). Since any break-through parasites progressing to the blood-stage sustain transmission, pre-erythrocytic vaccines alone may be insufficient to support complete protection or eradication. Additionally, the blood-stage of malaria is symptomatic of disease, highlighting the need to eradicate parasites at or before this stage.

One of the major challenges to designing an effective vaccine for malaria is the identification of appropriate antigen targets. Many candidates are polymorphic or poorly immunogenic, thus making them inadequate vaccine antigens. One group of potential blood-stage vaccine antigens are the merozoite surface proteins (MSP) (3). MSP1, MSP2, and MSP3 have been used in human vaccine trials alone or in combination vaccines (4–6) but demonstrate little protective efficacy (6). Similar results have been seen with other leading blood-stage proteins from the merozoite, such as AMA1 which has shown promising humoral immunogenicity (7, 8) but only modest protective efficacy (9). However, there have been very few trials assessing efficacy in humans, particularly in children for blood-stage vaccines and many more are needed. Vaccine development at this stage mainly focuses on generating a neutralizing antibody response to prevent erythrocyte invasion (similar to that seen with naturally acquired immunity) though inducing strong cellular responses may be just as important to promote protection. Therefore, it is important to identify the antigenic epitopes that are not only highly immunogenic but also protective.

MSP4 and MSP5 are candidates for blood-stage vaccines as they show limited antigenic diversity in both *P. falciparum* (10–12) and *P. vivax* (13, 14). MSP5 is largely conserved across both these strains, and also geographic locations of Plasmodium (15), with polymorphisms detected only in specific gene regions (16). Naturally acquired antibodies have been detected to MSP4 (17, 18) and high antibody levels have been associated with a protective role in subsequent malaria seasons (18), though the precise cause of protection in these cohorts is yet to be fully defined. Similarly, naturally acquired antibodies against MSP4 are associated with reduced clinical malaria cases (19) and low level frequency of cross reactive antibodies have been detected to both *P. falciparum* and *P. vivax* (20). Though possibly attributed to anti-MSP antibody production, the exact correlates of protection in these studies are yet to be identified, although it does indicate these antigens are good candidates for inclusion in vaccines. Importantly, functional MSP5 specific T cell responses have also been observed to *P. falciparum* and *P. vivax* (21). The low antigen diversity of MSP4 and MSP5 and correlation with protection makes them attractive vaccine candidates compared to the large number of other highly polymorphic antigens. In animal studies, the murine equivalent homolog of MSP4 and MSP5, MSP4/5, has shown protection using different vaccine formulations (22–25), and protection is enhanced when administered in combination with MSP1 (26). Most of these studies examine antibodies in the protective response, with less known about the protective role of the cellular immune response. One study showed that the selected adjuvant AFCo1 (synthetic cochleate structures) enhanced both antibodies and T cell responses against MSP4/5, attributable to the induced Th1-like immune responses (27). Thus, it is important for vaccine design to not only aim to induce antibody responses, but also cell mediated immunity.

One possible reason for the low protective responses seen in recent malaria vaccine trials may be due in part to adjuvant or vaccine delivery platform selection. Optimal antigen and adjuvant combinations are imperative for vaccine efficacy. Alum is currently one of the only licensed adjuvants for widespread human use (28) and the RTS, S vaccine in humans contains the proprietary adjuvant AS01, consisting of liposomes, monophosphoryl lipid A (MPLA, the non toxic derivative of LPS) and the saponin QS-21 (29). Both these adjuvants, as well as most adjuvants in development for human use, are pro-inflammatory (inducing cytokines such as interleukin [IL-6] and/or tumor necrosis factor [TNF]) (30). Recent literature suggests that such pro-inflammatory adjuvants could also promote the subsequent expansion of regulatory T cells (Treg) and myeloid derived suppressor cells (MDSC), which may be a natural mechanism aimed to turn off excessive inflammation (31). This property may limit the persistence of immunity, as well as potentially increase the frequency of cells such as TNFR2+ Treg associated with the development of severe malaria (32). It is therefore useful to explore whether non-inflammatory adjuvants and vaccine carriers, which do not induce Treg or MDSC, can also induce malaria specific immunity of sufficient type and magnitude to protect against a malaria challenge.

Viral sized 40–50 nm polystyrene nanoparticles (PSNPs) are non-inflammatory and when used as adjuvanting antigen carriers in experimental vaccines, induce high levels of CD4+ and CD8+ T cells, as well as antibodies (33–37). Though there are many different types of nanoparticles currently being used for malaria vaccines (38, 39) [reviewed in Powles et al. (40)], PSNPs in this size range (and negatively charged) can target antigen presenting cells (APCs) in the local lymph nodes to increase uptake and presentation of the vaccine antigen, leading to long lasting protective immune responses in murine studies (33, 34, 36). These PSNPs have been shown to induce high level CD8+ T cell responses when covalently coupled with malaria liver stage peptide epitopes, however not when simply "mixing" the PSNPs with the peptide (31, 41). Moreover, they have been confirmed to be "inert" in terms of failing to activate inflammatory cytokine or MAPK/ERK mediated inflammatory pathways (37, 42) and do not induce TNFR2+ Treg or MDSC (31). These inert and biocompatible PSNPs have repeatedly shown to be safe and well-tolerated in numerous animal models at both low and high doses (33, 36, 37, 43, 44), and can be coupled to different protein and peptide antigens with high efficiency and loading capacities (31, 37, 44). Additionally, recent pre-clinical studies progressing the translation of this approach as a cancer vaccine have seen no toxic or inflammatory effects when injecting similar PSNP doses in mice for up to 4 times at weekly intervals (44). Whilst the exact clearance mechanism of these PSNPs is unknown, it is known that nanoparticles in this viral size range allow their excretion from the body via hepatobiliary elimination and ultimately via feces (45).

Herein we assess both the immunogenicity and protective efficacy of blood-stage malaria vaccines in an animal model of malaria, formulated using PSNP antigen carriers using MSP4/5 as the target antigen and compared to formulations with MSP4/5 adjuvanted with Alum or the experimental adjuvant Complete Freund's Adjuvant (CFA).

MATERIALS AND METHODS

Mice

Six-to-eight-week-old BALB/c and IFN-γ gene knock out (KO) mice were purchased from the Austin Research Institute or Monash Animal Services. Austin Health and the Alfred Medical Research and Education Precinct (AMREP) Animal Ethics Committees approved the use of all animals and procedures.

Recombinant MSP4/5 Production

Recombinant MSP4/5 generated in *E. coli*, described in Kedzierski et al. (22), was kindly provided by Professor R. Coppel for use in these studies. The protein concentration of recombinant MSP4/5 was determined by Bicinchoninic Assay (BCA, Thermo Fisher) following manufacturer's instructions.

Conjugation of MSP4/5 to PSNPs

Conjugation of MSP4/5 to PSNPs was performed as described previously (35, 37). Briefly, 40–50 nm carboxylated polystyrene nanoparticles (PSNPs, Polysciences Inc, USA) at a final 1% solids ($\sim 1.9 \times 10^{14}$ PSNPs/ml, unless otherwise stated) were pre-activated using a 2-*N*-morpholino-ethanesulfonicacid buffered (MES; 50 mM final, pH 6.2) solution of 1-ethyl-3-(3-dimethylaminoproplyl) carbodiimide hydrochloride (EDC; 4 mg/ml final) (Sigma Aldrich) (with sulfo-NHS for some conjugations) for 15 minutes on a rotating wheel at room temperature (RT). MSP4/5 was added (target final concentration of 0.4 or 1 mg/ml) and further incubated for 2–3 hours (h) at RT. The conjugation reaction was stopped by the addition of glycine (7 mg/ml final) for a further 30 minutes at RT. Conjugation mixture was dialyzed using 100–300 kDa dialysis membrane overnight against phosphate buffered saline (PBS) at 4°C. Dialysis against 100–300 kDa cutoff membrane permits retention of the PSNPs conjugated to the antigen, and any remaining activating agents and unconjugated protein [MSP4/5 is ~36kDa (24)] are dialyzed out. This process also allows for buffer exchange into a physiological solution, such as PBS, for immunizations. Conjugated PSNPs were stored at 4°C and sonicated for 15 minutes before use to create a uniform and homogenous formulation for immunizations.

Vaccine Formulations and Immunizations

Mice were immunized intradermally (id) once or twice with the following vaccine formulations: 100 μl of either PSNPs conjugated to MSP4/5 or MSP4/5 with adjuvant, 2–3 weeks apart for immunogenicity studies. Adjuvanted vaccine formulations contained either Alum (Rehydragel HPA, General Chemical) at 0.3 g/ml with MSP4/5 in PBS, or a prime with MSP4/5 emulsified in CFA at a 1:1 v/v ratio and boost with Incomplete Freund's Adjuvant (IFA) at a 1:1 v/v ratio. Ten to fourteen days following the last immunization, mice were humanely sacrificed by CO_2 asphyxiation. Conjugated and adjuvanted MSP4/5 protein doses, immunization volume and route were matched per experiment, with specific vaccine formulations provided in each of the figure legends. For challenge experiments, mice were injected with parasitized red blood cells (pRBCs) 3 weeks following the last immunization (see detailed procedure below).

ELISpot

Splenocytes from immunized animals were isolated from 10 to 14 days following the last immunization and assessed by ELISpot for IFN-γ and IL-4 production. Ninety six well multiscreen plates (MAHA, MAIP or MSIP, Millipore) were coated overnight at 4°C with 5 μg/ml anti-mouse IFN-γ (AN18, Mabtech) or anti-mouse IL-4 (BVD4-1d11, Mabtech or BD Biosciences). All wells were washed 5 times with PBS and blocked with RPMI 1640 (Gibco, Life technologies) containing 10% FBS (further supplemented with 100 units/ml penicillin, 100 μg/ml streptomycin, 4 mM L-glutamine, 1 M Hepes, and 0.1 mM 2- mercaptoethanol, to make complete media) for 2 h at 37°C. Splenocytes were added at a final concentration of 0.5×10^6 or 1×10^6 cells per well and co-incubated with recall antigens (MSP4/5 at 15–25 μg/ml final for each recall antigen) in complete media for 12–16 h at 37°C. Media alone and positive control Concanavalin A (1 μg/ml final) wells were also added. Following incubation, plates were washed with PBS (MSIP plates) or PBS containing 0.05% Tween 20 (MAHA and MAIP plates) and 1 μg/ml anti-mouse IFN-γ-biotin (R4-6A2, Mabtech) or anti-mouse IL-4-biotin (BVD6-24G2, Mabtech or BD Biosciences) in 0.5% FBS/PBS was added for 2 h at RT. Plates were washed and 1 μg/ml Streptavidin-ALP or extravidin-ALP in 0.5% FBS/PBS was added for a further 1–2 h at RT. Plates were given a final wash with PBS followed by reverse osmosis water and spots were developed using an AP colorimetric kit (Bio-Rad). Once plates were dry, spots were counted using an AID ELISpot Reader system (AutoImmune Diagnostika, GmbH, Germany).

ELISA

Sera from immunized animals was collected at endpoint and assessed for antigen specific antibody production by ELISA. Ninety six well plates (polyvinyl chloride micro-titer plates, Costar, or Nunc Maxisorp plates) were coated with 5 μg/ml of MSP4/5 in carbonate/bicarbonate coating buffer overnight at 4°C. Plates were washed with 0.05% Tween 20/PBS and blocked with 2% bovine serum albumin (BSA)/PBS or 5% skim milk/PBS and incubated for 1 h at 37°C. Plates were washed as above and serial dilutions of sera added and incubated for 2 h at 37°C (or 4°C overnight). Plates were washed and horseradish peroxidase (HRP) conjugated anti-mouse total Ig or IgG antibodies (1/2000 dilution for total IgG/A/M, Zymed, and sheep anti-mouse IgG, Amersham Biosciences, UK) added for 1 h at 37°C. Where indicated HRP conjugated subclass antibodies were used as the secondary antibody and incubated for 1 h at 37°C (HRP-IgG1 at final 1/1,000, HRP-IgG2a at final 1/1,000 and IgG2b-biotin at final 1/250 dilution, BD Biosciences). Biotinylated secondary antibodies were followed with a further incubation of streptavidin-HRP (1/1,000, Amersham biosciences) for 1 h at 37°C. Plates were given a final wash and antibody detection was developed using ABTS or TMB substrate solution before being stopped with 1 M HCl. Absorbance was read at optical density (OD) 405–450 nm on a plate reader (Fluostar Optima, BMG lab technologies, or Multiscan GO, Thermo Fisher). Antibody end titers were calculated closest to the serum dilution at which the OD was equal to the mean of the naïve sera (averaged across naïve mice for all dilutions tested) plus 3 standard deviations.

Malaria Infection Challenge

Plasmodium yoelii parasites were cultured *in vivo* in naïve mice and pRBCs harvested when mice reached a required level of parasitemia (~4–5%). pRBCs were harvested from infected mice and experimental mice were infected with 5×10^4 or 5×10^5 pRBCs in PBS by intraperitoneal injection (total volume 100 μl, 50 μl either side of abdomen). Blood parasitemia levels were monitored every 1-2 days beginning from day 3 until ~21–25 days post-infection. Blood parasitemia levels were calculated by venous blood smears that were Giemsa stained and counted using a light microscope. A representative field at 100X magnification was chosen and the number of pRBCs including all ring, merozoite, and schizont stages calculated compared to the total number of RBCs in the field. Mice were humanely euthanized when blood parasitemia levels reached >70%, according to ethical approval, and parasitemia levels and number of surviving mice (% survival) at each time point calculated.

Statistics

Statistical analysis was performed as follows; One or two-way ANOVA with *post hoc* Tukey analysis was used to assess differences between groups for immunogenicity (ELISpot and ELISA) assays. Kaplan Meyer survival curves with log-rank (Mantel-Cox) test comparisons were used for survival analysis. All statistical analyses were performed using Graphpad Prism software (v.7.02) and statistical significance was set at $p < 0.05$. Data is expressed as mean ± standard deviation (SD) for each group, with group sizes and additional information indicated in the relevant figure legends.

RESULTS

Highly Immunogenic Vaccine Formulations of PSNPs Conjugated to MSP4/5 (PSNPs-MSP4/5) Induce Broad Immune Responses Including Th1 and Th2 Cells and Multiple Antibody Subclasses

Identifying an immunogenic and highly conserved protein for blood-stage malaria remains a challenge for vaccine development. MSP4 and MSP5 are promising blood-stage vaccine candidates in humans, as they are relatively conserved in different strains of Plasmodium compared to other highly polymorphic antigens. The murine equivalent *P. yoelii* MSP4/5 has been identified as a protective blood-stage antigen in prior murine studies (23, 25, 46), therefore, we wanted to assess this protein using our nanoparticle delivery system.

To assess the immunogenicity of PSNPs-MSP4/5 we compared this vaccine to one containing MSP4/5 mixed with the most widely used adjuvant, Alum. BALB/c mice were immunized twice intradermally at the base of tail and 14 days following the last immunization T cell (from whole splenocytes) and serum antibody responses were measured by ELISpot and ELISA, respectively. PSNPs-MSP4/5 immunization elicited high levels of antigen specific IFN-γ producing T cells, significantly higher than mice immunized with Alum and naïve controls (**Figure 1A**, $p < 0.0001$). Whilst Alum did not induce significantly higher IFN-γ producing T cells above control conditions, both the PSNPs-MSP4/5 and Alum + MSP4/5 groups induced similar levels of IL-4 producing T cells compared to naïve mice (**Figure 1B**, $p < 0.001$, $p < 0.01$, respectively). Alum is known to induce Th2 biased responses which is reflected in the above results. Furthermore, when looking at total antibody levels induced by vaccination, both Alum and PSNPs induced comparable levels of total Ig (**Figure 1C**) and similar levels of IgG1 antibodies (**Figure 1D**), the latter being classically associated with a Th2 response. Mice immunized with PSNPs-MSP4/5 developed higher IgG2a and IgG2b antibodies compared to either the Alum + MSP4/5 or the naïve groups but these responses were not significant (**Figures 1E, F**). These results indicate PSNPs induce a spectrum of IgG antibody subclasses as well as both IFN-γ-producing Th1 and IL-4-producing Th2 cells.

Comparable Immunogenicity of PSNPs-MSP4/5 Nanovaccines Against "Gold Standard" Experimental Vaccine Formulations of MSP4/5 in CFA/IFA

The immune responses generated by PSNPs-MSP4/5 immunizations were comparatively similar for Th2, and better for Th1 type responses, compared to the conventional adjuvant Alum. Therefore, we further tested the robustness of these responses against the strong experimental Th1 inducing adjuvant, CFA, followed by a boost with IFA, and compared against one or two immunizations with PSNPs-MSP4/5. MSP4/5 in CFA/IFA induced functional IFN-γ and IL-4 producing T cells, as well as IgG antibodies, significantly higher than naïve mice (**Figures 2A–C**, $p < 0.0001$, $p < 0.001$, $p < 0.01$, respectively). One immunization with PSNPs-MSP4/5 was comparable to MSP4/5 in CFA/IFA for both IFN-γ and IL-4 producing T cell immune responses (**Figures 2A,B**), and significantly higher than naïve responses (**Figures 2A,B**, $p < 0.0001$). Two immunizations with PSNPs-MSP4/5 elicited the highest levels of IFN-γ and IL-4 T cell responses, significantly higher than all other groups for IFN-γ producing T cells (**Figure 2A**, $p < 0.0001$ compared to naïve, $p < 0.001$ compared to CFA/IFA and $p < 0.01$ compared to one immunization with PSNPs-MSP4/5) and significantly higher than MSP4/5 in CFA/IFA and naïve groups for IL-4 producing T cell responses (**Figure 2B**, $p < 0.0001$ compared to naïve and $p < 0.01$ compared to CFA/ IFA). Antibody titers were also different when comparing one vs. two immunizations with PSNPs-MSP4/5. Two immunizations of PSNPs-MSP4/5 elicited

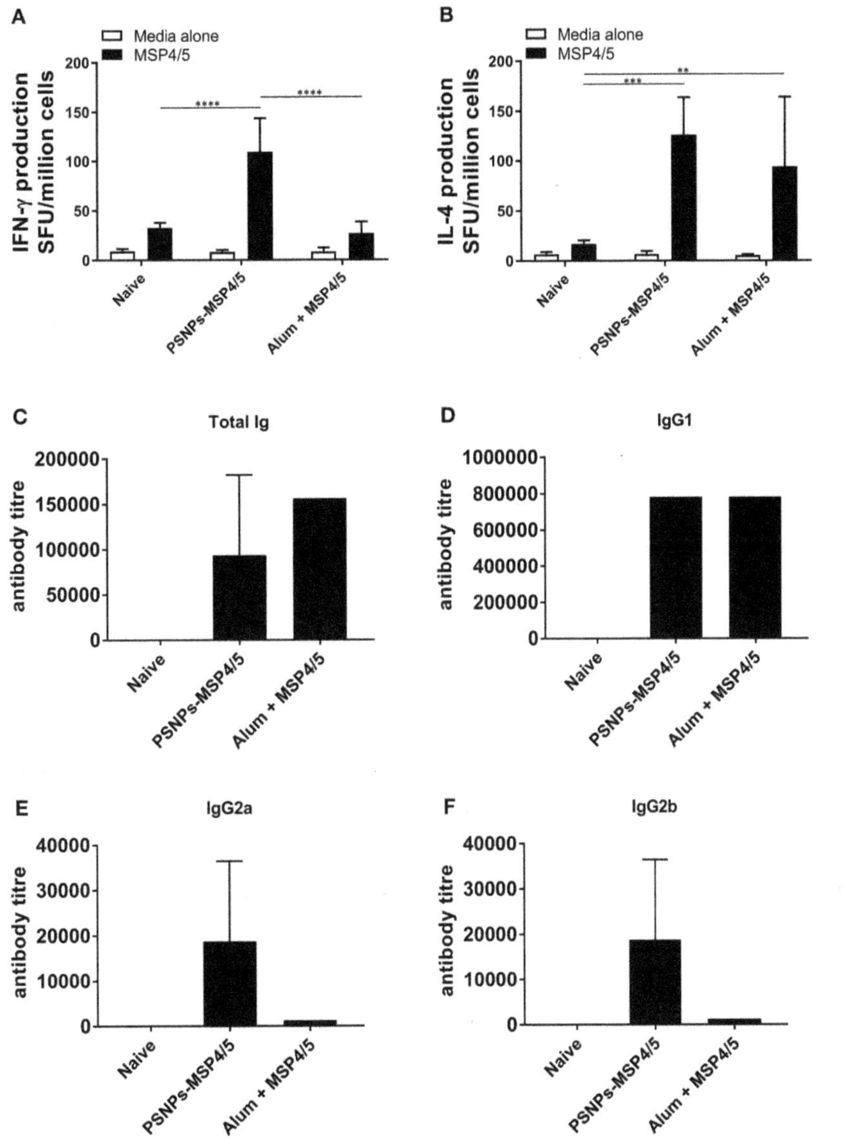

FIGURE 1 | Diverse Th1 and Th2 associated immunogenicity induced by PSNPs-MSP4/5 compared to Alum adjuvanted vaccines. BALB/c mice were immunized twice intradermally at the base of tail (100 µl/immunization), 14 days apart with PBS (Naive), PSNPs conjugated to MSP4/5 (PSNPs-MSP4/5, 40 µg/ml) or MSP4/5 in Alum (Alum + MSP4/5, 0.3 g/ml Alum and 40 µg/ml MSP4/5 in PBS). Fourteen days after the last immunization, mice were humanely sacrificed and splenocytes and serum collected for immunogenicity analysis. **(A)** IFN-γ and **(B)** IL-4 producing T cells were assessed by ELISpot and **(C)** Total IgG/A/M, **(D)** IgG1, **(E)** IgG2a, and **(F)** IgG2b anti-MSP4/5 antibody levels were measured by ELISA. Data is shown as mean spot forming units (SFU) ± SD for ELISpot and mean antibody titer ± SD of duplicate measurements of pooled sera per group for ELISA. $^{**}p < 0.01$, $^{***}p < 0.001$, $^{****}p < 0.0001$ by two-way ANOVA with *post hoc* Tukey analysis. $n = 4$ mice per group.

higher antibody titers compared to one immunization with PSNPs-MSP4/5 (**Figure 2C**, not significant) and comparable antibody titers to MSP4/5 in CFA/IFA (**Figure 2C**). MSP4/5 in CFA/IFA induced a significantly higher antibody end titre compared to only one immunization of PSNPs-MSP4/5 (**Figure 2C**, $p < 0.05$).

Immunization with PSNPs-MSP4/5 showed strong T cell and antibody responses, especially following a two-immunization regime, therefore, we next determined the effect of PSNP dose on the resulting immune response. De-escalating doses of PSNPs (2.1×10^{14}, 3.7×10^{13}, and 1.7×10^{13} PSNP/ml) conjugated to matched levels of MSP4/5 were used to assess the potential for dose-sparing of the vaccine preparation, for both immunogenicity and protection studies. As IFN-γ has been identified as the key protective cytokine (47), the effect of different doses of PSNPs (conjugated to the same amount of MSP4/5) were assessed for their ability to affect the resulting IFN-γ T cell response. De-escalating doses of the PSNPs were compared to CFA/IFA adjuvated formulations for IFN-γ T cell responses following two immunizations. As

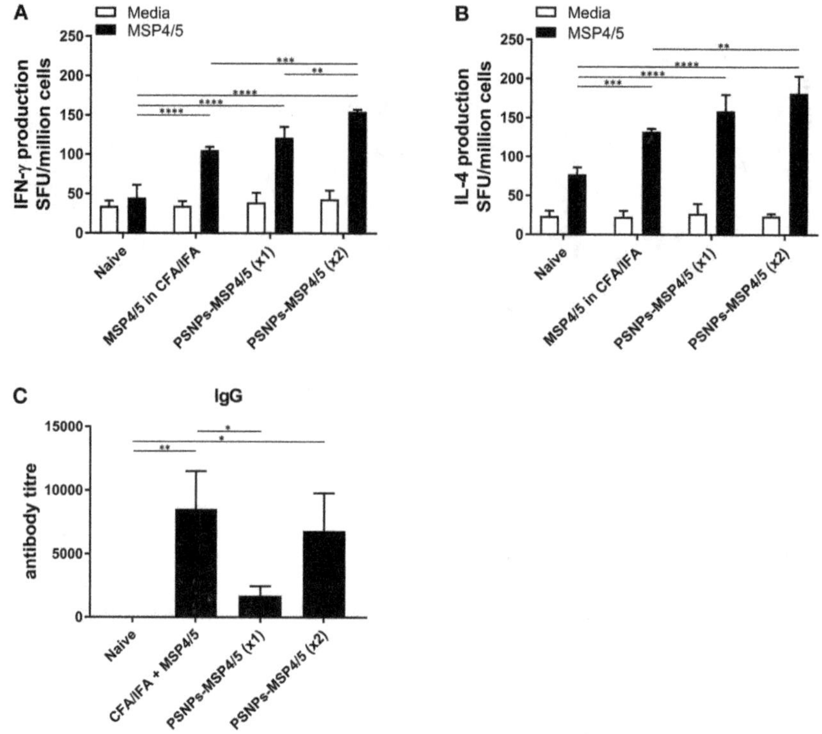

FIGURE 2 | Immunogenicity of PSNPs-MSP4/5 is comparable to CFA/IFA adjuvanted vaccines. BALB/c mice were immunized intradermally (100 μl per immunization) with one (PSNPs-MSP4/5 x1) or two (PSNPs-MSP4/5 x2) immunizations of PSNPs-MSP4/5 (100 μg/ml), or MSP4/5 in CFA (100 μg/ml MSP4/5 mixed 1:1 v/v in CFA) followed by MSP4/5 in IFA (100 μg/ml MSP4/5 mixed 1:1 v/v in IFA), or twice with PBS alone (Naïve). Ten days after the last immunization, mice were humanely sacrificed and splenocytes and serum collected for immunogenicity analysis. **(A)** IFNγ and **(B)** IL-4 producing T cells were assessed by ELISpot assay and **(C)** Total IgG antibody levels were measured by ELISA. Data is shown as mean SFU ± SD per group for ELISpot and mean antibody titer ± SD per group for ELISA. *$p < 0.05$, **$p < 0.01$, ***$p < 0.001$, ****$p < 0.0001$ by two-way ANOVA for ELISPOT and one-way ANOVA for ELISA analyses. $n = 6–8$ mice per group.

expected, MSP4/5 in CFA/IFA produced significantly higher T cell responses compared to controls (**Figure 3**, $p < 0.05$ compared to MSP4/5 alone and naïve). The three doses of PSNPs-MSP4/5 elicited differing IFN-γ T cell responses. Both the highest and lowest PSNP doses (2.1×10^{14} and 1.7×10^{13} PSNPs/ml-MSP4/5) induced IFN-γ producing T cell responses comparable to CFA/IFA adjuvanted vaccines and both significantly higher than control groups (**Figure 3**, $p < 0.0001$ 2.1×10^{14} PSNPs-MSP4/5 compared to MSP4/5 alone, $p < 0.001$ compared to naïve, $p < 0.001$ 1.7×10^{13} PSNPs-MSP4/5 compared to MSP4/5 alone, $p < 0.01$, compared to naïve). Unexpectedly, both the highest and lowest PSNP doses also induced significantly higher IFN-γ T cell responses compared to the 3.7×10^{13} PSNPs-MSP4/5 dose (**Figure 3**, $p < 0.01$ and $p < 0.05$, respectively), indicating no clear titratable effect of the PSNPs dose.

Immunization With PSNPs-MSP4/5 Induces Survival Against Blood-Stage Malaria Infection

Not only is it important to identify vaccine formulations that elicit strong T cell and antibody responses, they also need to translate into a clinical effect of blood-stage protection and/or enhanced survival. To investigate this, mice were immunized twice, 3 weeks apart with de-escalating doses of PSNPs-MSP4/5 and MSP4/5 in CFA/IFA. Two weeks following immunizations, mice were then challenged with *P. yoelii* parasites and monitored for parasitemia levels and overall survival. Mice reached end point when blood smears showed over 70% parasitemia levels. All groups survived significantly longer than naïve mice (**Figure 4A**, $p < 0.001$ for MSP4/5 in CFA/IFA and $p < 0.01$ for all doses PSNPs-MSP4/5, compared to naive mice) as shown on the Kaplan-Meyer survival curve. Despite observing different survival curve patterns, there were no significant differences between MSP4/5 in CFA/IFA and the three doses of PSNPs-MSP4/5 up until 21 days post-challenge, indicating these are comparably protective vaccine formulations. In terms of overall survival, the control naïve mice all reached endpoint parasitemia's (**Figure 4B**). All mice in the MSP3/5 in CFA/IFA group resolved their parasitemia levels 6/6 (**Figure 4C**), in comparison to 5/6 mice in both the 3.7×10^{13} and 1.7×10^{13} PSNPs-MSP4/5 groups (**Figures 4E,F**), and 3/6 mice in the 2.1×10^{14} PSNP-MSP4/5 group resolved their parasitemia levels (**Figure 4D**). This suggests the observed partial protection is not dependent on PSNP dose, regardless of significant differences in immune responses induced.

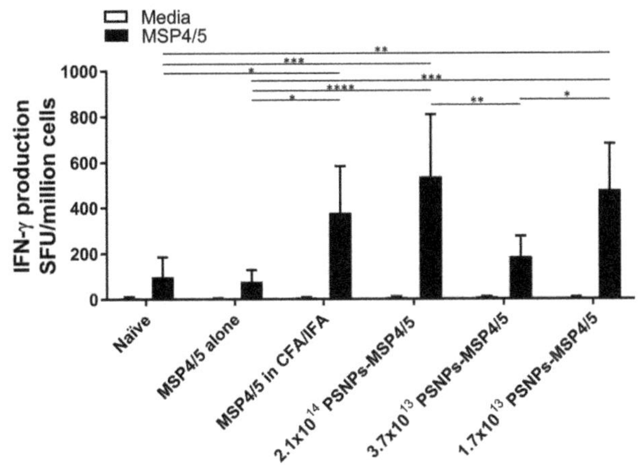

FIGURE 3 | IFN-γ producing T cell responses induced by de-escalating doses of PSNPs compared to CFA/IFA. BALB/c mice were immunized intradermally at the base of tail (100 μl/immunization) and boosted 3 weeks later with PBS alone (Naïve), MSP4/5 alone (80 μg per mouse), MSP4/5 in CFA (80 μg per mouse, 1:1 v/v with CFA) for the initial immunization and MSP4/5 in IFA (80 μg per mouse, 1:1 v/v with IFA) for the boost, or 3 different doses of PSNPs conjugated to MSP4/5 (2.1×10^{14}, 3.7×10^{13}, 1.7×10^{1} PSNPs/ml, 80 μg MSP4/5 per mouse). Fourteen days after the last immunization, mice were humanely sacrificed and splenocytes and serum collected for immunogenicity analysis. IFN-γ producing T cells were assessed by ELISpot. Data is shown as mean SFU ± SD per group for ELISpot $^{*}p < 0.05$, $^{**}p < 0.01$, $^{***}p < 0.001$, $^{****}p < 0.0001$ by two-way ANOVA with *post hoc* Tukey analysis. $n = 4$ mice per group.

Moderate Blood-Stage Malaria Protection Induced by PSNPs-MSP4/5 Is IFN-γ dependent

In the above studies, high levels of IFN-γ and IL-4 producing T cells were induced by PSNPs-MSP4/5 vaccine formulations, as well as antibody responses including diverse IgG subclasses. Generally, functional antibodies have been associated with protective responses in humans for blood-stage malaria, with few studies characterizing the T cell response (48, 49). IFN-γ has been reported to be protective in prior *P. yoelii* liver stage murine malaria models (50), and *P. chabaudi* blood-stage infections (51), therefore, we wanted to assess mechanistically the necessity of IFN-γ production in protecting mice from blood-stage malaria immunized with PSNPs-MSP4/5. Wild type (WT) or IFN-γ KO (IFN-γ KO) BALB/c mice were immunized twice, intradermally, 2 weeks apart, with PSNPs-MSP4/5 and 2 weeks following the last immunization, mice were challenged with *P. yoelii* parasites and monitored for survival and parasitemia levels. As expected, naïve WT mice reached parasitemias over 70% (**Figures 5A,B**). PSNPs-MSP4/5 immunized WT mice were significantly protected in comparison to naive WT mice (**Figure 5A**, $p < 0.01$), with 3/6 mice protected up to 25 days post-infection and resolving their parasitemia levels (**Figures 5A,C**). Both the naïve and PSNPs-MSP4/5 experimental groups reached parasitemias above 70% in the IFN-γ KO mice (**Figures 5A,D,E**). There was a significant difference in survival between the PSNPs-MSP4/5 immunized WT mice compared to PSNPs-MSP4/5 immunized IFN-γ KO mice (**Figure 5A**, $p < 0.01$) suggesting protection may be IFN-γ dependent. There was also a significant difference between the immunized WT mice compared to naive WT mice (**Figure 5A**, $p< 0.01$), but no significant difference between the immunized and naïve IFN-γ KO mice. Some naive IFN-γ KO mice survived for marginally longer than PSNPs-MSP4/5 immunized mice, though this result was not significant.

Furthermore, antibody responses pre-challenge demonstrated high levels of IgG1 antibodies in PSNPs-MSP4/5 immunized mice in both the WT and IFN-γ KO mice, with both inducing antibody titres significantly higher than WT naïve mice and IFN-γ KO naïve mice (**Figure 5F**, $p < 0.0001$). PSNPs-MSP4/5 immunized WT mice also induced significantly higher IgG1 antibody levels compared to PSNPs-MSP4/5 immunized IFN-γ KO mice (**Figure 5F**, $p < 0.05$). IgG2a and IgG2b induction was impaired in IFN-γ KO mice but not in WT mice when immunized with PSNPs-MSP4/5. IgG2a antibody levels elicited by PSNPs-MSP4/5 in WT mice were significantly higher than WT naïve mice and both IFN-γ KO naïve and immunized mice (**Figure 5G**, $p < 0.001$). IgG2b antibodies were also significantly higher in the WT PSNPs-MSP4/5 immunized mice compared to WT naïve and IFN-γ KO naïve mice (**Figure 5H**, $p < 0.001$) and PSNPs-MSP4/5 immunized IFN-γ KO mice (**Figure 5H**, $p < 0.01$). These results may be explained when considering IgG1 antibodies are induced by IL-4 and associated with Th2 responses and IgG2 antibodies are associated with Th1 responses a and dependent on IFN-γ.

DISCUSSION

The present study shows immune responses induced by a biocompatible nanoparticle carrier vaccine approach can induce immunity and moderate protection against blood-stage malaria comparable to the "gold standard" experimental adjuvant CFA. This finding adds to the repertoire of possible adjuvants and vaccine approaches in development, by showing that delivering a classical pro-inflammatory danger signal is not necessary to induce immune responses of sufficient magnitude, or of the type, necessary to protect against blood-stage malaria infection. We note, however, that associations of immune responses with protection do not necessarily imply causality. Nonetheless, the above results support the MSP4 and MSP5 families as candidate antigens for vaccine development when used with an appropriate delivery system.

PSNPs have repeatedly shown, in a range of disease models, to be non-inflammatory and capable of inducing robust immune responses without the addition of T helper epitopes or additional stimuli (31, 37, 42, 44, 52). Side by side comparisons of immunogenicity elicited by PSNPs-MSP4/5 showed them to be capable of producing superior cellular responses to MSP4/5 in Alum, inducing balanced Th1 and Th2 responses, as well as comparable responses to MSP4/5 in CFA/IFA vaccine formulations, the latter representing a gold standard level of immune responses in experimental models. Similar results were obtained with MSP4/5 with an alternative production system in *Saccharomyces cerevisiae* (unpublished).

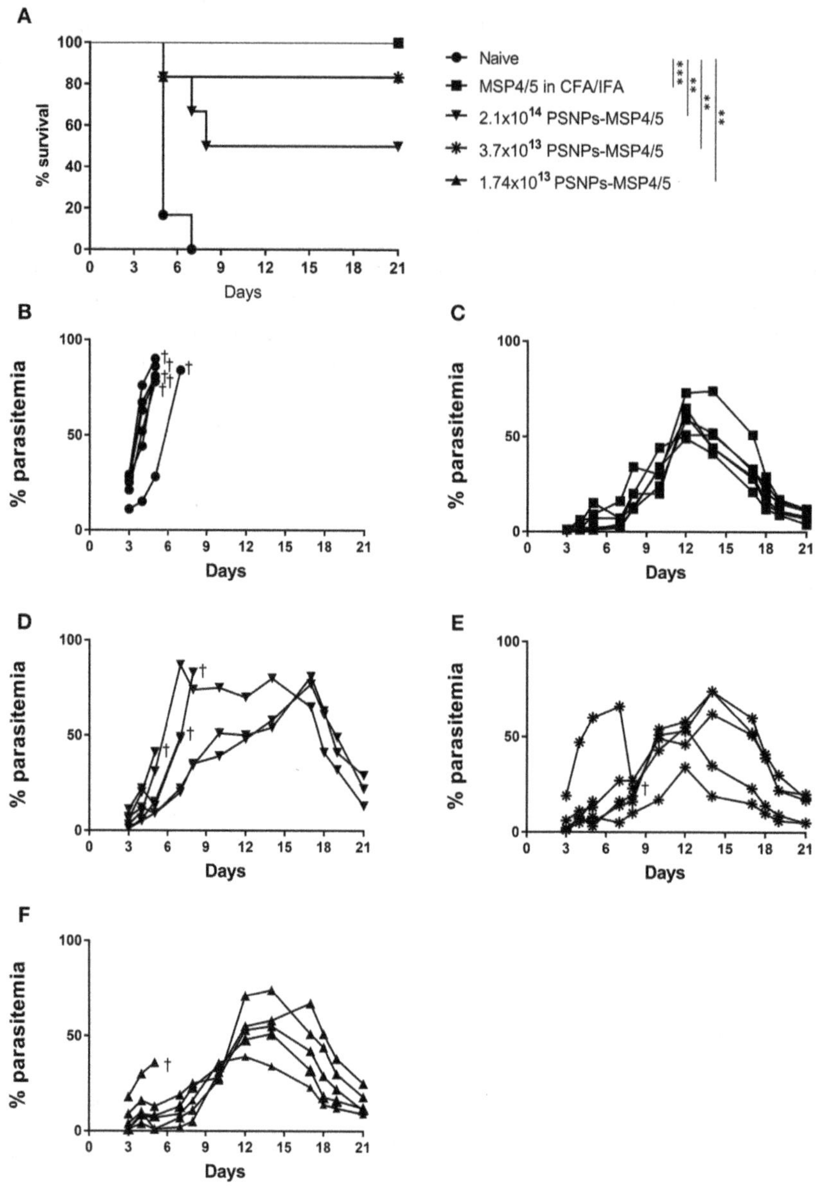

FIGURE 4 | Moderate survival against blood-stage malaria infection following immunization with de-escalating doses of PSNPs compared to CFA/IFA adjuvanted vaccines. BALB/c mice were immunized intradermally at the base of tail (100 μl/immunization) and then a boost 3 weeks later with PBS alone (Naïve), MSP4/5 in CFA (80 μg per mouse, first immunization) or MSP4/5 in IFA (80 μg per mouse, boost immunization) or 3 different doses of PSNPs-MSP4/5 (2.1×10^{14}, 3.7×10^{13}, 1.7×10^{13} PSNPs/ml). Fourteen days after the last immunization, mice were challenged intraperitoneally with 5×10^5 *P. yoelii* pRBCs and parasitemia levels were monitored starting at 3 days post-challenge. **(A)** Kaplan-Meier survival curve and percentage parasitemias of mice immunized with **(B)** Naïve -●-, **(C)** MSP4/5 in CFA/IFA -■-, **(D)** 2.1×10^{14} PSNPs-MSP4/5 -▼-, **(E)** 3.7×10^{13} PSNPs-MSP4/5 -✻- and **(F)** 1.74×10^{13} PSNPs-MSP4/5 -▲-. $^{**}p < 0.01$, $^{***}p < 0.001$, with Mantel Cox Log Rank Test. †Indicates mouse endpoint. Data shown are from 6 mice per experimental group.

Antigen specific IFN-γ production by T cells was predominantly measured in the present study, though as whole splenocytes were used in the assays there is a possibility that IFN-γ production from other cell types (i.e. NK cells) may also be measured, but unlikely to this protein antigen. The cells that respond in ELISpot assays are predominantly T cells, as shown by depletion assays (53–55). Dose-sparing of the PSNP formulations unexpectedly showed that the middle dose induced significantly lower IFN-γ producing T cell responses, compared to the highest and lowest PSNP doses. Therefore, it will be useful in future studies to explore the dose dependency of other types of immune responses.

PSNPs-MSP4/5 formulations showed substantial improvement over MSP4/5 in Alum formulations in the elicitation of specific antibody subclasses such as IgG2a and IgG2b, but not total Ig or IgG1. Although the antibody titers induced by PSNPs-MSP4/5 vaccines were lower than the "gold standard" MSP4/5 in CFA/IFA, PSNPs-MSP4/5 vaccines

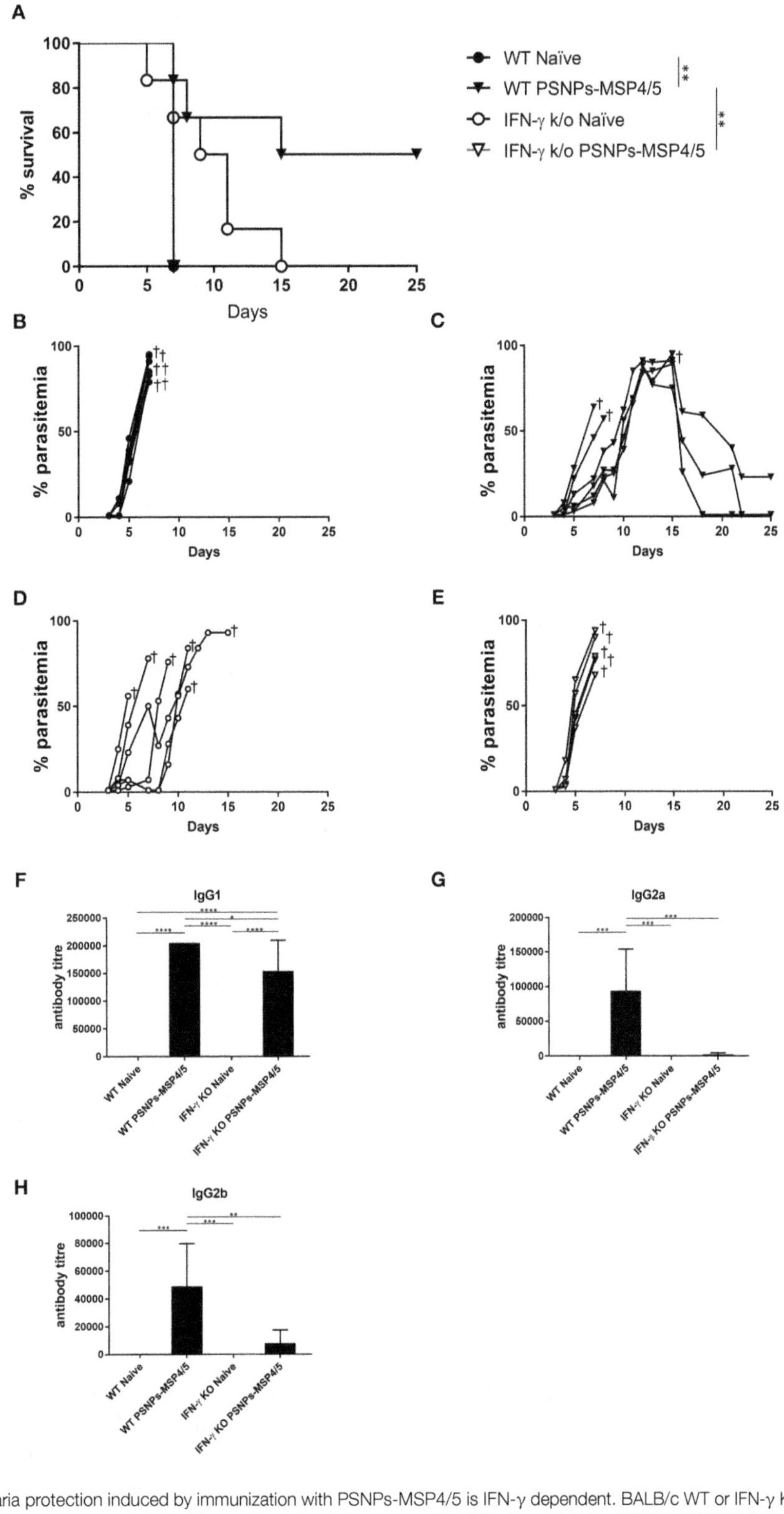

FIGURE 5 | Blood-stage malaria protection induced by immunization with PSNPs-MSP4/5 is IFN-γ dependent. BALB/c WT or IFN-γ KO BALB/c mice were immunized twice intradermally at the base of tail (100 μl/immunization), 14 days apart with PBS alone (Naïve) or PSNPs-MSP4/5 (100 μg/ml MSP4/5). Fourteen days following the boost immunization, mice were challenged intraperitoneally with 5×10^4 pRBCs from *P. yoelii* and survival parasitemia levels were monitored starting at 3 days post-challenge. **(A)** Kaplan-Meier survival curve and parasitemia levels of mice immunized with **(B)** WT Naïve -•-, **(C)** WT PSNPs-MSP4/5 -▼-, **(D)** IFNγ KO Naïve -○- and **(E)** IFNγ KO PSNPs-MSP4/5 -▽-. Pre-challenge **(F)** IgG1, **(G)** IgG2a, and **(H)** IgG2b anti-MSP4/5 antibody levels are also shown as mean antibody titer ± SD per group. $^{*}p < 0.05$, $^{**}p < 0.01$, $^{***}p < 0.001$, $^{****}p < 0.0001$ with Mantel Cox Log Rank Test for survival analysis and one-way ANOVA for antibody titer. †Indicates mouse endpoint. Data shown are from 5–6 mice per experimental group.

induced moderate protective immunity compared to CFA/IFA adjuvanted formulations. Though only CFA/IFA adjuvanted formulations achieved complete protection, it has been noted in this model that is difficult to observe complete protection (22, 24, 46). Surprisingly, there were no significant differences in the protection observed between the different PSNP doses, however there was a slightly lower survival rate in the group immunized with the highest dose of PSNPs. Overall, the partial protection observed with PSNPs in this model shows promise for current and future nanoparticle delivery platforms for blood-stage malaria.

Studying the mechanism of the protective immunity against malaria induced by PSNPs-MSP4/5, using knockout mice, demonstrated protection to be IFN-γ dependent. This is consistent with reports in the literature suggesting IFN-γ is the critical mediator of protection in erythrocytic stage infections (47), and for other strains of blood-stage Plasmodium infection (51), though the exact mechanism of protection has yet to be defined. Our results show a change in IgG subclasses elicited by the vaccine, with sustained IgG1 (Th2 associated) production but significantly decreased anti-MSP4/5 levels of IgG2a and IgG2b (Th1 associated) compared to non-immunized controls. These results indicate that the induction of IgG1 alone is not protective in this model (56), as the IFN-γ KO mice are still able to produce IgG1 but are not protected. Previous studies have shown that high levels of both IgG1 and IgG2a are required to mediate protection in the *P. yoelii* model (57, 58) however both Hirunpetcharat et al. (59) and Oakley et al. (60) showed that IgG1 alone correlates with protection against *P. yoelii* challenge (59, 60). In contrast, Adame-Gallegos et al. (61) showed that IgG1 did not mediate protection against *P. yoelii* (61).

One interesting finding in the knock out experiment was that the IFN-γ KO naïve mice had slightly better survival that the immunized KO mice (though this was not significant). Whilst it is possible that this is due to the potency of the parasites themselves, it may also be due to the differences in vaccine induced responses. As these mice do not have any vaccine induced responses, compared with the PSNPs vaccinated mice, there may be other mechanisms compensating for IFN-γ and contributing to the marginally increased survival. A potential cell type that has been identified as having a key role in clearing early parasitemia's are γδ T cells (62). It is possible that without the expansion of αβ T cells as would be expected in vaccinated animals, γδ T cells may expand instead, as well as there being a potential difference in cytokine profiles, especially from innate cells (63). Though it cannot be proven for the present study, the above hypothesis would be of interest to investigate further in this model in future studies. Indeed, in future studies it would be preferable to explore other immune responses induced by these PSNPs vaccines in the context of blood-stage malaria, including investigating other cytokines (i.e., TNF, IL-5, IL-17) in addition to the hallmark Th1 and Th2 cytokines IFN-γ and IL-4, respectively. Likewise, it would be beneficial to examine immune cell types such as B cells, γδ T cells, Th17, Tfh, Tr1, and T regulatory cells, as well as individual subsets within these populations to explore the different effector functions and cytokine profiles within cell subsets.

Plasmodium falciparum derived MSP4 and MSP5 are closely related to the MSP4/5 *P. yoelli* antigen used in this murine model of malaria. Their attractiveness as an antigen for target development came from the finding that they, and particularly MSP5, are largely conserved across malaria species, and show little polymorphism when analyzing within any single species of malaria parasites (10, 15). However, enthusiasm declined when it was shown that naturally found antibodies against MSP4 or MSP5 had little neutralizing capacity in *in vitro* red cell parasite growth inhibitory assays (GIA). Other MSP antigens were also shown to be associated with reduced incidence of malaria (64), and have been more widely studied. Although recent studies have shown association of both MSP4 and MSP5 antigens with decreased cases of malaria, specifically severe malaria (18, 19). The present study reinforces the contention that it is possible to deliver vaccine induced protection against malaria blood-stage, focusing on the induction of robust Th1 immunity, and not necessarily particular antibody functions. Of note is the fact that >60% humans naturally exposed to either acute *P. falciparum* (63%) or *P. vivax* (67%) malaria infection show IFN-γ responses to PfMSP5, suggesting it is (1) immunogenic in humans, (2) has the potential to be boosted by natural infection, and (3) is potentially a cross-reactive antigen between the two main stains of malaria found in many malaria endemic regions of the globe, including Asia (20). In agreement with previous studies, the current study suggests it is possible to design vaccines capable of inducing such potentially useful T cell responses. Moreover, we show it is possible to do so using carriers and adjuvants that do not need to deliver classical pro-inflammatory signals, a potentially important consideration when vaccinating infants in malaria endemic areas. Given our positive findings with PSNPs-MSP4/5, this supports the usefulness of further exploring other diverse nanoparticles as they are developed, as carriers for MSP antigens, beyond PSNPs. Conventional adjuvants carry the risk of damaging inflammatory responses, as well as data emerging from the literature suggesting that non-live adjuvanted vaccines may be directly associated with unhelpful non-specific effects (65). Overall, we hope the present study will spur further research into non-inflammatory vaccine carriers and adjuvants, as well as the potential for Th1 associated vaccine induced immunity in blood-stage malaria, which may help us re-examine from an additional perspective the nature of the antigens for inclusion in malaria vaccines.

AUTHOR CONTRIBUTIONS

MP designed and supervised all experiments and analyzed and interpreted all the data. KW designed and performed some of the experiments and analyzed some of the data. DP designed and performed some of the experiments and analyzed some of the data. JH and CM performed some of the experiments. SX designed and supervised some of the experiments and analyzed some of the data. RC planned some of the experiments. MP, KW, and DP wrote the manuscript and all authors contributed segments and editing to the manuscript preparation.

REFERENCES

1. WHO. *World Malaria Report*. 2017 (2017).
2. Penny MA, Pemberton-Ross P, Smith TA. The time-course of protection of the RTS,S vaccine against malaria infections and clinical disease. *Malar J.* (2015) 14:437. doi: 10.1186/s12936-015-0969-8
3. Beeson JG, Drew DR, Boyle MJ, Feng G, Fowkes FJ, Richards JS. Merozoite surface proteins in red blood cell invasion, immunity and vaccines against malaria. *FEMS Microbiol Rev.* (2016) 40:343–72. doi: 10.1093/femsre /fuw001
4. Genton B, Betuela I, Felger I, Al-Yaman F, Anders RF, Saul A, et al. A recombinant blood-stage malaria vaccine reduces *Plasmodium falciparum*. density and exerts selective pressure on parasite populations in a phase 1-2b trial in Papua New Guinea. *J Infect Dis.* (2002) 185:820–7. doi: 10.1086/339342
5. Chauhan VS, Yazdani SS, Gaur D. Malaria vaccine development based on merozoite surface proteins of *Plasmodium falciparum*. *Hum Vacc.* (2010) 6:757–62. doi: 10.4161/hv.6.9.12468
6. Sirima SB, Mordmuller B, Milligan P, Ngoa UA, Kironde F, Atuguba F, et al. A phase 2b randomized, controlled trial of the efficacy of the GMZ2 malaria vaccine in African children. *Vaccine.* (2016) 34:4536–42. doi: 10.1016/j.vaccine.2016.07.041
7. Thera MA, Doumbo OK, Coulibaly D, Diallo DA, Kone AK, Guindo AB, et al. Safety and immunogenicity of an AMA-1 malaria vaccine in Malian adults: results of a phase 1 randomized controlled trial. *PLoS ONE.* (2008) 3:e1465. doi: 10.1371/journal.pone.0001465
8. Thera MA, Doumbo OK, Coulibaly D, Laurens MB, Kone AK, Guindo AB, et al. Safety and immunogenicity of an AMA1 malaria vaccine in Malian children: results of a phase 1 randomized controlled trial. *PLoS ONE.* (2010) 5:e9041. doi: 10.1371/journal.pone.0009041
9. Thera MA, Doumbo OK, Coulibaly D, Laurens MB, Ouattara A, Kone AK, et al. A field trial to assess a blood-stage malaria vaccine. *N Engl J Med.* (2011) 365:1004–13. doi: 10.1056/NEJMoa1008115
10. Wu T, Black CG, Wang L, Hibbs AR, Coppel RL. Lack of sequence diversity in the gene encoding merozoite surface protein 5 of *Plasmodium falciparum*. *Mol Biochem Parasitol.* (1999) 103:243–50. doi: 10.1016/S0166-6851(99)00134-6
11. Wang L, Marshall VM, Coppel RL. Limited polymorphism of the vaccine candidate merozoite surface protein 4 of *Plasmodium falciparum*. *Mol Biochem Parasitol.* (2002) 120:301–3. doi: 10.1016/S0166-6851(01)00457-1
12. Polson HE, Conway DJ, Fandeur T, Mercereau-Puijalon O, Longacre S. Gene polymorphism of *Plasmodium falciparum* merozoite surface proteins 4 and 5. *Mol Biochem Parasitol.* (2005) 142:110–5. doi: 10.1016/j.molbiopara.2005.02.009
13. Martinez P, Suarez CF, Gomez A, Cardenas PP, Guerrero JE, Patarroyo MA. High level of conservation in *Plasmodium vivax* merozoite surface protein 4 (PvMSP4). *Infect Genet Evol.* (2005) 5:354–61. doi: 10.1016/j.meegid.2004.12.001
14. Putaporntip C, Jongwutiwes S, Ferreira MU, Kanbara H, Udomsangpetch R, Cui L. Limited global diversity of the *Plasmodium vivax* merozoite surface protein 4 gene. *Infect Genet Evol.* (2009) 9:821–6. doi: 10.1016/j.meegid.2009.04.017
15. Putaporntip C, Udomsangpetch R, Pattanawong U, Cui L, Jongwutiwes S. Genetic diversity of the *Plasmodium vivax* merozoite surface protein-5 locus from diverse geographic origins. *Gene.* (2010) 456:24–35. doi: 10.1016/j.gene.2010.02.007
16. Gomez A, Suarez CF, Martinez P, Saravia C, Patarroyo MA. High polymorphism in *Plasmodium vivax* merozoite surface protein-5 (MSP5). *Parasitology.* (2006) 133:661–72. doi: 10.1017/S0031182006001168
17. Wang L, Richie TL, Stowers A, Nhan DH, Coppel RL. Naturally acquired antibody responses to *Plasmodium falciparum* merozoite surface protein 4 in a population living in an area of endemicity in Vietnam. *Infect Immun.* (2001) 69:4390–7. doi: 10.1128/IAI.69.7.4390-4397.2001
18. Perraut R, Varela ML, Joos C, Diouf B, Sokhna C, Mbengue B, et al. Association of antibodies to *Plasmodium falciparum* merozoite surface protein-4 with protection against clinical malaria. *Vaccine.* (2017) 35:6720–6. doi: 10.1016/j.vaccine.2017.10.012
19. Perraut R, Joos C, Sokhna C, Polson HE, Trape JF, Tall A, et al. Association of antibody responses to the conserved *Plasmodium falciparum* merozoite surface protein 5 with protection against clinical malaria. *PLoS ONE.* (2014) 9:e101737. doi: 10.1371/journal.pone.0101737
20. Woodberry T, Minigo G, Piera KA, Hanley JC, De Silva HD, Salwati E, et al. Antibodies to *Plasmodium falciparum* and *Plasmodium vivax* merozoite surface protein 5 in Indonesia: species-specific and cross-reactive responses. *J Infect Dis.* (2008) 198:134–42. doi: 10.1086/588711
21. Salwati E, Minigo G, Woodberry T, Piera KA, De Silva HD, Kenangalem E, et al. Differential cellular recognition of antigens during acute *Plasmodium falciparum* and *Plasmodium vivax* malaria. *J Infect Dis.* (2011) 203:1192–9. doi: 10.1093/infdis/jiq166
22. Kedzierski L, Black CG, Coppel RL. Immunization with recombinant *Plasmodium yoelii* merozoite surface protein 4/5 protects mice against lethal challenge. *Infect Immun.* (2000) 68:6034–7. doi: 10.1128/IAI.68.10.6034-6037.2000
23. Kedzierski L, Black CG, Stowers AW, Goschnick MW, Kaslow DC, Coppel RL. Comparison of the protective efficacy of yeast-derived and *Escherichia coli*-derived recombinant merozoite surface protein 4/5 against lethal challenge by *Plasmodium yoelii*. *Vaccine.* (2001) 19:4661–8. doi: 10.1016/S0264-410X(01)00244-4
24. Rainczuk A, Smooker PM, Kedzierski L, Black CG, Coppel RL, Spithill TW. The protective efficacy of MSP4/5 against lethal *Plasmodium chabaudi* adami challenge is dependent on the type of DNA vaccine vector and vaccination protocol. *Vaccine.* (2003) 21:3030–42. doi: 10.1016/S0264-410X(03)00116-6
25. Goschnick MW, Black CG, Kedzierski L, Holder AA, Coppel RL. Merozoite surface protein 4/5 provides protection against lethal challenge with a heterologous malaria parasite strain. *Infect Immun.* (2004) 72:5840–9. doi: 10.1128/IAI.72.10.5840-5849.2004
26. Wang L, Goschnick MW, Coppel RL. Oral immunization with a combination of *Plasmodium yoelii* merozoite surface proteins 1 and 4/5 enhances protection against lethal malaria challenge. *Infect Immun.* (2004) 72:6172–5. doi: 10.1128/IAI.72.10.6172-6175.2004
27. Bracho G, Zayas C, Wang L, Coppel R, Perez O, Petrovsky N. AFCo1, a meningococcal B-derived cochleate adjuvant, strongly enhances antibody and T-cell immunity against *Plasmodium falciparum* merozoite surface protein 4 and 5. *Malar J.* (2009) 8:35. doi: 10.1186/1475-2875-8-35
28. Kool M, Fierens K, Lambrecht BN. Alum adjuvant: some of the tricks of the oldest adjuvant. *J Med Microbiol.* (2012) 61:927–34. doi: 10.1099/jmm.0.038943-0
29. Garcon N, Chomez P, Van Mechelen M. GlaxoSmithKline adjuvant systems in vaccines: concepts, achievements and perspectives. *Exp Rev Vacc.* (2007) 6:723–39. doi: 10.1586/14760584.6.5.723
30. Didierlaurent AM, Laupeze B, Di Pasquale A, Hergli N, Collignon C, Garcon N. Adjuvant system AS01: helping to overcome the challenges of modern vaccines. *Exp Rev Vacc.* (2017) 16:55–63. doi: 10.1080/14760584.2016.1213632
31. Wilson KL, Xiang SD, Plebanski M. Montanide, Poly I:C and nanoparticle based vaccines promote differential suppressor and effector cell expansion: a study of induction of CD8 T cells to a minimal *Plasmodium berghei* epitope. *Front Microbiol.* (2015) 6:29. doi: 10.3389/fmicb.2015.00029
32. Minigo G, Woodberry T, Piera KA, Salwati E, Tjitra E, Kenangalem E, et al. Parasite-dependent expansion of TNF receptor II-positive regulatory T cells with enhanced suppressive activity in adults with severe malaria. *PLoS Pathog.* (2009) 5:e1000402. doi: 10.1371/journal.ppat.1000402
33. Fifis T, Gamvrellis A, Crimeen-Irwin B, Pietersz GA, Li J, Mottram PL, et al. Size-dependent immunogenicity: therapeutic and protective properties of nano-vaccines against tumors. *J Immunol.* (2004) 173:3148–54. doi: 10.4049/jimmunol.173.5.3148
34. Fifis T, Mottram P, Bogdanoska V, Hanley J, Plebanski M. Short peptide sequences containing MHC class I and/or class II epitopes linked to nano-beads induce strong immunity and inhibition of growth of antigen-specific tumour challenge in mice. *Vaccine.* (2004) 23:258–66. doi: 10.1016/j.vaccine.2004.05.022
35. Kalkanidis M, Pietersz GA, Xiang SD, Mottram PL, Crimeen-Irwin B, Ardipradja K, et al. Methods for nano-particle based vaccine formulation and evaluation of their immunogenicity. *Methods.* (2006) 40:20–9. doi: 10.1016/j.ymeth.2006.05.018
36. Mottram PL, Leong D, Crimeen-Irwin B, Gloster S, Xiang SD, Meanger J, et al. Type 1 and 2 immunity following vaccination is influenced by nanoparticle

size: formulation of a model vaccine for respiratory syncytial virus. *Mol Pharm.* (2007) 4:73–84. doi: 10.1021/mp060096p
37. Xiang SD, Wilson K, Day S, Fuchsberger M, Plebanski M. Methods of effective conjugation of antigens to nanoparticles as non-inflammatory vaccine carriers. *Methods.* (2013) 60:232–41. doi: 10.1016/j.ymeth.2013.03.036
38. Scaria PV, Chen B, Rowe CG, Jones DS, Barnafo E, Fischer ER, et al. Protein-protein conjugate nanoparticles for malaria antigen delivery and enhanced immunogenicity. *PLoS ONE.* (2017) 12:e0190312. doi: 10.1371/journal.pone.0190312
39. Kaba SA, Karch CP, Seth L, Ferlez KMB, Storme CK, Pesavento DM, et al. Self-assembling protein nanoparticles with built-in flagellin domains increases protective efficacy of a *Plasmodium falciparum* based vaccine. *Vaccine.* (2018) 36:906–14. doi: 10.1016/j.vaccine.2017.12.001
40. Powles L, Xiang SD, Selomulya C, Plebanski M. The use of synthetic carriers in malaria vaccine design. *Vaccines.* (2015) 3:894–929. doi: 10.3390/vaccines3040894
41. Wilson KL, Xiang SD, Plebanski M. A model to study the impact of polymorphism driven liver-stage immune evasion by malaria parasites, to help design effective cross-reactive vaccines. *Front Microbiol.* (2016) 7:303. doi: 10.3389/fmicb.2016.00303
42. Karlson Tde L, Kong YY, Hardy CL, Xiang SD, Plebanski M. The signalling imprints of nanoparticle uptake by bone marrow derived dendritic cells. *Methods.* (2013) 60:275–83. doi: 10.1016/j.ymeth.2013.02.009
43. Gamvrellis A, Gloster S, Jefferies M, Mottram PL, Smooker P, Plebanski M, et al. Characterisation of local immune responses induced by a novel nano-particle based carrier-adjuvant in sheep. *Vet Immunol Immunopathol.* (2013) 155:21–9. doi: 10.1016/j.vetimm.2013.05.015
44. Xiang SD, Wilson KL, Goubier A, Heyerick A, Plebanski M. Design of peptide-based nanovaccines targeting leading antigens from gynecological cancers to induce HLA-A2.1 restricted CD8+ T cell responses. *Front Immunol.* (2018) 9:2968. doi: 10.3389/fimmu.2018.02968
45. Zhang YN, Poon W, Tavares AJ, Mcgilvray ID, Chan WCW. Nanoparticle-liver interactions: cellular uptake and hepatobiliary elimination. *J Control Release.* (2016) 240:332–48. doi: 10.1016/j.jconrel.2016.01.020
46. Kedzierski L, Black CG, Goschnick MW, Stowers AW, Coppel RL. Immunization with a combination of merozoite surface proteins 4/5 and 1 enhances protection against lethal challenge with *Plasmodium yoelii. Infect Immun.* (2002) 70:6606–13. doi: 10.1128/IAI.70.12.6606-6613.2002
47. Mccall MB, Sauerwein RW. Interferon-gamma–central mediator of protective immune responses against the pre-erythrocytic and blood stage of malaria. *J Leukoc Biol.* (2010) 88:1131–43. doi: 10.1189/jlb.0310137
48. Pouniotis DS, Proudfoot O, Minigo G, Hanley JL, Plebanski M. Malaria parasite interactions with the human host. *J Postgrad Med.* (2004) 50:30–4. Available online at: http://www.jpgmonline.com/
49. Pinzon-Charry A, Mcphun V, Kienzle V, Hirunpetcharat C, Engwerda C, Mccarthy J, et al. Low doses of killed parasite in CpG elicit vigorous CD4+ T cell responses against blood-stage malaria in mice. *J Clin Invest.* (2010) 120:2967–78. doi: 10.1172/JCI39222
50. Charoenvit Y, Majam VF, Corradin G, Sacci JB Jr, Wang R. CD4(+) T-cell- and gamma interferon-dependent protection against murine malaria by immunization with linear synthetic peptides from a *Plasmodium yoelii* 17-kilodalton hepatocyte erythrocyte protein. *Infect Immun.* (1999) 67:5604–14.
51. Su Z, Stevenson MM. Central role of endogenous gamma interferon in protective immunity against blood-stage *Plasmodium chabaudi* AS infection. *Infect Immun.* (2000) 68:4399–406. doi: 10.1128/IAI.68.8.4399-4406.2000
52. Hardy CL, Lemasurier JS, Belz GT, Scalzo-Inguanti K, Yao J, Xiang SD, et al. Inert 50-nm polystyrene nanoparticles that modify pulmonary dendritic cell function and inhibit allergic airway inflammation. *J Immunol.* (2012) 188:1431–41. doi: 10.4049/jimmunol.1100156
53. Yang J, Lemas VM, Flinn IW, Krone C, Ambinder RF. Application of the ELISPOT assay to the characterization of CD8(+) responses to Epstein-Barr virus antigens. *Blood.* (2000) 95:241–8. Available online at: http://www.bloodjournal.org
54. Calarota SA, Baldanti F. Enumeration and characterization of human memory T cells by enzyme-linked immunospot assays. *Clin Dev Immunol.* (2013) 2013:637649. doi: 10.1155/2013/637649
55. Ramirez M, Santos S, Martinez O, Rodriguez R, Miranda E, Ramos-Perez WD, et al. Characterization of the immune response elicited by the vaccinia virus L3 protein delivered as naked DNA. *Vaccine.* (2018) 36:2049–55. doi: 10.1016/j.vaccine.2018.02.033
56. Gazzinelli RT, Kalantari P, Fitzgerald KA, Golenbock DT. Innate sensing of malaria parasites. *Nat Rev Immunol.* (2014) 14:744–57. doi: 10.1038/nri3742
57. Llewellyn D, De Cassan SC, Williams AR, Douglas AD, Forbes EK, Adame-Gallegos JR, et al. Assessment of antibody-dependent respiratory burst activity from mouse neutrophils on *Plasmodium yoelii* malaria challenge outcome. *J Leukoc Biol.* (2014) 95:369–82. doi: 10.1189/jlb.0513274
58. Leite JA, Bargieri DY, Carvalho BO, Albrecht L, Lopes SC, Kayano AC, et al. Immunization with the MAEBL M2 domain protects against lethal *Plasmodium yoelii* infection. *Infect Immun.* (2015) 83:3781–92. doi: 10.1128/IAI.00262-15
59. Hirunpetcharat C, Mahakunkijcharoen Y, Jeamwattanalert P, Kittigul L, Mahannop P, Pichyangkul S. A single injection of 19 kda carboxy-terminal fragment of *Plasmodium yoelii* merozoite surface protein 1 [PyMSP1(19)] formulated with Montanide ISA and CpG ODN induces protective immune response in mice. *Asian Pac J Allergy Immunol.* (2011) 29:252–9. Available online at: http://apjai-journal.org/
60. Oakley MS, Sahu BR, Lotspeich-Cole L, Majam V, Thao Pham P, Sengupta Banerjee A, et al. T-bet modulates the antibody response and immune protection during murine malaria. *Eur J Immunol.* (2014) 44:2680–91. doi: 10.1002/eji.201344437
61. Adame-Gallegos JR, Shi J, Mcintosh RS, Pleass RJ. The generation and evaluation of two panels of epitope-matched mouse IgG1, IgG2a, IgG2b and IgG3 antibodies specific for *Plasmodium falciparum* and *Plasmodium yoelii* merozoite surface protein 1-19 (MSP1(19)). *Exp Parasitol.* (2012) 130:384–93. doi: 10.1016/j.exppara.2012.02.003
62. Dantzler KW, Jagannathan P. gammadelta T cells in antimalarial immunity: new insights into their diverse functions in protection and tolerance. *Front Immunol.* (2018) 9:2445. doi: 10.3389/fimmu.2018.02445
63. Mamedov MR, Scholzen A, Nair RV, Cumnock K, Kenkel JA, Oliveira JHM, et al. A macrophage colony-stimulating-factor-producing gammadelta T cell subset prevents malarial parasitemic recurrence. *Immunity.* (2018) 48:350–363.e357. doi: 10.1016/j.immuni.2018.01.009
64. Fowkes FJ, Richards JS, Simpson JA, Beeson JG. The relationship between anti-merozoite antibodies and incidence of *Plasmodium falciparum* malaria: a systematic review and meta-analysis. *PLoS Med.* (2010) 7:e1000218. doi: 10.1371/journal.pmed.1000218
65. Fish EN, Flanagan KL, Furman D, Klein SL, Kollmann TR, Jeppesen DL, et al. Changing oral vaccine to inactivated polio vaccine might increase mortality. *Lancet.* (2016) 387:1054–5. doi: 10.1016/S0140-6736(16)00661-9

2

KILchip v1.0: A Novel *Plasmodium falciparum* Merozoite Protein Microarray to Facilitate Malaria Vaccine Candidate Prioritization

Gathoni Kamuyu[1,2†], James Tuju[1,3†], Rinter Kimathi[1], Kennedy Mwai[1], James Mburu[1], Nelson Kibinge[1], Marisa Chong Kwan[4], Sam Hawkings[4], Reuben Yaa[1], Emily Chepsat[1], James M. Njunge[1], Timothy Chege[1], Fatuma Guleid[5], Micha Rosenkranz[2], Christopher K. Kariuki[6,7], Roland Frank[2], Samson M. Kinyanjui[1,3,8], Linda M. Murungi[1], Philip Bejon[1], Anna Färnert[9,10], Kevin K. A. Tetteh[11], James G. Beeson[12,13,14], David J. Conway[15], Kevin Marsh[1,8,16], Julian C. Rayner[17] and Faith H. A. Osier[1,2,3,8]*

[1] KEMRI-Wellcome Trust Research Programme, Centre for Geographic Medicine Research—Coast, Kilifi, Kenya, [2] Centre for Infectious Diseases, Parasitology, Heidelberg University Hospital, Heidelberg, Germany, [3] Department of Biochemistry, Pwani University, Kilifi, Kenya, [4] Arrayjet, Innovative Microarray Solutions, Edinburgh, United Kingdom, [5] Department of Pathology, University of Cape Town, Cape Town, South Africa, [6] Department of Tropical and Infectious Diseases, Institute of Primate Research, Nairobi, Kenya, [7] Cellular and Molecular Immunology, Vrije Universiteit Brussels, Brussels, Belgium, [8] Centre for Tropical Medicine and Global Health, Nuffield Department of Clinical Medicine, University of Oxford, Oxford, United Kingdom, [9] Division of Infectious Diseases, Department of Medicine Solna, Karolinska Institutet, Stockholm, Sweden, [10] Department of Infectious Diseases, Karolinska University Hospital, Stockholm, Sweden, [11] Immunology and Infection Department, London School of Hygiene and Tropical Medicine, London, United Kingdom, [12] Burnet Institute, Melbourne, VIC, Australia, [13] Central Clinical School, Monash University, Melbourne, VIC, Australia, [14] Department of Medicine, University of Melbourne, Melbourne, VIC, Australia, [15] Pathogen Molecular Biology Department, London School of Hygiene and Tropical Medicine, London, United Kingdom, [16] African Academy of Sciences, Nairobi, Kenya, [17] Wellcome Sanger Institute, Hinxton, Cambridge, United Kingdom

***Correspondence:**
Faith H. A. Osier
FOsier@kemri-wellcome.org;
faith.osier@med.uni-heidelberg.de

† These authors have contributed equally to this work

Passive transfer studies in humans clearly demonstrated the protective role of IgG antibodies against malaria. Identifying the precise parasite antigens that mediate immunity is essential for vaccine design, but has proved difficult. Completion of the *Plasmodium falciparum* genome revealed thousands of potential vaccine candidates, but a significant bottleneck remains in their validation and prioritization for further evaluation in clinical trials. Focusing initially on the *Plasmodium falciparum* merozoite proteome, we used peer-reviewed publications, multiple proteomic and bioinformatic approaches, to select and prioritize potential immune targets. We expressed 109 *P. falciparum* recombinant proteins, the majority of which were obtained using a mammalian expression system that has been shown to produce biologically functional extracellular proteins, and used them to create KILchip v1.0: a novel protein microarray to facilitate high-throughput multiplexed antibody detection from individual samples.

The microarray assay was highly specific; antibodies against *P. falciparum* proteins were detected exclusively in sera from malaria-exposed but not malaria-naïve individuals. The intensity of antibody reactivity varied as expected from strong to weak across well-studied antigens such as AMA1 and RH5 (Kruskal–Wallis H test for trend: $p < 0.0001$). The inter-assay and intra-assay variability was minimal, with reproducible results obtained in re-assays using the same chip over a duration of 3 months. Antibodies quantified using the multiplexed format in KILchip v1.0 were highly correlated with those measured in the gold-standard monoplex ELISA [median (range) Spearman's R of 0.84 (0.65–0.95)]. KILchip v1.0 is a robust, scalable and adaptable protein microarray that has broad applicability to studies of naturally acquired immunity against malaria by providing a standardized tool for the detection of antibody correlates of protection. It will facilitate rapid high-throughput validation and prioritization of potential *Plasmodium falciparum* merozoite-stage antigens paving the way for urgently needed clinical trials for the next generation of malaria vaccines.

Keywords: *Plasmodium falciparum*, merozoite, antibodies, vaccine candidates, protein microarray, bioinformatics

INTRODUCTION

Protein microarrays are increasingly used in the "omic" era of research in multiple formats that share the basic requirement to investigate interactions of tens to thousands of proteins simultaneously (1). They have had important translational applications in biomarker discovery to guide patient diagnosis, treatment and prognosis, as well as in drug discovery and vaccine antigen identification (2). Protein microarrays have facilitated a rapid, systematic and high-throughput approach to probing an entire pathogens' proteome or fraction thereof for immunoreactivity, in an approach that forms part of a reverse vaccinology workflow. These have aided in the discovery of potential diagnostic markers for *Mycobacterium tuberculosis* and *SARS-coronavirus* as well as potential vaccine candidates in over 30 human pathogens including *Plasmodium falciparum* (2, 3).

P. falciparum malaria causes ~450,000 deaths per year (4), and is of major public health importance to sub-Saharan Africa (5). Recent gains in reducing the burden appear to have stalled despite ongoing control efforts (4, 6). Efforts to design a highly effective vaccine that would protect against this disease have been hampered by the complexity of the organism and its' multi-stage life cycle: its genome encodes >5,300 proteins that are expressed variably in different tissues as the infection develops in the host (7). Coupled to this is an impressive array of strategies for generating protein polymorphisms or protein variants and redundant erythrocyte invasion pathways, which facilitate immune evasion (8–10). Consequently, although efforts to develop a highly effective malaria vaccine have been on-going for over a century, this goal has yet to be achieved. The current leading vaccine candidate against *P. falciparum* malaria has limited efficacy and induces only short-lived protective immunity (11, 12).

Multiple *P. falciparum* and/or *P. vivax* protein arrays have been designed over the past decade to help identify and prioritize potential malaria vaccine antigen candidates. The majority of these arrays have been manufactured using either the *E. coli*-based or the wheat germ cell free *in-vitro* transcription/translation expression system, with the largest to date including ~30% of the entire *P. falciparum* proteome (13–17). Protein selection was based on stage-specific transcription or protein expression, sub-cellular localization, secondary protein structures or documented immunogenicity in human and animal models. However, the *in-vitro* transcription/translation systems are relatively poor at generating functional surface proteins, which frequently require disulphide bonding and/or post-translational modification to attain their correct three-dimensional structure. Nevertheless, subsequent studies have down-selected proteins from this initial panel (18–31), indicating that essentially >75% of the parasite genome has yet to be evaluated in the context of immunity. A few additional proteins have been tested independently in smaller scale studies accounting for only a marginal increase in the proportion of the parasite proteome evaluated to date (32–34). These studies have rationally selected merozoite proteins that were established or plausible targets of antibodies, and evaluated antibody associations with protection in longitudinal studies using standard ELISA-based approaches (32, 33). They highlighted the importance of evaluating a broad repertoire of antigens and combinations of antibody responses in studies of acquired immunity. However, there still remains a need for a common platform with standardized protein expression and high-throughput antibody detection methods that can be applied widely across different clinical studies (35). This would accelerate identification of protective antibody targets and facilitate the comparisons between studies and populations.

To contribute to vaccine candidate discovery, as well as the validation and prioritization of existing candidates for clinical trials, we designed a novel protein microarray. We focused on the merozoite stage that is a target of immunity that can prevent or reduce the clinical symptoms of malaria. As per the case with other infectious diseases (36, 37), we hypothesized that proteins on or associated with the surface of the invasive *P. falciparum* merozoite would be accessible targets for protective antibodies (33). We mined the literature to identify multiple potential surface-associated merozoite proteins (32–34, 38–43) and added new proteins that were identified as immunogenic in adults from malaria-endemic countries and had proteomic and/or bioinformatic features suggestive of merozoite surface-localization, secretion and/or involvement in erythrocyte invasion (44). We expressed and purified these proteins and printed them on a custom microarray, which we refer to as KILchip v1.0 for its origin at the KEMRI-Wellcome Trust Research Programme in Kilifi, Kenya where the majority of the work was carried out. We demonstrate that KILchip v1.0 is highly specific, has minimal inter- and intra-assay variation, and is strongly correlated with equivalent data acquired using the gold-standard monoplex ELISA.

MATERIALS AND METHODS

Protein Selection

We aimed to design a microarray that would include proteins already considered as vaccine candidates, as well as novel proteins that had not been studied in the context of protective immunity. This would serve multiple purposes: (i) validation of existing vaccine candidates in new sample sets, (ii) identification of novel potential candidates and (iii) facilitation of head-to-head comparisons of all selected candidates in the same experiment. To this end, we selected a panel of antigens previously published in Zenonos et al. (38), Richards et al. (32), Crosnier et al. (39), Tetteh et al. (34), Raj et al. (43), Polley et al. (40, 45), Kimbi et al. (46), Metzger et al. (47), Taylor et al. (41), and Burghaus and Holder (48), for inclusion in the KILchip v1.0. These proteins are known or predicted to be anchored or associated with the surface of merozoites, secreted from its apical organelles or involved in erythrocyte invasion and have been shown to correlate with protection from clinical malaria (32, 33). We also included 28 novel proteins selected through a protein discovery pipeline that employed proteomic approaches for the detection of proteins that were either immunogenic or located on the surface of merozoites (44). Down-selection criteria for the novel proteins included either (i) the presence of a predicted N-terminal signal peptide and/or transmembrane domain(s), (ii) upregulated transcription at the late stages of the asexual life cycle, (iii) a predicted role in merozoite invasion (49) and (iv) novel with regards to a potential role in protective immunity.

Recombinant *P. falciparum* Protein Expression

Plasmids containing codon-optimized genes of interest were either obtained from the plasmid repository Addgene (https://www.addgene.org) or newly synthesized by GeneartAG as has been previously published (38, 39). Briefly, predicted signal peptides and transmembrane domains were excluded and the serine or threonine amino acid residues in all potential N-linked glycosylation sites (NXS/T) were substituted with alanine. Codon-optimized genes of interest were sub-cloned into a derivative of the pTT3 expression vector (also obtained from Addgene) that contained an N-terminal signal peptide derived from the mouse *kappa* light chain to drive secretion of antigen and a rat Cd4 domains 3 and 4 tag followed by a hexa-histidine tag for protein purification (39). Proteins were subsequently expressed using the Expi293 expression system (Invitrogen) according to manufacturer's instructions. Briefly, Expi293F cells were cultured to a density of 2.0×10^6 cells/ml and transfected with expression vectors using the Expifectamine 293 transfection reagent (Invitrogen). Cells were then incubated at 37°C with 8% CO_2 in an orbital shaker at 125 rpm. Culture supernatants were harvested 6 days post-transfection and proteins purified using Ni-NTA purification columns (Invitrogen). The majority of proteins included in KILchip v1.0 were expressed using the above mammalian expression system.

A minority of proteins were expressed in *E. coli* using pGEX-2T and pMAL-c2X vectors to produce fusion proteins with the carriers glutathione-S-transferase (GST) and maltose-binding protein (MBP), respectively. These were transformed into BL21 (DE3) *E. coli* cells and expressed as previously described (34, 40–42). The gene encoding *Pf*SEA1 protein was amplified from *P. falciparum* 3D7 cDNA using previously described primers (43). The PCR products were cloned into pEXP5-NT/TOPO expression vector and transformed into BL21 (DE3) pLysS *E.coli* cells. Cell expansion, induction of protein expression and subsequent purification was performed as previously published (34, 40–42). Purified recombinant proteins were dialysed into phosphate buffered saline and quantified using NanoDrop (Thermo scientific) before printing onto nitrocellulose slides. Further details are provided in the **Supplementary information**.

LC-MS/MS Analysis, Protein Validation, and Circular Dichroism Spectroscopy

Five to fifteen μg of purified recombinant proteins were denatured in 50 mM Tris-HCL pH 8.0 (Sigma) containing 8 M urea (Sigma). Proteins were reduced with 40 mM dithiothreitol (Sigma), alkylated with 80 mM iodoacetamide (Sigma) and precipitated using cold acetone. Pelleted proteins were resuspended in 15 μl of 6 M urea in 50 mM Tris-HCL pH 8.0 and digested with trypsin/Lys-C mix (Promega) according to manufacturer's instructions using the two step in-solution digestion. Peptides were desalted using P10 c18 pipette ZipTips (Millipore), dried using the Speedvac concentrator (Thermo Scientific) and resuspended in 15 μl of 99% H_20, 1% acetonitrile, and 0.1% formic acid. Peptides (5 μl) were loaded using a Dionex Ultimate 3,000 nano-flow ultra-high-pressure liquid chromatography system (Thermo Scientific) on to a 75 μm × 2 cm C18 trap column (Thermo Scientific). Chromatographic separation of peptides was carried out on a reverse-phase 50 cm-long column (Thermo Scientific) maintained at 40°C over a 60-min elution gradient (2–40% of mobile phase B; 80% acetonitrile with 0.1% formic acid) at a flow rate of 0.3 μl/min. Peptides were measured using LC instrumentation consisting of a Dionex Ultimate 3,000 nano-flow ultra-high-pressure liquid chromatography system (Thermo Scientific) coupled via a nano-electrospray ion source (Thermo Scientific) to a Q Exactive Orbitrap mass spectrometer (Thermo Scientific). The ms^1 settings were: Resolution, 70,000; Automatic gain control (AGC) target, 3e6; maximum injection time, 100 ms; scan range, 380–1600 m/z; while the ms^2 settings were: Resolution, 17,500; AGC target, 5e4; maximum injection time, 100 ms; isolation window, 1.6 m/z. The top 10 most intense ions were selected for ms^2 and fragmented with higher-energy collision fragmentation using normalized collision energy of 28 and these ions were subsequently excluded for the next 20 s. Mass spectrometry raw files were searched on Proteome Discoverer software version 1.3.0.339 (Thermo Scientific) using the Mascot server (Matrix Science) using a concatenated database of human and 3D7 *Plasmodium falciparum* protein FASTA sequences. Cysteine carbamidomethylation was set as a fixed modification and deamidation of asparagine or glutamine and methionine oxidation as variable modifications. The false discovery rate (FDR) was set to 0.01 for both proteins and peptides and a maximum of two missed cleavages were allowed in the database search. A minimum of two unique peptides for a protein was considered a positive identification.

Two proteins were selected for circular dichroism spectroscopy analysis (50). Briefly, phosphate buffer (50 mM NaH_2PO_4 pH 8.0, 0.1 M NaCl) and samples in phosphate buffer were degassed in a vacuum at room temperature and the CD spectra recorded on a J-715 spectropolarimeter (Jasco). Six accumulations were taken per protein with continuous scans taken using a 1 mm (0.1 cm) quartz cuvette, a scan rate of 50 nm/min, a band width of 1.0 nm and a resolution of 0.5 nm. The raw CD data (ellipticity θ in mDeg) were normalized for protein concentration and the number of residues yielding the mean residue ellipticity [θ] in mDeg·cm2·$dmol^{-1}$·res^{-1}.

Data Availability

The mass spectrometry raw files generated and analyzed in the current study have been deposited to the ProteomeXchange Consortium51 (PXD011746), via the MassIVE partner repository (MSV000083144), under the following title: KILchip v1.0 A novel *Plasmodium falciparum* merozoite protein microarray to facilitate malaria vaccine candidate prioritization. The FTP for the dataset is available here: ftp://massive.ucsd.edu/MSV000083144.

KILchip v1.0 Protein Microarray Assay

Overview

We designed our protein microarray to test 21 unique serum samples per slide with a customized barcode for slide identification. Four slides fitted into a 4 × 24 hybridization cassette (Arrayit Corporation ARYC), thus accommodating 84 samples per cassette and 336 samples per hybridization workstation (ARYC), each of which contains 4 hybridization cassettes (**Figure 1**).

Microarray Protein Map

Each slide contained 21 identical protein mini-arrays. Each mini-array had 384 features (printed spots) at a volume of 400 pl per spot. Recombinant *P. falciparum* proteins ($n = 111$) and controls ($n = 17$) were printed on each mini-array in triplicate, at the same concentration, using the same printer (Ultra Marathon micro-arrayer, ArrayJet) and printing protocol. The first control spots were Alexafluor[647] human IgG (Jackson ImmunoResearch) that served as landmarks demarcating the four edges of each mini-array (4 spots to match the edges of each mini-array). Purified human IgG (Jackson ImmunoResearch, 1 spot), served as the second control that confirmed the activity of the secondary antibody utilized in the assay. Protein printing buffer (30% glycerol/PBS, 9 spots) was used as the third set of controls that allowed for the monitoring of background reactivity and for the detection of any potential protein carryover during printing. The last sets of controls were the CD4, MBP, and GST proteins (1 spot each) to control for any potential antibody reactivity against the tags, each of which is present in one or more of the recombinant *P. falciparum* antigens. Thus, each mini-array contained a total of 384 features: 333 derived from 111 *P. falciparum* recombinant proteins (109 proteins, 2 of which were included twice) and 51 from 17 controls, all printed in triplicate.

Microarray Printing

We optimized the concentrations for individual proteins, serum samples and the secondary antibody by checkerboard titration. Proteins were printed on nitrocellulose slides (ONCYTE SuperNOVA, GraceBio) at a concentration of 250 μg/ml using the Ultra Marathon micro-arrayer (ArrayJet) with the Inkjet printing technology and the command center 1.5.0.1 (ArrayJet). Printing was carried out at 50% relative humidity and at 18°C. As a drying step, slides were incubated overnight at 18°C in the arrayer after printing, before storage in slide boxes with dessicant at 4°C until use. A salt scan was carried out at a high photomultiplier (PMT) at the 532 nm wavelength (green channel) to verify post-printing quality and at the 635 nm wavelength (red channel) to allow visualization of the landmark spots.

Antibody Detection

Printed slides were carefully assembled onto the hybridization cassette and sealed using silicone gaskets (ARYC) to form leak-proof individual wells. We modified a published protocol for the detection of antibodies (51). Briefly, wells were washed thrice with 0.1% Tween 20/HEPES buffered saline (1.4 M NaCl, 50 mM KCl, 20 mM $CaCl_2$, 10 mM $MgCl_2$, 100 mM HEPES; HBS) followed by HBS to remove any unbound proteins. Non-specific binding to the slide surface was prevented by blocking with 200 μl of 2% BSA/0.1% Tween 20/HBS for 2 h at room temperature while rotating on a microarray hybridization station (ARYC) at 350 rpm. Wells were subsequently washed thrice and incubated overnight at 4°C with 150 μl of serum diluted 1:400 and rotating at 350 rpm on the hybridization station. Thereafter, wells were washed as described above and incubated with 150 μl of donkey anti-human IgG-Fcγ fragment specific Alexafluor[647] for 3 h at room temperature followed by three washes. Slides were carefully disassembled from the hybridization cassettes, rinsed thrice in distilled water and dried by centrifugation at 300 g for 5 min using a combiSlide adapter (Eppendorf) and stored in slide boxes in the dark. Slides were scanned using a Genepix 4,000 B scanner coupled to the GenePix Pro & Microarray Acquisition and Analysis Software (Molecular Devices).

ELISA

A standard protocol for an indirect ELISA was performed as has been previously described (52–54). Briefly, a pre-determined concentration for each recombinant protein was either heat-treated at 80°C for 10 min or left untreated and coated overnight at 4°C on 96-microwell ELISA plates (Dynex 4HBX Immunolon). Wells were washed four times in PBST (phosphate-buffered saline/0.05 Tween 20) and blocked at room temperature with 1% skimmed milk (Marvel)/PBST for 5 h. Individual wells were washed and incubated with 100 μl of either test sera or a panel of monoclonal antibodies overnight at 4°C, before being washed four times in PBST and incubated for 3 h at room temperature with 100 μl of the respective horseradish peroxidase-conjugated secondary antibody diluted in 1%Marvel/PBST. Wells were washed four times in PBST and incubated at room temperature with 100 μl of substrate development buffer consisting of H_2O_2 and o-phenylenediamine

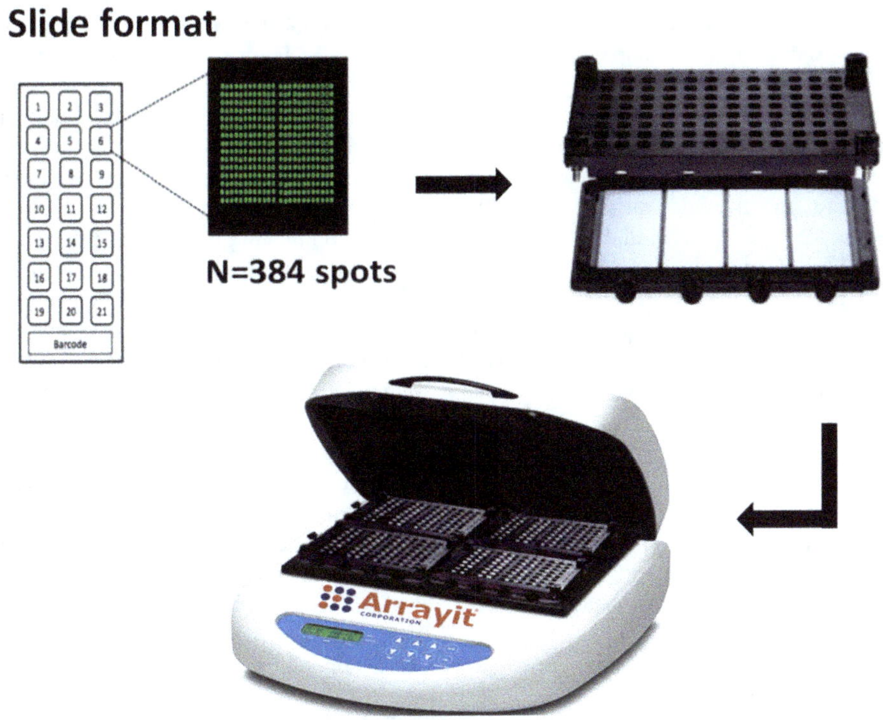

FIGURE 1 | Configuration of KILchip v1.0. Individual slides contain 21 identical mini-arrays comprised of protein spots and a barcode for identification. Each mini-array contains 384 individual spots that include proteins and controls printed in triplicate. Four slides are assembled onto a hybridization cassette, four of which are simultaneously processed in a microarray hybridization work-station (image from Arrayit Corporation, used with permission).

dihydrochloride (SigmaFAST). The reaction was stopped with 30μl of 2M H_2SO_4 per well and the absorbance read at 492 nm.

Serum Samples

Ethics Statement

This study was carried out in accordance with the recommendations of "the Declaration of Helsinki, and the Kenyan National Scientific and Ethical Review Unit (SERU)" with written informed consent from all subjects. The protocol was approved by SERU, reference number KEMRI/SERU/CGMR-C/001/3139.

Kilifi Adults

Samples from life-long adult residents of Junju in Kilifi, Kenya collected in 2008 were used for assay optimization ($n = 66$). These sera were assayed for antibody responses to well-studied recombinant merozoite proteins using monoplex ELISA assays, and the data compared with that generated from the same proteins printed on KILchip v1.0. Five serum samples from adults residing in Sweden who reported no travel to malaria-endemic regions and designated malaria naïve sera (MNS) were used as negative controls. Purified malaria immunoglobulins (MIG) were obtained from a pool of healthy Malawian adults and were used to generate a standard curve as previously described (54). An additional serum pool from Kenyan adult residents of Kilifi, Kenya was designated malaria immune sera (MIS) and served as a second positive control.

Statistical Analysis

Spot intensities were acquired using the GenePix scanner (Molecular Devices). Background, pre-scan and purification-tag intensities were subtracted (55) before analysis of within sample variability using the Coefficient of Variation (CV)

$$CV = \frac{\sigma}{\mu} \tag{1}$$

where σ is the standard deviation and μ the mean fluorescent intensity (MFI).

We used a two-step variance-stabilizing normalization to minimize the systematic variation commonly observed with this type of data. The first step was to handle the differences that could have occurred with different batches of data (machines or day) using the ComBat (SVA package in R). In the second step, variance-stabilizing normalization was used to minimize the systematic variation commonly observed with this type of data (55–58).

RESULTS

Recombinant Proteins

One hundred and ten *P. falciparum* merozoite proteins were selected from the literature based on their surface localization, known or predicted roles in erythrocyte invasion and associations with protective immunity (32–34, 38–42). Twenty-eight additional novel proteins were identified using a combination of immuno-proteomics and bioinformatics. Of these, 111 *P. falciparum* proteins, 21 of which were novel targets, were successfully printed onto KILchip v1.0 (**Figure 2** and **Supplementary Table 1**). These included 82 full-length ectodomains or the largest predicted extracellular loop of multi-membrane proteins and 29 protein fragments obtained from different regions of eight unique proteins. Thirteen protein fragments corresponded to polymorphic variants of MSP1 ($n = 7$), MSP2 ($n = 3$), MSP3 ($n = 1$) and SURFIN4.2 ($n = 2$) (**Figure 2** and **Supplementary Table 1**). All the remaining proteins were based on the *P. falciparum* 3D7 sequence and in total, 87 unique *P. falciparum* merozoite proteins are printed on KILchip v1.0. Two antigens (MSP2-CH150/9 and PF3D7_0424400) were printed twice to serve as additional internal controls.

Protein Quality

The quality of the majority of the recombinantly expressed proteins/protein fragments included in KILchip v1.0 have been validated elsewhere, including the demonstration of specific protein-protein interactions (34, 38–41, 43, 45–48). A subset of the well-studied proteins namely: AMA1, EBA175, MSP1, MSP4, and RH5 were evaluated using monoclonal antibodies targeting conformational and disulfide-constrained epitopes in these proteins. Recombinant proteins were tested against humAbAMA1 (59), mAb R217 (60), mAb R218 (60), mAb 2.44 (61), mAb 5.2 (62), mAb 2AC7 (63, 64), and mAb QA1 (64). As shown in **Figure 3A**, each monoclonal antibody was highly reactive with its respective antigen and showed no reactivity when the target antigen was heat-denatured, confirming the presence of conformational and disulfide-constrained epitopes in the panel of recombinant proteins. As expected, low or negligible reactivity was observed between monoclonal antibodies and off-target recombinant proteins. The presence of heat-labile epitopes was further confirmed by testing native and heat-denatured recombinant proteins for their reactivity with MIS. As shown in **Figure 3B**, a decrease in immunoreactivity was observed when the proteins were heat-denatured. However, for MSP4, only a minimal drop in immunoreactivity was observed, suggesting the presence of linear epitopes. Collectively, these results suggest that proteins included in KILchip v1.0 were folded correctly and contained heat-labile, conformational epitopes. In addition, circular dichroism analysis of MSP3 and SPATR indicated that these proteins appear to be folded (**Supplementary Figure 1**).

The novel proteins reported here were expressed using Expi293F cells under the same conditions, lending support to their quality with regards to post-translational modifications and disulfide bond formation. The purity of the novel proteins was assessed using reducing SDS gels and mass-spectrometry analysis. Nineteen (90%) of the novel proteins ($n = 21$)

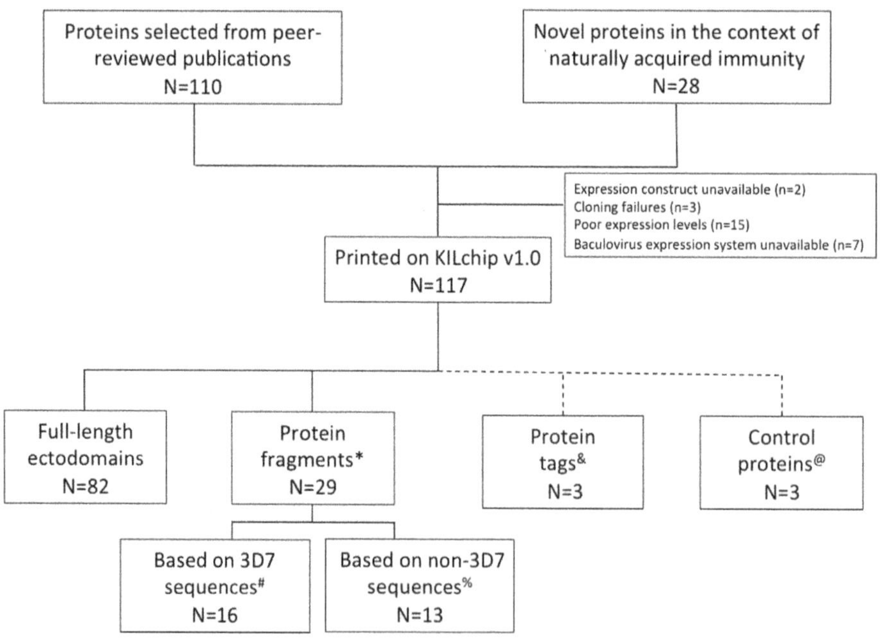

FIGURE 2 | *P. falciparum* merozoite protein panel included in KILchip v1.0. Proteins were either selected from the literature or from a combination of proteomics and bioinformatics analysis. Details of the parasite proteins are provided in **Supplementary Table 1**. *Protein fragments refers to specific amino acid regions selected from within a full-length protein ectodomain. #The protein fragments based on the 3D7 allele include MSP1-19 (Block 17), MSP1 Block 2 full, MSP1 Block 2 repeat, MSP3, MSPDBL1 N-terminus, MSPDBL1 C-terminus, MSPDBL2 N-terminus, MSPDBL2 C-terminus, 2 extracellular loops of PF3D7_0629500, *Pf*SEA1, SURFIN 4.2 3D7A, SURFIN 4.2 3D7B and the C-terminus of SURFIN 4.2. %Thirteen polymorphic variants of the *P. falciparum* merozoite proteins MSP1, MSP2, MSP3, and SURFIN 4.2 were included in KILchip v1.0. These included MSP1 Block 2 from the K1, MAD20, PaloAlto, Wellcome and RO33 alleles, the CH150/9 and DD2 alleles of MSP2, the K1 allele of MSP3 and the K1A and K1B alleles of SURFIN 4.2. &Protein tags refer to specific amino acids or polypeptides fused to target proteins to facilitate their subsequent affinity purification. These include the CD4 hexa-histidine, MBP and GST tags. @Technical controls for the assay included Alexafluor^{647} human IgG, purified human IgG and protein printing buffer.

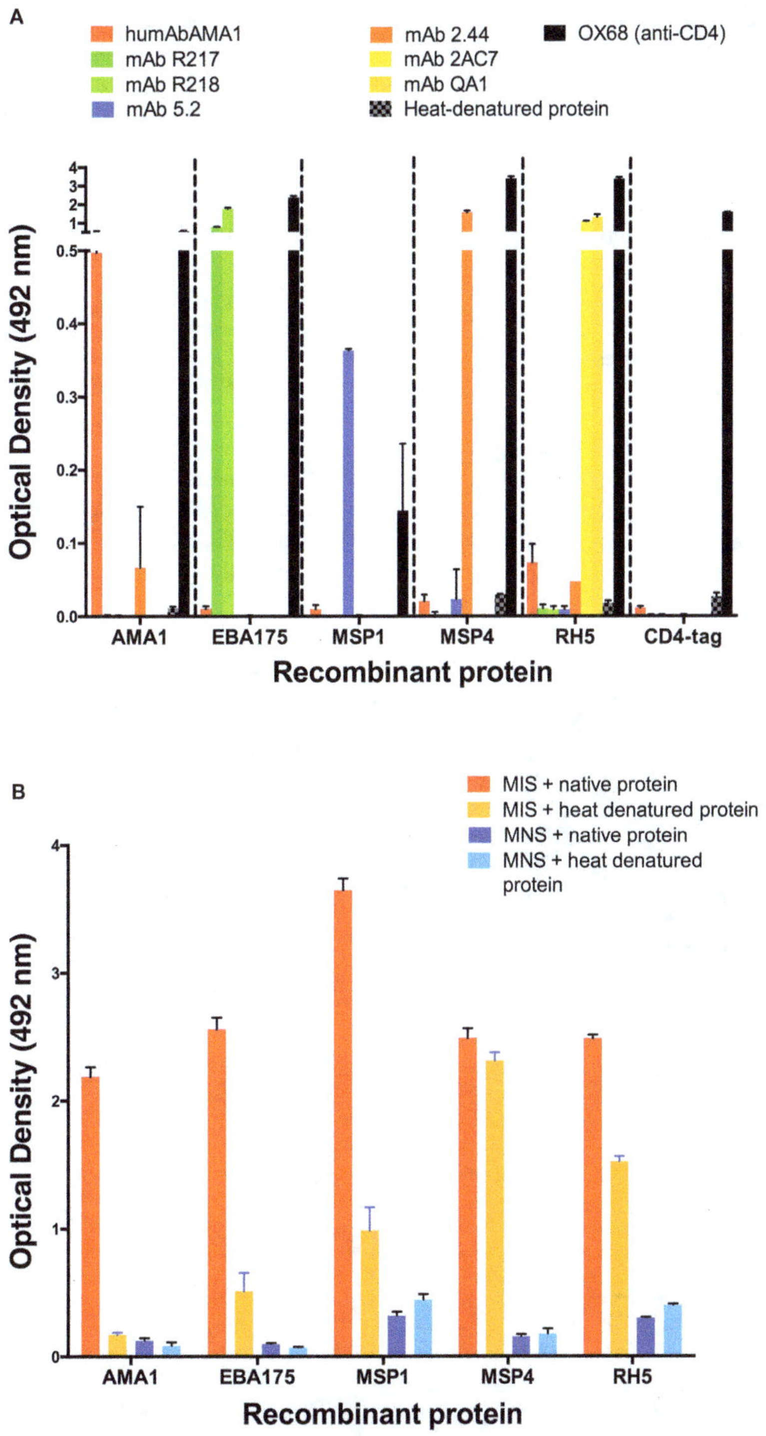

FIGURE 3 | Detection of heat-labile and conformational epitopes in a subset of recombinant proteins. Native and heat-denatured recombinant proteins were tested for reactivity against malaria immune sera (MIS), malaria naïve sera (MNS) and 5 monoclonal antibodies targeting conformational-dependent epitopes. **(A)** The monoclonal antibodies targeting conformational and disulfide-constrained epitopes on AMA1 (humAbAMA1), the F2 domain of EBA175 region II (mAb R217), the F1 domain of EBA175 region II (mAb R218), MSP1 (mAb 5.2), MSP4 (mAb 2.44), RH5 (mAb QA1 and mAb 2AC7) and rat CD4 domain (OX68) were used to measure reactivity against recombinant proteins by ELISA. All recombinant proteins demonstrated high reactivity with their respective monoclonal antibodies only. Low/negligible reactivity was observed after heat-denaturation of the recombinant proteins. **(B)** High antibody reactivity was detected with native recombinant protein. Decreased reactivity was observed with the heat-denatured proteins. Low reactivity was detected with malaria naïve sera (MNS) in both native and heat-denatured proteins.

included in KILchip v1.0 were readily detectable on Coomassie stained SDS gels and migrated at a size compatible with their predicted molecular weights (**Supplementary Figure 2**). Mass-spectrometry analysis confirmed the identity of the majority of recombinant proteins (**Supplementary Table 2**).

KILchip v1.0

Specificity

To confirm the specificity of antibody detection, individual mini-arrays were probed with the following positive and negative controls: (i) malaria immune sera (MIS), (ii) malaria naïve sera (MNS) and (iii) sample buffer consisting of 2% BSA/0.1% Tween 20/HBS. As expected, strong fluorescence was detected on each mini-array for the landmarks (blue) and commercial human IgG (green), whilst none was detected against the printing buffer (yellow) (**Figure 4A**, all panels). When probed with MIS, high levels of antibody reactivity against multiple *P. falciparum* proteins were clearly visible (**Figure 4A**, panel 1). In contrast, when probed with MNS, negligible antibody reactivity was observed. Similarly, when probed with sample buffer, nil or minimal reactivity was observed against *P. falciparum* proteins (**Figure 4A**, panel 2 and 3 respectively).

We further explored the specificity by comparing antibody reactivity to selected, previously characterized proteins in individual samples from Kenyan adults ($n = 66$) and malaria naïve Swedes ($n = 5$). The intensity of antibody reactivity varied between these selected proteins in the order AMA1 > MSP2 > MSP3 > *Pf*RH5 > RIPR (**Figure 4B** and **Supplementary Figure 3**). The median (minimum-maximum) fluorescence intensity (MFI) responses to AMA1, MSP2, and MSP3 were 23629 (1426-64840), 4762 (733-37025), and 2105 (72-4069), respectively in the Kenyan adults. MFI responses to RH5 and RIPR were low at 44 (4-914) and 28 (-2-994), respectively (**Figure 4B**). In contrast, reactivity against all *P. falciparum* proteins was low or negligible when probed with the non-malaria exposed serum from Swedish adults (**Figure 4C** and **Supplementary Figure 3**). AMA1, MSP2, and MSP3 are well-characterized immunodominant merozoite antigens while RH5 and RIPR appear to not be primary targets of naturally acquired antibody responses in some studies (32, 33, 65, 66).

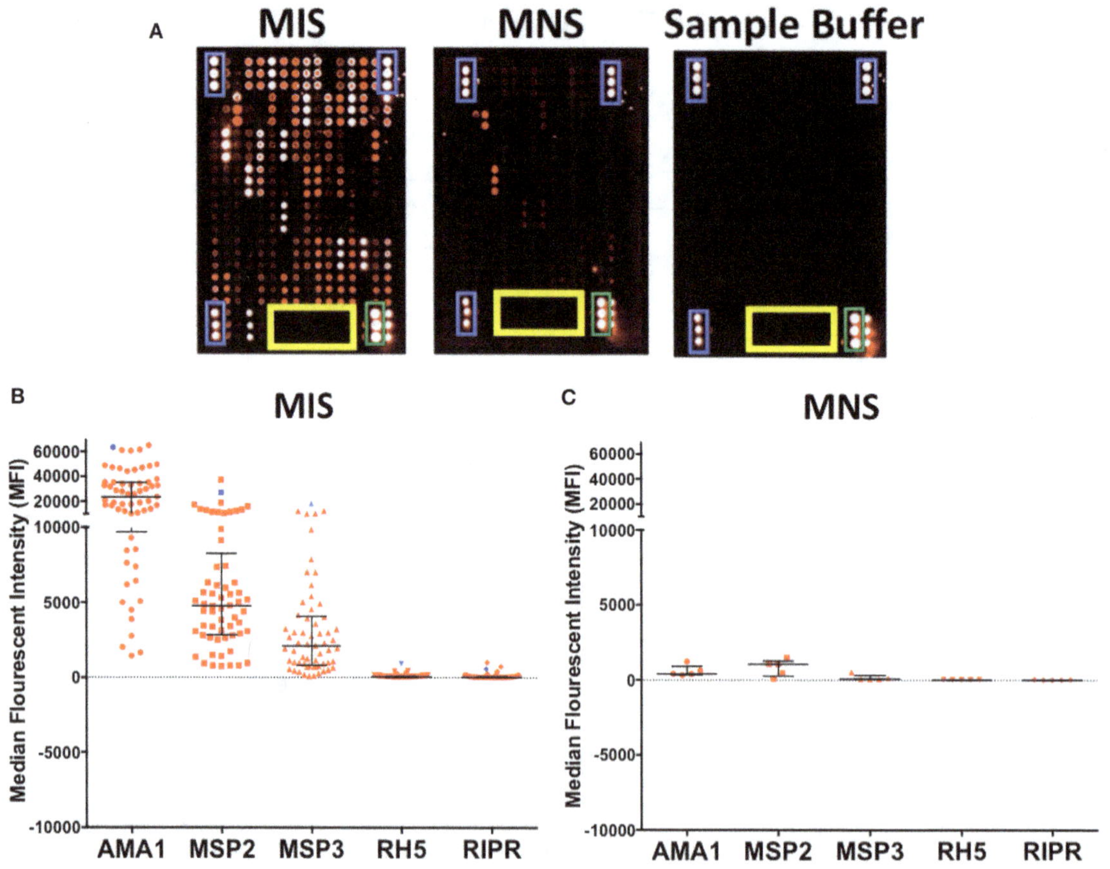

FIGURE 4 | Specificity of KILchip v1.0. Positive and negative controls were used to confirm specificity. **(A)** High antibody reactivity was detected using malaria immune sera (MIS) and low or negligible reactivity was observed with malaria naïve sera (MNS). No reactivity was observed with the sample buffer with the exception of the technical controls. Blue, landmarks; green, commercial human IgG and yellow, printing buffer. **(B)** Antibody reactivity to selected well-characterized merozoite antigens AMA1, MSP2 (3D7), MSP3 (3D7), Rh5, and RIPR varied as expected in MIS (blue) and serum samples from adult residents of Kilifi. Kenya (red). High reactivity to AMA1, MSP2 (3D7), and MSP3 (3D7) and low reactivity to Rh5 and RIPR was observed in the serum samples. **(C)** Antibody reactivity to well-characterized antigens AMA1, MSP2, MSP3, Rh5, and RIPR were all low/negligible when tested in serum samples from Swedish residents.

A direct comparison of antibody responses to multiple antigens can be evaluated using KILchip v1.0 as each protein was printed at the same concentration (250 μg/ml), and would be tested simultaneously with the same sera, providing information on the relative immunogenicity of this panel of merozoite antigens (**Supplementary Figure 4**).

Intra- and Inter-assay Variability

Intra-assay variability was tested using 66 serum samples obtained from Kenyan adults resident in Kilifi. Antibody measurements between protein spot replicates tested in the same assay and on the same day were strongly positively correlated, Spearman's R > 0.9770, $p < 0.0001$ (**Figure 5**). Inter-assay variability was tested using the positive and negative control sera. Antibody reactivity was measured repeatedly on five separate microarray slides printed over five consecutive days using identical printing conditions. As shown in **Figure 6**, the average signal intensities against individual proteins were highly reproducible.

Protein Stability on KILchip v1.0

To determine the durability of the microarray slides, we measured responses to the same batch of slides over a 3 months period using the reference reagent, MIG. These slides were printed on the same day, with identical printing conditions and

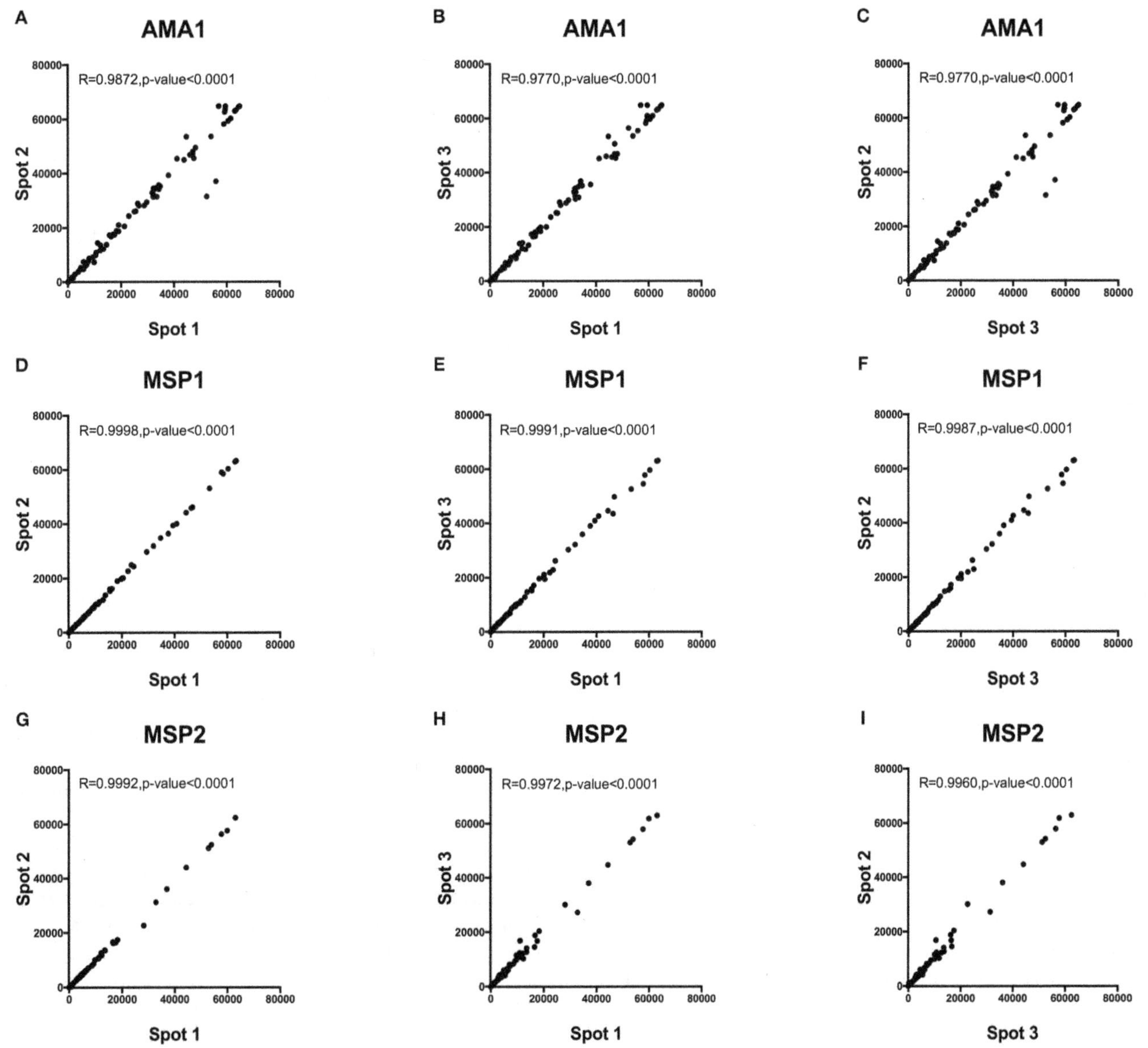

FIGURE 5 | Intra-assay variability of antibody detection by KILchip v1.0. A comparison of antibody responses to triplicate readings of AMA1, MSP1, and MSP2 was measured in 66 serum samples from adults living in the malaria endemic region of Kilifi, Kenya. A strong positive correlation of >0.98 was observed in all three-way scatter plots tested for the three antigens. Correlation between triplicate readings for recombinant AMA1 **(A–C)**, MSP1 **(D–F)** and MSP2 **(G–I)**.

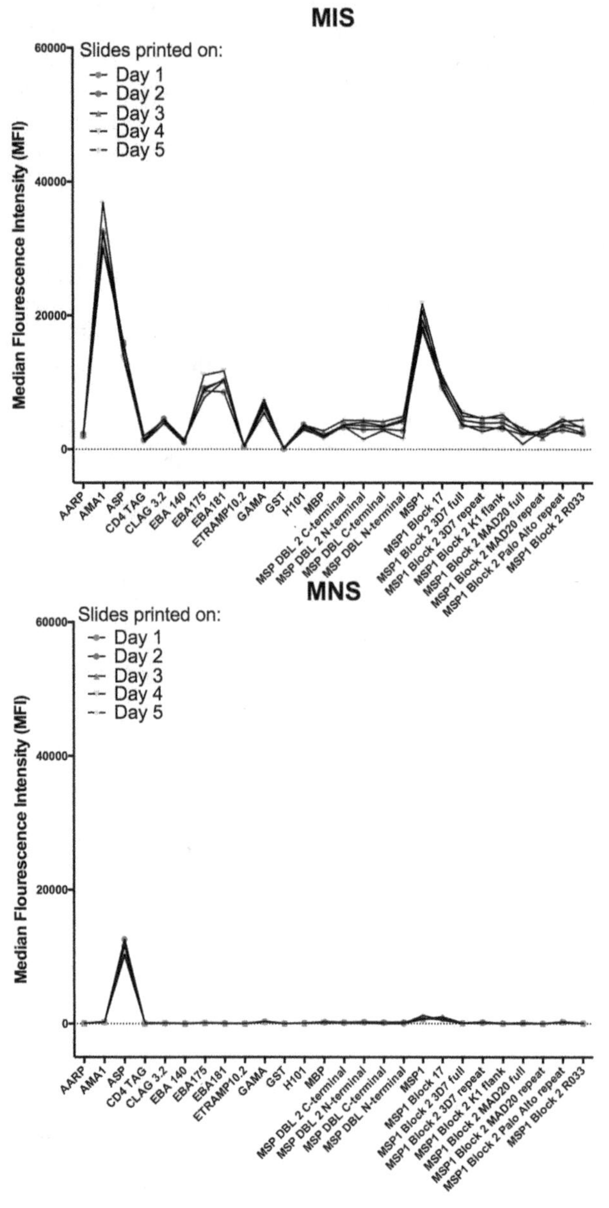

FIGURE 6 | Inter-assay variability of antibody detection by KILchip v1.0. Positive and negative controls were used to measure antibody responses to 5 protein arrays printed on 5 consecutive days using identical printing conditions and the same batch of recombinant proteins. Data presented are the mean MFI values of triplicate readings obtained with MIS (top graph) and MNS (bottom graph) to a subset of the proteins ($n = 26$) printed on each mini-array. Individual proteins are represented as dots and lines have been included to aid visualization.

the same batch of recombinant proteins. A tripling dilution of MIG was used to measure responses to each protein and to generate a standard curve. We performed a pairwise comparison of the slopes for each of the sigmoidal 5-parameter curves generated for each antigen over the 3-months period ($n =$ 4 sigmoidal curves; 6 pairwise comparisons per antigen) (67, 68). We observed no significant differences in the slopes for all 6 pairwise comparisons for 79/111 (71%) proteins (T-test; $p > 0.05$). Of the 32 proteins whose slopes differed significantly from each other, eight proteins had a single curve that differed while 24 proteins had 2 or more significantly different slopes. Results from 12/111 (10%) of the proteins printed on the array are shown in **Figure 7** and demonstrate that the curves to the majority of proteins were comparable indicating the detection of responses up to 3 months post printing without significant variation.

Strong Correlations Between KILchip v1.0 and the Monoplex ELISA

We compared measurements obtained using 12/111 proteins (representing ~10% of the *P. falciparum* proteins included in the array) printed on KILchip v1.0 vs. the identical proteins using our standardized ELISA in 66 samples from Kenyan adults. As shown in **Figures 8A–L**, a strong positive Spearman's correlation coefficient R of between 0.65 and 0.95 was observed between antibodies measured by KILchip v1.0 and by the standard ELISA, $P < 0.0001$. Sixty-seven percent of the proteins tested had a correlation coefficient R above 0.8 (**Figures 8A–H**). A wider dynamic range of antibody measurement was evident in the protein array assay as observed for AMA1 (**Figure 8B**), where a subset of samples whose MFI values ranged from 40,000 to 60,000 all had an optical density value of 4.0 (red box), the upper limit detectable by ELISA.

DISCUSSION

KILchip v1.0 is a new protein microarray designed to simultaneously quantify antibodies against multiple *P. falciparum* merozoite proteins and is currently configured to include >100 proteins, the majority of which are full-length ectodomains from secreted and surface exposed proteins. This facilitates the standardized measurement of antibodies against multiple merozoite proteins in cohort studies or in controlled human malaria infections, both of which are currently used to identify and prioritize potential vaccine candidates. It can be utilized to evaluate antibody dynamics and to monitor antibody decay or longevity. The chip is flexible and can be adapted to include fewer or more proteins, allelic variants of selected proteins, full-length proteins or functionally relevant domains of proteins of interest. Adaptations of the chip could expand from the current species-specific focus on *P. falciparum* in KILchip v1.0, and be designed to test additional *Plasmodium* species singly or in parallel. Of particular importance to the research setting in sub-Saharan Africa, the chip is durable, easily stored and transported, and can be shared between partnering laboratories. With modest investments, this tool could transform the pace at which *P. falciparum* antibody response data is generated across the African continent and the same principles could be applied to other infections, ultimately contributing to improvements in health through the development of diagnostics and vaccines.

Although other protein microarrays have been in existence since the early 2,000 s, none has been designed and developed from Africa specifically to study naturally acquired immunity

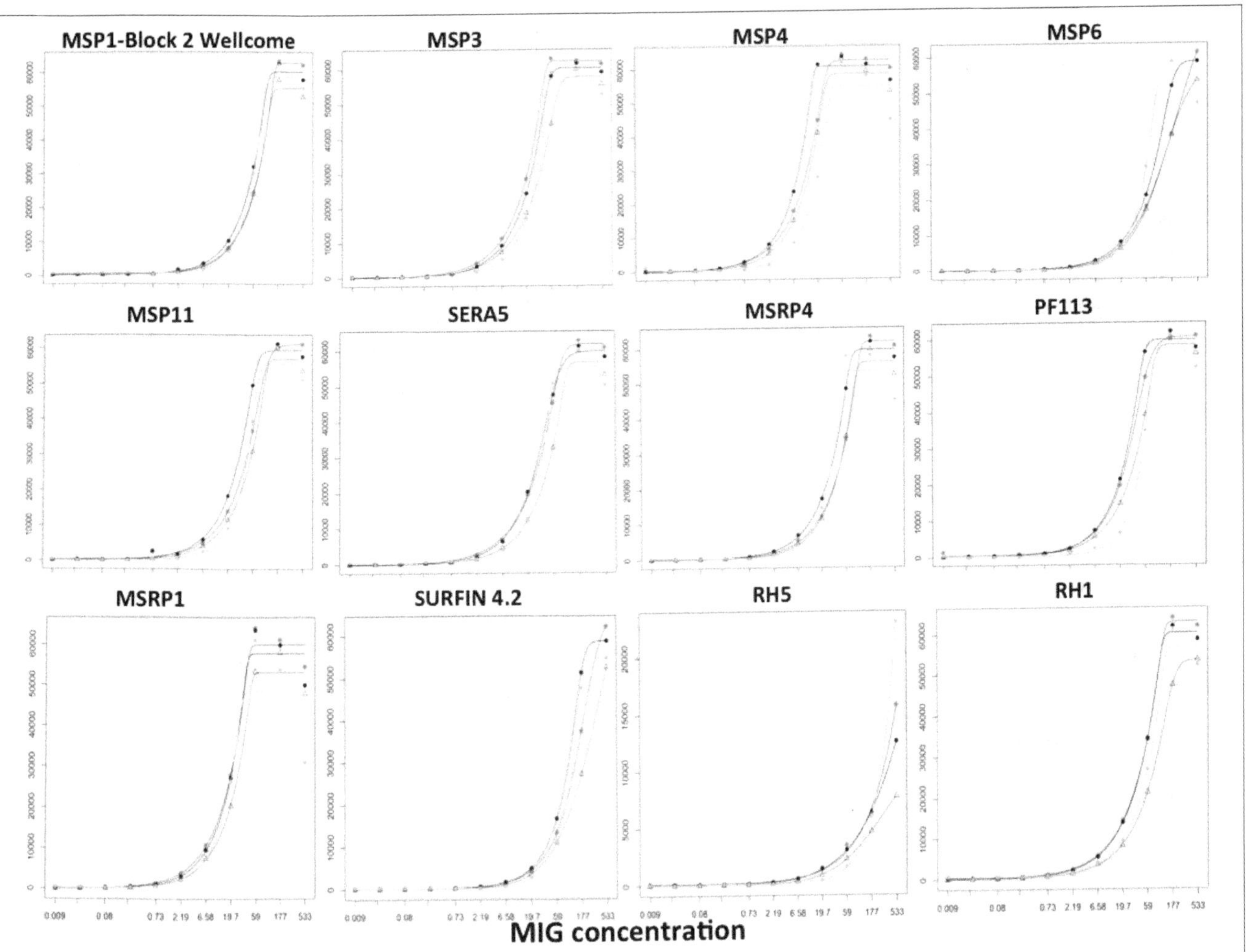

FIGURE 7 | Stability of KILchip v1.0. A reference reagent, MIG, consisting of purified immunoglobulins (98% Total IgG) was used to generate a standard curve by testing a tripling dilution against all antigens printed on the protein array. A batch of slides printed at the same time was tested 24, 40, 54, and 86 days post printing. The standard curve showed good concordance without significant variation. Red, blue, black, and green lines were obtained from measurements obtained on day 24, day 40, day 54, and day 86 post printing of the slides.

against *P. falciparum* malaria merozoites (13, 15, 69, 70). In addition, KILchip v1.0 consists predominantly of merozoite specific proteins, the majority of which were full-length ectodomains, a considerable improvement from evaluating segments of proteins, as is the case for other pre-existing protein microarrays available for *P. falciparum*. This was enabled by the use of a recently published method for transient protein expression of *P. falciparum* surface proteins in mammalian cells (39). Many of the proteins included in KILchip v1.0 are known to be immunogenic to varying degrees during natural exposure to malaria parasites, but have only been evaluated in a handful of cohort studies (32, 33). Typically, the exact nature, size and quality of antigens tested in these studies vary considerably, making it difficult to accurately compare results (35). Consequently, although some antigens have been studied for nearly 30 years, it is still not clear which proteins should be prioritized as vaccine candidates in clinical trials. KILchip v1.0 now provides a standardized tool that enables head-to-head comparisons of the immunoreactivity of a large number of proteins in multiple cohorts. One such study is already underway in which samples from at least 15 distinct geographical locations spread across 7 African countries have been tested using KILchip v1.0 (SMART: South-South Malaria Antigen Research Partnership) (71) and highlights the potential strength of KILchip v1.0.

We demonstrate that KILchip v1.0 is a sensitive tool for the detection of *P. falciparum* specific antibody responses. It is highly reproducible within and between assays and a strong concordance with the gold-standard monoplex ELISA was observed, comparable to the results reported for the different *P. falciparum* microarrays currently in use (13). Crucially, antibody measurements were stable on KILchip v1.0 up to 3 months post-printing, providing a suitable time frame for the testing of multiple samples. This is probably due to the addition of 60% glycerol to the recombinant proteins at the time of printing which

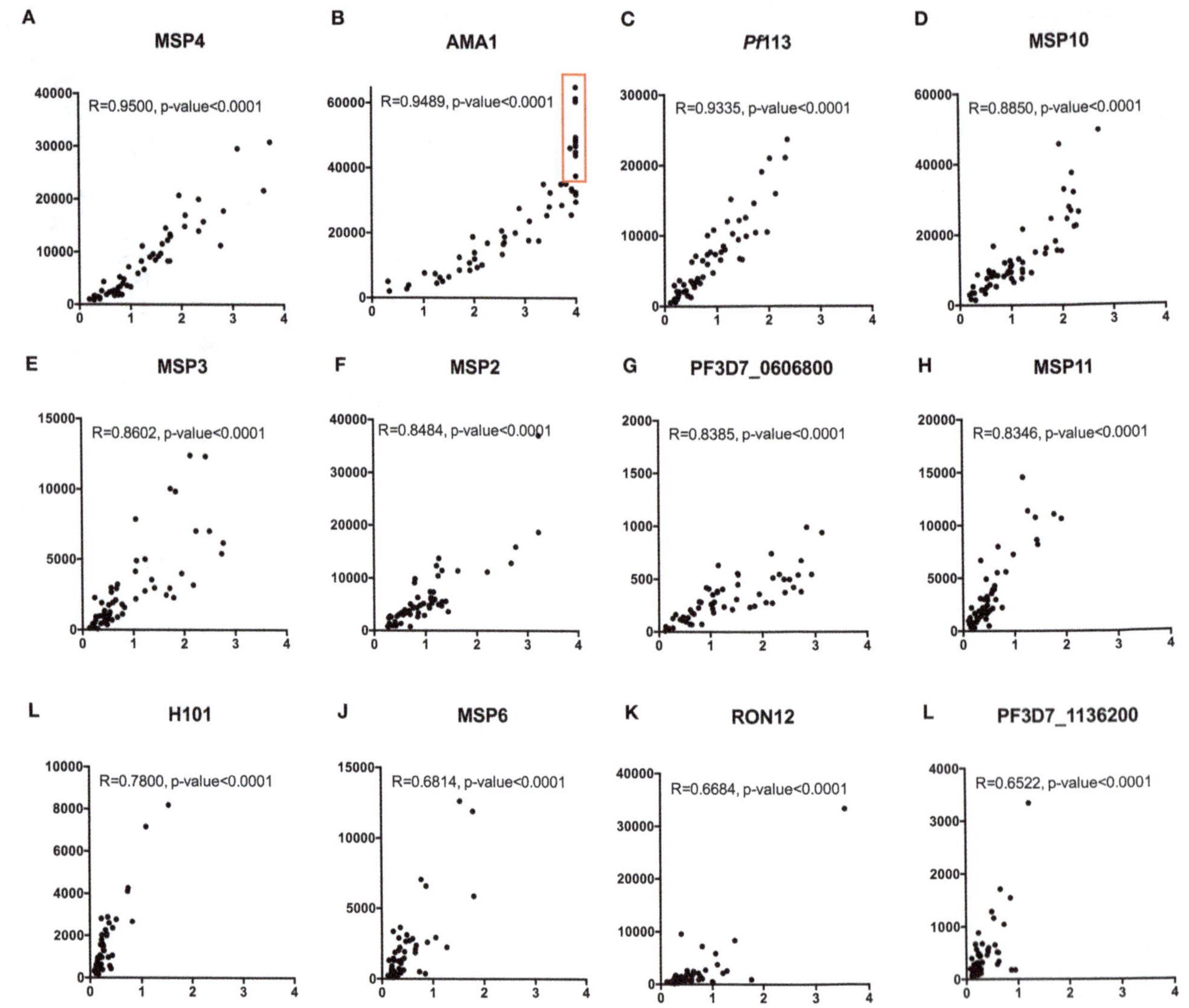

FIGURE 8 | Concordance between KILchip v1.0 and the gold standard ELISA. A comparison of antibody responses to 12 antigens measured simultaneously in KILchip v1.0 and individually by ELISA. Sixty-six serum samples from adults living in the malaria endemic region of Kilifi, Kenya were used to facilitate comparisons. A strong positive correlation of >0.8 was observed in 8 of the antigens **(A–H)** while four antigens **(I–L)** showed a correlation coefficient between 0.65 and 0.78. Red box - serum samples in which antibody responses reached the upper limit of detection when measured by ELISA, yet distinguishable by microarray with MFI values ranging from 40,000 to 60,000.

provides a stabilizing effect on proteins preventing degradation (72). Slides are conveniently stored with desiccant at 4°C.

In comparison to our standard ELISA protocol (52, 54), our microarray utilized 0.375 μl of serum to measure responses to all proteins simultaneously, compared to 23 μl required for ELISA assays of the same number of proteins. Similarly, over 100-fold less recombinant protein was required and the laser scanning and data acquisition by the GenePix 4,000 B scanner allowed for much wider dynamic ranges of antibody measurement. Lastly, this is a custom microarray format that could be scaled upwards or downwards and can be adapted to meet specific requirements. In the current version of KILchip v1.0, a single slide has 21 mini-arrays each containing 384 protein spots. This can be re-designed to include more or less proteins, to focus on allelic versions of specific proteins or to facilitate the simultaneous characterization of stage or species-specific antibody responses.

Although we selected 138 proteins/protein fragments for inclusion in KILchip v1.0, we were unable to obtain recombinant protein for 27 targets due to challenges in protein expression. These include targets such as RH4, RAP1-2, RhopH3, GLURP, SERA1, and SERA6 that have also been reported to be difficult to obtain in recombinant form in previous studies (38, 39). Also, the DBL domains of MSPDBL1 and MSPDBL2 have been previously obtained in soluble recombinant form using the baculovirus expression system but this has not yet been established within our laboratories (34). We also observed low antibody responses to some of the merozoite proteins such as RH5 and RIPR, similar to responses measured in adults from Kenya (65) and Mali (66). However, a higher response to these proteins expressed in the wheat germ cell-free expression system has been reported in children in Papua New Guinea (73), suggesting that the protein expression system used may influence the antibody responses measured. Another limitation of the KILchip v1.0 is that the majority of proteins are based on the 3D7 *P. falciparum* isolate which may underestimate responses to highly polymorphic proteins and limit the evaluation of antigenic diversity on humoral responses and immunity. Efforts are underway to generate an additional protein array that will include allelic variants of specific proteins that warrant further study. Lastly, adsorption of proteins onto nitrocellulose-coated slides may interfere with protein structure and consequently with the detection of conformation-dependent antibody responses (74). However, these and other solid-surface platforms such as in ELISAs are widely utilized for antibody detection for vaccine candidate discovery and prioritization in multiple infectious and non-infectious diseases.

Current and future versions of KILchip v1.0 will be essential to multi-center prospective cohort studies designed to identify correlates of protection, allowing the research community to rapidly compare results head-to-head, and fast track the prioritization of new and old potential vaccine candidates. This would bridge an important gap for the urgently needed evidence base that could guide the development of the next generation of malaria vaccines. Efforts are underway to make this a resource that could be provided at a minimal cost to the malaria research community.

AUTHOR CONTRIBUTIONS

FO, JR, and KevM conceived the study. GK and JT designed the array. GK, JT, RK, MC, SH, JN, CK, MR, RF, RY, EC, TC, JM, and FG performed the experiments, GK wrote the paper with contributions from JT, KenM, NK, and FO. SK, LM, and PB provided helpful discussions. AF, KT, JB, and DC provided reagents for the array design and testing. All authors read and approved the final manuscript.

FUNDING

This work was supported by an MRC/DFID African Research Leader Award jointly funded by the UK Medical Research Council (MRC) and the UK Department for International Development (DFID) under the MRC/DFID Concordat agreement (MR/L00450X/1); an EDCTP Senior Fellowship (TMA 2015 SF1001); and a Sofja Kovalevskaja Award from the Alexander von Humboldt Foundation (3.2 - 1184811 - KEN - SKP) awarded to FHAO. JB was supported by a Senior Research Fellowship from the National Health and Medical Research Council of Australia. Additional support was obtained from TIBA (Tackling Infections to Benefit Africa, Project Number is 16/136/33) in collaboration with the IDeAL and DELTAS Africa Initiative [DEL-15-003]. The DELTAS Africa Initiative is an independent funding scheme of the African Academy of Sciences (AAS)'s Alliance for Accelerating Excellence in Science in Africa (AESA) and supported by the New Partnership for Africa's Development Planning and Coordinating Agency (NEPAD Agency) with funding from the Wellcome Trust [107769/Z/10/Z] and the UK government. The views expressed in this publication are those of the author(s) and not necessarily those of AAS, NEPAD Agency, Wellcome Trust or the UK government.

ACKNOWLEDGMENTS

This work was published with permission from the office of the Director of KEMRI. We thank Dr. Gavin Wright and Dr. Cecile Crosnier of the Wellcome Trust Sanger Institute and Prof. Ray Owens of The Oxford Protein Production Facility (OPPP) in Oxford, UK for helpful discussions and training on transient protein expression. We are grateful to Dr. Rolf Fendel of Fraunhofer IME, Aachen and the Institute of Tropical Medicine (ITM), Tübingen, Germany and Dr. Torsten Klockenbring of Fraunhofer IME, Aachen, Germany, who provided the HumAbAMA1 and mAb 2.44 monoclonal antibodies. We thank Prof. Simon Draper of the Jenner Institute, University of Oxford, United Kingdom who provided the mAb 2AC7 and mAb QA1 monoclonal antibodies. Monoclonal antibody R217 and R218 were obtained through BEI resources, and were contributed by EntreMed/NIAID. We thank Prof Stefan Magez of Vrije Universiteit Brussels and Ghent University Global Campus, and Dr. Yann Sterckx of Universiteit Antwerpen, for helpful discussions on the circular dichroism spectroscopy experiments.

SUPPLEMENTARY MATERIAL

Supplementary Table 1 | List of P. falciparum merozoite proteins included in KILchip v1.0. The details of the P. falciparum merozoite proteins provided include the expression system used, the region of the protein expressed, the P. falciparum strain the protein was based on and the recombinant expression levels achieved. The expression levels were categorized as low, intermediate and high based on the concentration of purified protein obtained following transfection of a standard concentration of 50.0 × 10^6 Expi293F cells. The protein concentration following purification and concentration of low, intermediate and high expressors were <100 μg/ml, 100–250 μg/ml, and >250 μg/ml, respectively. The expression levels are given as guide only given the variability that may be observed with different expression batches. We observed no differences in the background signals when malaria naïve sera were tested against recombinant proteins grouped according to their expression levels (Kruskal-Wallis H Test for trend: p-value = 0.5975) (data not shown).

Supplementary Table 2 | Mass-spectrometry confirmation of novel Plasmodium falciparum recombinant proteins. Mass-spectrometry confirmation of the novel Plasmodium falciparum recombinant proteins included in KILchip v1.0. Data for PF3D7_0830500, PF3D7_1025300, PF3D7_1229300, PF3D7_1252300, PF3D7_1237900, PF3D7_1343700, and PF3D7_0629500_SEG2 are not yet available.

Supplementary Figure 1 | Circular dichroism spectroscopy on recombinant SPATR and MSP3. Circular Dichroism (CD) spectra graphs for SPATR (A) and MSP3 (B) proteins are plotted from mean residual ellipticity [θ] (mDeg ·

cm2·dmol−1·res−1) as a function of the wavelength, λ (nM). The ellipticity for the blank (phosphate buffer (50mM NaH2PO4 pH 8.0, 0.1M NaCl)) was subtracted from the ellipticity for the protein samples before calculation of the mean residue ellipticity [θ].

Supplementary Figure 2 | Purity of novel Plasmodium falciparum proteins. Coomassie stained SDS gels showing 19 purified recombinant proteins. The numbers in bracket indicate the predicted molecular masses (in KDa) for each protein. Protein bands for PF3D7_1343700 and PF3D7_0629500_SEG2 were not readily visible on a coomassie stained SDS gel. Protein bands for AMA1 and CD4-hexa-histidine tags were included as controls.

Supplementary Figure 3 | Antibody responses to previously characterized merozoite proteins. The protein spots corresponding to previously characterized merozoite antigens AMA1, MSP2 (3D7), MSP3 (3D7), Rh5, and RIPR are shown in protein arrays probed with MIS and MNS sera. Red-AMA1, Yellow-MSP2, Blue-MSP3, Orange-RH5, and Green-RIPR.

Supplementary Figure 4 | Immunoreactivity of all the recombinant proteins printed on KILchip v1.0 measured using a pool of sera from naturally exposed adults. The immunoreactivity of the 111 novel proteins was tested using malaria immune sera (MIS, red bars) and malaria naïve sera (MNS, blue bars). Bar charts show mean plus standard deviation; $n = 2$.

REFERENCES

1. Kingsmore SF. Multiplexed protein measurement: technologies and applications of protein and antibody arrays. *Nat Rev Drug Discov.* (2006) 5:310–20. doi: 10.1038/nrd2006
2. Yu X, Petritis B, LaBaer J. Advancing translational research with next-generation protein microarrays. *Proteomics* (2016) 16:1238–50. doi: 10.1002/pmic.201500374
3. Davies DH, Duffy P, Bodmer JL, Felgner PL, Doolan DL. Large screen approaches to identify novel malaria vaccine candidates. *Vaccine* (2015) 33:7496–505. doi: 10.1016/j.vaccine.2015.09.059
4. Davies DH, Duffy P, Bodmer JL, Felgner PL, Doolan DL. *World Malaria Report 2017.* WHO (2017).
5. Nkumama IN, O'Meara WP, Osier FHA. Changes in malaria epidemiology in africa and new challenges for elimination. *Trends Parasitol.* (2016) 33:128–40. doi: 10.1016/j.pt.2016.11.006
6. Snow RW, Sartorius B, Kyalo D, Maina J, Amratia P, Mundia CW, et al. The prevalence of Plasmodium falciparum in sub-Saharan Africa since 1900. *Nature* (2017) 550:515–8. doi: 10.1038/nature24059
7. Gardner MJ, Hall N, Fung E, White O, Berriman M, Hyman RW, et al. Genome sequence of the human malaria parasite Plasmodium falciparum. *Nature* (2002) 419:498–511. doi: 10.1038/nature01097
8. Rénia L, Goh YS. Malaria Parasites: the great escape. *Front Immunol.* (2016) 7:463. doi: 10.3389/fimmu.2016.00463
9. Gomes PS, Bhardwaj J, Rivera-Correa J, Freire-De-Lima CG, Morrot A. Immune escape strategies of malaria parasites. *Front Microbiol.* (2016) 7:1617. doi: 10.3389/fmicb.2016.01617
10. Persson KE, McCallum FJ, Reiling L, Lister NA, Stubbs J, Cowman AF, et al. Variation in use of erythrocyte invasion pathways by *Plasmodium falciparum* mediates evasion of human inhibitory antibodies. *J Clin Invest.* (2008) 118:342–51. doi: 10.1172/JCI32138
11. RTS, S. Clinical Trials Partnership. Efficacy and safety of RTS,S/AS01 malaria vaccine with or without a booster dose in infants and children in Africa: final results of a phase 3, individually randomised, controlled trial. *Lancet* (2015) 386:31–45. doi: 10.1016/S0140-6736(15)60721-8
12. Olotu A, Fegan G, Wambua J, Nyangweso G, Leach A, Lievens M, et al. Seven-year efficacy of RTS,S/AS01 malaria vaccine among young african children. *N Engl J Med.* (2016) 374:2519–29. doi: 10.1056/NEJMoa1515257
13. Crompton PD, Kayala MA, Traore B, Kayentao K, Ongoiba A, Weiss GE, et al. A prospective analysis of the Ab response to Plasmodium falciparum before and after a malaria season by protein microarray. *Proc Natl Acad Sci USA.* (2010) 107:6958–63. doi: 10.1073/pnas.1001323107
14. Trieu A, Kayala MA, Burk C, Molina DM, Freilich DA, Richie TL, et al. Sterile protective immunity to malaria is associated with a panel of novel P. falciparum antigens. *Mol Cell Proteomics* (2011) 10:M111 007948. doi: 10.1074/mcp.M111.007948
15. Finney OC, Danziger SA, Molina DM, Vignali M, Takagi A, Ji M, et al. Predicting antidisease immunity using proteome arrays and sera from children naturally exposed to malaria. *Mol Cell Proteomics* (2014) 13:2646–60. doi: 10.1074/mcp.M113.036632
16. Kanoi BN, Takashima E, Morita M, White MT, Palacpac NM, Ntege EH, et al. Antibody profiles to wheat germ cell-free system synthesized Plasmodium falciparum proteins correlate with protection from symptomatic malaria in Uganda. *Vaccine* (2017) 35:873–81. doi: 10.1016/j.vaccine.2017.01.001
17. Morita M, Takashima E, Ito D, Miura K, Thongkukiatkul A, Diouf A, et al. Immunoscreening of Plasmodium falciparum proteins expressed in a wheat germ cell-free system reveals a novel malaria vaccine candidate. *Sci Rep.* (2017) 7:46086. doi: 10.1038/srep46086
18. Tan X, Traore B, Kayentao K, Ongoiba A, Doumbo S, Waisberg M, et al. Hemoglobin S and C heterozygosity enhances neither the magnitude nor breadth of antibody responses to a diverse array of Plasmodium falciparum antigens. *J Infect Dis.* (2011) 204:1750–61. doi: 10.1093/infdis/jir638
19. Nnedu ON, O'Leary MP, Mutua D, Mutai B, Kalantari-Dehaghi M, Jasinskas A, et al. Humoral immune responses to Plasmodium falciparum among HIV-1-infected Kenyan adults. *Proteomics Clin Appl.* (2011) 5:613–23. doi: 10.1002/prca.201100021
20. Baum E, Badu K, Molina DM, Liang X, Felgner PL, Yan G. Protein microarray analysis of antibody responses to Plasmodium falciparum in western Kenyan highland sites with differing transmission levels. *PLoS ONE* (2013) 8:e82246. doi: 10.1371/journal.pone.0082246
21. Felgner PL, Roestenberg M, Liang L, Hung C, Jain A, Pablo J, et al. Pre-erythrocytic antibody profiles induced by controlled human malaria infections in healthy volunteers under chloroquine prophylaxis. *Sci Rep.* (2013) 3:3549. doi: 10.1038/srep03549
22. Arama C, Skinner J, Doumtabe D, Portugal S, Tran TM, Jain A, et al. Genetic resistance to malaria is associated with greater enhancement of immunoglobulin (Ig)M than IgG responses to a broad array of plasmodium falciparum antigens. *Open Forum Infect Dis.* (2015) 2:ofv118. doi: 10.1093/ofid/ofv118
23. Campo JJ, Aponte JJ, Skinner J, Nakajima R, Molina DM, Liang L, et al. RTS,S vaccination is associated with serologic evidence of decreased exposure to Plasmodium falciparum liver- and blood-stage parasites. *Mol Cell Proteomics* (2015) 14:519–31. doi: 10.1074/mcp.M114.044677
24. Helb DA, Tetteh KK, Felgner PL, Skinner J, Hubbard A, Arinaitwe E, et al. Novel serologic biomarkers provide accurate estimates of recent Plasmodium falciparum exposure for individuals and communities. *Proc Natl Acad Sci USA.* (2015) 112:E4438–47. doi: 10.1073/pnas.1501705112
25. Baum E, Sattabongkot J, Sirichaisinthop J, Kiattibutr K, Davies DH, Jain A, et al. Submicroscopic and asymptomatic Plasmodium falciparum and Plasmodium vivax infections are common in western Thailand - molecular and serological evidence. *Malar J.* (2015) 14:95. doi: 10.1186/s12936-015-0611-9
26. Torres KJ, Castrillon CE, Moss EL, Saito M, Tenorio R, Molina DM, et al. Genome-level determination of Plasmodium falciparum blood-stage targets of malarial clinical immunity in the Peruvian Amazon. *J Infect Dis.* (2015) 211:1342–51. doi: 10.1093/infdis/jiu614
27. Dent AE, Nakajima R, Liang L, Baum E, Moormann AM, Sumba PO, et al. Plasmodium falciparum protein microarray antibody profiles correlate with protection from symptomatic malaria in kenya. *J Infect Dis.* (2015) 212:1429–38. doi: 10.1093/infdis/jiv224
28. Baum E, Sattabongkot J, Sirichaisinthop J, Kiattibutr K, Jain A, Taghavian O, et al. Common asymptomatic and submicroscopic malaria infections in Western Thailand revealed in longitudinal molecular and serological studies: a challenge to malaria elimination. *Malar J.* (2016) 15:333. doi: 10.1186/s12936-016-1393-4
29. King CL, Davies DH, Felgner P, Baum E, Jain A, Randall A, et al. Biosignatures of Exposure/Transmission and immunity. *Am J Trop Med Hyg.* (2015) 93(3 Suppl.):16–27. doi: 10.4269/ajtmh.15-0037

30. Portugal S, et al. Treatment of chronic asymptomatic plasmodium falciparum infection does not increase the risk of clinical malaria upon reinfection. *Clin Infect Dis.* (2017) 64:645–53. doi: 10.1093/cid/ciw849
31. Uplekar S, Rao PN, Ramanathapuram L, Awasthi V, Verma K, Sutton P, et al. Characterizing antibody responses to plasmodium vivax and plasmodium falciparum antigens in india using genome-scale protein microarrays. *PLoS Negl Trop Dis.* (2017) 11:e0005323. doi: 10.1371/journal.pntd.0005323
32. Richards JS, Arumugam TU, Reiling L, Healer J, Hodder AN, Fowkes FJ, et al. Identification and prioritization of merozoite antigens as targets of protective human immunity to Plasmodium falciparum malaria for vaccine and biomarker development. *J Immunol.* (2013) 191:795–809. doi: 10.4049/jimmunol.1300778
33. Osier FH, Mackinnon MJ, Crosnier C, Fegan G, Kamuyu G, Wanaguru M, et al. New antigens for a multicomponent blood-stage malaria vaccine. *Sci Transl Med.* (2014) 6:247ra102. doi: 10.1126/scitranslmed.3008705
34. Tetteh KK, Osier FH, Salanti A, Kamuyu G, Drought L, Failly M, et al. Analysis of antibodies to newly described Plasmodium falciparum merozoite antigens supports MSPDBL2 as a predicted target of naturally acquired immunity. *Infect Immun.* (2013) 81:3835–42. doi: 10.1128/IAI.00301-13
35. Fowkes FJ, Richards JS, Simpson JA, Beeson JG. The relationship between anti-merozoite antibodies and incidence of Plasmodium falciparum malaria: a systematic review and meta-analysis. *PLoS Med.* (2010) 7:e1000218. doi: 10.1371/journal.pmed.1000218
36. Pizza M, Scarlato V, Masignani V, Giuliani MM, Aricò B, Comanducci M, et al. Identification of vaccine candidates against serogroup B meningococcus by whole-genome sequencing. *Science* (2000) 287:1816–20. doi: 10.1126/science.287.5459.1816
37. Rodríguez-Ortega MJ, Norais N, Bensi G, Liberatori S, Capo S, Mora M, et al. Characterization and identification of vaccine candidate proteins through analysis of the group A Streptococcus surface proteome. *Nat Biotechnol.* (2006) 24:191–7. doi: 10.1038/nbt1179
38. Zenonos ZA, Rayner JC, Wright GJ. Towards a comprehensive Plasmodium falciparum merozoite cell surface and secreted recombinant protein library. *Malar J.* (2014) 13:93. doi: 10.1186/1475-2875-13-93
39. Crosnier C, Wanaguru M, McDade B, Osier FH, Marsh K, Rayner JC, et al. A library of functional recombinant cell-surface and secreted P. falciparum merozoite proteins. *Mol Cell Proteomics* (2013) 12:3976–86. doi: 10.1074/mcp.O113.028357
40. Polley SD, Tetteh KK, Lloyd JM, Akpogheneta OJ, Greenwood BM, Bojang KA, et al. Plasmodium falciparum merozoite surface protein 3 is a target of allele-specific immunity and alleles are maintained by natural selection. *J Infect Dis.* (2007) 195:279–87. doi: 10.1086/509806
41. Taylor RR, Smith DB, Robinson VJ, McBride JS, Riley EM. Human antibody response to Plasmodium falciparum merozoite surface protein 2 is serogroup specific and predominantly of the immunoglobulin G3 subclass. *Infect Immun.* (1995) 63:4382–8.
42. Cavanagh DR, McBride JS. Antigenicity of recombinant proteins derived from Plasmodium falciparum merozoite surface protein 1. *Mol Biochem Parasitol.* (1997) 85:197–211. doi: 10.1016/S0166-6851(96)02826-5
43. Raj DK, Nixon CP, Nixon CE, Dvorin JD, DiPetrillo CG, Pond-Tor S, et al. Antibodies to PfSEA-1 block parasite egress from RBCs and protect against malaria infection. *Science* (2014) 344:871–7. doi: 10.1126/science.1254417
44. Kamuyu G. *Identifying the Merozoite Targets of Protective Immunity to Plasmodium Falciparum Malaria.* PhD thesis The Open University (2017).
45. Polley SD, Tetteh KK, Cavanagh DR, Pearce RJ, Lloyd JM, Bojang KA, et al. Repeat sequences in block 2 of Plasmodium falciparum merozoite surface protein 1 are targets of antibodies associated with protection from malaria. *Infect Immun.* (2003) 71:1833–42. doi: 10.1128/IAI.71.4.1833-1842.2003
46. Kimbi HK, Tetteh KK, Polley SD, Conway DJ. Cross-sectional study of specific antibodies to a polymorphic Plasmodium falciparum antigen and of parasite antigen genotypes in school children on the slope of Mount Cameroon. *Trans R Soc Trop Med Hyg.* (2004) 98:284–9. doi: 10.1016/S0035-9203(03)00068-3
47. Metzger WG, Okenu DM, Cavanagh DR, Robinson JV, Bojang KA, Weiss HA, et al. Serum IgG3 to the Plasmodium falciparum merozoite surface protein 2 is strongly associated with a reduced prospective risk of malaria. *Parasite Immunol.* (2003) 25:307–12. doi: 10.1046/j.1365-3024.2003.00636.x
48. Burghaus PA, Holder AA. Expression of the 19-kilodalton carboxy-terminal fragment of the Plasmodium falciparum merozoite surface protein-1 in Escherichia coli as a correctly folded protein. *Mol Biochem Parasitol.* (1994) 64:165–9. doi: 10.1016/0166-6851(94)90144-9
49. Hu G, Cabrera A, Kono M, Mok S, Chaal BK, Haase S, et al. Transcriptional profiling of growth perturbations of the human malaria parasite Plasmodium falciparum. *Nat Biotechnol.* (2010) 28:91–8. doi: 10.1038/nbt.1597
50. Greenfield NJ. Using circular dichroism spectra to estimate protein secondary structure. *Nat Protoc.* (2006) 1:2876–90. doi: 10.1038/nprot.2006.202
51. Sun Y, Gallagher-Jones M, Barker C, Wright GJ. A benchmarked protein microarray-based platform for the identification of novel low-affinity extracellular protein interactions. *Anal Biochem.* (2012) 424:45–53. doi: 10.1016/j.ab.2012.01.034
52. Osier FH, Fegan G, Polley SD, Murungi L, Verra F, Tetteh KK, et al. Breadth and magnitude of antibody responses to multiple Plasmodium falciparum merozoite antigens are associated with protection from clinical malaria. *Infect Immun.* (2008) 76:2240–8. doi: 10.1128/IAI.01585-07
53. Rono J, Färnert A, Murungi L, Ojal J, Kamuyu G, Guleid F, et al. Multiple clinical episodes of Plasmodium falciparum malaria in a low transmission intensity setting: exposure versus immunity. *BMC Med.* (2015) 13:114. doi: 10.1186/s12916-015-0354-z
54. Murungi LM, Kamuyu G, Lowe B, Bejon P, Theisen M, Kinyanjui SM, et al. A threshold concentration of anti-merozoite antibodies is required for protection from clinical episodes of malaria. *Vaccine* (2013) 31:3936–42. doi: 10.1016/j.vaccine.2013.06.042
55. Sundaresh S, Doolan DL, Hirst S, Mu Y, Unal B, Davies DH, et al. Identification of humoral immune responses in protein microarrays using DNA microarray data analysis techniques. *Bioinformatics* (2006) 22:1760–6. doi: 10.1093/bioinformatics/btl162
56. Sboner A, Karpikov A, Chen G, Smith M, Mattoon D, Freeman-Cook L, et al. Robust-linear-model normalization to reduce technical variability in functional protein microarrays. *J Proteome Res.* (2009) 8:5451–64. doi: 10.1021/pr900412k
57. Huber W, von Heydebreck A, Sültmann H, Poustka A, Vingron M. Variance stabilization applied to microarray data calibration and to the quantification of differential expression. *Bioinformatics* (2002) 18(Suppl. 1):S96–104. doi: 10.1093/bioinformatics/18.suppl_1.S96
58. Johnson WE, Li C, Rabinovic A. Adjusting batch effects in microarray expression data using empirical Bayes methods. *Biostatistics* (2007) 8:118–27. doi: 10.1093/biostatistics/kxj037
59. Maskus DJ, Królik M, Bethke S, Spiegel H, Kapelski S, Seidel M, et al. Characterization of a novel inhibitory human monoclonal antibody directed against Plasmodium falciparum Apical Membrane Antigen 1. *Sci Rep.* (2016) 6:39462. doi: 10.1038/srep39462
60. Sim BK, Narum DL, Chattopadhyay R, Ahumada A, Haynes JD, Fuhrmann SR, et al. Delineation of stage specific expression of Plasmodium falciparum EBA−175 by biologically functional region II monoclonal antibodies. *PLoS ONE* (2011) 6:e18393. doi: 10.1371/journal.pone.0018393
61. Kapelski S, Boes A, Spiegel H, de Almeida M, Klockenbring T, Reimann A, et al. Fast track antibody V-gene rescue, recombinant expression in plants and characterization of a PfMSP4-specific antibody. *Malar J.* (2015) 14:50. doi: 10.1186/s12936-015-0577-7
62. Chang SP, Gibson HL, Lee-Ng CT, Barr PJ, Hui GS. A carboxyl-terminal fragment of Plasmodium falciparum gp195 expressed by a recombinant baculovirus induces antibodies that completely inhibit parasite growth. *J Immunol.* (1992) 149:548–55.
63. Douglas AD, Williams AR, Knuepfer E, Illingworth JJ, Furze JM, Crosnier C, et al. Neutralization of Plasmodium falciparum merozoites by antibodies against PfRH5. *J Immunol.* (2014) 192:245–58. doi: 10.4049/jimmunol.1302045
64. Wright KE, Hjerrild KA, Bartlett J, Douglas AD, Jin J, Brown RE, et al. Structure of malaria invasion protein RH5 with erythrocyte basigin and blocking antibodies. *Nature* (2014) 515:427–30. doi: 10.1038/nature13715
65. Douglas AD, Williams AR, Illingworth JJ, Kamuyu G, Biswas S, Goodman AL, et al. The blood-stage malaria antigen PfRH5 is susceptible to vaccine-inducible cross-strain neutralizing antibody. *Nat Commun.* (2011) 2:601. doi: 10.1038/ncomms1615
66. Tran TM, Ongoiba A, Coursen J, Crosnier C, Diouf A, Huang CY, et al. Naturally acquired antibodies specific for Plasmodium falciparum reticulocyte-binding protein homologue 5 inhibit parasite growth

and predict protection from malaria. *J Infect Dis.* (2014) 209:789–98. doi: 10.1093/infdis/jit553
67. Ritz C, Streibig JC. Bioassay analysis using R. *J Stat Softw.* (2005) 12:30764. doi: 10.18637/jss.v012.i05
68. Jensen SM, Ritz C, Baty F, Gerhard D. Dose response analysis using R. *PLoS ONE* (2015) 10:e0146021. doi: 10.1371/journal.pone.0146021
69. Gray JC, Corran PH, Mangia E, Gaunt MW, Li Q, Tetteh KK, et al. Profiling the antibody immune response against blood stage malaria vaccine candidates. *Clin Chem.* (2007) 53:1244–53. doi: 10.1373/clinchem.2006.081695
70. Fan YT, Wang Y, Ju C, Zhang T, Xu B, Hu W, et al. Systematic analysis of natural antibody responses to P. falciparum merozoite antigens by protein arrays. *J Proteomics* (2013) 78:148–58. doi: 10.1016/j.jprot.2012.11.020
71. SMART. Availabe online at: https://www.smartpartnership.net/
72. Vagenende V, Yap MG, Trout BL. Mechanisms of protein stabilization and prevention of protein aggregation by glycerol. *Biochemistry* (2009) 48:11084–96. doi: 10.1021/bi900649t
73. Weaver R, Reiling L, Feng G, Drew DR, Mueller I, Siba PM, et al. The association between naturally acquired IgG subclass specific antibodies to the PfRH5 invasion complex and protection from Plasmodium falciparum malaria. *Sci Rep.* (2016) 6:33094. doi: 10.1038/srep33094
74. Fici DA, McCormick W, Brown DW, Herrmann JE, Kumar V, Awdeh ZL. A protein multiplex microarray substrate with high sensitivity and specificity. *J Immunol Methods* (2010) 363:60–6. doi: 10.1016/j.jim.2010.10.005

3

The Development of Whole Sporozoite Vaccines for *Plasmodium falciparum* Malaria

Leslie S. Itsara[1†], *Yaxian Zhou*[1], *Julie Do*[1], *Alexis M. Grieser*[1], *Ashley M. Vaughan*[2] *and Anil K. Ghosh*[1*]

[1] MalarVx, Inc., Seattle, WA, United States, [2] Seattle Children's Research Institute, Seattle, WA, United States

***Correspondence:**
Anil K. Ghosh
Aghosh@malarvx.com

†Present Address:
Leslie S. Itsara,
National Institutes of Health (NIH),
Bethesda, MD, United States

Each year malaria kills hundreds of thousands of people and infects hundreds of millions of people despite current control measures. An effective malaria vaccine will likely be necessary to aid in malaria eradication. Vaccination using whole sporozoites provides an increased repertoire of immunogens compared to subunit vaccines across at least two life cycle stages of the parasite, the extracellular sporozoite, and intracellular liver stage. Three potential whole sporozoite vaccine approaches are under development and include genetically attenuated parasites, radiation attenuated sporozoites, and wild-type sporozoites administered in combination with chemoprophylaxis. Pre-clinical and clinical studies have demonstrated whole sporozoite vaccine immunogenicity, including humoral and cellular immunity and a range of vaccine efficacy that depends on the pre-exposure of vaccinated individuals. While whole sporozoite vaccines can provide protection against malaria in some cases, more recent studies in malaria-endemic regions demonstrate the need for improvements. Moreover, challenges remain in manufacturing large quantities of sporozoites for vaccine commercialization. A promising solution to the whole sporozoite manufacturing challenge is *in vitro* culturing methodology, which has been described for several *Plasmodium* species, including the major disease-causing human malaria parasite, *Plasmodium falciparum*. Here, we review whole sporozoite vaccine immunogenicity and *in vitro* culturing platforms for sporozoite production.

Keywords: *Plasmodium falciparum*, malaria, whole sporozoite vaccines, genetically attenuated parasite, radiation attenuated sporozoite, *in vitro* culturing

INTRODUCTION

According to the 2016 World Malaria Report by the World Health Organization (WHO), nearly half of the world's population live in areas at risk of malaria transmission (1). The people most impacted by malaria are children under the age of five and pregnant women living in sub-Saharan Africa. In 2016, *Plasmodium falciparum* (Pf) caused the majority of the 445 thousand deaths and more than 200 million clinical cases, despite recent progress in malaria control efforts, which include vector control with insecticidal bed-nets and insecticide spray and chemoprevention with anti-malarial drugs (1). While these efforts have reduced morbidity and mortality caused by the disease, their impact has declined since the number of deaths and clinical cases have remained constant in the recent years highlighting the need for an effective vaccine. Vaccines represent the most effective form of control for certain infectious disease as demonstrated by the eradication of smallpox and near eradication of polio. However, vaccine development against

Plasmodium has proved more challenging than vaccine development against simpler bacteria or viruses. *Plasmodia* are complex eukaryotic parasites with large genomes (5,300 genes) and transform through multiple life cycle stages with stage-specific gene (antigen) expression (2). Thus, malaria vaccine development has been more challenging. For example, RTS, S/AS-01 (RTS, S) the most developed malaria vaccine candidate, which elicits antibodies against the major sporozoite (SPZ) surface protein, circumsporozoite protein (CSP), only provides partial efficacy (3, 4).

WHOLE SPOROZOITE MALARIA VACCINES IN DEVELOPMENT

Whole sporozoite vaccines (WSV) have demonstrated a range of vaccine efficacy that depends on prior exposure to malaria and ranges from ~35 to 100% efficacy, in which malaria naïve volunteers are better protected. WSV in development include radiation attenuated sporozoites (RAS), genetically attenuated parasites (GAP), and WT sporozoites administered under drug cover (known as CPS–chemical prophylaxis with SPZ, ITV–infection treatment vaccination, or CVac–using Sanaria's injectable SPZ; hereafter referred to as CPS) (**Figure 1**). These live SPZ infect hepatocytes but do not lead to an established blood stage infection either by arresting in liver stage development (RAS and GAP) or by being eliminated during the initial stages of red blood cell (RBC) infection (CPS). WSV elicit immunity during two stages of the parasite life cycle, extracellular SPZ and intracellular liver stage for GAP and RAS and up to the initial stages of RBC infection for CPS. Thus, WSV can elicit immunity without causing clinical malaria symptoms. RAS delivered by bites of irradiated mosquitoes were first tested in humans in 1973 and protected humans from *Pf* malaria challenge (5). Since then, Hoffman and colleagues have made significant progress to produce vialed SPZ from aseptic mosquitoes for clinical testing of RAS (PfSPZ Vaccine) and CVac [Reviewed in (6)]. A recent PfSPZ study involving malaria-experienced individuals in Mali, in which 66% of the Malian vaccine group developed malaria infection, demonstrated reduced efficacy compared to trials involving malaria-naïve individuals (7). Thus, the PfSPZ vaccine failed to provide adequate protection in pre-exposed individuals. This study highlights the need for an improved dosing strategy, immunogenicity enhancement, and/or alternative vaccine approach for populations in malarious regions.

Alternative approaches include other WSV types described here and immunogenicity enhancement of WSV and subunit vaccines described in the following section (Whole Sporozoite Vaccine Immunogenicity). Current GAP in clinical development include early-arresting liver stage parasites that arrest at a similar developmental stage as RAS (<24 h) (8, 9). More recent *P. yoelii* pre-clinical GAP studies have engineered late-arresting liver stage GAP (2–3 days) (10–12). Whole parasites that arrest later in liver stage development (late-arresting GAP) or progress to the blood stage (CPS), provide a larger biomass and broader repertoire of immunogens, permitting lower SPZ doses for protection. For example, clinical CPS studies showed volunteers required 10- to 100-fold fewer parasites than RAS to achieve complete protection against malaria challenge, and pre-clinical late-arresting GAP studies showed that at least 10-fold fewer parasites could provide sterilizing protection and also protect against blood stage challenge (12, 13). Broad protection of late-arresting GAP was demonstrated by immunization with late-arresting *P. yoelii* GAP, which protected against cross-species challenge using *P. berghei* SPZ (11); however, heterologous challenge after CPS vaccination resulted in only modest protection after challenge (14). *Pf* GAP3KO safety has been demonstrated in a human clinical trial in which parasites arrested during liver stage development as all ten volunteers remained blood stage negative (8). However, in a previous safety trial using the first developed GAP, GAP2KO (*p36*$^-$ and *p52*$^-$) one in six volunteers showed patent blood stage infection (15). GAP2KO arrest later in liver stage development compared to GAP3KO (16), thus highlighting the challenge in developing a late-arresting GAP that is also completely liver-stage attenuated. Nevertheless, several groups are working on the development of late-arresting GAP due to their potential benefits.

Abbreviations: CHMI, controlled human malaria infection; CPS, chemoprophylaxis with *Pf* sporozoites; CSP, circumsporozoite protein; CVac, CPS using Sanaria's injectable sporozoites; GAP, genetically attenuated parasite; IFN-γ, interferon-γ; IL-2, interleuken-2; ITV, infection treatment vaccination; IVS, *in vitro* sporozoite; NHP, non-human primate; *Pf, Plasmodium falciparum*; PMBC, peripheral blood mononuclear cells; RAS, radiation attenuated sporozoite; RBC, red blood cell; SPZ, sporozoite; RPMI, Roswell Park Memorial Institute; RTS, S, RTS, S/AS-01; SPZ, sporozoite; TNF-α, transcription factor α; WHO, World Health Organization; WSV, whole sporozoite vaccine.

WHOLE SPOROZOITE VACCINE IMMUNOGENICITY

Pre-clinical and clinical studies using GAP, RAS, and CPS have demonstrated safety of vaccination with WSV, immunogenicity, and vaccine efficacy [(17); Reviewed in (6, 8, 18)]. WSV immunogenicity data supports CD8$^+$ T cells as playing a critical role in protection. CD4$^+$ T cells, γδ T cells, and antibodies are also elicited after immunization, but their roles in the protective immune response are less clear. Complete reviews focused on WSV immunogenicity and potential clinical correlates of protection are discussed elsewhere (19, 20).

Cellular Immunity: CD8$^+$, and γδ T Cells

Numerous studies support roles for cellular immunity in WSV protection, including CD8$^+$, γδ, and CD4$^+$ T cells. The strongest immunological data supports roles for cytokine-producing CD8$^+$ T cells, liver resident CD8$^+$ T cells, and γδ T cells as possible WSV immune correlates during liver stage infection. For example, in rodents, depletion of interferon-gamma (IFN-γ) or CD8$^+$ T cells blocked RAS mediated sterile immunity (21). Subsequent studies were performed to analyze cellular responses and cytokine production after immunization by obtaining peripheral blood mononuclear cells (PBMC) and stimulating with *Pf* specific antigens, whole SPZ, or infected RBC. For *Pf*GAP2KO studies, interferon-γ (IFN-γ) producing CD8$^+$ T cell responses increased after immunization (15). For PfSPZ Vaccine immunization, levels of CD8$^+$ T cells that

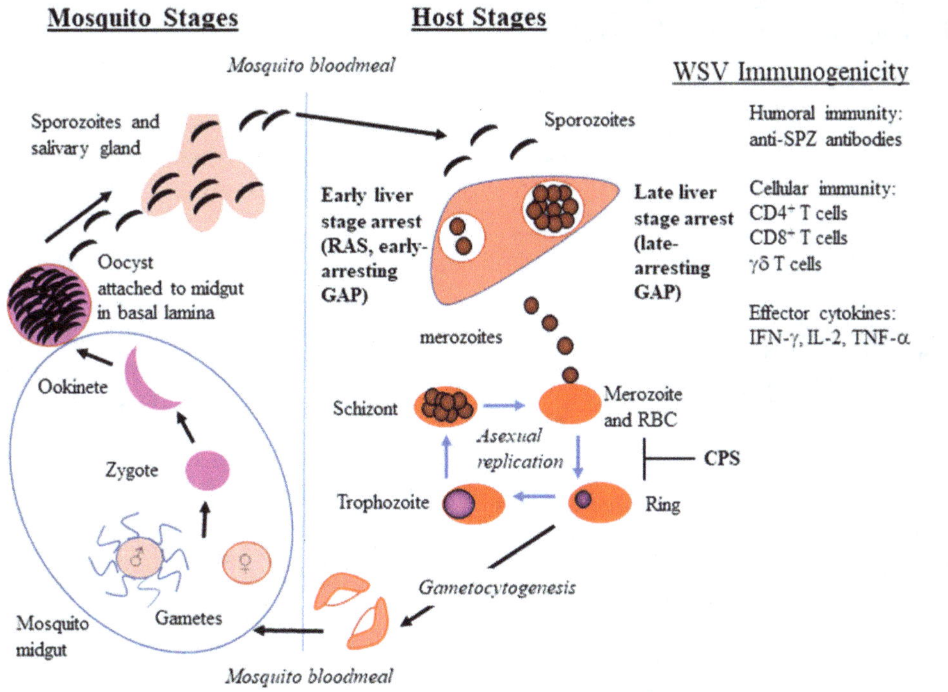

FIGURE 1 | *Plasmodium* life cycle in mosquitoes and vertebrate hosts. The whole sporozite vaccine (WSV) strategy for radiation attenuated sporozoites (RAS), genetically attenuated parasites (GAP), and chemoprophylaxis with WT sporozoites (CPS) is shown in bold. The WSV immunogenicity provided by WSV administration is also listed.

produced effector cytokine molecules [IFN-γ, interleuken-2 (IL-2), or transcription factor-alpha (TNF-α)] increased compared to pre-vaccination (22, 23). However, cytokine-producing T cell responses did not correlate with protection (22, 23).

Non-recirculating liver resident $CD8^+$ T cells represent an immunological marker that cannot be sampled in peripherally circulating cell populations (e.g., PBMC) from human clinical trials. Several studies support liver-resident and IFN-γ-producing $CD8^+$ T cells in providing protection after WSV administration. First, a PfSPZ immunization study was performed and involved different vaccine administration routes in mice, non-human primates (NHP), and humans (24). The greatest protection after CHMI was provided by IV vaccination compared to intradermal or intramuscular. Also, animal studies in mice and NHP identified IFN-γ-producing $CD8^+$ T cells in the liver, which correlated with protection by IV administration (24). Subsequent parabiosis experiments in mice confirmed the existence of liver-resident $CD8^+$ T cells (25), which provided RAS-induced malaria immunity (26). Further PfSPZ vaccination studies of NHP support liver resident IFN-γ-producing $CD8^+$ T cells in providing immunity as these cell levels were ~100-fold higher in liver than in blood (27). Finally, several pre-clinical and clinical PfSPZ and CVac studies have also identified γδ T cells as possible correlates of protection that increase after subsequent vaccinations (22, 23, 27, 28).

While WSV have reduced immunogenicity and efficacy in some pre-exposed individuals (7, 29), vaccination strategies are underway to improve WSV immunogenicity. This work was motivated by numerous studies that support liver-resident $CD8^+$ T cells as primary mediators of long-term pre-erythrocytic immunity. Several groups are developing either "prime and target" or "prime and trap" approaches in which peripheral $CD8^+$ T cells are first primed and then targeting to the liver by high expression of *Plasmodium* subunit antigens or RAS infection (30, 31). These methods lead to higher levels of liver-resident $CD8^+$ T cells and improved RAS or subunit vaccine efficacy compared to RAS or subunit alone (30, 31). Further clinical studies will determine whether these pre-clinical results translate to protect diverse populations of humans, especially in malarious regions.

Additional WSV immunogenicity studies must be performed to identify strong immune correlates for the purpose of guiding clinical trials, including dose and regimen strategies. These studies may be focused on identifying antigen specificity of important T cell populations (γδ and liver resident $CD8^+$ T cells). For example, sequencing studies of T-cell receptors that bind malaria-specific antigens may identify strong correlates of protection. Moreover, since liver resident T-cells cannot be studied using PBMC from human clinical trials, future studies using NHP will prove valuable in identifying strong immune correlates of protection provided by WSV.

In vitro Sporozoites for *Pf* Malaria Vaccines

While WSV are the most effective vaccines against *Pf* malaria, major hurdles prevent the manufacturing of sufficient quantities at a commercial scale. Current methods of vaccination with SPZ include delivery by mosquito bite or by injection after technically challenging and laborious mosquito dissections. Neither approach is practical for large-scale or cost-effective vaccination, which is required for commercialization. Culturing systems that produce infective SPZ independent of mosquitoes would enable scalable production of *Pf* SPZ for WSV.

Plasmodium Stage Development in Mosquitoes

Continuous culture of blood stage malaria parasites (asexual and sexual) has been established for decades (32–35). However, the *in vitro* culturing of mosquito stages has proven extremely challenging. To culture SPZ, one must understand *Pf* development within the mosquito and recapitulate this in culture. *Pf* develops through five sequential stages in mosquitoes: gamete, zygote, ookinete, oocyst, and SPZ (**Figure 1**). Prior to mosquito stages, gametocytes are ingested by mosquitoes during a blood meal. After ingestion, gametocytes within the mosquito midgut emerge and transform into gametes that fuse to form a zygote. The zygote undergoes DNA replication and maturation into a motile and invasive ookinete that traverses the mosquito peritrophic membrane and midgut epithelium, and finally embeds into the basal lamina on the midgut periphery. The interaction between the ookinete and the mosquito midgut basal lamina is thought to trigger the transformation into the early oocyst (36–38). The sessile oocyst is the site of SPZ development (up to several thousand SPZ per mature oocyst). Once released, SPZ travel to the salivary glands through the hemocoel where they can be inoculated into a host during a mosquito blood meal (39).

As *Plasmodium* develops through multiple life cycle stages, studies indicate that transitions are driven by coordinated changes in stage-specific gene expression controlled by the apicomplexan Apetala2 (AP2) family of transcription factors (TFs) (40, 41). The 26 AP2 TFs represent the only known family of *Plasmodia* TFs and contain at least one AP2 DNA-binding domain (42). TFs controlling stage transitions include AP2-O, AP2-O2, AP2-O3, and AP2-O4 for ookinetes and oocysts (41, 43, 44), AP2-Sp, AP2-Sp2, and AP2-Sp3 for mature oocysts and/or SPZ (41, 45), AP2-G, and AP2-G2 for gametocytes (41, 46, 47), and AP2-L for liver stages (48). These TFs co-regulate expression of genes with common *cis* promoter elements enabling control of the *Plasmodium* life cycle (41). Understanding stage transition through gene regulation could improve SPZ culturing systems. Other culturing system improvements could include applying knowledge of the parasite's environment while developing in mosquitoes.

Plasmodium in vitro Sporozoite Culturing Systems

Although several publications already exist that describe *in vitro* culturing of *Plasmodium* SPZ for the mouse (*P. berghei*, *P. yoelii*), avian (*P. gallinaceum*), and human (*Pf*) species (49–52), there is only a single publication outlining culturing methods for each species and SPZ characterization. Specific details on the different *Plasmodium* culturing systems are provided in **Table 1**. Culturing system factors that likely support production of SPZ include co-culturing with *Drosophila* support cells (L2/S2), an optimal medium (Roswell Park Memorial Institute [RPMI] or Schneider's), and culturing on a gel-like surrogate for the mosquito basal lamina. All culturing systems required *Drosophila* co-culturing or using conditioned media (spent media) from L2/S2 cells. *Drosophila* cells may provide nutrients for the developing oocyst and/or oocyst capsule, including soluble nutrients, growth/signaling factors and/or extracellular matrix molecules that are normally present in the mosquito midgut basal lamina or hemolymph. For culturing media, the avian and human culturing systems utilized RPMI, which is also used for *Pf* blood stage culture. Subsequent studies on culturing the murine-specific *Plasmodia* determined that Schneider's media optimally supported *Drosophila* cell growth (49). Finally, for the basal lamina, all culturing systems except the *P. yoelii* system found the necessity of Matrigel, which is a basal lamina-like gel derived from murine Engleberth-Holm-Swarm tumor cells and consists of laminin, collagen type IV, heparan sulfate proteoglycan, entactin, and growth factors. Laminin and collagen IV are known components of the mosquito basal lamina and are considered important for ookinete binding and oocyst transformation for mosquito and *in vitro* development (36–38, 56). In sum, there are shared characteristics of the *Plasmodium in vitro* sporozoite (IVS) culturing systems that reveal important factors supporting axenic SPZ development, including *Drosophila* cells, Schneider's media, and Matrigel or a similar basal lamina.

Characterization of Cultured Oocysts and Sporozoites

For the different *Plasmodium* culturing systems, oocyst, and SPZ development have been characterized to varying degrees (**Table 1**). The study that describes *Pf* culturing demonstrated that IVS morphology was similar to mosquito-derived SPZ and that IVS expressed the major SPZ surface protein, CSP (52). However, IVS functionality in terms of motility or hepatocyte traversal/invasion/infection was not analyzed. Similarly, for *P. gallinaceum*, only morphology and CSP expression were described (51). Separate studies on the rodent malaria parasites, *P. berghei* (49), and *P. yoelii* (50) analyzed morphology and sporozoite invasion of hepatocytes in mice. For *P. berghei*, IVS were produced with similar morphology and mouse infectivity compared to mosquito-derived SPZ, and blood stage infection was also observed (49). For *P. yoelii*, IVS infected primary hepatocytes in culture at a low rate (1/10,000) and hepatocytes in mice but infectivity was reduced compared to mosquito-derived SPZ. Furthermore, blood stage parasites were only seen in 1/15 infected mice (50).

While these studies demonstrate the feasibility of producing IVS that are capable of hepatocyte infection, many researchers have failed to replicate mosquito-stage culturing of *Pf* and other *Plasmodium* species due to the complexity of *Plasmodium* mosquito stage development and the extreme scientific and technical challenges of establishing culturing systems. We and

TABLE 1 | Characteristics of *in vitro* sporozoite culturing systems for *Plasmodium gallinaceum*, *falciparum*, *berghei* and *yoelli*.

***Plasmodium* species (reference)**	**Oocyst /SPZ culture conditions**	**Basal lamina requirement**	**Oocyst diameter**	**Ookinete to oocyst conversion *in vitro* (early or mature) / *in vivo* provided for comparison**	**SPZ days observed**	**SPZ characterization**
P. gallinaceum	*Drosophila* cells required	Matrigel	Day 3–7 mm for elongate	10–30% (mature)	Days 10 to 22 peaking on Day 16	Morphology with anti-CSP staining
(51)	In RPMI media		Days 5 to 7–up to 30 mm for spherical and up to 40 mm for elongated	1–21%* (53)		
P. falciparum	*Drosophila* cells required	Matrigel	Day 7–15 to 20 mm	N.D.	Days 12 to 16	Morphology with anti-CSP staining
(52)	In RPMI media		Days 10 to 12–25 to 40 mm	0.4–1.3%* (54)		
P. berghei	*Drosophila* cells required	Matrigel	Day 15–up to 40 mm	68% (mature)	Days 15 to 28	Morphology with Giemsa staining; Infectivity in hepatocytes of mice observed with subsequent blood stage transition and then mosquito infection
(49)	In Schneider's media			0–18%* (53)		
P. yoelii	*Drosophila* cells or conditioned media required	Matrigel not required	Day 3–4 mm	7.1% (early)	Days 6 to 30	Morphology with anti-CSP staining; Infectivity of primary mouse hepatocytes and hepatocytes of mice observed with subsequent blood stage transition
(50)	In Scheider's media		Days 6 to 7–10 mm	0–75%* (55)		

The features, including culture conditions, parasites observed, conversion frequency from ookinete to oocyst, and details of SPZ characterization are outlined and compared between culturing systems. For oocyst diameter, the observed oocysts were spherical unless otherwise noted. N.D, not described; RPMI, Roswell Park Memorial Institute.

**The range is due to differences in Anopheles mosquito species tested.*

others, including Sanaria, have made further improvements on developing *Pf* IVS culturing systems to ultimately produce SPZ for use in WSV development. For example, our *Pf* culturing system uses the unique nutrient, insect (silk-worm) hemolymph (56). Oocysts and maturing SPZ may receive soluble nutrients, growth factors, and/or signaling factors from the insect hemolymph as from the mosquito hemolymph. Successful *in vitro Pf* conversion frequencies compared to mosquito development have been achieved for life cycle stages up to the mature oocyst stage (56). Current developing approaches are focused on improving conversion to the mature oocyst and SPZ stages by using 3-dimensional culturing on non-Matrigel basal lamina-like substrates. Matrigel presents challenges for cGMP vaccine production as it is tumor-derived and may vary between batches.

Summary and Future Considerations

Future hurdles for the production of IVS to use in WSV include demonstrating equivalent functionality compared to mosquito-derived SPZ in terms of hepatocyte invasion/infection using cell lines and human-liver chimeric mouse models (57). While *P. berghei* IVS exhibit infectivity comparable to mosquito-derived SPZ, *P. yoelii* IVS have decreased infectivity, and hepatocyte infectivity was not assessed for *Pf* or *P. gallinaceum* IVS. IVS may resemble immature mosquito midgut SPZ more so than fully infectious mosquito salivary gland SPZ, which further develop in the mosquito hemocoel and salivary gland (58). Additional cues may be necessary for the IVS culturing systems to produce fully infectious, mature SPZ for use as a WSV. Moreover, GAP or RAS IVS will also need to satisfy safety requirements in terms of liver stage arrest and demonstrate absence of toxins, pathogens, or other contaminants. Thus, hurdles must be overcome in the purification of IVS from the 3D basal lamina and from *Drosophila* cells while maintaining IVS functionality. If these issues can be solved, culturing of SPZ would provide scalable production of WSV for further development as *Pf* malaria vaccines.

AUTHOR CONTRIBUTIONS

LSI, YZ, JD, AMG, AMV, and AKG developed the manuscript. LSI and AKG drafted the manuscript. All authors read and approved the final manuscript.

FUNDING

The manuscript was supported by private funds from MalarVx, Inc.

ACKNOWLEDGMENTS

The authors acknowledge Mr. James W. Davie for supporting this manuscript.

REFERENCES

1. WHO, World Health Organization. *World Malaria Report,* 2016. WHO (2017).
2. Gardner MJ, Hall N, Fung E, White O, Berriman M, Hyman RW, et al. Genome sequence of the human malaria parasite *Plasmodium falciparum. Nature* (2002) 419:498–511. doi: 10.1038/nature01097
3. White MT, Verity R, Griffin JT, Asante KP, Owusu-Agyei S, Greenwood B, et al. Immunogenicity of the RTS,S/AS01 malaria vaccine and implications for duration of vaccine efficacy: secondary analysis of data from a phase 3 randomised controlled trial. *Lancet Infect Dis.* (2015) 15:1450–8. doi: 10.1016/S1473-3099(15)00239-X
4. RTSS Clinical Trials Partnership. Efficacy and safety of RTS,S/AS01 malaria vaccine with or without a booster dose in infants and children in Africa: final results of a phase 3, individually randomised, controlled trial. *Lancet* (2015) 386:31–45. doi: 10.1016/S0140-6736(15)60721-8
5. Clyde DF, Most H, McCarthy VC, Vanderberg JP. Immunization of man against sporozoite-induced falciparum malaria. *Am J Med Sci.* (1973) 266:169–77. doi: 10.1097/00000441-197309000-00002
6. Hoffman SL, Vekemans J, Richie TL, Duffy PE. The march toward malaria vaccines. *Vaccine* (2015) 33:13–23. doi: 10.1016/j.vaccine.2015.07.091
7. Sissoko MS, Healy SA, Katile A, Omaswa F, Zaidi I, Gabriel EE, et al. Safety and efficacy of PfSPZ vaccine against *Plasmodium falciparum* via direct venous inoculation in healthy malaria-exposed adults in Mali: a randomised, double-blind phase 1 trial. *Lancet Infect Dis.* (2017) 17:498–509. doi: 10.1016/S1473-3099(17)30104-4
8. Kublin JG, Sack BK, Fishbaugher ME, Seilie A, Shelton L, VonGoedert T, et al. Complete attenuation of genetically engineered Plasmodium falciparum sporozoites in human subjects. *Sci Transl Med.* (2017) 9:1–11. doi: 10.1126/scitranslmed.aad9099
9. van Schaijk BC, Ploemen IH, Annoura T, Vos MW, Foquet L, van Gemert GJ, et al. A genetically attenuated malaria vaccine candidate based on P. falciparum b9/slarp gene-deficient sporozoites. *Elife* (2014) 3:e03582. doi: 10.7554/eLife.03582
10. Vaughan AM, O'Neill MT, Tarun AS, Camargo N, Phuong TM, Aly ASI, et al. Type II fatty acid synthesis is essential only for malaria parasite late liver stage development. *Cell Microbiol.* (2009) 11:506–20. doi: 10.1111/j.1462-5822.2008.01270.x.
11. Butler NS, Schmidt NW, Vaughan AM, Aly AS, Kappe SH, Harty JT. Superior antimalarial immunity after vaccination with late liver stage-arresting genetically attenuated parasites. *Cell Host Microbe* (2011) 9:451–62. doi: 10.1016/j.chom.2011.05.008
12. Vaughan AM, Sack BK, Dankwa D, Minkah N, Nguyen T, Cardamone H, et al. A plasmodium parasite with complete late liver stage arrest protects against preerythrocytic and erythrocytic stage infection in mice. *Infect Immun.* (2018) 86:e00088-18. doi: 10.1128/IAI.00088-18
13. Bijker EM, Bastiaens GJ, Teirlinck AC, van Gemert GJ, Graumans W, van de Vegte-Bolmer M, et al. Protection against malaria after immunization by chloroquine prophylaxis and sporozoites is mediated by preerythrocytic immunity. *Proc Natl Acad Sci USA.* (2013) 110:7862–7. doi: 10.1073/pnas.1220360110
14. Walk J, Reuling IJ, Behet MC, Meerstein-Kessel L, Graumans W, van Gemert GJ, et al. Modest heterologous protection after Plasmodium falciparum sporozoite immunization: a double-blind randomized controlled clinical trial. *BMC Med.* (2017) 15:168. doi: 10.1186/s12916-017-0923-4
15. Spring M, Murphy J, Nielsen R, Dowler M, Bennett JW, Zarling S, et al. First-in human evaluation of genetically attenuated *Plasmodium falciparum* sporozoites administered by bite of Anopheles Mosquitoes to adult volunteers. *Vaccine* (2013) 31:4975–83. doi: 10.1016/j.vaccine.2013.08.007
16. VanBuskirk KM, O'Neill MT, De La Vega P, Maier AG, Krzych U, Williams J, et al. Preerythrocytic, live-attenuated *Plasmodium falciparum* vaccine candidates by design. *Proc Natl Acad Sci USA.* (2009) 106:13004–9. doi: 10.1073/pnas.0906387106
17. Mikolajczak SA, Lakshmanan V, Fishbaugher M, Camargo N, Harupa A, Kaushansky A, et al. A next-generation genetically attenuated *Plasmodium falciparum* parasite created by triple gene deletion. *Mol Ther.* (2014) 22:1707–15. doi: 10.1038/mt.2014.85
18. Mordmüller B, Surat G, Lagler H, Chakravarty S, Ishizuka AS, Lalremruata A, et al. Sterile protection against human malaria by chemoattenuated PfSPZ vaccine. *Nature* (2017) 542:445–9. doi: 10.1038/nature21060
19. Doll KL, Harty JT. Correlates of protective immunity following whole sporozoite vaccination against malaria. *Immunol Res.* (2014) 59:166–76. doi: 10.1007/s12026-014-8525-0
20. Draper SJ, Sack BK, King CR, Nielsen CM, Rayner JC, Higgins MK, et al. Malaria vaccines: recent advances and new horizons. *Cell Host Microbe* (2018) 24:43–56. doi: 10.1016/j.chom.2018.06.008
21. Schofield L, Villaquiran J, Ferreira A, Schellekens H, Nussenzweig R, Nussenzweig V. Gamma interferon, $CD8^+$ T cells and antibodies required for immunity to malaria sporozoites. *Nature* (1987) 330:664–6.
22. Seder RA, Chang LJ, Enama ME, Zephir KL, Sarwar UN, Gordon IJ, et al. Protection against malaria by intravenous immunization with a nonreplicating sporozoite vaccine. *Science* (2013) 341:1359–65. doi: 10.1126/science.1241800
23. Lyke KE, Ishizuka AS, Berry AA, Chakravarty S, DeZure A, Enama ME, et al. Attenuated PfSPZ vaccine induces strain-transcending T cells and durable protection against heterologous controlled human malaria infection. *Proc Natl Acad Sci USA.* (2017) 114:2711–6. doi: 10.1073/pnas.1615324114
24. Epstein JE, Tewari K, Lyke KE, Sim BK, Billingsley PF, Laurens MB, et al. Live attenuated malaria vaccine designed to protect through hepatic $CD8^+$ T cell immunity. *Science* (2011) 334:475–80. doi: 10.1126/science.1211548
25. Steinert EM, Schenkel JM, Fraser KA, Beura LK, Manlove LS, Igyártó BZ, et al. Quantifying memory CD8 T cells reveals regionalization of immunosurveillance. *Cell* (2015) 161:737–49. doi: 10.1016/j.cell.2015.03.031
26. Fernandez-Ruiz D, Ng WY, Holz LE, Ma JZ, Zaid A, Wong YC, et al. Liver-resident memory $CD8^+$ T cells form a front-line defense against malaria liver-stage infection. *Immunity* (2016) 45:889–902. doi: 10.1016/j.immuni.2016.08.011
27. Ishizuka AS, Lyke KE, DeZure A, Berry AA, Richie TL, Mendoza FH, et al. Protection against malaria at 1 year and immune correlates following PfSPZ vaccination. *Nat Med.* (2016) 22:614–23. doi: 10.1038/nm.4110
28. Zaidi I, Diallo H, Conteh S, Robbins Y, Kolasny J, Orr-Gonzalez S, et al. $\gamma\delta$ T Cells Are required for the induction of sterile immunity during irradiated sporozoite vaccinations. *J Immunol.* (2017) 199:3781–8. doi: 10.4049/jimmunol.1700314
29. Olotu A, Urbano V, Hamad A, Eka M, Chemba M, Nyakarungu E, et al. Advancing global health through development and clinical trials partnerships: a randomized, placebo-controlled, double-blind assessment of safety, tolerability, and immunogenicity of PfSPZ vaccine for malaria in healthy Equatoguinean men. *Am J Trop Med Hyg.* (2018) 98:308–18. doi: 10.4269/ajtmh.17-0449
30. Gola A, Silman D, Walters AA, Sridhar S, Uderhardt S, Salman AM, et al. Prime and target immunization protects against liver-stage malaria in mice. *Sci Transl Med.* (2018) 10:eaap9128. doi: 10.1126/scitranslmed.aap9128
31. Olsen TM, Stone BC, Chuenchob V, Murphy SC. Prime-and-trap malaria vaccination to generate protective $CD8^+$ liver-resident memory T cells. *J Immunol.* (2018) 201:1984–93. doi: 10.4049/jimmunol.1800740
32. Haynes DJ, Diggs CL, Hines FA, Desjardins RE. Culture of human malaria parasites *Plasmodium falciparum. Nature* (1976) 263:767–9. doi: 10.1038/263767a0
33. Ifediba T, Vanderberg JP. Complete *in vitro* maturation of *Plasmodium falciparum* gametocytes. *Nature* (1981) 294:364–6. doi: 10.1038/294364a0
34. Ponnudurai T, Meuwissen JH, Leeuwenberg AD, Verhave JP, Lensen AH. The production of mature gametocytes of *Plasmodium falciparum* in continuous cultures of different isolates infective to mosquitoes. *Trans R Soc Trop Med Hyg.* (1982) 76:242–50. doi: 10.1016/0035-9203(82)90289-9
35. Trager W, Jensen JB. Human malaria parasites in continuous culture. *Science* (1976) 193:673–5.
36. Arrighi RB, Hurd H. The role of Plasmodium berghei ookinete proteins in binding to basal lamina components and transformation into oocysts. *Int J Parasitol.* (2002) 32:91–8. doi: 10.1016/S0020-7519(01)00298-3
37. Adini A, Warburg A. Interaction of *Plasmodium gallinaceum* ookinetes and oocysts with extracellular matrix proteins. *Parasitology* (1999) 119:331–6. doi: 10.1017/S0031182099004874

38. Vlachou D, Lycett G, Siden-Kiamos I, Blass C, Sinden RE, Louis C. Anopheles gambiae laminin interacts with the P25 surface protein of Plasmodium berghei ookinetes. *Mol Biochem Parasitol.* (2001) 112:229–37. doi: 10.1016/S0166-6851(00)00371-6
39. Sinden RE. The biology of Plasmodium in the mosquito. *Experientia* (1984) 40:1330–43. doi: 10.1007/BF01951886
40. Zhou Y, Ramachandran V, Kumar KA, Westenberger S, Refour P, Zhou B, et al. Evidence-based annotation of the malaria parasite's genome using comparative expression profiling. *PLoS ONE* (2008) 3:e1570.
41. Modrzynska K, Pfander C, Chappell L, Yu L, Suarez C, Dundas K, et al. A knockout screen of ApiAP2 genes reveals networks of interacting transcriptional regulators controlling the plasmodium life cycle. *Cell Host Microbe* (2017) 21:11–22. doi: 10.1016/j.chom.2016.12.003
42. Balaji S, Babu MM, Iyer LM, Aravind L. Discovery of the principal specific transcription factors of Apicomplexa and their implication for the evolution of the AP2-integrase DNA binding domains. *Nucleic Acids Res.* (2005) 33:3994–4006. doi: 10.1093/nar/gki709
43. Yuda M, Iwanaga S, Shigenobu S, Mair GR, Janse CJ, Waters AP, et al. Identification of a transcription factor in the mosquito-invasive stage of malaria parasites. *Mol Microbiol.* (2009) 71:1402–14. doi: 10.1111/j.1365-2958.2009.06609.x
44. Kaneko I, Iwanaga S, Kato T, Kobayashi I, Yuda M. Genome-wide identification of the target genes of AP2-O, a plasmodium AP2-family transcription factor. *PLoS Pathog.* (2015) 11:e1004905. doi: 10.1371/journal.ppat.1004905
45. Yuda M, Iwanaga S, Shigenobu S, Kato T, Kaneko I. Transcription factor AP2-Sp and its target genes in malarial sporozoites. *Mol Microbiol.* (2010) 75:854–63. doi: 10.1111/j.1365-2958.2009.07005.x
46. Kafsack BFC, Rovira-Graells N, Clark TG, Bancells C, Crowley VM, Campino SG, et al. A transcriptional switch underlies commitment to sexual development in malaria parasites. *Nature* (2014) 507:248–52. doi: 10.1038/nature12920
47. Sinha A, Hughes KR, Modrzynska KK, Otto TD, Pfander C, Dickens NJ, et al. A cascade of DNA-binding proteins for sexual commitment and development in Plasmodium. *Nature* (2014) 507:253–7. doi: 10.1038/nature 12970
48. Iwanaga S, Kaneko I, Kato T, Yuda M. Identification of an AP2-family protein that is critical for malaria liver stage development. *PLoS ONE* (2012) 7:e47557. doi: 10.1371/journal.pone.0047557
49. Al-Olayan EM, Beetsma AL, Butcher GA, Sinden RE, Hurd H. Complete development of mosquito phases of the malaria parasite *in vitro*. *Science* (2002) 295:677–9. doi: 10.1126/science.1067159
50. Porter-Kelley JM, Dinglasan RR, Alam U, Ndeta GA, Sacci JB, Jr, Azad AF. *Plasmodium yoelii*: axenic development of the parasite mosquito stages. *Exp Parasitol.* (2006) 112:99–108. doi: 10.1016/j.exppara.2005.09.011
51. Warburg A, Miller LH. Sporogonic Development of a malaria parasite *in vitro*. *Science* (1992) 255:448–50. doi: 10.1126/science.1734521
52. Warburg A, Schneider I. *In vitro* culture of the mosquito stages of *Plasmodium falciparum*. *Exp Parasitol.* (1993) 76:121–6. doi: 10.1006/expr.1993.1014
53. Alavi Y, Arai M, Mendoza J, Tufet-Bayona M, Sinha R, Fowler K, et al. The dynamics of interactions between Plasmodium and the mosquito: a study of the infectivity of *Plasmodium berghei* and *Plasmodium gallinaceum* and their transmission by *Anopheles stephensi*, *Anopheles gambiae* and *Aedes aegypti*. *Int J Parasitol.* (2003) 33:933–43. doi: 10.1016/s0020-7519(03)00112-7
54. Vaughan JA, Noden BH, Beier JC. Sporogonic development of cultured *Plasmodium falciparum* in six species of laboratory-reared *Anopheles mosquitoes*. *Am J Trop Med Hyg.* (1994) 51:233–43. doi: 10.4269/ajtmh.1994.51.233
55. Vaughan JA, Hensley L, Beier JC. Sporogonic development of *Plasmodium yoelii* in five anopheline species. *J Parasitol.* (1994) 80:674–81. doi: 10.2307/3283245
56. Itsara LS, Zhou Y, Do J, Dungel S, Fishbaugher ME, Betz WW, et al. PfCap380 as a marker for *Plasmodium falciparum* oocyst development *in vivo* and *in vitro*. *Malar J.* (2018). 17:135. doi: 10.1186/s12936-018-2277-6
57. Vaughan AM, Mikolajczak SA, Camargo N, Lakshmanan V, Kennedy M, Lindner SE, et al. A transgenic *Plasmodium falciparum* NF54 strain that expresses GFP-luciferase throughout the parasite life cycle. *Mol Biochem Parasitol.* (2012) 186:143–7. doi: 10.1016/j.molbiopara.2012.10.004
58. Matuschewski K, Ross J, Brown SM, Kaiser K, Nussenzweig V, Kappe SH. Infectivity-associated changes in the transcriptional repertoire of the malaria parasite sporozoite stage. *J Biol Chem.* (2002) 277:41948–53.

4

Combination of RTS,S and Pfs25-IMX313 Induces a Functional Antibody Response Against Malaria Infection and Transmission in Mice

Florian Brod[1*], *Kazutoyo Miura*[2], *Iona Taylor*[1], *Yuanyuan Li*[1], *Arianna Marini*[1], *Ahmed M. Salman*[1], *Alexandra J. Spencer*[1], *Carole A. Long*[2] *and Sumi Biswas*[1*]

[1] *Jenner Institute, University of Oxford, Oxford, United Kingdom,* [2] *Laboratory of Malaria and Vector Research, National Institute of Allergy and Infectious Disease, National Institutes of Health, Rockville, MD, United States*

Correspondence:
Florian Brod
florian.brod87@gmail.com
Sumi Biswas
sumi.biswas@ndm.ox.ac.uk

The last two decades saw a dramatic reduction in malaria incidence rates, but this decrease has been stalling recently, indicating control measures are starting to fail. An effective vaccine, particularly one with a marked effect on disease transmission, would undoubtedly be an invaluable tool for efforts to control and eliminate malaria. RTS,S/AS01, the most advanced malaria vaccine to date, targets the parasite before it invades the liver and has the potential to prevent malaria disease as well as transmission by preventing blood stage infection and therefore gametocytogenesis. Unfortunately efficacy in a phase III clinical trial was limited and it is widely believed that a malaria vaccine needed to contain multiple antigens from different life-cycle stages to have a realistic chance of success. A recent study in mice has shown that partially efficacious interventions targeting the pre-erythrocytic and the sexual lifecycle stage synergise in eliminating malaria from a population over multiple generations. Hence, the combination of RTS,S/AS01 with a transmission blocking vaccine (TBV) is highly appealing as a pragmatic and powerful way to increase vaccine efficacy. Here we demonstrate that combining Pfs25-IMX313, one of the TBV candidates currently in clinical development, with RTS,S/AS01 readily induces a functional immune response against both antigens in outbred CD1 mice. Formulation of Pfs25-IMX313 in AS01 significantly increased antibody titres when compared to formulation in Alhydrogel, resulting in improved transmission reducing activity in standard membrane feeding assays (SMFA). Upon co-formulation of Pfs25-IMX313 with RTS,S/AS01, the immunogenicity of both vaccines was maintained, and functional assessment of the induced antibody response by SMFA and inhibition of sporozoite invasion assay (ISI) showed no reduction in biological activity against parasites of both lifecycle stages. Should this findings be translatable to human vaccination this could greatly aid efforts to eliminate and eventually eradicate malaria.

Keywords: malaria, vaccine, transmission blocking, pre-erythrocytic, synergy

INTRODUCTION

Malaria is caused by parasites of the genus *Plasmodium*, and it is one of the world's oldest and deadliest diseases. According to estimates in the World Health Organisation (WHO) world malaria report 2017 (1) the global number of malaria deaths reached 445,000 in 2016, and there were a total of 216 million malaria cases, an increase of 5 million cases over 2015. This is the first time since 2010 that case numbers increased with respect to the estimates of the previous year indicating that current control measures, which helped to drastically reduce malaria prevalence over the last decade are starting to fail and novel interventions are necessary if malaria eradication is to be achieved (2).

Vaccines are undoubtedly one of the most successful public heath interventions of all time, and played an essential role in the control or eradication of a number of diseases. An efficacious vaccine would be of immense value to all efforts to contain and eventually eradicate malaria. As outlined in the malaria vaccine technology (MVT) roadmap, as well as the malERA research agenda for malaria eradication (3, 4), an ideal malaria vaccine would have two characteristics; it would protect a vaccinated individual from illness as well as have an impact on malaria transmission (5). *Plasmodium* parasites have an exquisitely complex lifecycle with obligate developmental steps in the human host as well as in the mosquito vector. Roughly, it can be broken down in three different stages, the pre-erythrocytic stage, the erythrocytic stage or asexual blood stage and the sexual or sporogonic stage. Vaccines with an impact on malaria transmission are often referred to as VIMTs (vaccines that interrupt malaria transmission), and include classic TBVs that target the sexual life-cycle stage of the parasite in the mosquito vector as well as pre-erythrocytic vaccines (PEVs) that prevent blood stage infection and therefore gametocytogenesis. The impact of vaccines targeting the asexual blood stage, which also is the target of naturally acquired immunity, is likely to be more limited. The most advanced malaria vaccine candidate to date RTS,S/AS01 targets the pre-erythrocytic stage antigen circumsporozoite protein (CSP) of *P. falciparum*, the causative agent of the most severe form of human malaria, with the aim to interrupt the parasite's lifecycle before the establishment of liver stage infection. It is the only malaria vaccine to have completed Phase III clinical trials (6–9) and to have obtained a positive scientific opinion from the European Medicines Agency (EMA) (10). As RTS,S/AS01 targets a stage in the lifecycle before the emergence of symptomatic and transmissible stages, it has the potential to prevent disease as well as transmission. However, efficacy of RTS,S/AS01 in the recently concluded Phase III clinical trial, stayed below the targets formulated in the MVT roadmap (8, 9).

One way to build on the substantial efforts that led to development of RTS,S/AS01 is to combine it with other malaria vaccines currently in development, and indeed consensus is now that a vaccine containing multiple antigens from different life-cycle stages has the most realistic chance of success (11, 12). A recent study using two monoclonal antibodies targeting CSP and the sexual stage antigen Pfs25 at partially efficacious concentrations showed that pre-erythrocytic and sexual stage interventions synergise over multiple generations as the efficacy of PEVs is sensitively dependent on the sporozoite load of an infectious mosquito and TBVs can reduce the number of oocysts that develop in the mosquito midgut and therefore reduce the number of sporozoites that reach the mosquito's salivary gland (13). Therefore, combination of RTS,S/AS01 with a TBV, targeting the sexual stage of the parasite, is particularly attractive. Furthermore, addition of RTS,S/AS01 to a TBV could overcome one of the perceived drawbacks of TBVs, which is the absence of a direct protective effect on the vaccinee, while addition of a TBV to RTS,S/AS01 could increase the effect RTS,S has on malaria transmission, as well as reduce the emergence of escape mutants.

The most advanced candidate antigen for a transmission blocking malaria vaccine is Pfs25. It has been extensively tested in mouse models where immunization with Pfs25 containing vaccines can induce an antibody response that completely blocks parasite transmission to mosquitoes (14). Pfs25, as well as its *P. vivax* ortholog Pvs25, has been tested in clinical trials (15, 16) making it, alongside Pfs230, one of only two *P. falciparum* transmission blocking antigens to be tested in humans. This showed that antibodies against Pfs25 reduce malaria transmission in SMFA (15, 17) and that the transmission reducing activity (TRA) is correlated with the induced antibody titres. Unfortunately repeated immunizations resulted in above 50% TRA in only 9 out of 11 volunteers, and this was reduced to 2 out of 11 6 weeks later (17). Similar observations were made in early clinical trials with vaccines targeting CSP, where limited vaccine efficacy correlated with a moderate antibody response. This triggered the research and evaluation of improved vaccine candidates which eventually led to the development of RTS,S/AS01 (18–20). Consequently a number of strategies have been applied to increase the antibody response induced by vaccines targeting Pfs25 (14). These included conjugating Pfs25 to the exoprotein A of *Pseudomonas aeruginosa* (EPA), which substantially increase antibody titres against Pfs25 in mice (21), but clinical trials using Pfs25-EPA formulated in Allhydrogel found only limited and short lived serum transmission blocking activity in vacinees (16, 17). The shortcoming of Pfs25-EPA/Allhydrogel in clinical trials suggests that further antigen/adjuvant combinations need to be assessed to improve TRA of vaccines targeting Pfs25. One alternative antigen, currently under clinical development, is generated by multimerisation of Pfs25 by fusion to the nanoparticle platform IMX313 (Pfs25-IMX313). This resulted in increased antibody titres and TRA in mice after immunization, either when encoded in viral vectors or as protein in adjuvant formulations (22). Furthermore, RTS,S, the antigenic component of the RTS,S/AS01 vaccine, is delivered with a highly potent adjuvant (AS01) specifically developed to induce very high antibody responses. In this study we show that formulation of Pfs25-IMX313 with AS01 increases antibody responses against Pfs25 in mice. We also show that RTS,S and Pfs25-IMX313 can be combined without any immunological interference in mice, maintaining the level of antibody immunogenicity and functional activity induced by the individual vaccines. This is the first proof of concept of the compatibility of combining RTS,S with a TBV, which could be of great value, particularly in local malaria eradication campaigns.

RESULTS

AS01 Increases Induced Antibody Titres After Immunization With Pfs25-IMX313

Pfs25-IMX313 was purified and expressed as previously described (22), formulated in adjuvant and administered to mice, to assess whether the antibody response induced after vaccination with Pfs25-IMX313 could be improved further by using AS01 instead of Alhydrogel as the adjuvant. Three doses of Pfs25-IMX313 were tested in order to measure if there was a dose sparing effect. Ten CD-1 mice per group were immunized on day 0 and day 28 (**Figure 1A**). Blood samples were collected at day 27 and day 42 and anti-Pfs25 IgG titres assessed by ELISA (**Figures 1B,C**). On day 27 after primary immunization, only vaccine formulations containing 4 μg of Pfs25-IMX313 induced a detectable antibody response in all mice. The next lower dose, 0.4 μg of Pfs25-IMX313 in AS01 induced a detectable immune response in 9 out of 10 mice, but the induced antibody titres were significantly lower than those induced by 4 μg of Pfs25-IMX313 in AS01 ($p = 0.0118$, Dunn's multiple comparison test). The lowest dose tested, 0.04 μg of Pfs25-IMX313 in AS01, induced a detectable anti-Pfs25 IgG response only in 1 out of 10 mice, and the induced antibody titres were significantly lower than those induced by both formulations containing 4 μg of Pfs25-IMX313 (4 μg of Pfs25-IMX313 in AS01 $p < 0.0001$, 4 μg of Pfs25-IMX313 in Alhydrogel $p = 0.0006$, Dunn's multiple comparison test).

After boosting, all vaccine formulations induced a detectable immune response in all mice on day 42, while no detectable immune response was induced in the mice immunized with PBS/AS01. The two highest doses of Pfs25-IMX313 in AS01 induced the highest anti-Pfs25 IgG titres. 4 μg of Pfs25-IMX313 in Alhydrogel induced significantly lower titres than the same vaccine dose in AS01 ($p = 0.0014$). Titres induced by 0.04 μg of Pfs25-IMX313 in AS01 were significantly lower than those induced by the two higher doses in the same adjuvant (4 μg of Pfs25-IMX313 in AS01 $p < 0.0001$, 0.4 μg of Pfs25-IMX313 in AS01 $p = 0.004$, Dunn's multiple comparison test), but not than those induced by the 100-fold higher dose of 4 μg of Pfs25-IMX313 in Alhydrogel. Formulation of Pfs25-IMX313 in AS01 therefore clearly increases the vaccine's immunogenicity, but while there is a dose sparing effect when compared to formulation in Alhydrogel, the highest antibody titres are achieved by immunization with the highest tested dose.

Antibodies Induced by Pfs25-IMX313/AS01 Are Functionally Active

Functional activity of the induced antibodies after the second immunization was assessed by SMFA. Live mosquitoes were fed with a mixture of *P. falciparum* gametocyte-infected blood and purified IgG from each group, and the number of oocysts which developed in the midgut was determined after dissection (**Figure 2**). Functional efficacy was calculated as transmission reducing activity (TRA), the reduction in the number of oocysts compared to the negative control group. In a first feed, total IgG concentrations of 750, 150, and 30 μg/ml were tested. All groups apart from the one that received 0.04 μg Pfs25-IMX313/AS01 induced statistically significant TRA when compared to the negative control at the two highest IgG concentrations, but only 4 μg Pfs25-IMX313/AS01 induced statistically significant TRA at 30 μg/ml. To further dissect differences between groups at lower IgG concentrations a second feed was performed using 250, 83.3, and 27.8 μg/ml IgG. This confirmed results from the first feed with only 4 μg Pfs25-IMX313/AS01 inducing statistically significant TRA at all three IgG concentrations, suggesting the high antibody titres observed in this group correlate with improved TRA.

Adjuvant and Vaccine Dose do Not Affect Antibody Quality

As a means to assess whether differences in TRA between groups were caused by a qualitative or a quantitative difference in the antibody response, the SMFA results were correlated with the amount of Pfs25 specific IgG in the feeder (**Figure 2C**). Datasets for 4 μg Pfs25-IMX313/Alhydrogel, 4 μg Pfs25-IMX313/AS01 and 0.4 μg Pfs25-IMX313/AS01 were analyzed by linear regression. The 0.04 μg Pfs25-IMX313/AS01 group was excluded from the analyses due to the absence of any statistically significant TRA in this group. To determine the transmission reducing efficacy per anti-Pfs25 AU, anti-Pfs25 AU and vaccine groups were used as explanatory variables in a multiple linear regression analysis. The overall fit to the linear regression model was $R^2 = 0.78$, and anti-Pfs25 AU ($p < 0.001$) but not vaccine groups ($p = 0.1625$) showed a significant effect. TRA in all three groups is therefore dependent on the amount of IgG used in SMFA but not on the dose or adjuvant the vaccine was administered in, suggesting that there is no qualitative difference between the antibody responses induced by the different vaccine regimens. This, as well as the differences in the induced antibody titres measured by ELISA (**Figure 1C**), suggests that the difference in induced TRA is due to an quantitative, not a qualitative difference in the antibody response. To confirm this, a similar linear regression analysis as before was performed using the reciprocal dilution factor of the serum pool as one of the explanatory variables, instead of anti-Pfs25 AU (**Figure 2D**). This allows an indirect analysis of the antibody response's efficacy in the undiluted mouse serum from each group, therefore providing a combined assessment of antibody quantity and quality. The overall fit to the linear regression model was $R^2 = 0.68$ and the serum dilution factor ($p < 0.001$) as well as the vaccine group ($p = 0.0001$) showed significant effects. When three groups were compared, 4 μg Pfs25-IMX313/Alhydrogel and 0.4 μg Pfs25-IMX313/AS01, which had both induced a similar antibody titres also appeared to have induced a similarly efficacious response ($p = 0.0924$), while both of these vaccine formulations induced a significantly less efficacious antibody response than 4 μg Pfs25-IMX313/AS01 ($p < 0.001$ and $p = 0.0026$, respectively), which had induced a significantly higher antibody titer. This analysis therefore confirms the observation from the antibody quality analysis, that the observed difference in SMFA and the superior performance of the 4 μg Pfs25-IMX313/AS01 vaccine formulation is due to a quantitative but not a qualitative difference in the induced antibody response.

A

Group	Day 0 (Prime)	Day 27	Day 28 (Boost)	Day 42
1	4μg Pfs25-IMX313/Alhydrogel	Blood sampling for Post Prime ELISA	4μg Pfs25-IMX313/Alhydrogel	Blood sampling for Post Boost ELISA and SMFA
2	4μg Pfs25-IMX313/AS01		4μg Pfs25-IMX313/AS01	
3	0.4μg Pfs25-IMX313/AS01		0.4μg Pfs25-IMX313/AS01	
4	0.04μg Pfs25-IMX313/AS01		0.04μg Pfs25-IMX313/AS01	
5	PBS/AS01		PBS/AS01	

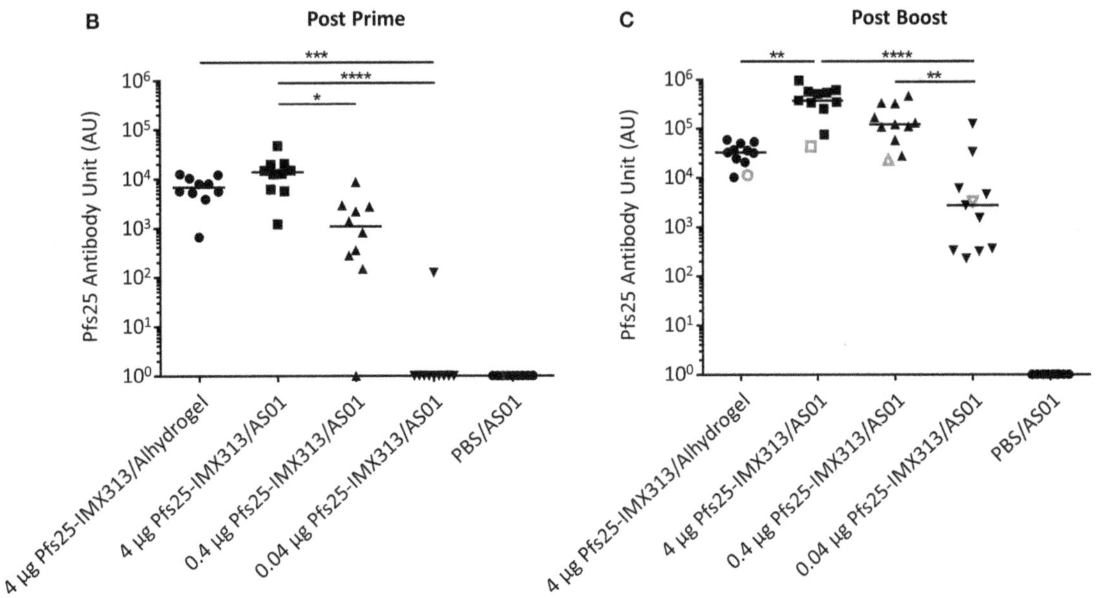

FIGURE 1 | Immunogenicity of Pfs25-IMX313 in AlhydrogelFigure or AS01. **(A)** CD1 mice ($n = 10$) were vaccinated twice with 4 μg Pfs25-IMX313 in Alhydrogel or with decreasing doses (4 μg, 0.4 μg and 0.04 μg) of Pfs25-IMX313 in AS01. BC Anti-Pfs25 IgG titres were measured by ELISA at 4 weeks post prime **(B)** and 2 weeks post boost **(C)**. Empty gray shapes show the antibody units of a 1 mg/ml dilution of purified IgG. Data points show antibody titres in individual mice, lines show the median. $^{*}p \leq 0.05$, $^{**}p \leq 0.005$, $^{***}p \leq 0.001$, $^{****}p \leq 0.0001$, Dunn's multiple comparison test.

Pfs25-IMX313 can be Combined With RTS,S Without Immunological Interference

Having established that AS01 increases the immunogenicity and efficacy of Pfs25-IMX313 as well as determined an optimal dose, we assessed whether Pfs25-IMX313 could be combined with RTS,S/AS01 as a multi-antigen, multi-stage malaria vaccine. Ten CD1 mice per group were immunized on day 0 and day 28 (**Figure 3A**). The mixed vaccine group was immunized with RTS,S/AS01 and Pfs25-IMX313 combined into a single injection, while the co-administered group received both vaccines separately into the left and the right hind leg, respectively. In the latter group, each injection was formulated with only half a dose of AS01, to keep the total amount of administered adjuvant constant. Blood samples were collected at day 27 and day 42 and anti-Pfs25 and anti-CSP IgG titres were assessed by ELISA (**Figure 3**). All Pfs25-IMX313 containing vaccine formulations induced strong anti-Pfs25 antibody responses and all RTS,S containing vaccine formulations induced strong anti-CSP antibody responses. Mixing or co-administration of the two vaccines did not result in any significant reduction in antibody titres when compared to the groups that had received Pfs25-IMX313/AS01 or RTS,S/AS01 alone, suggesting that there is no immune competition between the two vaccines.

Combination of Pfs25-IMX313 With RTS,S Does not Reduce the Functional Activity of Anti-Pfs25 IgG

Functional activity of anti-Pfs25 IgG was assessed by SMFA (**Figure 4**). In a first feed, IgGs from all Pfs25-IMX313 containing groups were tested at 750, 250, and 83.3 μg/ml, groups that had received RTS,S/AS01 or PBS/AS01 were tested at 750 μg/ml only. Significant TRA was observed for all groups that received Pfs25-IMX313 at all the tested concentrations. Immunization with RTS,S/AS01 had no statistically significant effect on oocyst intensity. In a second feed we therefore tested lower IgG concentrations (250, 83.3, and 27.8 μg/ml) to assess for differences between groups at these lower concentrations. As

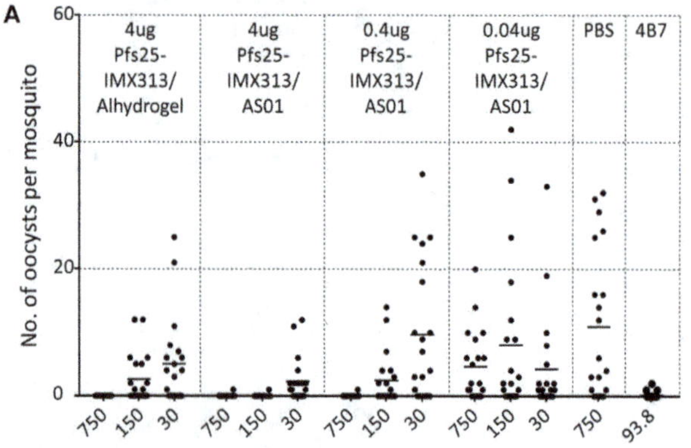

Sample	IgG conc [µg/ml][a]	Mean Oocysts[b]	% inhibition[c]	p-value[d]
4ug Pfs25-IMX313/ Alhydrogel	750	0	100 (98.8, 100)	<0.001
	150	2.6	76.3 (30.7, 91.9)	0.007
	30	5.05	53.9 (-31.6, 83.8)	0.165
4ug Pfs25-IMX313/AS01	750	0.05	99.5 (97, 100)	<0.001
	150	0.05	99.5 (98.2, 100)	<0.001
	30	2.3	79 (35.8, 93)	0.009
0.4ug Pfs25-IMX313/AS01	750	0.05	99.5 (98.4, 100)	<0.001
	150	2.45	77.6 (35.7, 92.9)	0.006
	30	9.75	11 (-165.5, 69)	0.850
0.04ug Pfs25-IMX313/AS01	750	4.65	57.5 (-30, 85.9)	0.144
	150	8.1	26 (-112.7, 74.2)	0.569
	30	4.25	61.2 (-11.7, 87.3)	0.072
PBS /AS01	750	10.95	N/A	N/A
4B7	93.8	0.2	99.1 (97.1, 99.8)	<0.001

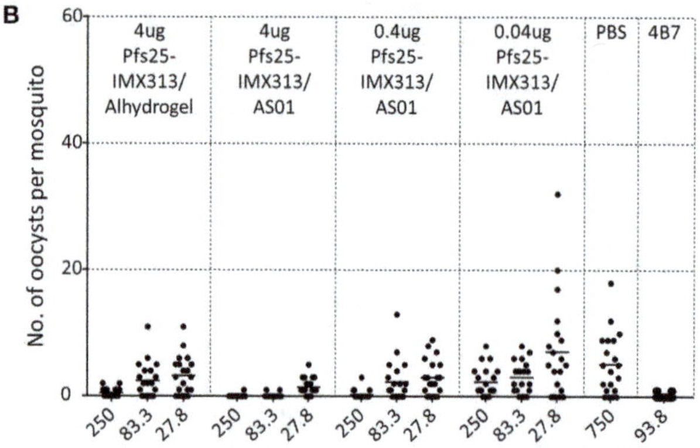

Sample	IgG conc [µg/ml][a]	Mean Oocysts[b]	% inhibition[c]	p-value[d]
4ug Pfs25-IMX313/ Alhydrogel	250	0.5	90.3 (77.5, 96.2)	<0.001
	83.3	2.45	52.4 (-28.6, 84.4)	0.125
	27.8	3.25	36.9 (-47.7, 72.1)	0.302
4ug Pfs25-IMX313/AS01	250	0.05	99 (92.3, 100)	<0.001
	83.3	0.1	98.1 (90, 100)	<0.001
	27.8	1.45	71.8 (33.7, 88.1)	0.004
0.4ug Pfs25-IMX313/AS01	250	0.3	94.2 (85.3, 98)	<0.001
	83.3	2.3	55.3 (-16.2, 84.1)	0.083
	27.8	3	41.7 (-39.5, 76.5)	0.195
0.04ug Pfs25-IMX313/AS01	250	2.3	55.3 (-6.5, 82.2)	0.072
	83.3	3.05	40.8 (-63.2, 80)	0.297
	27.8	7.1	-37.9 (-222.4, 39.1)	0.429
PBS/AS01	750	5.15	N/A	N/A
4B7	93.8	0.2	95.2 (87.4, 98.5)	<0.001

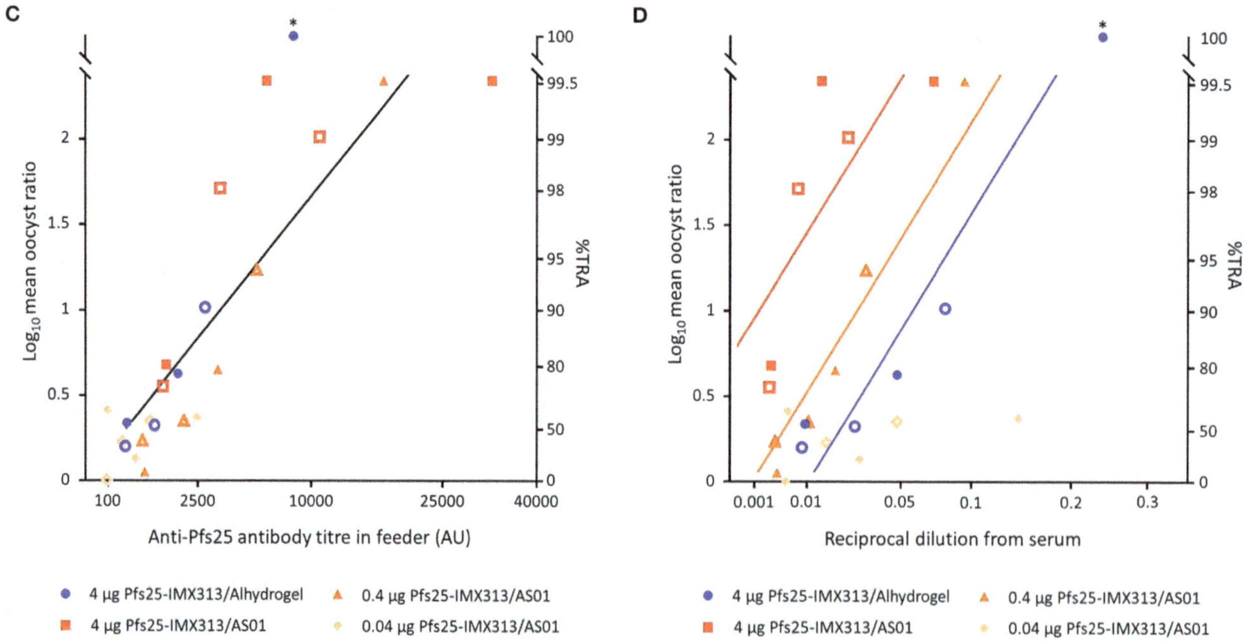

FIGURE 2 | Transmission blocking activity of anti Pfs25-IgG induced by immunization with Pfs25-IMX313 in Alhydrogel or AS01. **(A,B)** Total IgG, purified from pooled serum of each group (2 weeks post boost) was tested in SMFA in two independent experiments, one using total IgG concentrations of 750, 150 and 30 µg/ml **(A)** and one using total IgG concentrations of 250, 83.3, and 27.7 µg/ml **(B)**. The transmission blocking monoclonal anti-Pfs25 antibody 4B7 was used as a positive control. Data

(Continued)

FIGURE 2 | points represent the number of oocysts in individual mosquitoes and the lines show the arithmetic mean. X-axis values are μg/ml total IgG in the assay. The results of the two feeds are summarized in the tables. [a]IgG concentration (μg/ml) in feeder. [b]Arithmetic mean of oocyst intensity from 20 mosquitoes. [c]Percent inhibition of mean oocyst intensity and the 95% confidence interval (95% CI). [d]Two-sided *p*-values testing whether % inhibition is significantly different from zero. **(C,D)** The quality of the anti-Pfs25-IgG used in the SMFA was assessed by linear two regression analyses, correlating the Log10-transformed ratios of mean oocyst counts in control and test samples (log-mean ratio, LMR) with the anti-Pfs25 specific IgG level in the feeder **(C)** or the reciprocal dilution factor from the original serum pool **(D)**. LMR is plotted on the left y-axis. The right y-axis shows the correspondent %TRA. Values on the x-axis are plotted on a square root scale. The black line shows the shared linear fit for IgG from groups of mice immunized with 4 μg Pfs25-IMX313 in Alhydrogel or with 4 μg and 0.4 μg of Pfs25-IMX313 in AS01. Colored lines show linear fits for individual groups. Filled and unfilled shapes show data points from two independent SMFA experiments. Data points marked with an asterisk were excluded from the analysis as they showed 100% TRA (upper plateau level of dose response).

before, at IgG concentrations of 250 and 83.3 μg/ml all groups that had received Pfs25-IMX313 showed significant TRA, while immunization with RTS,S/AS01 had no statistically significant effect when compared to immunization with PBS/AS01. At the lowest tested concentration of 27.8 μg/ml, only the Pfs25-IMX313 alone group showed significant TRA. Correlation of antibody titres in the feeder with the SMFA results, however, did not indicate a difference in antibody quality between combination and individually administered vaccine (**Figure 4C**). The overall fit to the linear regression model was $R^2 = 0.68$, and again anti-Pfs25 AU ($p = 0.0012$) but not vaccine groups ($p = 0.7322$) showed a significant effect. Correlation of SMFA results with reciprocal serum dilutions furthermore confirmed the quantification of the antibody response by ELISA (**Figure 3C**) in indicating there was no quantitative difference in the IgG response between the groups ($R^2 = 0.69$, serum dilution factor: $p = 0.001$, group: $p = 0.1275$). The observed difference in SMFA is therefore most likely due to a higher concentration of Pfs25-specific IgG in the purified total IgG from the Pfs25-IMX313 alone group, than in the total IgG purified from the groups that received both vaccines ($\log_{10}$ antibody titer of 1 mg/ml purified IgG: mixed = 3.76, co-administered: 3.75, Pfs25-IMX313 alone: 4.06). This is however not reflective of the amount of Pfs25-specific IgG in serum of immunized mice, which was similar in all three groups (arithmetic mean $\log_{10}$ antibody titer: mixed = 4.83 AU, co-administered =4.81 AU, Pfs25-IMX313 alone = 4.86 AU).

Combination of RTS,S With Pfs25-IMX313 Does not Reduce the Functional Activity of Induced Anti-CSP Antibodies

Functional activity of anti-CSP antibodies was assessed by ISI assay using *P.berghei* sporozoites expressing PfCSP under the PbCSP promoter (**Figure 5**). Sporozoites were obtained from the salivary glands of infected *A. stephensi* mosquitoes and added to Huh7 hepatoma cells in the presence of test and control serum. At 1% serum concentration inhibition of sporozoite invasion is detectable in all groups that received RTS,S. There is no statistically significant difference between groups immunized with RTS,S/AS01 alone or mixed or co-administered with Pfs25-IMX313, but all groups that received RTS,S inhibit sporozoite invasion above the assay's limit of sensitivity and inhibition was significantly higher than in the group that had been immunized with Pfs25-IMX313 (mixed $p = 0.0011$, co-administered $p = 0.0154$, RTS,S alone $p = 0.0015$, Dunn's multiple comparison test). To further characterize the anti-CSP antibody response induced by the different vaccine formulations containing RTS,S the log transformed mean ratio of infected hepatocytes in the vaccinated and PBS control groups was plotted against the square root of the anti-CSP endpoint titer in the hepatocyte growth medium, as had been done to analyse SMFA results. For all vaccine groups there was a significant correlation between increased LMR and higher anti-CSP AU (one-tailed Spearman correlation, mixed $r = 0.9273$, $p = 0.0002$, co-administered $r = 0.612$, $p = 0.0334$, RTS,S alone $r = 0.8601$, $p = 0.0036$. In a multiple linear regression analysis anti-CSP AU and vaccine groups were used as explanatory variables. The overall fit to the linear regression model was $R^2 = 0.55$, and anti-CSP AU ($p < 0.001$) but not vaccine groups ($p = 0.7913$) showed a significant effect on the inhibition of sporozoite invasion, indicating that there is no loss of quality in the antibody response when RTS,S is combined with Pfs25-IMX313 rather than administered alone.

DISCUSSION

The modest efficacy of recent clinical trials using single antigen subunit vaccines support the development of multi-antigen vaccines targeting multiple stages of malaria. Mixing vaccines in a multi-component formulation is an easy process that does not require developing a new product. This means that it is possible to draw from previous experience in product development and clinical trials. This experience is particularly rich in the case of RTS,S the most advanced malaria vaccine candidate to date. Pfs25-IMX313 is a TBV candidate that we developed specifically to overcome the low antibody titres induced by vaccines targeting Pfs25 in past clinical trials (15, 17). Encoded in viral vectors it has now been tested in a clinical trial (ClinicalTrials.gov Identifier: NCT02532049), and it is currently being produced as a nanoparticle to GMP standards to be tested in clinical trials as a protein in adjuvant formulation, which in mice induced higher antibody titres than viral vectors (22). Here we showed that Pfs25-IMX313 can be formulated in AS01, which results in increased antibody titres when compared to formulation in Alhydrogel as well as increased TRA in SMFA. The functional activity of the induced antibodies per AU is similar for both adjuvants, but the overall stronger antibody response induced by Pfs25-IMX313/AS01 results in a substantially improved efficacy over Pfs25-IMX313/Alhydrogel.

This study also shows that RTS,S and Pfs25-IMX313 can be combined successfully maintaining both the antibody titres

A

Group	Day 0 (Prime)	Day 27	Day 28 (Boost)	Day 42
1	4μg Pfs25-IMX313 + 5μg RTS,S/AS01 **(mixed)**	Blood sampling for Post Prime ELISA	4μg Pfs25-IMX313 + 5μg RTS,S/AS01 **(mixed)**	Blood sampling for Post Boost ELISA and SMFA
2	4μg Pfs25-IMX313 + 5μg RTS,S/AS01 **(co-administered)**		4μg Pfs25-IMX313 + 5μg RTS,S/AS01 **(co-administered)**	
3	5μg RTS,S/AS01		5μg RTS,S/AS01	
4	4μg Pfs25-IMX313/AS01		4μg Pfs25-IMX313/AS01	
5	PBS/AS01		PBS/AS01	

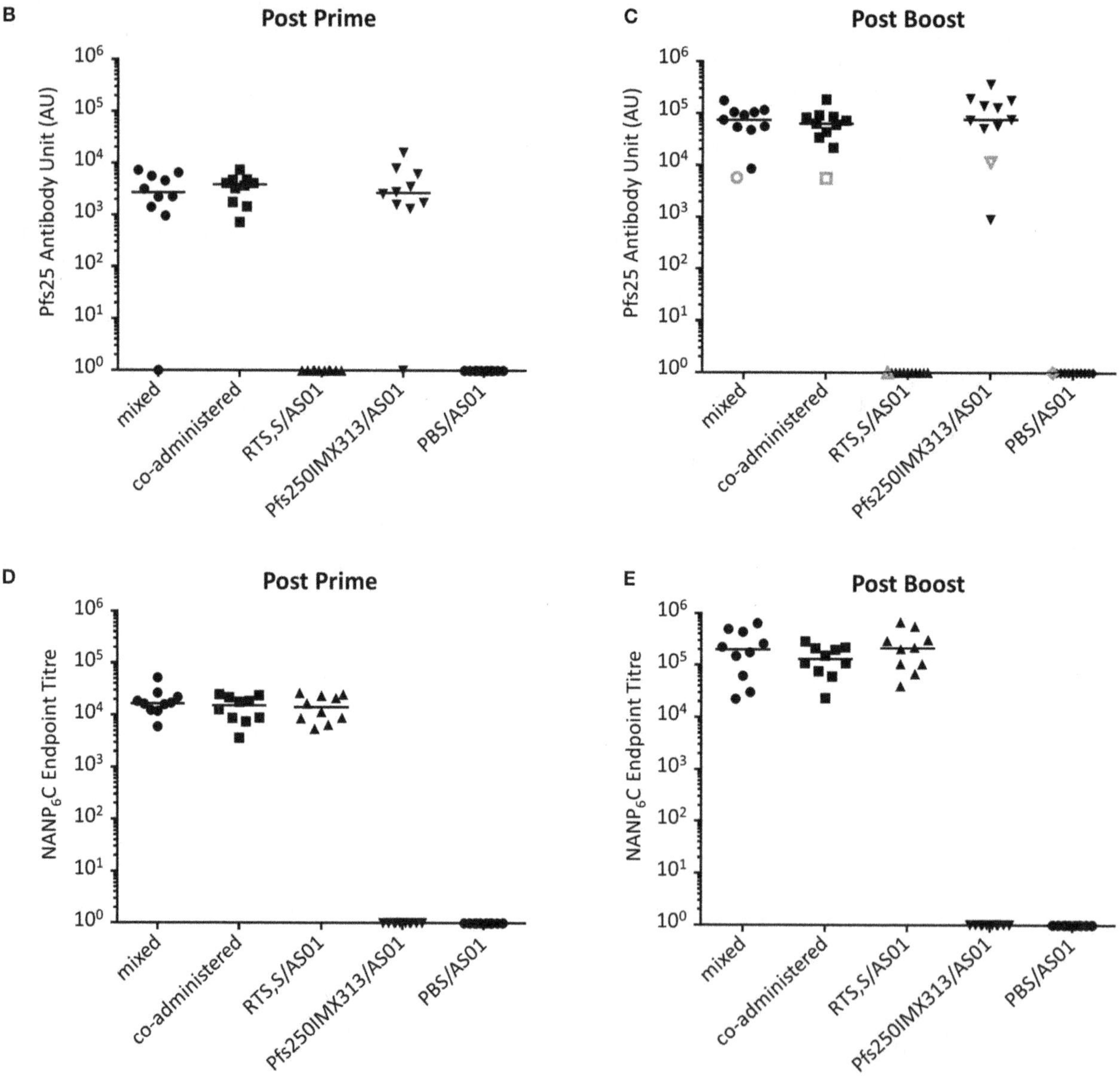

FIGURE 3 | Immunogenicity of Pfs25-IMX313 and RTS,S alone or when combined. **(A)** CD1 mice ($n = 10$) were vaccinated twice with (1) a mixture of 4 μg Pfs25-IMX313 and 5 μg RTS,S/AS01, (2) 4 μg Pfs25-IMX313/AS01 and 5 μg RTS,S/AS01, administered separately in individual hind legs, (3) 5 μg RTS,S/AS01 and (4) 4 μg Pfs25-IMX313/AS01. A control group (5) was immunized with PBS + AS01. **(B,C)** Anti-Pfs25 IgG titres were measured by ELISA at 4 weeks post prime

(Continued)

FIGURE 3 | (B) and 2 weeks post boost **(C)**. Empty shapes show the antibody units of a 1 mg/ml dilution of purified IgG. **(D,E)** Anti-NANP6C IgG endpoint titres were measured by ELISA at 4 weeks post prime **(D)** and 2 weeks post boost **(E)**. Data points show antibody titres in individual mice, lines show the median.

and functional activity of antibodies against CSP and Pfs25 compared to the individual vaccines. The perceived lower activity in SMFA of the combined vaccines is explained by the higher amount of antigen specific IgG in the total IgG preparation of the Pfs25-IMX313 alone group (**Figure 3C**), and not an inferior antibody quality in the groups that received both vaccines (**Figure 4C**). Quantification of anti-Pfs25 serum antibody titres by ELISA (**Figure 3C**) and correlation of TRA with reciprocal serum dilutions (**Figure 4D**) showed that a similar amount of anti-Pfs25 specific IgG had been generated in all three groups. However, in the groups that received RTS,S as well as Pfs25-IMX313 there is an additional strong antibody response against the CSP component in RTS,S. A fixed amount of total IgG from these groups will therefore contain a significant amount of anti-CSP antibodies not present in a total IgG preparation from mice that had been immunized with Pfs25-IMX313 alone, and hence a smaller amount of anti-Pfs25 specific IgG. A trend for increased oocyst intensity after immunization with RTS,S/AS01 (**Figure 4**) is not statistically significant, and most likely due to the high variability of the assay at lower inhibition range, rather than to an enhancing effect of RTS,S/AS01 on parasite transmission. This strongly suggests that there is no negative effect on the TRA induced by immunization with Pfs25-IMX313 when the vaccine is either mixed or co-administered with RTS,S/AS01.

The successful combination of the two vaccines contrasts with previous studies where the combination of different viral vectored malaria vaccines did result in strong immune interference (23, 24) and the combination of RTS,S/AS01 with a viral vector PEV (ChAd63/MVA ME-TRAP) failed to improve vaccine efficacy when compared to the two vaccines administered individually and reduced immunogenicity and efficacy against malaria (25). This success might be attributed to shared characteristics and modes of action of RTS,S/AS01 and Pfs25-IMX313. Both vaccines target antigens that are expressed with high abundance on the surface of the sporozoites and zygotes/ookinetes, respectively, both vaccines are produced in yeast and both vaccines use a particulate platform to array the antigen in order to induce a strong antibody response.

The combination of RTS,S/AS01 and Pfs25-IMX313, as we demonstrated here, is of particular interest, for combining a TBV with a vaccine that protects from clinical disease creates a vaccine which reduces disease as well as malaria transmission, as called for in the MVT roadmap and the malERA research agenda for malaria eradication (malERA 3; 5; malERA 4). Furthermore, a recent study in mice, using monoclonal antibodies against CSP and Pfs25, suggests that partially efficacious PEVs and TBVs could be synergistic within a population (13), as the protective efficacy of PEVs is negatively correlated with the parasite density within an infectious mosquito (26), which can be reduced through the presence of anti-Pfs25 antibodies in the human host (27). Finally, not being a target of naturally acquired immunity against malaria and therefore not under immune pressure, the sequence of Pfs25 is highly conserved (28). The selection of *P. falciparum* variants less affected by anti-CSP antibodies induced by RTS,S/AS01 can therefore likely be reduced through the presence of anti-Pfs25 which reduce the human-to-mosquito transmission of such escape variants. The advanced stage of RTS,S/AS01 and Pfs25-IMX313 as malaria vaccine candidates harbors the intriguing prospect of being able to test these hypothesis, with their potentially far reaching consequences for malaria control, in human clinical trials.

MATERIAL AND METHODS

Vaccines and Adjuvants

RTS,S and AS01 were provided by GSK. Pfs25-IMX313 was expressed and purified as described previously (22). In brief: Pfs25-IMX313 was expressed in *Pichia pastoris* under the control of the methanol inducible promoter AOX1. N-terminal fusion to the alpha-mating factor secretion signal sequence allowed secretion into the culture media. Following expression, nanoparticles were purified from the culture supernatant using a 5 ml CaptureSelect^{TM} C-tag affinity matrix column.

Immunizations

All animal experiments and procedures were performed according to the UK Animals (Scientific Procedures) Act Project License (PPL 30/2889) and approved by the Oxford University Local Ethical Review Committee. Age-matched female CD1 mice (Envigo, United Kingdom), housed in specific pathogen-free environments, were vaccinated with 50 μl of vaccine formulation in one leg intramuscularly (IM). Protein-in-Alhydrogel was formulated as follows: 85 μg Alhydrogel (Brenntag) per dose was mixed with TBS at room temperature for 15 min, antigen was then added and incubated for a further 60 min at room temperature. AS01E was supplied pre-mixed by GSK to be at 1-fold concentration upon mixing with an appropriate amount of antigen. Total protein per dose for each group is detailed in the tables in **Figures 1**, **3**. Animals were immunized on days 0 and 28, and blood samples were collected on days 27 (4 weeks post prime) and 42 (2 weeks post boost). The samples were allowed to clot at 4°C overnight before centrifugation at 13,000 × *g* in a benchtop centrifuge and serum was collected for testing.

ELISA

Standardized Pfs25 total IgG ELISAs were carried out as described previously (29). In brief, Nunc-Immuno Maxisorp 96 well plates (Thermo Scientific, UK) were coated with 1μg/ml Pfs25 in carbonate-bicarbonate coating buffer (Sigma Aldrich, UK) overnight at 4°C. Plates were washed with PBS-Tween and blocked with 5% milk in PBS-Tween. Sera were diluted to reach an OD405 in the linear range of the standard curve at the same time an internal control reaches an OD405 of 1. Samples were added in triplicates. An internal control was added

A

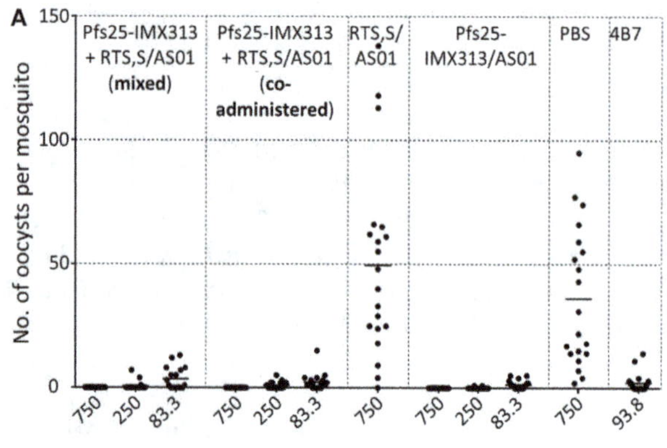

Sample	IgG conc [μg/ml][a]	Mean Oocysts[b]	% inhibition[c]	p-value[d]
Pfs25-IMX313 + RTS,S/AS01 (mixed)	750	0	100 (99.7, 100)	<0.001
	250	0.6	98.3 (96.3, 99.3)	<0.001
	83.3	3.5	90.3 (78.1, 95.8)	<0.001
Pfs25-IMX313 + RTS,S/AS01 (co-administered)	750	0	100 (99.8, 100)	<0.001
	250	0.95	97.4 (92.6, 99.6)	<0.001
	83.3	2.25	93.8 (85.5, 97.4)	<0.001
RTS,S/AS01	750	49.6	-37 (-223.6, 40)	0.443
Pfs25-IMX313/AS01	750	0	100 (99.6, 100)	<0.001
	250	0.1	99.7 (99.2, 100)	<0.001
	83.3	1.4	96.1 (90.9, 98.5)	<0.001
PBS/AS01	750	36.2	N/A	N/A
4B7	93.8	2.15	94.1 (83.6, 98.1)	<0.001

B

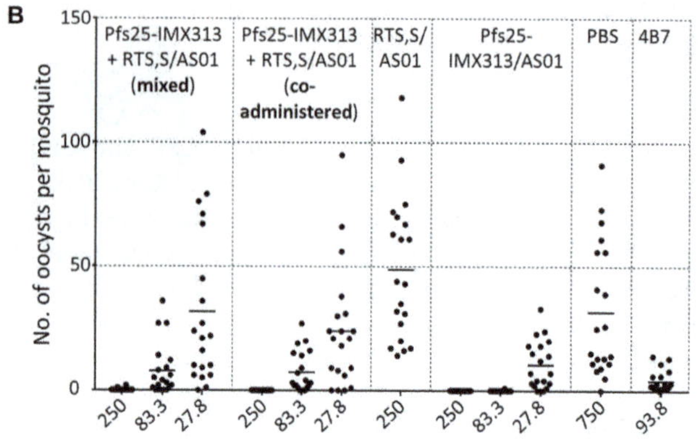

Sample	IgG conc [μg/ml][a]	Mean Oocysts[b]	% inhibition[c]	p-value[d]
Pfs25-IMX313 + RTS,S/AS01 (mixed)	250	0.15	99.5 (98.7, 99.9)	<0.001
	83.3	7.85	75.3 (41.6, 89.6)	0.003
	27.8	31.75	0 (-132.3, 56)	0.988
Pfs25-IMX313 + RTS,S/AS01 (co-administered)	250	0	100 (99.7, 100)	<0.001
	83.3	7.25	77.2 (49.4, 90.2)	<0.001
	27.8	24.05	24.3 (-72.3, 68.4)	0.499
RTS,S/AS01	250	48.8	-53.7 (-244.7, 30.8)	0.274
Pfs25-IMX313/AS01	250	0	100 (99.6, 100)	<0.001
	83.3	0.05	99.8 (99.6, 100)	<0.001
	27.8	10.4	67.2 (26.6, 86.5)	0.01
PBS/AS01	750	31.75	N/A	N/A
4B7	93.8	4	89.7 (76.2, 95.4)	<0.001

C

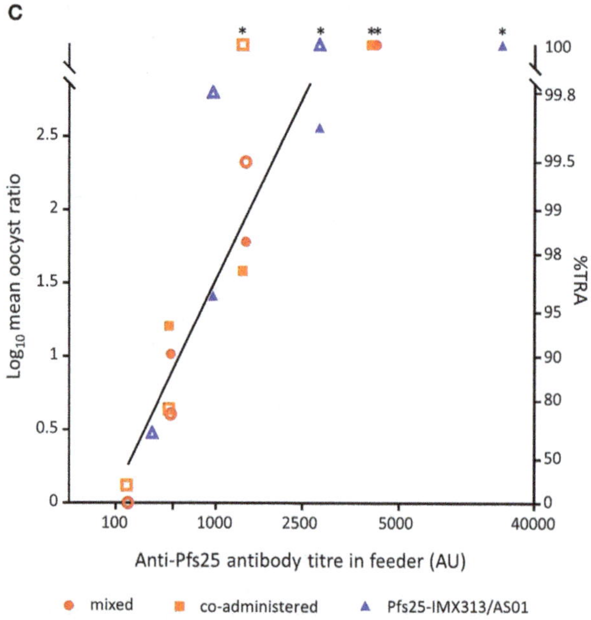

D

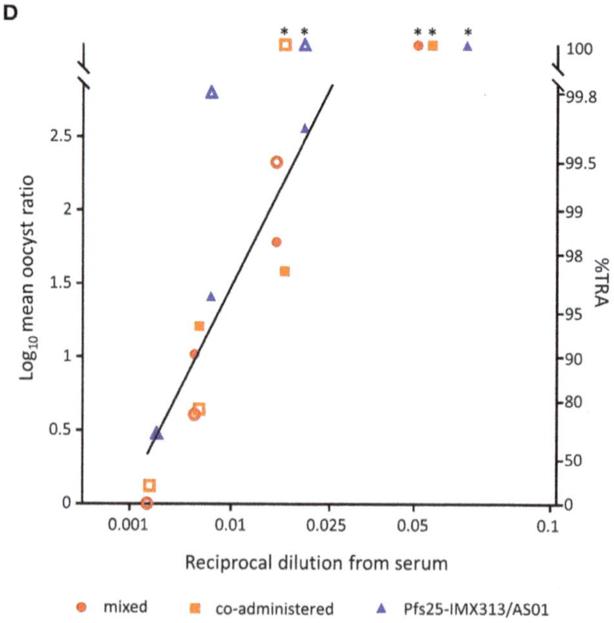

FIGURE 4 | Transmission blocking activity of anti Pfs25-IgG induced by immunization with Pfs25-IMX313 alone or in combination with RTS,S. **(A,B)** Total IgG, purified from pooled serum of each group (2 weeks post boost) was tested in SMFA in two independent experiments, one using total IgG concentrations of 750, 250 and 83.3 μg/ml **(A)** and one using total IgG concentrations of 250, 83.3, and 27.7 μg/ml. The transmission blocking monoclonal anti-Pfs25 antibody 4B7

(Continued)

FIGURE 4 | was used as a positive control. Data points represent the number of oocysts in individual mosquitoes and the lines show the arithmetic mean. X-axis values are μg/ml total IgG in the assay. The results of the two feeds are summarized in the tables. [a]IgG concentration (μg/ml) in feeder. [b]Arithmetic mean of oocyst intensity from 20 mosquitoes. [c]Percent inhibition of mean oocyst intensity and the 95% confidence interval (95% CI). [d]Two-sided *p*-values testing whether % inhibition is significantly different from zero. **(C,D)** The quality of the anti-Pfs25-IgG used in the SMFA was assessed by linear two regression analyses, correlating the Log10-transformed ratios of mean oocyst counts in control and test samples (log-mean ratio, LMR) with the anti-Pfs25 specific IgG level in the feeder **(C)** or the reciprocal dilution factor from the original serum pool **(D)**. LMR is plotted on the left y-axis. The right y-axis shows the correspondent %TRA. Values on the x-axis are plotted on a square root scale. The black line shows the shared linear fit for IgG from all groups. Filled and unfilled shapes show data points from the two independent SMFA experiments. Data points marked with an asterisk were excluded from the analysis as they showed 100% TRA (upper plateau level of dose response).

in six replicates. A standard curve was added in duplicates, starting with a 1:1,000 dilution of reference sera diluted down the plate in 1:2 steps 10 times. Plates were incubated for 2 h at room temperature and then washed as before. Goat anti-mouse whole IgG conjugated to alkaline phosphatase (Sigma Aldrich, UK) was added for 1 h at room temperature. Following a final wash, plates were developed by adding p-nitrophenylphosphate at 1 mg/mL in diethanolamine buffer (Pierce, UK) and optical density (OD) was read at 405 nm. Antibody units (AU) were defined as the dilution of a serum sample at which it had the same OD as the internal control. AUs were extrapolated from the samples OD on the linear range of the standard curve.

NANP-repeat endpoint total IgG ELISAs were carried out as described previously (30). Nunc-Immuno Maxisorp 96 well plates (Thermo Scientific, United Kingdom) were coated with 2 μg/ml NANP6C peptide in carbonate-bicarbonate coating buffer (Sigma Aldrich, United Kingdom) overnight at 4°C. Plates were washed with PBS-Tween and blocked with 10% Casein Block (Thermo Scientific, United Kingdom). Sera were diluted at a starting concentration of 1:1,000, added in duplicate, and serially diluted 3-fold. Plates were incubated for 2 h at room temperature and then washed as before. Goat anti-mouse whole IgG conjugated to alkaline phosphatase (Sigma Aldrich, United Kingdom) was added for 1 h at room temperature. Following a final wash, plates were developed by adding p-nitrophenylphosphate at 1 mg/mL in diethanolamine buffer (Pierce, UK) and optical density (OD) was read at 405 nm. Serum antibody endpoint titres were taken as the x-axis intercept of the dilution curve at an absorbance value of 0.15. A monoclonal antibody against CSP (2A10) was included in each assay as a reference control.

SMFA

The ability of vaccine-induced antibodies to block the development of *P. falciparum* NF54 strain oocysts in the mosquito midgut was evaluated by SMFA as described previously (31). Stage V gametocytes from a mature gametocyte culture were mixed with normal human serum and normal red blood cells to make a feeding mixture with 0.15–0.2% stage V gametocytemia. Purified IgG was added to these at the concentrations shown in the figures and then fed to 3–6 day old starved female *Anopheles stephensi* (SDA 500) via a parafilm® membrane. The mosquitoes were maintained for 8 days and then dissected to count the number of oocysts per midgut in 20 mosquitos. The transmission blocking, Pfs25 specific monoclonal antibody 4B7 was used as a positive control (31). Percent reduction in infection intensity was calculated relative to the respective control IgG tested in the same assay.

Parasite Production

To produce parasites for the ISI assay, donor mice were intraperitoneally injected with a parasite bloodstock. Parasitaemia was monitored through blood sampling by tail tip amputation and thin film preparation. As soon as the parasitaemia exceeded 5%, the mouse was anesthetized by intra muscular injection of ketamine and placed on top of a pot containing approximately 50 female *A. stephensi* mosquitoes. Mosquitoes were allowed to feed through the mesh covering the pots for at least 10 min. Seven to ten days after the blood meal mosquitoes were allowed to feed on an uninfected mouse, as this had been shown to increase the number of parasites per mosquito. Twenty-one days after the initial feed salivary glands were dissected from the mosquitoes to obtain sporozoites.

ISI

Functional activity of anti-sporozoite antibodies was assessed by ISI using transgenic *Plasmodium berghei* parasites expressing PfCSP under the PbCSP promoter, at the PbCSP locus, replacing the PbCSP gene, as well as GFP to allow detection of infected cells by flow cytometry (Salman, in preparation). This strain of transgenic parasites has been validated for use in ISI (32) and in murine malaria challenge models (33). One day prior to mosquito dissection for isolation of sporozoites, HuH7 cells were seeded in a 96 well plate at a concentration of 300,000 cells/ml in a volume of 100 μl/well, resulting in a concentration of 30,000 cells per well. One day later mosquitoes were dissected and salivary glands collected in ice cold RPMI. Sporozoites were released from salivary glands by tissue disruption using a pestle and mortar, and counted in a hemocytometer. Sera were diluted to double the required concentration in 120 μl complete RPMI. The medium was removed from the HuH7 cells seeded the day before, and 50 μl of diluted serum was added to the wells in duplicates. Sporozoites were then diluted to 300,000 sporozoites per ml in complete RPMI and 50 μl were added to each well, resulting in 15,000 sporozoites per well and a ratio of cells to sporozoites of 2:1. To aid sporozoite invasion of the cells, the plate was centrifuged at 500 × g for 5 min before incubation at 37°C and 5% CO_2 overnight in a tissue culture incubator. After 24 h of incubation, cells were detached from the plate by removing medium from the plate and then adding 100 μl of TrypLE ™ Express (Gibco) to the wells and incubation for 5 min

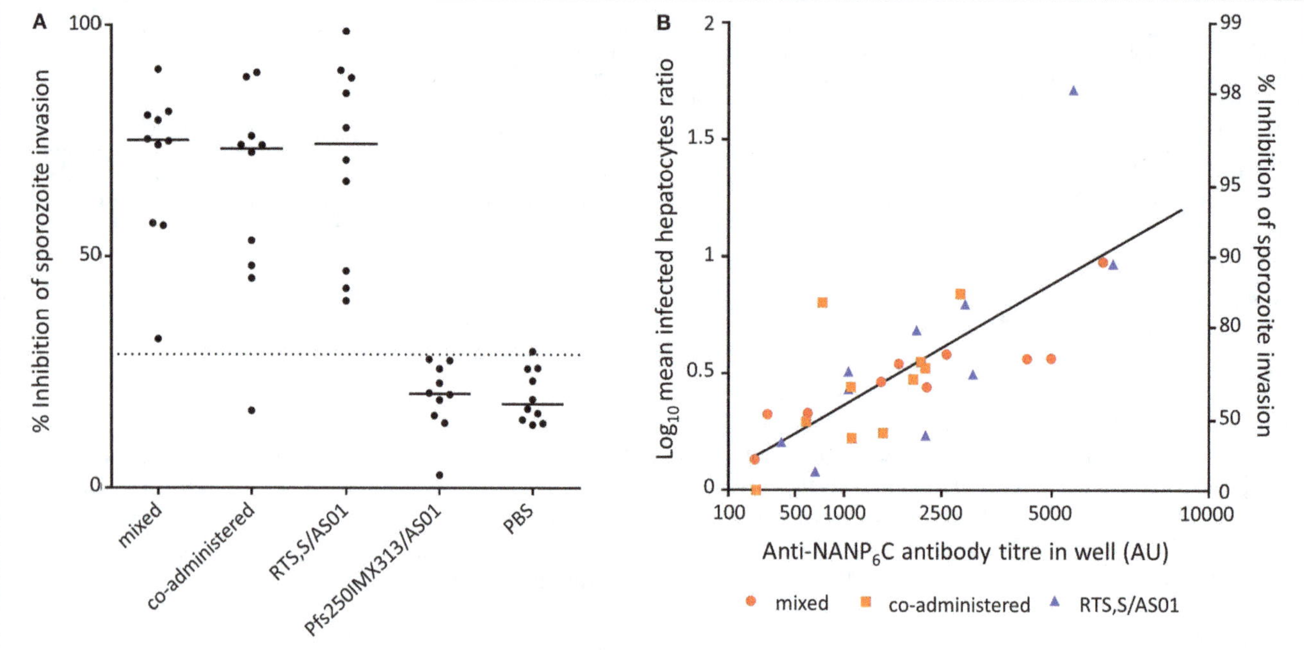

C

mouse #	Pfs25-IMX313 + RTS,S/AS01 (mixed)		Pfs25-IMX313 + RTS,S/AS01 (co-administered)		RTS,S/AS01	
	endpoint titre[a]	% inhibition[b]	endpoint titre[a]	% inhibition[b]	endpoint titre[a]	% inhibition[b]
1	5.8	90	5.0	45	5.3	47
2	4.3	32	5.3	73	5.0	66
3	4.8	57	5.3	74	5.5	71
4	4.5	57	4.8	53	4.6	43
5	5.6	75	5.2	48	5.8	90
6	5.7	81	5.0	74	5.0	78
7	5.3	74	5.3	76	5.5	89
8	5.2	75	5.5	90	4.8	40
9	5.2	79	4.4	17	5.3	85
10	5.4	81	4.9	89	5.7	99

FIGURE 5 | Inhibition of sporozoite invasion by anti CSP-serum induced by immunization with RTS,S alone or in combination with Pfs25-IMX313. **(A)** Serum from individual mice (2 weeks post boost) was mixed with *P. berghei* sporozoites from mosquito salivary gland dissections, and the inhibition of sporozoite invasion was assessed. Data points show inhibition of sporozoite invasion by serum from individual mice, lines show the median, the dotted line shows the limit of sensitivity. **(B)** The quality of anti-CSP serum induced in individual mice was assessed by linear regression analysis, correlating the anti-CSP IgG endpoint titres in the culture medium with the log-transformed ratios of infected hepatocytes in control and test samples (log-mean ratio, LMR). LMR is plotted on the left y-axis. The right y-axis shows the correspondent %ISI. Values on the x-axis are plotted on a square root scale. The black line shows the shared linear fit for IgG from all groups. **(C)** The induced anti-NANP endpoint titres and the correlating %ISI in individual mice are detailed in the table. [a]Log10-transformed NANP6C endpoint titres as determined by ELISA. [b]% Inhibition of sporozoite invasion by 1% serum in culture medium.

at 37°C and then transferred into cluster tubes. The empty wells were washed twice with 200 μl FACS buffer (PBS +0.5% BSA +0.05% Azide). Both washes were added to the cluster tubes. Cells were pelleted in the cluster tubes by centrifuging at 2,000 rpm for 2 min and the supernatant discarded. Cells were then resuspended in 80 μl FACS buffer. Directly before running cells on an LSR II flow cytometer (BD Biosciences), DAPI was added to the cells to a final concentration of 1 μg/ml, which allowed the separation of live from dead cells. Samples were acquired with a LSR II flow cytometer (BD Biosciences) using FACSDIVA software V 6.2 (BD Biosciences). *P. berghei* infected cells were identified by gating on viability and size, removing doublets and gating on GFP positive but PE (autofluorescene) negative cells (32).

Statistical Analysis

Comparison of antibody titers and ISI results was performed using a Kruskal-Wallis test, which was followed up by a Dunn's multiple comparison test.

TRA was calculated from SMFA data, as 100 × [1- (mean number of oocysts in test/mean number of oocysts in control)] and 95% confidence intervals (95%CIs) of % inhibition in oocyst density from a single or multiple feeding experiments for each test antibody at each concentration were calculated using a zero inflation negative binomial model, as described previously (31).

ISI was calculated from cytometer acquisitions files (.fcs) using FlowJo.V 9.7.6 (Tree Star). The percentage of sporozoite inhibition was calculated as a reduction in the percentage of infected cells observed in untreated wells (average) compared to the percentage of infected cells observed in the presence of serum. The sensitivity limit of the assay was defined as the mean of the negative control + 1.645 standard deviations, i.e., 95% of observed values in the negative control, assuming a Gausian distribution.

A linear regression model was used to evaluate differences in functional activity among vaccine groups. The $\log_{10}$ transformed ratio of the mean oocyst count in control and test samples for SMFA, or the ratio of the percentage of viable, GFP positive hepatoma cells in control and test sample for ISI, was the dependent variable, and the square root of anti-Pfs25 and anti-CSP AU, respectively, were independent variables in the model. In another linear regression analysis, reciprocal of dilution (in a square root scale) from the original pooled serum to the tested IgG in a feeder was utilized as the independent variable, instead of anti-Pfs25 AU. Since the ratio of anti-Pfs25-specific IgG to entire IgG in a sample is considered to be stable before (i.e., in the original pooled serum) and after (i.e., in the purified IgG) protein G affinity purification, the anti-Pfs25 AU in the original pooled serum and in the purified IgG were used to calculate the dilution factor of each test IgG at each test concentration. Differences within the linear regression analyses were determined using Tukeys HSD.

Statistical tests were performed using Prism 6 (GraphPad Software Inc, United States), JMP11 (SAS Institute Inc, United States) or R (version 3.4.1). $P < 0.05$ were considered significant.

AUTHOR CONTRIBUTIONS

FB and SB: conceived and planned the study and wrote the manuscript. YL: prepared Pfs25-IMX313 vaccine for immunization. FB: performed mouse experiments. FB, IT, and AM: performed ELISAs. KM and CL: performed SMFAs. AMS: generated parasites for the ISI assay. FB and AJS: conducted the ISI assay. KM and FB: performed statistical analyses of the SMFA and ISI results. All authors read and commented on the manuscript.

FUNDING

This work was funded by a Wellcome-Trust 4-years Ph.D. grant (102051/Z/13/Z) to FB. The SMFA activity was supported by the intramural program of the National Institute of Allergy and Infectious Disease / NIH and by PATH's Malaria Vaccine Initiative.

ACKNOWLEDGMENTS

We would like to thank David Franco as well as Lucile Warter, Danielle Morelle, and Ulrike Krause at GSK for supplying the RTS,S and AS01 used in this study as well as for their help in the study design. The authors are also to Fergal Hill and Alexandre Levert at OSIVAX for their support in respect to the IMX313 nanoparticle platform.

REFERENCES

1. World-Health-Organisation. *"World Malaria Report 2017"*. Geneva. (2017).
2. Walker PG, Griffin JT, Ferguson NM, Ghani AC. Estimating the most efficient allocation of interventions to achieve reductions in *Plasmodium falciparum* malaria burden and transmission in Africa: a modelling study. *Lancet Glob Health* (2016) 4:e474–84. doi: 10.1016/S2214-109X(16)30073-0
3. malERA Consultative Group on Vaccines. A research agenda for malaria eradication: vaccines. *PLoS Med* (2011) 8:e1000398. doi: 10.1371/journal.pmed.1000398
4. malERA Refresh Consultative Panel on Tools for Malaria Elimination. malERA: an updated research agenda for diagnostics, drugs, vaccines, and vector control in malaria elimination and eradication. *PLoS Med* (2017) 14:e1002455. doi: 10.1371/journal.pmed.1002455
5. World-Health-Organisation. *"Malaria Vaccine Technology Roadmap"*. Geneva (2013).
6. Leach A, Vekemans J, Lievens M, Ofori-Anyinam O, Cahill C, Owusu-Agyei S, et al. Design of a phase III multicenter trial to evaluate the efficacy of the RTS,S/AS01 malaria vaccine in children across diverse transmission settings in Africa. *Malar J* (2011) 10:224. doi: 10.1186/1475-2875-10-224
7. RTS,S Clinical Trials Partnership, Agnandji ST, Lell B, Fernandes JF, Abossolo BP, et al. A phase 3 trial of RTS,S/AS01 malaria vaccine in African infants. *N Engl J Med.* (2012) 367:2284–2295. doi: 10.1056/NEJMoa1208394
8. RTS,S Clinical Trials Partnership. Efficacy and safety of the RTS,S/AS01 malaria vaccine during 18 months after vaccination: a phase 3 randomized, controlled trial in children and young infants at 11 African sites. *PLoS Med.* (2014) 11:e1001685. doi: 10.1371/journal.pmed.1001685
9. RTS,S Clinical Trials Partnership. Efficacy and safety of RTS,S/AS01 malaria vaccine with or without a booster dose in infants and children in Africa: final results of a phase 3, individually randomised,

controlled trial. *Lancet* (2015) 386:31–45. doi: 10.1016/S.0140-6736(15)60721-8

10. European Medicines Agency. *First Malaria Vaccine Receives Positive Scientific Opinion From EMA*. London, UK: European Medicines Agenecy (EMA). (2015).
11. Hill AV, Biswas S, Draper S, Rampling T, Reyes-Sandoval A. Towards a multi-antigen multi-stage malaria vaccine. *Malaria J.* (2014) 13:O31. doi: 10.1186/1475-2875-13-S1-O31
12. Tran TM, Portugal S, Draper SJ, Crompton PD. Malaria vaccines: moving forward after encouraging first steps. *Curr Trop Med Rep.* (2015) 2:1–3. doi: 10.1007/s40475-015-0041-3
13. Sherrard-Smith E, Sala KA, Betancourt M, Upton LM, Angrisano F, Morin MJ, et al. Synergy in anti-malarial pre-erythrocytic and transmission-blocking antibodies is achieved by reducing parasite density. *Elife* (2018) 7:e35213. doi: 10.7554/eLife.35213
14. Nikolaeva D, Draper SJ, Biswas S. Toward the development of effective transmission-blocking vaccines for malaria. *Expert Rev Vaccines* (2015) 14:653–80. doi: 10.1586/14760584.2015.993383
15. Wu Y, Ellis RD, Shaffer D, Fontes E, Malkin EM, Mahanty S, et al. Phase 1 trial of malaria transmission blocking vaccine candidates Pfs25 and Pvs25 formulated with montanide ISA 51. *PLoS ONE* (2008) 3:e2636. doi: 10.1371/journal.pone.0002636
16. Sagara I, Healy SA, Assadou MH, Gabriel EE, Kone M, Sissoko K, et al. Safety and immunogenicity of Pfs25H-EPA/Alhydrogel, a transmission-blocking vaccine against *Plasmodium falciparum*: a randomised, double-blind, comparator-controlled, dose-escalation study in healthy Malian adults. *Lancet Infect Dis.* (2018) 18:969–82. doi: 10.1016/S1473-3099(18)30344-X
17. Talaat KR, Ellis RD, Hurd J, Hentrich A, Gabriel E, Hynes NA, et al. Safety and Immunogenicity of Pfs25-EPA/Alhydrogel(R), a transmission blocking vaccine against *Plasmodium falciparum*: an open label study in malaria naive adults. *PLoS ONE* (2016) 11:e0163144. doi: 10.1371/journal.pone.0163144
18. Rutgers T, Gordon D, Gathoye AM, Hollingdale M, Hockmeyer W, Rosenberg M, et al. Hepatitis B surface antigen as carrier matrix for the repetitive epitope of the circumsporozoite protein of *Plasmodium Falciparum*. *Bio/Technology* (1988) 6:1065. doi: 10.1038/nbt0988-1065
19. Sherwood JA, Copeland RS, Taylor KA, Abok K, Oloo AJ, Were JB, et al. *Plasmodium falciparum* circumsporozoite vaccine immunogenicity and efficacy trial with natural challenge quantitation in an area of endemic human malaria of Kenya. *Vaccine* (1996) 14:817–27. doi: 10.1016/0264-410X(95)00221-L
20. Cohen J, Nussenzweig V, Nussenzweig R, Vekemans J, Leach A. From the circumsporozoite protein to the RTS, S/AS candidate vaccine. *Hum Vaccine* (2010) 6:90–6. doi: 10.4161/hv.6.1.9677
21. Shimp RLJr, Rowe C, Reiter K, Chen B, Nguyen V, Aebig J, et al. Development of a Pfs25-EPA malaria transmission blocking vaccine as a chemically conjugated nanoparticle. *Vaccine* (2013) 31:2954–62. doi: 10.1016/j.vaccine.2013.04.034
22. Li Y, Leneghan DB, Miura K, Nikolaeva D, Brian IJ, Dicks MD, et al. Enhancing immunogenicity and transmission-blocking activity of malaria vaccines by fusing Pfs25 to IMX313 multimerization technology. *Sci Rep.* (2016) 6:18848. doi: 10.1038/srep18848
23. Sheehy SH, Duncan CJ, Elias SC, Choudhary P, Biswas S, Halstead FD, et al. ChAd63-MVA-vectored blood-stage malaria vaccines targeting MSP1 and AMA1: assessment of efficacy against mosquito bite challenge in humans. *Mol Ther.* (2012) 20:2355–68. doi: 10.1038/mt.2012.223
24. Elias SC, Collins KA, Halstead FD, Choudhary P, Bliss CM, Ewer KJ, et al. Assessment of immune interference, antagonism, and diversion following human immunization with biallelic blood-stage malaria viral-vectored vaccines and controlled malaria infection. *J Immunol.* (2013) 190:1135–47. doi: 10.4049/jimmunol.1201455
25. Bowyer G, Grobbelaar A, Rampling T, Venkatraman N, Morelle D, Ballou RW, et al. CXCR3+ T follicular helper cells induced by co-administration of RTS,S/AS01B and viral-vectored vaccines are associated with reduced immunogenicity and efficacy against malaria. *Front Immunol.* (2018) 9:1660. doi: 10.3389/fimmu.2018.01660
26. Churcher TS, Sinden RE, Edwards NJ, Poulton ID, Rampling TW, Brock PM, et al. Probability of transmission of malaria from mosquito to human is regulated by mosquito parasite density in naive and vaccinated hosts. *PLoS Pathog.* (2017) 13:e1006108. doi: 10.1371/journal.ppat.1006108
27. Bompard A, Da DF, Yerbanga RS, Biswas S, Kapulu M, Bousema T, et al. Evaluation of two lead malaria transmission blocking vaccine candidate antibodies in natural parasite-vector combinations. *Sci Rep.* (2017) 7:6766. doi: 10.1038/s41598-017-06130-1
28. Niederwieser I, Felger I, Beck HP. Limited polymorphism in *Plasmodium falciparum* sexual-stage antigens. *Am J Trop Med Hyg.* (2001) 64:9–11. doi: 10.4269/ajtmh.2001.64.9
29. Miura K, Orcutt AC, Muratova OV, Miller LH, Saul A, Long CA. Development and characterization of a standardized ELISA including a reference serum on each plate to detect antibodies induced by experimental malaria vaccines. *Vaccine* (2008) 26:193–200. doi: 10.1016/j.vaccine.2007.10.064
30. Collins KA, Snaith R, Cottingham MG, Gilbert SC, Hill AVS. Enhancing protective immunity to malaria with a highly immunogenic virus-like particle vaccine. *Sci Rep.* (2017) 7:46621. doi: 10.1038/srep46621
31. Miura K, Deng B, Tullo G, Diouf A, Moretz SE, Locke E, et al. Qualification of standard membrane-feeding assay with *Plasmodium falciparum* malaria and potential improvements for future assays. *PLoS ONE* (2013) 8:e57909. doi: 10.1371/journal.pone.0057909
32. Rodriguez-Galan A, Salman AM, Bowyer G, Collins KA, Longley RJ, Brod F, et al. An *in vitro* assay to measure antibody-mediated inhibition of *P. berghei* sporozoite invasion against *P falciparum* antigens. *Sci Rep.* (2017) 7:17011. doi: 10.1038/s,41598-017-17274-5
33. Triller G, Scally SW, Costa G, Pissarev M, Kreschel C, Bosch A, et al. Natural parasite exposure induces protective human anti-malarial antibodies. *Immunity* (2017) 47:1197–209.e10. doi: 10.1016/j.immuni.2017.11.007

5

Vaccination with Sporozoites: Models and Correlates of Protection

Yun Shan Goh[1]*, *Daniel McGuire*[1,2] and *Laurent Rénia*[1,2,3]

[1] *Singapore Immunology Network (SIgN), Agency for Science, Technology and Research (A*STAR), Biopolis, Singapore, Singapore,* [2] *School of Biological Sciences, Nanyang Technological University, Singapore, Singapore,* [3] *Department of Microbiology and Immunology, Yong Loo Lin School of Medicine, National University of Singapore, Singapore, Singapore*

Correspondence:
Yun Shan Goh
goh_yun_shan@immunol.a-star.edu.sg

Despite continuous efforts, the century-old goal of eradicating malaria still remains. Multiple control interventions need to be in place simultaneously to achieve this goal. In addition to effective control measures, drug therapies and insecticides, vaccines are critical to reduce mortality and morbidity. Hence, there are numerous studies investigating various malaria vaccine candidates. Most of the malaria vaccine candidates are subunit vaccines. However, they have shown limited efficacy in Phase II and III studies. To date, only whole parasite formulations have been shown to induce sterile immunity in human. In this article, we review and discuss the recent developments in vaccination with sporozoites and the mechanisms of protection involved.

Keywords: ***Plasmodium falciparum*, malaria, sporozoites, protection, vaccine, models, correlates**

INTRODUCTION

Malaria is one of the deadliest diseases, causing a major public health problem with high mortality and morbidity. In 2017, the World Health Organization reported 219 million clinical cases and 435,000 deaths (1). The use of different control interventions such as insecticide-treated bed nets, combination drug therapies and early diagnostics has greatly reduced malaria mortality worldwide (2). However, with increasing drug resistance and insecticide resistance, these efforts are insufficient to eradicate malaria globally (3, 4). It has become increasingly clear that there is no control intervention that can singly eradicate malaria. Multiple control interventions need to be in place simultaneously and a malaria vaccine is integral to global malaria eradication (5).

PARASITE LIFE CYCLE

Plasmodium parasites have a complex life cycle, infecting two hosts, the human and the mosquito. In the human host, the *Plasmodium* life cycle consists of two stages, the liver stage and the blood stage. Infected female *Anopheles* mosquitoes inject sporozoites into the dermis of their mammalian host upon feeding. Sporozoites then enter the bloodstream and migrate to the liver, where the liver stage begins. The sporozoites multiply in hepatocytes, eventually forming merozoites in vesicles called merosomes. These vesicles rupture and release the merozoites into the bloodstream, commencing the blood stage by infecting red blood cells (RBCs). It is the continual cycling of malaria parasites within the RBCs, and the immune responses directed against this stage of the parasite, that causes most of the pathologies observed in malaria infections. The malaria parasites are then transmitted back to the mosquito following blood feeding by a female mosquito. The sexual forms of the blood stage parasites, gametocytes, develop into male and female gametes which fertilize each other, eventually forming oocysts in the mosquito's midgut wall. The oocysts then lyse to release sporozoites, which migrate to the mosquito's salivary glands. When the *Anopheles* mosquito takes a blood meal on another human, the injected sporozoites migrate from the dermis to the liver, thereby beginning a new cycle of infection.

VACCINES AGAINST MALARIA

The development of vaccines for malaria has been met with many difficulties. Despite decades of research efforts, there is still no available vaccine for human use. This has led to the development of a wide range of approaches, in the search for an efficacious malaria vaccine. These approaches can be broadly divided into three main categories: (1) whole parasite-based vaccines, (2) subunit vaccines, and (3) viral, bacterial and parasite vectors as delivery vectors.

Whole Parasite-Based Vaccines

Whole parasite-based vaccines have had considerably more success than other vaccines. Whole parasite-based vaccines contain all parasitic antigens. This approach allows the development of different types of immune responses. Whole parasites used for the vaccines are obtained by dissecting sporozoites from mosquitoes or harvesting asexual blood stages from culture. There are many technical, logistical, and regulatory hurdles associated with large scale production and delivery of whole parasite vaccines in the field. However, recent sporozoite vaccine trials have shown considerable progress in overcoming these hurdles (6, 7).

History

The development of malaria vaccines began with whole parasite-based vaccines more than a 100 years ago when the Sergent brothers used heat-inactivated *P. relictum* sporozoites to immunize canaries and obtained partial protection (8). This was followed by the work of Russell and Mohan where both cellular and humoral responses against malaria were induced in immunized domestic fowls (9). In 1946, Jules Freund invented the Freund adjuvant and formulated the vaccine by combining the adjuvant with formalin-inactivated-blood infected with *P. lophurae*, an avian malaria parasite, or *P. knowlesi*, a monkey malaria parasite (10, 11). The formulations showed promising efficacy. However, the toxic side effects of the Freund adjuvant have prevented its use in humans. The first attempt in humans was done by Heidelberger et al., using formalin-inactivated *P. vivax*-infected blood to immunize volunteers, however no protection was induced (12). These initial studies, though suboptimal, have paved the way for future whole parasite-based vaccine development.

Vaccination With Sporozoites

Among the whole parasite-based vaccine candidates, there is considerable research on the pre-erythrocytic parasites. The pre-erythrocytic stage is an asymptomatic phase. Very few sporozoites are injected and subsequently developed in the hepatocytes during natural infection in human volunteers (13). The idea of inducing an immune response that can neutralize sporozoites in the skin and circulation and prevent the penetration of a low number of sporozoites into hepatocytes or destroy a low number of infected hepatocytes during the asymptomatic phase make pre-erythrocytic stage vaccines attractive. By preventing the pre-erythrocytic stage development, the vaccines would prevent blood stage infection, hence preventing pathology. In addition, the pre-erythrocytic stage vaccines have had more success than the other stages, which provides more support for their development.

Whole sporozoite-based vaccines developed thus far in human include (1) irradiated parasites (6, 14), (2) genetically-attenuated parasites (15, 16), and (3) drug-infection-treatment vaccination (17, 18).

Vaccination with irradiated sporozoites

Irradiated sporozoite vaccine is the most clinically developed whole parasite-based vaccine, and also the most clinically developed pre-erythrocytic vaccine (17). The first few studies that showed definitive protective immunity with irradiated sporozoites were done in chicks and subsequently in mice (18, 19). This was later demonstrated in humans, where vaccination with irradiated sporozoites, *via* infective mosquito bites, protected 92% of the volunteers from infection (20–22). However, >1,000 mosquito bites are required to introduce sufficient irradiated sporozoites to induce the high level of efficacy. This prevented the development of this approach for mass vaccination.

More recently, delivery of cyropreserved irradiated sporozoites into the host by direct venous inoculation *via* needle and syringe, has been tested in humans and showed promising efficacy data (6, 17, 23). While four doses only protected 33% of the individuals (6), five doses protected 100% of the individuals (6). More studies to perfect the vaccination regimes would allow direct venous inoculation *via* needle and syringe to replace mosquito bites as a delivery system. Another hurdle with irradiated sporozoite vaccines is the need for a high dose of irradiated parasites. Vaccine dosage, vaccination regimen, and route of administration have been investigated in malaria-naive adults (24). In the study, administration of higher doses may further enhance protection— four intravenous immunizations with a higher dose of 2.7×10^5 irradiated sporozoites was found to be the most optimal, where 55% of vaccinated subjects remained uninfected following controlled human malaria infections (CHMI) 21 weeks after immunization. The timing of the CHMI following vaccination has also been found to be important, with vaccine efficacy being higher when CHMI was performed 3 weeks after immunization, instead of 21 weeks. While vaccination with irradiated sporozoites led to sterile protection in 100% (6/6) of vaccinated malaria naïve volunteers (6), irradiated sporozoites vaccination in malaria-endemic Mali yielded a lower protection (14). There are fundamental differences between the two studies, such as the first study examines protection against homologous challenge and the latter study examines protection against heterologous challenge. Naturally transmitted parasites are often different from the vaccine strain. Twenty-four weeks after final immunization regimen, five doses of 2.7×10^5 irradiated sporozoites protected 7 of 10 against homologous CHMI, but only 1 of 10 against heterologous CHMI (25), showing that the vaccine efficacy against heterologous infection is markedly reduced. In addition, the findings also suggest that pre-exposure to the malaria parasites may prevent the establishment of a protective immune response since blood stage infection is able to induce immune suppression (26). This also further highlights the need for optimization of the required dose and regime in the target population to achieve robust and sterile protection.

The irradiation of parasites is a delicate process that requires the sporozoites to retain a certain degree of viability. Similar to heat-inactivated and frozen-thawed sporozoites, over-irradiated sporozoites do not induce protection (27, 28). Irradiating the sporozoites leads to DNA damage in the sporozoites with no or limited reduction on hepatocyte infectivity (29, 30). Although irradiation results in an inhibition of parasite DNA replication, ultrastructure modification and alteration in gene expression (31, 32), eventually leading to developmental arrest of the liver stage within hepatocytes (33, 34), it still allows for parasite antigen presentation and priming of immune responses.

Vaccination with genetically-attenuated sporozoites

Non-irradiated sporozoites have been postulated to be more efficacious as whole parasite-based vaccines because, as compared to irradiated sporozoites, they are able to progress to a later stage of pre-erythrocytic development, (35). By doing so, the host immune system is exposed to a wide repertoire of malarial antigens and thus able to target more of the pre-erythrocytic stage. To this end, research efforts have focused on developing ways, other than irradiation, to attenuate the growth of the parasite. Recent advances in *Plasmodium* research such as genetic manipulation have brought forward a new approach to attenuate parasites. Genetically-attenuated parasites are modified by deleting key essential genes that result in developmental arrest of the liver stage after hepatocyte infection, but do not affect parasite viability, mosquito infectivity, and sporozoite production in animal models (36). Inactivation of UIS3, UIS4, or P36p prevented the attenuated parasites from developing beyond the early pre-erythrocytic stage in mice (37–39). Vaccination of these live genetically-attenuated parasites offered sterile protection against a challenge with a wild type isolate. While promising, one of the major concerns for the development of genetically-attenuated parasites as vaccines is the possible occurrence of breakthrough infections. The first clinical trial using live genetically-attenuated parasites that lack the two genes, p52 and p36, led to breakthrough infections (15). Breakthrough infections in mice have also been observed for UIS4- and P36p-deficient parasites (37, 39). However, great progress has been made recently. Live genetically-attenuated parasites lacking three genes (p52–/p36–/sap1–; "PfGAP3KO") arrest early in liver-stage development, and were safe with no observed breakthrough infection following administration into human subjects by infective mosquito bites (16). Compared to irradiated sporozoite vaccine and early liver stage-arresting genetically-attenuated parasites, second generation genetically-attenuated parasites that arrest late liver stages have shown to demonstrate superior anti-malarial immunity following vaccination in mice by having a greater antigen repertoire (40, 41). These candidate vaccines could also have greater efficacy in humans, but this remains to be demonstrated.

Drug-infection-treatment vaccination

Drug-infection-treatment vaccination is the last approach. It involves vaccination with live wild-type parasites under drug prophylaxis, where the drug targets and eliminates the blood stage parasites. This approach allows full liver development and a limited initial blood stage development, thereby focusing immunity toward the liver stages. Pioneer mouse studies have, indeed, shown greater efficacy when the mice were vaccinated with live *P. berghei* or *P. yoelii* sporozoites under drug prophylaxis than when the mice were vaccinated with irradiated sporozoites—fewer inoculations and less sporozoites were required to induce sterile protection (42–44). Vaccination with live sporozoites under chloroquine prophylaxis is the most investigated vaccine formulation under this approach, and it has shown very promising efficacy data. The first study in humans examined the efficacy of the vaccine where the live sporozoites were introduced into the volunteers *via* infective mosquito bites (45). The study utilized CHMI and demonstrated sterile protection, where 100% of the volunteers were protected from infection following a wild-type sporozoite challenge. A subsequent CHMI study investigated the efficacy of the vaccine where the live sporozoites were intravenously inoculated *via* a needle and syringe. In this study, a dose-dependent protection was observed, where only three doses of 5.12×10^4 sporozoites were sufficient to protect all volunteers from the challenge (46). In addition to chloroquine, vaccination with live wild-type parasites under prophylaxis of other antimalarials has also been investigated. Primaquine (47), mefloquine (48) and artemisinin derivatives such as artesunate (49) have been used in place of chloroquine and vaccination with live wild-type parasites under prophylaxis of these antimalarials has demonstrated protective immunity against a homologous sporozoite challenge in mice and in humans.

However, there are various challenges with this approach such as the technical and logistical issues associated with generating sporozoites at large scale and field deployment. There are also concerns that the sporozoite injections might not be properly followed with antimalarial treatment, which could lead to sickness. In addition, while sterile immunity can be achieved against a homologous sporozoite challenge, protection was suboptimal when immunized volunteers were challenged with a heterologous strain (50, 51), suggesting that the protective immune mechanisms target polymorphic antigens. Nevertheless, the current published findings have demonstrated very encouraging efficacy data and suggest that vaccination with live sporozoites under chloroquine prophylaxis, following vaccination regime optimization, could potentially be the most efficacious sporozoite vaccine until date.

Subunit Vaccines

Subunit vaccines allow rational design of the vaccine to induce the desired immune effectors against the parasite. In addition, subunit vaccines are safe and generally easy to produce at large scale and to administer in the field. Hence, efficacious subunit vaccines that offer long term protection are the preferred vaccines of choice.

Peptides and Recombinant Proteins

Subunit vaccines have been developed either as peptides, multi-peptide constructs or recombinant proteins. They can be based on a single parasite antigen or a combination of multiple parasite antigens, and often in a formulation that includes adjuvants. Most constructs have been designed for the circumsporozoite protein (CSP), a major sporozoite surface protein (52), as it is the first cloned malaria antigen (53, 54). Both peptides and multi-peptide constructs containing either the B epitope alone or both B and T epitopes induced protection in mouse models (55–58). However, when tested in humans, the peptide constructs did not induce significant protection (59). The main reason for the failure in humans is that the immune response to these constructs was genetically restricted by major histocompatibility gene (60) and thus could not induce an efficient immune response in most volunteers.

To ameliorate immunogenicity and protective efficacy, peptides and proteins have been designed to contain T cell epitopes from the parasites or an unrelated proteins recognized by many MHC genes (61), coupled to diverse chemical backbones, or fused with other proteins to create particle vaccines to be used with or without various adjuvants (62–67). All these new constructs demonstrated a high efficacy in mouse models but have yet to be validated in humans.

Of all the subunit vaccines, RTS,S, a CSP-based subunit vaccine, is the current most clinically-advanced malaria vaccine, being the only malaria vaccine to have progressed to the pivotal Phase III clinical trials (68). Enormous resources have been spent on rationally improving RTS,S efficacy, which include developing novel adjuvant systems. Multiple studies have demonstrated a need for RTS,S be formulated with adjuvants such as monophosphoryl lipid A and QS21, to achieve immunogenicity (69–71). This was followed up by a series of clinical trials, where significant progress has been made to improve immunogenicity and efficacy (72, 73). The RTS,S vaccine has been designed to inhibit the liver stage and prevent blood stage infection. RTS,S is, ultimately, formulated with a chimeric molecule based on CSP, fused to the S antigen of the hepatitis B virus, together with a potent adjuvant, AS01. The first Phase IIb trials performed in adult volunteers in the USA showed ~50% protection against clinical malaria (69, 70, 74).

When tested in the endemic regions, RTS,S's efficacy against infection was less impressive and was of short-duration (<3 months) (75, 76). What is encouraging is that RTS,S/AS01 vaccination has been found to induce a significant reduction (~60%) in the incidence of clinical infections in children in the same study (76). This finding encouraged GlaxoSmithKline and the Malaria Vaccine initiative, with financial support from the Bill and Melinda Gates Foundation, to further develop this vaccine for infants and young children in Africa. However, RTS,S efficacy against clinical malaria was later found to be suboptimal in malaria-endemic populations, with a vaccine efficacy against clinical infection of 36.3% in young children and 25.9% in infants (77–81). One possible explanation is that the CSP used in the vaccine contains several T cell epitopes, which are all highly polymorphic in parasite population in the field. Neafsey et al. elegantly demonstrated that the overall vaccine efficacy was very low in field settings with minimal matching of the CSP alleles in the field with the CSP allele in RTS,S (80).

Another explanation for the limited efficacy of the CSP-based vaccines is that it may not be the best antigen to induce protection. It is likely that other antigens may be better vaccine candidates, alone or in combination with the CSP. This hypothesis was supported by various studies, which showed that the sterile protection against a sporozoite challenge obtained in mice immunized with irradiated sporozoites was independent of the immune response against the CSP (82–85).

With the limited success of subunit vaccines developed thus far, there have been many efforts to identify new pre-erythrocytic (liver) targets for vaccine development using various approaches (86–90). These new antigens have shown encouraging efficacy data in animal models either alone (91, 92) or in combinations (93, 94), however efficacy in humans has yet to be demonstrated (95).

DNA Vaccines

DNA has been identified as a vaccine delivery system in the 1990s (96). This approach was quickly taken up, and DNA vaccines against CSP were developed and tested in human (97–99). Although the CSP-based constructs induced high levels of protection in mice (100), they had poor immunogenicity in humans (101). DNA constructs encoding multiple genes (102, 103) or epitopes were also developed (104). However, none of these constructs induced high level of protection against a sporozoite challenge (104, 105). To enhance the immune responses, malaria DNA vaccines were developed in combination with DNA constructs encoding for cytokines such as GM-CSF. Although some of these constructs had increased immunogenicity and efficacy in murine models (106), they did not induce protection against sporozoite challenge in human (105).

Viral, Bacterial, and Parasite Vectors as Delivery Vectors

Viral, bacterial and parasite vectors have been developed as delivery vectors for malaria vaccines. As these vectors are based on whole organisms, they usually do not need to be adjuvanted to stimulate the innate immune system which is necessary for the development of an optimal adaptive immune response (107). However, in some studies, various adjuvants have also been used to increase vector constructs immunogenicity (108).

The use of viral vectors as delivery vectors for malaria vaccines is the most common (109). Recombinant influenza viruses (110), pox viruses such as vaccinia virus (110, 111), Sindbis virus (112), yellow fever virus (113, 114), adenovirus (115), human cytomegalovirus (116) as delivery vectors have shown promising efficacy in animal models. Bacterial vectors such as *Salmonella* (117, 118), Bacille-Calmette Guerin (BCG) (119), *Shigella flexneri* 2A strain (120) as delivery vectors have also shown good immunogenicity and efficacy against sporozoite challenge in mice. Currently, only *Salmonella* vectors as delivery vectors have been examined in humans, showing good safety profile and immunogenicity (121). Parasites such as *Leishmania* (122) and *Toxoplasma* (123, 124) as delivery vectors were also able to induce partial protection in mice. However, it remains to be seen if these vectors can induce protection in human.

Prime-Boost Combinations

To enhance humoral and T cell responses, various prime-boost strategies have been developed using combinations of different vaccine approaches. Vaccination with subunits or DNA constructs, followed by viral vectors or combination of viral vectors encoding one or multiple malaria antigens has been examined and efficacy has been demonstrated in mouse models (125–129). However, of all these combinations, only a few have shown significant efficacy in humans (104, 109, 130–133). Recent strategies, prime-and-target (134) and prime-and-trap (135), have shown that the best combination, that can induce high level of protection in mice, depends on the capacity to induce and maintain tissue-resident memory cells in the liver.

MODEL SYSTEMS

The use of experimental models has an important role in the development of vaccines. It is essential for the first assessments of safety, immunogenicity and potential protective efficacy of vaccine candidates. The early studies of malaria candidate vaccines utilized avian models, despite being a poor alternative to study pathogens with mammalian hosts. The eventual establishment of other malaria models has brought new insights and greatly facilitated malaria vaccine research. Current models used include: (1) mouse, (2) non-human primates (NHP), (3) humanized mice, and (4) human volunteers (CHMI).

Mouse Models

Until date, the traditional mouse model still remains the most commonly used model as it is less costly and more easily available. *P. berghei* and *P. yoelii* are two of the more commonly used rodent malaria species for *in vivo* and *in vitro* studies. It is often the starting ground for *in vivo* studies examining the development of pre-erythrocytic stage and whole sporozoite vaccine candidates. Human parasites such as *P. falciparum* and *P. vivax*, which contribute to the majority of the malaria global disease burden, display highly restricted host-cell tropism—they cannot establish an infection and develop the pre-erythrocytic stages effectively *in vitro* easily. A reproducible model of full development of the pre-erythrocytic stage has only been described in primary human hepatocytes (136). The mouse model allows the examination of the parasite infection in the liver *in vivo*, and the effectiveness of the whole sporozoite vaccine candidates to protect the host from infection. While vaccine efficacy in the mice does not necessarily predict vaccine efficacy in humans, there have not been any examples where an absence of vaccine efficacy in mice was contradicted by vaccine efficacy in humans. Quite a number of whole sporozoite vaccine candidates that are first identified to be protective in mouse models (19, 42, 44) have went on to be validated in humans (22, 45). The first study demonstrating that vaccination with a whole sporozoite vaccine candidate, irradiated sporozoites, can induce sterile protection from infective sporozoite challenge was in a *P. berghei* mouse model (19). This has been established as the gold standard as human volunteers vaccinated with irradiated *P. falciparum* sporozoites were found to develop protective immunity (22). Similarly, vaccination with live sporozoites under drug prophylaxis was also first identified to have promising efficacy in the *P. berghei* and *P. yoelii* mouse models (42, 44), before demonstrating sterile protection in all vaccinated human volunteers (45). A new approach to chemically attenuate sporozoites has been identified using the *P. berghei* model. This was performed by treating sporozoites with centanamycin, a DNA alkylating agent (137–139). This may also offer protection in humans, however further studies to validate its efficacy are still pending.

With the development of transgenic rodent malaria parasites, knock-in (KI) parasites expressing *P. falciparum* (140) or *P. vivax* (141) genes have been generated. These KI parasites allow the examination of the efficacy of immunogens (142–144) or antibodies against human malaria pre-erythrocytic antigens *in vivo* (145, 146).

While the mouse models have greatly contributed to the development of malaria vaccines, there are limitations. It is still largely unknown how relevant the mouse models are for the human parasite. The ability to interpret and draw conclusion from the mouse and translate it to the human remains unclear. There are major fundamental differences, both at genetic and proteomic levels, between the rodent and human malaria species, with the rodent parasite genomes missing orthologs for more than 730 *P. falciparum* genes (147, 148). In addition, there are differences in the both the liver and blood stages of infection. While the mouse parasites, *P. berghei* and *P. yoelii*, emerge from the liver after 2–3 days of infection, the human parasites, *P. falciparum* and *P. vivax*, require 7–10 days of pre-erythrocytic stage development (149). The formation of dormant pre-erythrocytic stages in *P. vivax* infections, which is a hallmark of *P. vivax* infections (150), is also not present in *P. berghei* and *P. yoelii* infections in mice, although liver forms of *P. yoelii* have been observed in the liver of their natural host, *Thamnomys gazellae*, at least 8 months post-sporozoite infection (151). Lastly, most murine studies are performed with genetically homogenous inbred mice with a limited MHC gene repertoire, which do not mimic the large genetic diversity of the human population. Laboratory mice are maintained in clean specific-pathogen—free facilities, hence the absence of the effect of environment (e.g., microbiome) on the mouse immune system may bias infection and vaccine studies (152). Taken together, while it is a powerful experiment tool, the traditional mouse model is not an ideal model, especially for studying pre-erythrocytic malaria vaccines.

Non-human Primates

Due to the limitations of the traditional mouse models, there have been substantial efforts to develop alternative animal models that are able to generate adequate parallels in an *in vivo* approach of the human immune system. Historically, non-human primates (NHP) have been used as the alternative model. Compared to the mouse, NHP share a lot more similarities with the human.

Simian *Plasmodium* species can infect various NHP species. In particular, human parasites can be adapted to NHP and some NHP can even support direct infection with *P. falciparum* and *P. vivax* (153). The *Aotus* monkeys have served as a valuable model. They can be infected by *P. falciparum* and *P. vivax* (154, 155). The NHP models are particularly important for assessments of *P. vivax* pre-erythrocytic stage vaccines (156), due to the formation of dormant pre-erythrocytic stages in *P. vivax* infections, which cannot be recapitulated in the mouse models. Simian malaria parasites, such as *P knowlesi* or *P. cynomolgi* in macaques, have also been used for immune and vaccine studies (157, 158). Vaccination with live sporozoites under chloroquine prophylaxis has shown promising efficacy data in Toque monkeys immunized with *P. cynomolgi* (159). However, the lack of availability, the high costs to maintain a colony and the restriction of utilization due to ethical issues limit the use of NHP, especially where large numbers are required.

Humanized Mouse

In the more recent years, the development of a humanized mouse as an animal model (160, 161) has greatly facilitated the study of human malaria research. These models mainly arise from the xenotransplantation of human hepatopoietic cells and/or tissues, allowing the long-term establishment of components of human immunity in permissive immunodeficient mice.

Using a human liver chimeric SCID/Alb-uPA mouse, studies on the pre-erythrocytic stages can be performed (162, 163). While it has been shown to be a viable model to study *P. falciparum* pre-erythrocytic stage development, the study of human malaria in this model is limited to the pre-erythrocytic stage as *P. falciparum* cannot transit from the pre-erythrocytic stages to the blood stages in this model (164). Other drawbacks include infertility of the mice due to the SCID/Alb-uPA immunodeficient background (165), and hepatotoxicity and high neonatal mortality due to the uPA transgene expression (166). These have made the generation of large number of the mice extremely costly and difficult.

Due to these drawbacks, an alternative, a human liver chimeric FAH$^{-/-}$Rag2$^{-/-}$IL2Rγ^{null} (FRG) mouse, has been developed. These mice can be bred relatively easily and do not suffer from hepatotoxicity. In addition, this model has been shown to support robust pre-erythrocytic stage infection and development (149). When human RBCs were transplanted into these mice, the new model supported the transition from a pre-erythrocytic infection to a blood stage infection (167). The NOD mice deficient for the IL2Rγ gene and transgenic for the thymidine kinase gene (TK-NOG) is another model that has also been developed. These mice do not suffer from liver failure. A transient injection of the drug gancyclovir induces a controlled ablation of the mouse hepatocytes. Treated mice are easily repopulated with human hepatocytes (168). These mice can also be doubly engrafted with human red blood cells and this allows the full development of *P. falciparum* in the liver and the transition to the blood stage. Interestingly, this model also supported the liver stage development of another human parasite, *P. ovale* (169).These findings are extremely encouraging as this raises the possibility of using these models to study a liver stage infection and also a combined liver and blood stage infection. While the use of the humanized mice offers many new possibilities to study human malaria biology in a non-human model *in vivo*, it is worth noting that these mice are immuno-compromised, which makes them unsuitable for vaccine immunogenicity and efficacy studies. Nonetheless, they have shown to be useful in passive transfer experiments to test antibody efficacy (170–172).

Studies on the development of humanized mice with a fully reconstituted immune system are underway (173). In fact, humanized mice that possess the human immune system (HIS) have been established for malaria research, using recombinant adeno-associated virus (AAV)-based gene transfer technologies (174). With functional human CD4 T cells and B cells (HIS-CD4/B mice), these HIS mice were able to produce a significant level of human IgG against *P. falciparum* CSP upon immunization (175). The HIS-CD4/B mice were also protected against infection from an *in vivo* challenge with transgenic *P. berghei* sporozoites expressing the PfCSP protein following immunization. While these models are essential pre-clinical models to understand immune responses against human malaria, it is worth noting that these HIS mice still retain mouse myeloid compartments that are likely to influence antigen presentation and immune cell residency, and *in vivo* vaccine efficacy can only be examined using transgenic rodent malaria parasites expressing selected *P. falciparum* proteins. New iterations of humanized mice that possess the humanization of the liver, bone marrow, lymphoid compartments, and human erythrocytes would be the ideal mouse model and would greatly help to understand human malaria parasite infection and immunology. It would be an essential tool in providing a more accurate initial assessment of the safety profile and vaccine efficacy of malaria vaccine candidates before moving onto human studies.

Human Volunteers

The most relevant model is the human host itself. The establishment of the CHMI model has greatly helped malaria research. The CHMI model involves exposing healthy human volunteers to the parasite *via* infective mosquito bites, monitoring the volunteers closely for signs and symptoms of malaria infection, and treating the volunteers with drug upon detection of fever and/or detection of parasites (45, 176).

The CHMI model uses the most relevant host-parasite pair. While CHMI has been performed *via* other routes such as intravenously and intramuscularly, it is more commonly done *via* infective mosquito bites. The use of infective mosquito bites in the model mimics the natural route of infection, offering advantages in the prediction of the potential efficacy of vaccine candidate against natural infections. However, it also has its limitations. The CHMI model is often performed with one parasite strain, while there are many antigenically diverse heterologous parasites in the field. Infection in the CHMI model is controlled and the parasite load is administered at one single time, whereas high parasite load at one single time is uncommon in natural field setting. Despite the limitations, CHMI studies with no observed efficacy could halt the pursuit of large and expensive clinical trials in malaria-endemic areas in time. CHMI studies with partial efficacy could provide insights on how protective efficacy could be improved by alterations in vaccination regimes such as the number of doses and number of immunizations. In particular, through a series of CHMI studies, the company Sanaria was able to optimize their PfSPZ vaccine, which is composed of radiation-attenuated, aseptic, purified, cryopreserved *P. falciparum* sporozoites, to induce sterile protection against homologous challenge for at least 59 weeks (24) and heterologous challenge for at least 33 weeks (51) in malaria-naïve individuals. The vaccination also prevented naturally transmitted heterogeneous *P. falciparum* in malaria-endemic adults in Mali for at least 24 weeks (vaccine efficacy of 29%) (14). Further CHMI studies to optimize dosage and vaccination regimes could improve the vaccine efficacy.

Immunity and Correlates of Protection Against the Pre-erythrocytic Stage

The malaria parasite has a complex life cycle. Depending on the stage of development in its mammalian host, the parasite can be extracellular or intracellular. They can also infect different cell types. Hence, various innate and adaptive immune mechanisms are needed for parasite control and elimination. In order to develop an efficacious pre-erythrocytic stage vaccine, it is important to know the protective immune mechanisms to induce (**Table 1**).

In addition, through better understanding of the mechanisms involved in the protection, we could potentially identify correlates of protection. The identification of correlates of protection is particularly important to the vaccine development as it helps to assess vaccine efficacy and design better immunogens. Through various animal models, we are beginning to tease out the potential correlates of protective immunity.

Innate Immunity

Upon infection, the innate immunity is triggered by the malaria parasites. Immune responses initiated by the innate immune system in response to parasites play key roles in protective immunity development. Early pro-inflammatory responses regulate anti-parasitic Th1 development and promote effector cell function for efficiently clearing infections. The use of a proper adjuvant is necessary to trigger the adequate innate pathway.

Cytokines

Cytokines play an important role in the protection against malaria. Upon infection, the RNA of the parasites is recognized by the cytosolic pathogen-recognition receptors of mouse hepatocytes. As a result, type I interferon pathway is induced, which can inhibit late stage parasites. Type I interferon leads to the recruitment of leukocytes that inhibit late liver forms through IFNγ (179, 212). IFNγ can inhibit the development of *P. yoelii* and *P. berghei in vitro* and *in vivo* in mice (177, 178), *P. falciparum* in human hepatocytes *in vitro* (213) and *P. vivax* infected chimpanzees *in vivo* (214). The effect of IFNγ is through the induction of the inducible nitric oxide synthase enzyme in hepatocyte which generates high of toxic nitric oxide (180–182).

In addition to IFNγ, IL6, and TNFα have also been implicated in protection. TNFα is able to inhibit parasite liver stage indirectly through induction of yet-to-be-identified mediators secreted by hepatocytes (215) or through IL-6 on non-parenchymal cells (216). IL-6 inhibits liver stage development through the induction of iNOS (217, 218).

NK and NKT Cells

NK and NKT cells are abundant in the liver, and interact with the parasites to initiate liver-stage cell-mediated immunity. Following the activation of the type I interferon pathway, the hepatocytes produce chemokines to recruit macrophages, neutrophils, lymphocytes, NK and NKT cells to the site of infection in mice (179, 219). This eventually leads to the killing of late liver stage parasites by NKT cells. NK cells have also been shown to inhibit the development of the liver stages in the hepatocytes, limiting the infection and/or reinfection in mice (185). NK cells also play an important role in CD4 T cell priming during murine malaria infections (186, 187), bridging between the innate and adaptive immunity.

γδ T Cells

Similar to NK T cells, γδ T cells are innate-like T cells that have been postulated to bridge the gap between innate and adaptive immunity (220). Early production of IFNγ by γδ T cells was detected following *in vitro* exposure of *P. falciparum*-infected RBCs to PBMCs from malaria-naïve donors (188). In mice, γδ T cells induced by whole sporozoites vaccination can inhibit intrahepatic parasitic development (190). γδ T cells are also important for the induction of early immunity against malaria (191). γδ T cell-deficient mice immunized with irradiated sporozoites were more susceptible to liver stage infection 42 h following a sporozoite challenge (191). γδ T cells can also directly prime CD4 and CD8 T cell responses *in vitro* (192, 193).

Sterile protection in mice following vaccination with irradiated sporozoites requires γδ T cells (194). Without γδ T cells, protective CD8 T cell responses were impaired (194). γδ T cells have been postulated to act either as effector cells that operate in the absence of αβ T cells, or as accessory cells for appropriate protective responses from other cells (194). In humans, γδ T cells have also been shown to recognize malaria antigens and proliferate, conferring immunity against clinical malaria in children from Uganda (221). In addition to influencing the protective CD8 T cell response, γδ T cells can also influence cytokine production. Higher frequencies and higher cytokine production by γδ T cells correlate with protection against subsequent infection in children living in endemic settings (189, 222). Recent studies on irradiated sporozoite vaccines have shown that γδ T cells expanded in a dose-dependent manner in immunized malaria-naïve subjects (6, 24), and were associated with protection (24). Hence, γδ T cells could be a potential correlate of protection, and further studies to better define a most appropriate outcome to represent a measurable positive correlation of γδ T cells with protection would be advantageous for vaccine development.

CD8α Dendritic Cells

Early adaptive immunity is triggered as early as a few hours post an infective mosquito bite, with T cell activation being observed in the skin draining lymph nodes in the murine model

TABLE 1 | Immunity against pre-erythrocytic stage parasites.

Immune response	Mode of action	References
Innate type I interferon response	*Plasmodium* RNA as a pathogen-associated molecular pattern (PAMP) to activate a type I IFN response, which in turn reduce the liver parasite load	(177–179)
Cytokines	IFNγ induces the inducible nitric oxide enzyme to produce nitric oxide to kill the sporozoites	(180–182)
	TNFα increases the capacity of monocytes and macrophages to phagocytose parasite to limit parasite infection	(183, 184)
NK cells	Inhibit liver stage development to limit liver parasite load CD4 T cell priming	(185–187)
γδ T cells	IFN-γ production Inhibit intrahepatic parasitic development Prime CD4 and CD8 T cell responses	(188–194)
CD8α dendritic cells	CD8 T cell priming	(195–197)
CD8 T cells	Lysis of infected hepatocytes by perforin and granzymes	(184, 198–200)
	Indirectly through the action of pro-inflammatory cytokines such as IFN-γ to mediate anti-parasite effects	(180–182, 201–204)
CD4 T cells	B cell development to produce antibodies against the liver stage	(198)
	Survival of protective effector and memory CD8 T cells	(205, 206)
	Can be induced to expresses CD107a, a marker for cytotoxic degranulation, to mediate protection	(48)
Antibodies	Inhibit sporozoite motility in the liver Mediate cytotoxicity against sporozoites in the host skin	(207, 208)
	Opsonize sporozoites for the subsequent sporozoite phagocytosis by monocytes or macrophages	(208, 209)
	Inhibit sporozoite invasion into hepatocytes	(210)
	Inhibit sporozoite development inside the hepatocytes	(210)
	Bind to parasite neo-antigens such as heat shock protein expressed at the surface of infected hepatocytes to induce liver parasite killing through an antibody-dependent cell-mediated mechanism	(211)

(196). After dermal inoculation, a fraction of sporozoites actively migrates to the draining lymph nodes (195). There is a direct uptake of the parasites by lymph-node resident CD8α dendritic cells followed by CD8 T cell-dendritic cell cluster formation in the draining lymph nodes (223). CD8α dendritic cells are also shown to be essential for the development of the protective immunity induced by intravenous injection of irradiated sporozoites since mice depleted of these subsets are not protected against a sporozoite challenge (224, 225). A subsequent study showed that splenic but not liver CD8α dendritic cells are the main cells involved in effector parasite specific-T cell priming (226). It was also shown recently that monocyte-derived CD11c cells infiltrated the liver after infection, acquired parasite-derived antigens and primed protective CD8 T cells (227). The role and functions of other dendritic subsets is controversial and remains to be determined (199, 228, 229).

Adaptive Immunity

As with any vaccination, the focus has been to trigger the adaptive immunity to induce an efficacious and long-lasting immunity. Various arms of the adaptive immunity are required to act in concert to provide protection against malaria.

CD8 T Cells

CD8 T cells have been implicated as the principal effector cells, central to protection against malaria. The importance of CD8 T cells in protective immunity was first demonstrated in mice vaccinated with irradiated sporozoites (177). The sterile immunity induced by the vaccination was abolished when CD8 T cells were depleted (177, 178). CD8 T cells can kill the parasites in mice (200) either directly through lysis of infected hepatocytes by perforin and granzymes (184, 230) or indirectly through IFNγ-mediated protection (180–182, 201–204). It must be stressed that while leukocytes and, in particular, CD8 T cells can kill liver parasites by these mechanisms, they differ depending of the host/parasite combinations (231).

Given the central role of CD8 T cells in protection, it is one potential correlate of protective immunity. In humans, CD8 T cells have been shown to be associated with protection from severe malaria (232), and a few of the identified CD8 T cell responses are directed against pre-erythrocytic stage antigens such as LSA1 and CSP (233, 234). However, vaccination studies, where human volunteers were immunized with irradiated sporozoites, showed that, while CD8 T cell response were also detected against various pre-erythrocytic stage antigens, the responses were not found to be associated with protection (235). More recently, a human trial where human volunteers were immunized with irradiated sporozoites showed seemingly contradicting data, where sterile protection correlated with the numbers of IFNγ-producing CD8 T cells in isolated PBMCs (6). This is also evident in animal studies on irradiated sporozoite vaccines, where high frequency of parasite-specific

CD8 T cells was observed in the liver of non-human primates and mice, and was associated with protection in mice (236). The differences are likely due to the differences in the vaccination regimes and the methods to detect/quantify T cells. Indeed, in humans, T cell activity is measured in peripheral blood, whereas, in mice, T cell activity is usually measured in spleen or liver.

Central memory T cells

Memory T cells provide long-term protection. Upon re-infection, these cells rapidly gain effector functions including cytokine production and lytic activity. There are three subsets of memory T cells: (1) central memory T cells, which predominantly reside in lymphoid tissues, (2) effector memory T cells, which reside in the spleen and peripheral tissues, and (3) tissue-resident memory T cells, which reside in the tissues and do not recirculate. The role of central memory T cells in protection against malaria is limited. While central memory T cells can produce IFN-γ after *in vitro* stimulation (201), their presence has not been associated with protection. Despite having a large proportion of central memory T cell, mice that were vaccinated with modified vaccinia ANKARA expressing the multiple epitope string and thrombospondin-related adhesion protein (ME-TRAP) were not protected from malaria challenge (237).

CD8 effector memory T cells

In contrast to the central memory T cells, the presence of effector memory T cells has been associated with sterile protection in the murine model, although large numbers are required for protection against malaria (238). Long-term sterile protection was only observed in mice when the parasite-specific CD8 T cells made up >1% of the total peripheral blood CD8 T cell population (238). Degree of protection in mice correlated with the frequencies of CD8 effector memory T cells present in liver, and failure to achieve the protective threshold frequency of these cells might make the host susceptible to infection (203).

CD8 tissue-resident memory T cells

More recently, a new subset of memory T cells, with a distinct gene expression profile, has been characterized (202). The liver tissue-resident memory T cells develop naturally during the course of an immune response following TCR stimulation, with rapidly expanding population due to the liver infection or inflammation in mice (239). These cells are found to be patrolling within the liver sinusoids, a process dependent on LFA-1–ICAM-1 interactions (240). Tissue-resident memory T cells were essential for sterile protection against sporozoite infection in mice following immunization with irradiated sporozoites (241).

CD4 T Cells

In contrast to CD8 T cells, the role of CD4 T cells in protection against malaria is not well understood. Despite this, it is clear that the development and maturation of an effective CD8T cell response is dependent on CD4 T cells help. CD4 T cells are activated to amplify the anti-pathogen response by driving B cell germinal responses and supporting CD8 T cell activation. Mouse hepatocytes express MHC Class I and Class II molecules that can be loaded with parasite antigen-derived epitopes following the TAP or the endosomal pathways (242–245). CD4 T cells are required to prime effective immunity. CD4 T cells recognizing CSP have been shown to protect against a *P. yoelii* sporozoite challenge in mice (243, 246). Pre-immunization but not pre-challenge depletion of CD4 T cells also resulted in a loss of protection in mice immunized with sporozoites, suggesting that CD4 T cells might provide signals for efficient maturation of effector CD8 T cells (247). In mice, CD4 T cells were essential to ensure survival of protective effector and memory CD8 T cell induced by irradiated sporozoites (205, 206). In humans, many studies have described a CSP-specific CD4 T cell response that is associated with protection against natural infection and disease (248), and is able to inhibit pre-erythrocytic stage development (249). CD4 T cells have also been shown to correlate with sterile protection in humans following immunization with live sporozoites under chloroquine prophylaxis. CSP-specific CD4 T cells were induced to express CD107a, a marker for cytotoxic degranulation, after immunizations with live sporozoites under chloroquine prophylaxis in humans, and these cytotoxic markers has been shown to be associated with sterile protection against the pre-erythrocytic stages (48). In addition to being crucial for B cell development to produce antibodies, CD4 T cells are also important for CD8 T cell responses.

While it is clear that CD4 T cells are involved in protective immunity against malaria, its use as a potential correlate of protection needs further validation. Together with CD8 T cells, the definitive role of CD4 T cells in protection requires more unraveling and the information will be critical to the development of a validated T cell-based correlate of protection for vaccine efficacy assessment.

Antibodies

Lastly, in addition to inducing an effective CD8 T cell response, the development of many malaria candidate vaccines also aims at being able to induce an effective antibody response. Antibodies are often the first host immune response being studied. Antibodies against the pre-erythrocytic stage can mediate protection by limiting pre-erythrocytic stage infection and development. More specifically, the antibodies do so by (1) inhibiting sporozoite motility in the dermis and liver (207), (2) mediating cytotoxicity against sporozoites in the host skin (208, 250), (3) opsonizing the sporozoites and subsequently facilitating sporozoite phagocytosis by monocytes or macrophages in the spleen or the liver (208, 209), (4) inhibiting sporozoite invasion into hepatocytes (210), (5) inhibiting sporozoite development inside the hepatocytes (210), and (6) binding to parasite neo-antigens such as heat shock protein expressed at the surface of infected hepatocytes and eventually inducing liver parasite killing through an antibody-dependent cell-mediated mechanism that is likely to involve Kupffer cells or NK cells (211).

Antibodies are potential correlates of protection. Passive transfer of RTS,S-induced human anti-CSP monoclonal antibodies into humanized mice at concentrations within the range observed in human, protected the mice against *P. falciparum* challenge (170). Immunization with genetically-attenuated sporozoites that arrest late in the liver stage development elicited protection against both a sporozoite challenge and a direct blood stage challenge by inducing the production of stage-transcending protective antibodies in mice (251). Sporozoite-specific antibodies induced by vaccination with irradiated sporozoites (252) or genetically-attenuated sporozoites (253) have also been shown to inhibit sporozoite invasion into human hepatocytes *in vitro* and correlate with protection in human individuals (254–256). However, a recent human study examining protection following vaccination with irradiated sporozoites in malaria-naïve individuals has found no significant correlation of antibody response with protection (46). In addition, there is no distinct antibody profile that allows differentiation of protected individuals from the susceptible individuals (257) following RTS,S vaccination. There is increasing awareness that, in addition of high level of antibodies, the quality of the antibodies is also important. *In vitro* assays to examine the functionality of the induced antibodies following vaccination of pre-erythrocytic stage vaccine have been developed. These assays include gliding motility assays (258), sporozoite traversal and invasion inhibition assays (6, 253, 259), and pre-erythrocytic stage development inhibition assays (136, 260). Recently, human monoclonal antibodies have been derived from volunteers immunized with irradiated sporozoites. These antibodies recognized an important epitope at the junction of the N terminal part and the repeat regions of the CSP. This can lead to the design of better CSP-based vaccines (146, 261). Further studies to draw parallels between the readouts of these assays and the protection in the field are necessary to develop a validated antibody-based correlate of protection for vaccine efficacy assessment.

CONCLUDING REMARKS

In contrast to the limited efficacy of RTS,S and other subunit vaccines, vaccination with sporozoites has had more success. In addition to promising efficacy data, a series of recent clinical trials on sporozoite-based vaccines has demonstrated formidable advances in overcoming issues in vaccine manufacturing and delivery (6, 14, 23, 46). Furthermore, there are now data showing that sporozoite vaccines are safe and tolerated in malaria-endemic areas (14, 23). While the vaccine efficacy is markedly reduced against heterologous CHMI (as compared with homologous CHMI), it is encouraging that it offers some protection against heterologous CHMI (25). Further studies to optimize the immunization regimen could potentially improve the vaccine efficacy. Here, we reviewed the various types of vaccination strategies with sporozoites and the different animal models being used for the vaccination studies. We also discussed the mechanisms of protection against the pre-erythrocytic parasites. While the mechanisms of protection are slowly being unraveled, the establishment of validated correlates of protection for assessment of vaccine efficacy has proved to be challenging. Half of the world population is at risk of a malaria infection. The target population is highly diverse, with individuals from different age groups (infants, adults and elderly), different exposed status (endemic and non-endemic), and different immunological background (immunocompromised and pregnant). The presence of co-infections in some populations in malaria-endemic regions adds further complexity. In addition, the complexity of the parasite and the diversity of its genome also makes it difficult to definitively establish correlates of protection. Depending on which part of the parasite life cycle the malaria vaccine candidates target, different forms of immunity are induced. As it is still unclear if the ultimate goal of a malaria vaccine should be to protect against infection or simply to protect against disease, different clinical endpoints have been used to measure vaccine efficacy. Vaccine-induced immune responses that correlate with protection against one endpoint may not necessarily correlate with protection against a different endpoint. Hence, until date, there is no validated correlate of protection. A concerted effort to develop/refine relevant animal models, investigate the definitive mechanisms of protection and identify validated correlates of protection would greatly help to inform critical decisions in human vaccine clinical trial, which will accelerate future progress in the development of an efficacious malaria vaccine.

AUTHOR CONTRIBUTIONS

All authors listed have made a substantial, direct and intellectual contribution to the work, and approved it for publication.

FUNDING

This work was supported by the Agency for Science Technology and Research (A*STAR).

REFERENCES

1. WHO. *Malaria Fact Sheet. [online]*. Available online at: http://www.who.int/mediacentre/factsheets/fs094/en/ (accessed January, 2019) (Online) (2018).
2. Bhatt S, Weiss DJ, Cameron E, Bisanzio D, Mappin B, Dalrymple U, et al. The effect of malaria control on *Plasmodium falciparum* in Africa between 2000 and 2015. *Nature.* (2015) 526:207–11. doi: 10.1038/nature15535
3. Hemingway J, Ranson H, Magill A, Kolaczinski J, Fornadel C, Gimnig J, et al. Averting a malaria disaster: will insecticide resistance derail malaria control? *Lancet.* (2016) 387:1785–8. doi: 10.1016/S0140-6736(15)00417-1
4. Wiebe A, Longbottom J, Gleave K, Shearer FM, Sinka ME, Massey NC, et al. Geographical distributions of African malaria vector sibling species and evidence for insecticide resistance. *Malar J.* (2017) 16:85. doi: 10.1186/s12936-017-1734-y
5. Healer J, Cowman AF, Kaslow DC, Birkett AJ. Vaccines to accelerate malaria elimination and eventual eradication. *Cold Spring Harb Perspect Med.* (2017) 7:a025627. doi: 10.1101/cshperspect.a025627
6. Seder RA, Chang LJ, Enama ME, Zephir KL, Sarwar UN, Gordon IJ, et al. Protection against malaria by intravenous immunization with a nonreplicating sporozoite vaccine. *Science.* (2013) 341:1359–65. doi: 10.1126/science.1241800
7. Jongo SA, Shekalaghe SA, Church LWP, Ruben AJ, Schindler T, Zenklusen I, et al. Safety, immunogenicity, and protective efficacy against controlled human malaria infection of *Plasmodium falciparum* sporozoite

vaccine in Tanzanian adults. *Am J Trop Med Hyg.* (2018) 99:338–49. doi: 10.4269/ajtmh.17-1014
8. Sergent E, Sergent E. Sur l'immunite sdans le paludismedes oiseaux. Conservation *in vitro* des sporozoites de plasmodium de *Plasmodium relictum* immmunite relative obtenue par inoculations de ces sporozoites. *C R Acad Sci.* (1910) 151:407–9.
9. Russell PF, Mohan BN. The immunization of fowls against mosquito-borne *Plasmodium gallinaceum* by injections of serum and of inactivated homologous sporozoites. *J Exp Med.* (1942) 76:477–95. doi: 10.1084/jem.76.5.477
10. Freund J, Sommer HE, Walter AW. Immunization against malaria: vaccination of ducks with killed parasites incorporated with adjuvants. *Science.* (1945) 102:200–2. doi: 10.1126/science.102.2643.200
11. Freund J, Thomson KJ, Sommer HE, Walter AW, Schenkein EL. Immunization of rhesus monkeys against malarial infection (*P. Knowlesi*) with killed parasites and adjuvants. *Science.* (1945) 102:202–4. doi: 10.1126/science.102.2643.202
12. Heidelberger M, Mayer MM, Demarest CR. Studies in human malaria; the preparation of vaccines and suspensions containing plasmodia. *J Immunol.* (1946) 52:325–30.
13. Rosenberg R. Ejection of malaria sporozoites by feeding mosquitoes. *Trans R Soc Trop Med Hyg.* (1992) 86:109. doi: 10.1016/0035-9203(92)90466-P
14. Sissoko MS, Healy SA, Katile A, Omaswa F, Zaidi I, Gabriel EE, et al. Safety and efficacy of PfSPZ vaccine against *Plasmodium falciparum* via direct venous inoculation in healthy malaria-exposed adults in Mali: a randomised, double-blind phase 1 trial. *Lancet Infect Dis.* (2017) 17:498–509. doi: 10.1016/S1473-3099(17)30104-4
15. Spring M, Murphy J, Nielsen R, Dowler M, Bennett JW, Zarling S, et al. First-in-human evaluation of genetically attenuated *Plasmodium falciparum* sporozoites administered by bite of anopheles mosquitoes to adult volunteers. *Vaccine.* (2013) 31:4975–83. doi: 10.1016/j.vaccine.2013.08.007
16. Kublin JG, Mikolajczak SA, Sack BK, Fishbaugher ME, Seilie A, Shelton L, et al. Complete attenuation of genetically engineered *Plasmodium falciparum* sporozoites in human subjects. *Sci Transl Med.* (2017) 9:eaad9099. doi: 10.1126/scitranslmed.aad9099
17. Richie TL, Billingsley PF, Sim BK, James ER, Chakravarty S, Epstein JE, et al. Progress with *Plasmodium falciparum* sporozoite (PfSPZ)-based malaria vaccines. *Vaccine.* (2015) 33:7452–61. doi: 10.1016/j.vaccine.2015.09.096
18. Richards WH. Active immunization of chicks against *Plasmodium gallinaceum* by inactivated homologous sporozoites and erythrocytic parasites. *Nature.* (1966) 212:1492–4. doi: 10.1038/2121492a0
19. Nussenzweig RS, Vanderberg J, Most H, Orton C. Protective immunity produced by the injection of x-irradiated sporozoites of *Plasmodium berghei. Nature.* (1967) 216:160–2. doi: 10.1038/216160a0
20. Clyde DF, Mccarthy VC, Miller RM, Hornick RB. Specificity of protection of man immunized against sporozoite-induced *Falciparum malaria. Am J Med Sci.* (1973) 266:398–403. doi: 10.1097/00000441-197312000-00001
21. Rieckmann KH, Carson PE, Beaudoin RL, Cassells JS, Sell KW. Letter: sporozoite induced immunity in man against an Ethiopian strain of *Plasmodium falciparum. Trans R Soc Trop Med Hyg.* (1974) 68:258–9. doi: 10.1016/0035-9203(74)90129-1
22. Hoffman SL, Goh LM, Luke TC, Schneider I, Le TP, Doolan DL, et al. Protection of humans against malaria by immunization with radiation-attenuated *Plasmodium falciparum* sporozoites. *J Infect Dis.* (2002) 185:1155–64. doi: 10.1086/339409
23. Hickey BW, Lumsden JM, Reyes S, Sedegah M, Hollingdale MR, Freilich DA, et al. Mosquito bite immunization with radiation-attenuated *Plasmodium falciparum* sporozoites: safety, tolerability, protective efficacy and humoral immunogenicity. *Malar J.* (2016) 15:377. doi: 10.1186/s12936-016-1 435-y
24. Ishizuka AS, Lyke KE, Dezure A, Berry AA, Richie TL, Mendoza FH, et al. Protection against malaria at 1 year and immune correlates following PfSPZ vaccination. *Nat Med.* (2016) 22:614–23. doi: 10.1038/nm.4110
25. Epstein JE, Paolino KM, Richie TL, Sedegah M, Singer A, Ruben AJ, et al. Protection against *Plasmodium falciparum* malaria by PfSPZ vaccine. *JCI Insight.* (2017) 2:e89154. doi: 10.1172/jci.insight.89154
26. Renia L, Goh YS. Malaria parasites: the great escape. *Front Immunol.* (2016) 7:463. doi: 10.3389/fimmu.2016.00463
27. Vanderberg JP, Nussenzweig RS, Most H, Orton CG. Protective immunity produced by the injection of x-irradiated sporozoites of *Plasmodium berghei.* II Effects of radiation on sporozoites. *J Parasitol.* (1968) 54:1175–80. doi: 10.2307/3276987
28. Spitalny GL, Nussenzweig RS. Effect of various routes of immunization and methods of parasite attenuation on development of protection against sporozoite-induced rodent malaria. *Proc Helminthol Soc Wash.* (1972) 39:506–14.
29. Nussler A, Follezou JY, Miltgen F, Mazier D. Effect of irradiation on Plasmodium sporozoites depends on the species of hepatocyte infected. *Trop Med Parasitol.* (1989) 40:468–9.
30. Mellouk S, Lunel F, Sedegah M, Beaudoin RL, Druilhe P. Protection against malaria induced by irradiated sporozoites. *Lancet.* (1990) 335:721. doi: 10.1016/0140-6736(90)90832-P
31. Hoffman BU, Chattopadhyay R. *Plasmodium falciparum*: effect of radiation on levels of gene transcripts in sporozoites. *Exp Parasitol.* (2008) 118:247–52. doi: 10.1016/j.exppara.2007.08.014
32. Oakley MS, Verma N, Zheng H, Anantharaman V, Takeda K, Gao Y, et al. Molecular markers of radiation induced attenuation in intrahepatic *Plasmodium falciparum* parasites. *PLoS ONE.* (2016) 11:e0166814. doi: 10.1371/journal.pone.0166814
33. Suhrbier A, Winger LA, Castellano E, Sinden RE. Survival and antigenic profile of irradiated malarial sporozoites in infected liver cells. *Infect Immun.* (1990) 58:2834–9.
34. Silvie O, Semblat JP, Franetich JF, Hannoun L, Eling W, Mazier D. Effects of irradiation on *Plasmodium falciparum* sporozoite hepatic development: implications for the design of pre-erythrocytic malaria vaccines. *Parasite Immunol.* (2002) 24:221–3. doi: 10.1046/j.1365-3024.2002.00450.x
35. Renia L, Gruner AC, Mauduit M, Snounou G. Vaccination against malaria with live parasites. *Expert Rev Vaccines.* (2006) 5:473–81. doi: 10.1586/14760584.5.4.473
36. Vaughan AM, Wang R, Kappe SH. Genetically engineered, attenuated whole-cell vaccine approaches for malaria. *Hum Vaccin.* (2010) 6:107–13. doi: 10.4161/hv.6.1.9654
37. Mueller AK, Camargo N, Kaiser K, Andorfer C, Frevert U, Matuschewski K, et al. Plasmodium liver stage developmental arrest by depletion of a protein at the parasite-host interface. *Proc Natl Acad Sci USA.* (2005) 102:3022–7. doi: 10.1073/pnas.0408442102
38. Mueller AK, Labaied M, Kappe SH, Matuschewski K. Genetically modified Plasmodium parasites as a protective experimental malaria vaccine. *Nature.* (2005) 433:164–7. doi: 10.1038/nature03188
39. van Dijk MR, Douradinha B, Franke-Fayard B, Heussler V, Van Dooren MW, Van Schaijk B, et al. Genetically attenuated, P36p-deficient malarial sporozoites induce protective immunity and apoptosis of infected liver cells. *Proc Natl Acad Sci USA.* (2005) 102:12194–9. doi: 10.1073/pnas.0500925102
40. Butler NS, Schmidt NW, Vaughan AM, Aly AS, Kappe SH, Harty JT. Superior antimalarial immunity after vaccination with late liver stage-arresting genetically attenuated parasites. *Cell Host Microbe.* (2011) 9:451–62. doi: 10.1016/j.chom.2011.05.008
41. Vaughan AM, Sack BK, Dankwa D, Minkah N, Nguyen T, Cardamone H, et al. A plasmodium parasite with complete late liver stage arrest protects against preerythrocytic and erythrocytic stage infection in mice. *Infect Immun.* (2018) 86:e00088-18. doi: 10.1128/IAI.00088-18
42. Beaudoin RL, Strome CP, Mitchell F, Tubergen TA. *Plasmodium berghei*: immunization of mice against the ANKA strain using the unaltered sporozoite as an antigen. *Exp Parasitol.* (1977) 42:1–5. doi: 10.1016/0014-4894(77)90054-6
43. Orjih AU, Cochrane AH, Nussenzweig RS. Comparative studies on the immunogenicity of infective and attenuated sporozoites of *Plasmodium berghei. Trans R Soc Trop Med Hyg.* (1982) 76:57–61. doi: 10.1016/0035-9203(82)90019-0
44. Belnoue E, Costa FT, Frankenberg T, Vigario AM, Voza T, Leroy N, et al. Protective T cell immunity against malaria liver stage after vaccination with live sporozoites under chloroquine treatment. *J Immunol.* (2004) 172:2487–95. doi: 10.4049/jimmunol.172.4.2487
45. Roestenberg M, Mccall M, Hopman J, Wiersma J, Luty AJ, Van Gemert GJ, et al. Protection against a malaria challenge by sporozoite inoculation. *N Engl J Med.* (2009) 361:468–77. doi: 10.1056/NEJMoa0805832

46. Mordmuller B, Surat G, Lagler H, Chakravarty S, Ishizuka AS, Lalremruata A, et al. Sterile protection against human malaria by chemoattenuated PfSPZ vaccine. *Nature.* (2017) 542:445–9. doi: 10.1038/nature21060
47. Friesen J, Silvie O, Putrianti ED, Hafalla JC, Matuschewski K, Borrmann S. Natural immunization against malaria: causal prophylaxis with antibiotics. *Sci Transl Med.* (2010) 2:40ra49. doi: 10.1126/scitranslmed.3001058
48. Bijker EM, Teirlinck AC, Schats R, Van Gemert GJ, Van De Vegte-Bolmer M, Van Lieshout L, et al. Cytotoxic markers associate with protection against malaria in human volunteers immunized with *Plasmodium falciparum* sporozoites. *J Infect Dis.* (2014) 210:1605–15. doi: 10.1093/infdis/jiu293
49. Peng X, Keitany GJ, Vignali M, Chen L, Gibson C, Choi K, et al. Artesunate versus chloroquine infection-treatment-vaccination defines stage-specific immune responses associated with prolonged sterile protection against both pre-erythrocytic and erythrocytic *Plasmodium yoelii* infection. *J Immunol.* (2014) 193:1268–77. doi: 10.4049/jimmunol.1400296
50. Schats R, Bijker EM, Van Gemert GJ, Graumans W, Van De Vegte-Bolmer M, Van Lieshout L, et al. Heterologous protection against malaria after immunization with *Plasmodium falciparum* sporozoites. *PLoS ONE.* (2015) 10:e0124243. doi: 10.1371/journal.pone.0124243
51. Lyke KE, Ishizuka AS, Berry AA, Chakravarty S, Dezure A, Enama ME, et al. Attenuated PfSPZ vaccine induces strain-transcending T cells and durable protection against heterologous controlled human malaria infection. *Proc Natl Acad Sci USA.* (2017) 114:2711–6. doi: 10.1073/pnas.1615324114
52. Yoshida N, Nussenzweig RS, Potocnjak P, Nussenzweig V, Aikawa M. Hybridoma produces protective antibodies directed against the sporozoite stage of malaria parasite. *Science.* (1980) 207:71–3. doi: 10.1126/science.6985745
53. Dame JB, Williams JL, Mccutchan TF, Weber JL, Wirtz RA, Hockmeyer WT, et al. Structure of the gene encoding the immunodominant surface antigen on the sporozoite of the human malaria parasite *Plasmodium falciparum. Science.* (1984) 225:593–9. doi: 10.1126/science.6204383
54. Enea V, Ellis J, Zavala F, Arnot DE, Asavanich A, Masuda A, et al. DNA cloning of *Plasmodium falciparum* circumsporozoite gene: amino acid sequence of repetitive epitope. *Science.* (1984) 225:628–30. doi: 10.1126/science.6204384
55. Egan JE, Weber JL, Ballou WR, Hollingdale MR, Majarian WR, Gordon DM, et al. Efficacy of murine malaria sporozoite vaccines: implications for human vaccine development. *Science.* (1987) 236:453–6. doi: 10.1126/science.3551073
56. Zavala F, Tam JP, Barr PJ, Romero PJ, Ley V, Nussenzweig RS, et al. Synthetic peptide vaccine confers protection against murine malaria. *J Exp Med.* (1987) 166:1591–6. doi: 10.1084/jem.166.5.1591
57. Tam JP, Clavijo P, Lu YA, Nussenzweig V, Nussenzweig R, Zavala F. Incorporation of T and B epitopes of the circumsporozoite protein in a chemically defined synthetic vaccine against malaria. *J Exp Med.* (1990) 171:299–306. doi: 10.1084/jem.171.1.299
58. Marussig M, Renia L, Motard A, Miltgen F, Petour P, Chauhan V, et al. Linear and multiple antigen peptides containing defined T and B epitopes of the Plasmodium yoelii circumsporozoite protein: antibody-mediated protection and boosting by sporozoite infection. *Int Immunol.* (1997) 9:1817–24. doi: 10.1093/intimm/9.12.1817
59. Herrington DA, Clyde DF, Losonsky G, Cortesia M, Murphy JR, Davis J, et al. Safety and immunogenicity in man of a synthetic peptide malaria vaccine against *Plasmodium falciparum* sporozoites. *Nature.* (1987) 328:257–9. doi: 10.1038/328257a0
60. Good MF, Berzofsky JA, Maloy WL, Hayashi Y, Fujii N, Hockmeyer WT, et al. Genetic control of the immune response in mice to a *Plasmodium falciparum* sporozoite vaccine. Widespread nonresponsiveness to single malaria T epitope in highly repetitive vaccine. *J Exp Med.* (1986) 164:655–60. doi: 10.1084/jem.164.2.655
61. Sinigaglia F, Guttinger M, Kilgus J, Doran DM, Matile H, Etlinger H, et al. A malaria T-cell epitope recognized in association with most mouse and human MHC class II molecules. *Nature.* (1988) 336:778–80. doi: 10.1038/336778a0
62. Schodel F, Wirtz R, Peterson D, Hughes J, Warren R, Sadoff J, et al. Immunity to malaria elicited by hybrid hepatitis B virus core particles carrying circumsporozoite protein epitopes. *J Exp Med.* (1994) 180:1037–46. doi: 10.1084/jem.180.3.1037
63. Kubler-Kielb J, Majadly F, Biesova Z, Mocca CP, Guo C, Nussenzweig R, et al. A bicomponent *Plasmodium falciparum* investigational vaccine composed of protein-peptide conjugates. *Proc Natl Acad Sci USA.* (2010) 107:1172–7. doi: 10.1073/pnas.0913374107
64. Powell TJ, Tang J, Derome ME, Mitchell RA, Jacobs A, Deng Y, et al. *Plasmodium falciparum* synthetic LbL microparticle vaccine elicits protective neutralizing antibody and parasite-specific cellular immune responses. *Vaccine.* (2013) 31:1898–904. doi: 10.1016/j.vaccine.2013.02.027
65. Collins KA, Snaith R, Cottingham MG, Gilbert SC, Hill AVS. Enhancing protective immunity to malaria with a highly immunogenic virus-like particle vaccine. *Sci Rep.* (2017) 7:46621. doi: 10.1038/srep46621
66. Espinosa DA, Christensen D, Munoz C, Singh S, Locke E, Andersen P, et al. Robust antibody and CD8(+) T-cell responses induced by *P. falciparum* CSP adsorbed to cationic liposomal adjuvant CAF09 confer sterilizing immunity against experimental rodent malaria infection. *NPJ Vaccines.* (2017) 2:10. doi: 10.1038/s41541-017-0011-y
67. Kaba SA, Karch CP, Seth L, Ferlez KMB, Storme CK, Pesavento DM, et al. Self-assembling protein nanoparticles with built-in flagellin domains increases protective efficacy of a Plasmodium falciparum based vaccine. *Vaccine.* (2018) 36:906–14. doi: 10.1016/j.vaccine.2017.12.001
68. Cohen J, Nussenzweig V, Nussenzweig R, Vekemans J, Leach A. From the circumsporozoite protein to the RTS, S/AS candidate vaccine. *Hum Vaccin.* (2010) 6:90–6. doi: 10.4161/hv.6.1.9677
69. Gordon DM, Mcgovern TW, Krzych U, Cohen JC, Schneider I, Lachance R, et al. Safety, immunogenicity, and efficacy of a recombinantly produced *Plasmodium falciparum* circumsporozoite protein-hepatitis B surface antigen subunit vaccine. *J Infect Dis.* (1995) 171:1576–85. doi: 10.1093/infdis/171.6.1576
70. Stoute JA, Slaoui M, Heppner DG, Momin P, Kester KE, Desmons P, et al. A preliminary evaluation of a recombinant circumsporozoite protein vaccine against *Plasmodium falciparum* malaria. RTS,S malaria vaccine evaluation group. *N Engl J Med.* (1997) 336:86–91. doi: 10.1056/NEJM199701093360202
71. Kester KE, Mckinney DA, Tornieporth N, Ockenhouse CF, Heppner DG, Hall T, et al. Efficacy of recombinant circumsporozoite protein vaccine regimens against experimental *Plasmodium falciparum* malaria. *J Infect Dis.* (2001) 183:640–7. doi: 10.1086/318534
72. Garcon N, Chomez P, Van Mechelen M. GlaxoSmithKline adjuvant systems in vaccines: concepts, achievements and perspectives. *Expert Rev Vaccines.* (2007) 6:723–39. doi: 10.1586/14760584.6.5.723
73. Kester KE, Cummings JF, Ofori-Anyinam O, Ockenhouse CF, Krzych U, Moris P, et al. Randomized, double-blind, phase 2a trial of falciparum malaria vaccines RTS,S/AS01B and RTS,S/AS02A in malaria-naive adults: safety, efficacy, and immunologic associates of protection. *J Infect Dis.* (2009) 200:337–46. doi: 10.1086/600120
74. Heppner DG Jr, Walsh DS, Uthaimongkol N, Tang DB, Tulyayon S, Permpanich B, et al. Randomized, controlled, double-blind trial of daily oral azithromycin in adults for the prophylaxis of *Plasmodium vivax* malaria in Western Thailand. *Am J Trop Med Hyg.* (2005) 73:842–9. doi: 10.4269/ajtmh.2005.73.842
75. Bojang KA, Milligan PJ, Pinder M, Vigneron L, Alloueche A, Kester KE, et al. Efficacy of RTS,S/AS02 malaria vaccine against *Plasmodium falciparum* infection in semi-immune adult men in the Gambia: a randomised trial. *Lancet.* (2001) 358:1927–34. doi: 10.1016/S0140-6736(01)06957-4
76. Alonso PL, Sacarlal J, Aponte JJ, Leach A, Macete E, Milman J, et al. Efficacy of the RTS,S/AS02A vaccine against *Plasmodium falciparum* infection and disease in young African children: randomised controlled trial. *Lancet.* (2004) 364:1411–20. doi: 10.1016/S0140-6736(04)17223-1
77. Olotu A, Moris P, Mwacharo J, Vekemans J, Kimani D, Janssens M, et al. Circumsporozoite-specific T cell responses in children vaccinated with RTS,S/AS01E and protection against P falciparum clinical malaria. *PLoS ONE.* (2011) 6:e25786. doi: 10.1371/journal.pone.0025786
78. Rts SCTP, Agnandji ST, Lell B, Fernandes JF, Abossolo BP, Methogo BG, et al. A phase 3 trial of RTS,S/AS01 malaria vaccine in African infants. *N Engl J Med.* (2012) 367:2284–95. doi: 10.1056/NEJMoa1208394
79. Kaslow DC, Biernaux S. RTS,S: toward a first landmark on the malaria vaccine technology roadmap. *Vaccine.* (2015) 33:7425–32. doi: 10.1016/j.vaccine.2015.09.061

80. Neafsey DE, Juraska M, Bedford T, Benkeser D, Valim C, Griggs A, et al. Genetic diversity and protective efficacy of the RTS,S/AS01 malaria vaccine. *N Engl J Med.* (2015) 373:2025–37. doi: 10.1056/NEJMoa1505819
81. Rts SCTP. Efficacy and safety of RTS,S/AS01 malaria vaccine with or without a booster dose in infants and children in Africa: final results of a phase 3, individually randomised, controlled trial. *Lancet.* (2015) 386:31–45. doi: 10.1016/S0140-6736(15)60721-8
82. Kumar KA, Sano G, Boscardin S, Nussenzweig RS, Nussenzweig MC, Zavala F, et al. The circumsporozoite protein is an immunodominant protective antigen in irradiated sporozoites. *Nature.* (2006) 444:937–40. doi: 10.1038/nature05361
83. Gruner AC, Mauduit M, Tewari R, Romero JF, Depinay N, Kayibanda M, et al. Sterile protection against malaria is independent of immune responses to the circumsporozoite protein. *PLoS ONE.* (2007) 2:e1371. doi: 10.1371/journal.pone.0001371
84. Mauduit M, Gruner AC, Tewari R, Depinay N, Kayibanda M, Chavatte JM, et al. A role for immune responses against non-CS components in the cross-species protection induced by immunization with irradiated malaria sporozoites. *PLoS ONE.* (2009) 4:e7717. doi: 10.1371/journal.pone.0007717
85. Mauduit M, Tewari R, Depinay N, Kayibanda M, Lallemand E, Chavatte JM, et al. Minimal role for the circumsporozoite protein in the induction of sterile immunity by vaccination with live rodent malaria sporozoites. *Infect Immun.* (2010) 78:2182–8. doi: 10.1128/IAI.01415-09
86. Tarun AS, Peng X, Dumpit RF, Ogata Y, Silva-Rivera H, Camargo N, et al. A combined transcriptome and proteome survey of malaria parasite liver stages. *Proc Natl Acad Sci USA.* (2008) 105:305–10. doi: 10.1073/pnas.0710780104
87. Trieu A, Kayala MA, Burk C, Molina DM, Freilich DA, Richie TL, et al. Sterile protective immunity to malaria is associated with a panel of novel *P. falciparum* antigens. *Mol Cell Proteomics.* (2011) 10:M111.007948. doi: 10.1074/mcp.M111.007948
88. Duffy PE, Sahu T, Akue A, Milman N, Anderson C. Pre-erythrocytic malaria vaccines: identifying the targets. *Expert Rev Vaccines.* (2012) 11:1261–80. doi: 10.1586/erv.12.92
89. Peng K, Goh YS, Siau A, Franetich JF, Chia WN, Ong AS, et al. Breadth of humoral response and antigenic targets of sporozoite-inhibitory antibodies associated with sterile protection induced by controlled human malaria infection. *Cell Microbiol.* (2016) 18:1739–50. doi: 10.1111/cmi.12608
90. Schussek S, Trieu A, Apte SH, Sidney J, Sette A, Doolan DL. Novel *Plasmodium antigens* identified via genome-based antibody screen induce protection associated with polyfunctional T cell responses. *Sci Rep.* (2017) 7:15053. doi: 10.1038/s41598-017-15354-0
91. Wang R, Charoenvit Y, Corradin G, De La Vega P, Franke ED, Hoffman SL. Protection against malaria by *Plasmodium yoelii* sporozoite surface protein 2 linear peptide induction of CD4+ T cell- and IFN-gamma-dependent elimination of infected hepatocytes. *J Immunol.* (1996) 157:4061–7.
92. Daubersies P, Thomas AW, Millet P, Brahimi K, Langermans JA, Ollomo B, et al. Protection against *Plasmodium falciparum* malaria in chimpanzees by immunization with the conserved pre-erythrocytic liver-stage antigen 3. *Nat Med.* (2000) 6:1258–63. doi: 10.1038/81366
93. Speake C, Pichugin A, Sahu T, Malkov V, Morrison R, Pei Y, et al. Identification of novel pre-erythrocytic malaria antigen candidates for combination vaccines with circumsporozoite protein. *PLoS ONE.* (2016) 11:e0159449. doi: 10.1371/journal.pone.0159449
94. Bruder JT, Chen P, Ekberg G, Smith EC, Lazarski CA, Myers BA, et al. Profiling the targets of protective CD8(+) T cell responses to infection. *Mol Ther Methods Clin Dev.* (2017) 7:20–31. doi: 10.1016/j.omtm.2017.08.003
95. Cummings JF, Spring MD, Schwenk RJ, Ockenhouse CF, Kester KE, Polhemus ME, et al. Recombinant liver stage antigen-1 (LSA-1) formulated with AS01 or AS02 is safe, elicits high titer antibody and induces IFN-gamma/IL-2 CD4+ T cells but does not protect against experimental *Plasmodium falciparum* infection. *Vaccine.* (2010) 28:5135–44. doi: 10.1016/j.vaccine.2009.08.046
96. Ulmer JB, Donnelly JJ, Parker SE, Rhodes GH, Felgner PL, Dwarki VJ, et al. Heterologous protection against influenza by injection of DNA encoding a viral protein. *Science.* (1993) 259:1745–9. doi: 10.1126/science.8456302
97. Wang R, Doolan DL, Le TP, Hedstrom RC, Coonan KM, Charoenvit Y, et al. Induction of antigen-specific cytotoxic T lymphocytes in humans by a malaria DNA vaccine. *Science.* (1998) 282:476–80. doi: 10.1126/science.282.5388.476
98. Le TP, Coonan KM, Hedstrom RC, Charoenvit Y, Sedegah M, Epstein JE, et al. Safety, tolerability and humoral immune responses after intramuscular administration of a malaria DNA vaccine to healthy adult volunteers. *Vaccine.* (2000) 18:1893–901. doi: 10.1016/S0264-410X(99)00407-7
99. Wang R, Epstein J, Baraceros FM, Gorak EJ, Charoenvit Y, Carucci DJ, et al. Induction of CD4(+) T cell-dependent CD8(+) type 1 responses in humans by a malaria DNA vaccine. *Proc Natl Acad Sci USA.* (2001) 98:10817–22. doi: 10.1073/pnas.181123498
100. Hedstrom RC, Sedegah M, Hoffman SL. Prospects and strategies for development of DNA vaccines against malaria. *Res Immunol.* (1994) 145:476–83. doi: 10.1016/S0923-2494(94)80179-7
101. Vuola JM, Keating S, Webster DP, Berthoud T, Dunachie S, Gilbert SC, et al. Differential immunogenicity of various heterologous prime-boost vaccine regimens using DNA and viral vectors in healthy volunteers. *J Immunol.* (2005) 174:449–55. doi: 10.4049/jimmunol.174.1.449
102. Wang R, Doolan DL, Charoenvit Y, Hedstrom RC, Gardner MJ, Hobart P, et al. Simultaneous induction of multiple antigen-specific cytotoxic T lymphocytes in nonhuman primates by immunization with a mixture of four *Plasmodium falciparum* DNA plasmids. *Infect Immun.* (1998) 66:4193–202.
103. Haddad D, Bilcikova E, Witney AA, Carlton JM, White CE, Blair PL, et al. Novel antigen identification method for discovery of protective malaria antigens by rapid testing of DNA vaccines encoding exons from the parasite genome. *Infect Immun.* (2004) 72:1594–602. doi: 10.1128/IAI.72.3.1594-1602.2004
104. McConkey SJ, Reece WH, Moorthy VS, Webster D, Dunachie S, Butcher G, et al. Enhanced T-cell immunogenicity of plasmid DNA vaccines boosted by recombinant modified vaccinia virus Ankara in humans. *Nat Med.* (2003) 9:729–35. doi: 10.1038/nm881
105. Richie TL, Charoenvit Y, Wang R, Epstein JE, Hedstrom RC, Kumar S, et al. Clinical trial in healthy malaria-naive adults to evaluate the safety, tolerability, immunogenicity and efficacy of MuStDO5, a five-gene, sporozoite/hepatic stage *Plasmodium falciparum* DNA vaccine combined with escalating dose human GM-CSF DNA. *Hum Vaccin Immunother.* (2012) 8:1564–84. doi: 10.4161/hv.22129
106. Weiss WR, Ishii KJ, Hedstrom RC, Sedegah M, Ichino M, Barnhart K, et al. A plasmid encoding murine granulocyte-macrophage colony-stimulating factor increases protection conferred by a malaria DNA vaccine. *J Immunol.* (1998) 161:2325–32.
107. Iwasaki A, Medzhitov R. Control of adaptive immunity by the innate immune system. *Nat Immunol.* (2015) 16:343–53. doi: 10.1038/ni.3123
108. Cabral-Miranda G, Heath MD, Gomes AC, Mohsen MO, Montoya-Diaz E, Salman AM, et al. Microcrystalline tyrosine (MCT®): a depot adjuvant in licensed allergy immunotherapy offers new opportunities in malaria. *Vaccines.* (2017) 5:E32. doi: 10.3390/vaccines5040032
109. Ewer KJ, Sierra-Davidson K, Salman AM, Illingworth JJ, Draper SJ, Biswas S, et al. Progress with viral vectored malaria vaccines: a multi-stage approach involving "unnatural immunity". *Vaccine.* (2015) 33:7444–51. doi: 10.1016/j.vaccine.2015.09.094
110. Rodrigues M, Li S, Murata K, Rodriguez D, Rodriguez JR, Bacik I, et al. Influenza and vaccinia viruses expressing malaria CD8+ T and B cell epitopes. Comparison of their immunogenicity and capacity to induce protective immunity. *J Immunol.* (1994) 153:4636–48.
111. Tine JA, Lanar DE, Smith DM, Wellde BT, Schultheiss P, Ware LA, et al. NYVAC-Pf7: a poxvirus-vectored, multiantigen, multistage vaccine candidate for *Plasmodium falciparum* malaria. *Infect Immun.* (1996) 64:3833–44.
112. Tsuji M, Bergmann CC, Takita-Sonoda Y, Murata K, Rodrigues EG, Nussenzweig RS, et al. Recombinant Sindbis viruses expressing a cytotoxic T-lymphocyte epitope of a malaria parasite or of influenza virus elicit protection against the corresponding pathogen in mice. *J Virol.* (1998) 72:6907–10.
113. Bonaldo MC, Garratt RC, Caufour PS, Freire MS, Rodrigues MM, Nussenzweig RS, et al. Surface expression of an immunodominant malaria protein B cell epitope by yellow fever virus. *J Mol Biol.* (2002) 315:873–85. doi: 10.1006/jmbi.2001.5258

114. Stoyanov CT, Boscardin SB, Deroubaix S, Barba-Spaeth G, Franco D, Nussenzweig RS, et al. Immunogenicity and protective efficacy of a recombinant yellow fever vaccine against the murine malarial parasite *Plasmodium yoelii*. *Vaccine.* (2010) 28:4644–52. doi: 10.1016/j.vaccine.2010.04.071
115. Hollingdale MR, Sedegah M, Limbach K. Development of replication-deficient adenovirus malaria vaccines. *Expert Rev Vaccines.* (2017) 16:261–71. doi: 10.1080/14760584.2016.1228454
116. Hansen SG, Womack J, Scholz I, Renner A, Edgel KA, Xu G, et al. Cytomegalovirus vectors expressing *Plasmodium knowlesi* antigens induce immune responses that delay parasitemia upon sporozoite challenge. *PLoS ONE.* (2019) 14:e0210252. doi: 10.1371/journal.pone.0210252
117. Sadoff JC, Ballou WR, Baron LS, Majarian WR, Brey RN, Hockmeyer WT, et al. Oral *Salmonella typhimurium* vaccine expressing circumsporozoite protein protects against malaria. *Science.* (1988) 240:336–8. doi: 10.1126/science.3281260
118. Aggarwal A, Kumar S, Jaffe R, Hone D, Gross M, Sadoff J. Oral *Salmonella: malaria* circumsporozoite recombinants induce specific CD8+ cytotoxic T cells. *J Exp Med.* (1990) 172:1083–90. doi: 10.1084/jem.172.4.1083
119. Arama C, Assefaw-Redda Y, Rodriguez A, Fernandez C, Corradin G, Kaufmann SH, et al. Heterologous prime-boost regimen adenovector 35-circumsporozoite protein vaccine/recombinant bacillus calmette-guerin expressing the *Plasmodium falciparum* circumsporozoite induces enhanced long-term memory immunity in BALB/c mice. *Vaccine.* (2012) 30:4040–5. doi: 10.1016/j.vaccine.2012.04.029
120. Bergmann-Leitner ES, Hosie H, Trichilo J, Deriso E, Ranallo RT, Alefantis T, et al. Self-adjuvanting bacterial vectors expressing pre-erythrocytic antigens induce sterile protection against malaria. *Front Immunol.* (2013) 4:176. doi: 10.3389/fimmu.2013.00176
121. Gonzalez C, Hone D, Noriega FR, Tacket CO, Davis JR, Losonsky G, et al. *Salmonella typhi* vaccine strain CVD 908 expressing the circumsporozoite protein of *Plasmodium falciparum*: strain construction and safety and immunogenicity in humans. *J Infect Dis.* (1994) 169:927–31. doi: 10.1093/infdis/169.4.927
122. Wang HH, Rogers WO, Kang YH, Sedegah M, Hoffman SL. Partial protection against malaria by immunization with *Leishmania enriettii* expressing the *Plasmodium yoelii* circumsporozoite protein. *Mol Biochem Parasitol.* (1995) 69:139–48. doi: 10.1016/0166-6851(94)00159-K
123. Di Cristina M, Ghouze F, Kocken CH, Naitza S, Cellini P, Soldati D, et al. Transformed *Toxoplasma gondii* tachyzoites expressing the circumsporozoite protein of *Plasmodium knowlesi* elicit a specific immune response in rhesus monkeys. *Infect Immun.* (1999) 67:1677–82.
124. Charest H, Sedegah M, Yap GS, Gazzinelli RT, Caspar P, Hoffman SL, et al. Recombinant attenuated *Toxoplasma gondii* expressing the *Plasmodium yoelii* circumsporozoite protein provides highly effective priming for CD8+ T cell-dependent protective immunity against malaria. *J Immunol.* (2000) 165:2084–92. doi: 10.4049/jimmunol.165.4.2084
125. Sedegah M, Jones TR, Kaur M, Hedstrom R, Hobart P, Tine JA, et al. Boosting with recombinant vaccinia increases immunogenicity and protective efficacy of malaria DNA vaccine. *Proc Natl Acad Sci USA.* (1998) 95:7648–53. doi: 10.1073/pnas.95.13.7648
126. Bruna-Romero O, Hafalla JC, Gonzalez-Aseguinolaza G, Sano G, Tsuji M, Zavala F. Detection of malaria liver-stages in mice infected through the bite of a single *Anopheles mosquito* using a highly sensitive real-time PCR. *Int J Parasitol.* (2001) 31:1499–502. doi: 10.1016/S0020-7519(01)00265-X
127. Hill AV, Reyes-Sandoval A, O'hara G, Ewer K, Lawrie A, Goodman A, et al. Prime-boost vectored malaria vaccines: progress and prospects. *Hum Vaccin.* (2010) 6:78–83. doi: 10.4161/hv.6.1.10116
128. Bliss CM, Bowyer G, Anagnostou NA, Havelock T, Snudden CM, Davies H, et al. Assessment of novel vaccination regimens using viral vectored liver stage malaria vaccines encoding ME-TRAP. *Sci Rep.* (2018) 8:3390. doi: 10.1038/s41598-018-21630-4
129. de Camargo TM, De Freitas EO, Gimenez AM, Lima LC, De Almeida Caramico K, Francoso KS, et al. Prime-boost vaccination with recombinant protein and adenovirus-vector expressing *Plasmodium vivax* circumsporozoite protein (CSP) partially protects mice against Pb/Pv sporozoite challenge. *Sci Rep.* (2018) 8:1118. doi: 10.1038/s41598-017-19063-6
130. Webster DP, Dunachie S, Vuola JM, Berthoud T, Keating S, Laidlaw SM, et al. Enhanced T cell-mediated protection against malaria in human challenges by using the recombinant poxviruses FP9 and modified vaccinia virus Ankara. *Proc Natl Acad Sci USA.* (2005) 102:4836–41. doi: 10.1073/pnas.0406381102
131. Hodgson SH, Juma E, Salim A, Magiri C, Njenga D, Molyneux S, et al. Lessons learnt from the first controlled human malaria infection study conducted in Nairobi, Kenya. *Malar J.* (2015) 14:182. doi: 10.1186/s12936-015-0671-x
132. Ogwang C, Kimani D, Edwards NJ, Roberts R, Mwacharo J, Bowyer G, et al. Prime-boost vaccination with chimpanzee adenovirus and modified vaccinia Ankara encoding TRAP provides partial protection against *Plasmodium falciparum* infection in Kenyan adults. *Sci Transl Med.* (2015) 7:286re285. doi: 10.1126/scitranslmed.aaa2373
133. Rampling T, Ewer KJ, Bowyer G, Bliss CM, Edwards NJ, Wright D, et al. Safety and high level efficacy of the combination malaria vaccine regimen of RTS,S/AS01B with chimpanzee adenovirus 63 and modified vaccinia ankara vectored vaccines expressing ME-TRAP. *J Infect Dis.* (2016) 214:772–81. doi: 10.1093/infdis/jiw244
134. Gola A, Silman D, Walters AA, Sridhar S, Uderhardt S, Salman AM, et al. Prime and target immunization protects against liver-stage malaria in mice. *Sci Transl Med.* (2018) 10:eaap9128. doi: 10.1126/scitranslmed.aap9128
135. Olsen TM, Stone BC, Chuenchob V, Murphy SC. Prime-and-trap malaria vaccination to generate protective CD8(+) liver-resident memory T cells. *J Immunol.* (2018) 201:1984–93. doi: 10.4049/jimmunol.1800740
136. Mazier D, Beaudoin RL, Mellouk S, Druilhe P, Texier B, Trosper J, et al. Complete development of hepatic stages of *Plasmodium falciparum in vitro*. *Science.* (1985) 227:440–2. doi: 10.1126/science.3880923
137. Purcell LA, Wong KA, Yanow SK, Lee M, Spithill TW, Rodriguez A. Chemically attenuated *Plasmodium sporozoites* induce specific immune responses, sterile immunity and cross-protection against heterologous challenge. *Vaccine.* (2008) 26:4880–4. doi: 10.1016/j.vaccine.2008.07.017
138. Purcell LA, Yanow SK, Lee M, Spithill TW, Rodriguez A. Chemical attenuation of Plasmodium berghei sporozoites induces sterile immunity in mice. *Infect Immun.* (2008) 76:1193–9. doi: 10.1128/IAI.01399-07
139. Raja AI, Stanisic DI, Good MF. Chemical attenuation in the development of a whole-organism malaria vaccine. *Infect Immun.* (2017) 85:e00062-17. doi: 10.1128/IAI.00062-17
140. Tewari R, Spaccapelo R, Bistoni F, Holder AA, Crisanti A. Function of region I and II adhesive motifs of *Plasmodium falciparum* circumsporozoite protein in sporozoite motility and infectivity. *J Biol Chem.* (2002) 277:47613–8. doi: 10.1074/jbc.M208453200
141. Espinosa DA, Yadava A, Angov E, Maurizio PL, Ockenhouse CF, Zavala F. Development of a chimeric *Plasmodium berghei* strain expressing the repeat region of the *P. vivax* circumsporozoite protein for *in vivo* evaluation of vaccine efficacy. *Infect Immun.* (2013) 81:2882–7. doi: 10.1128/IAI.00461-13
142. Kastenmuller K, Espinosa DA, Trager L, Stoyanov C, Salazar AM, Pokalwar S, et al. Full-length *Plasmodium falciparum* circumsporozoite protein administered with long-chain poly(I.C) or the Toll-like receptor 4 agonist glucopyranosyl lipid adjuvant-stable emulsion elicits potent antibody and CD4+ T cell immunity and protection in mice. *Infect Immun.* (2013) 81:789–800. doi: 10.1128/IAI.01108-12
143. Bauza K, Malinauskas T, Pfander C, Anar B, Jones EY, Billker O, et al. Efficacy of a *Plasmodium vivax* malaria vaccine using ChAd63 and modified vaccinia Ankara expressing thrombospondin-related anonymous protein as assessed with transgenic *Plasmodium berghei* parasites. *Infect Immun.* (2014) 82:1277–86. doi: 10.1128/IAI.01187-13
144. Deal C, Balazs AB, Espinosa DA, Zavala F, Baltimore D, Ketner G. Vectored antibody gene delivery protects against *Plasmodium falciparum* sporozoite challenge in mice. *Proc Natl Acad Sci USA.* (2014) 111:12528–32. doi: 10.1073/pnas.1407362111
145. Espinosa DA, Gutierrez GM, Rojas-Lopez M, Noe AR, Shi L, Tse SW, et al. Proteolytic cleavage of the *Plasmodium falciparum* circumsporozoite protein is a target of protective antibodies. *J Infect Dis.* (2015) 212:1111–9. doi: 10.1093/infdis/jiv154
146. Kisalu NK, Idris AH, Weidle C, Flores-Garcia Y, Flynn BJ, Sack BK, et al. A human monoclonal antibody prevents malaria infection by targeting a new site of vulnerability on the parasite. *Nat Med.* (2018) 24:408–16. doi: 10.1038/nm.4512

147. Carlton JM, Angiuoli SV, Suh BB, Kooij TW, Pertea M, Silva JC, et al. Genome sequence and comparative analysis of the model rodent malaria parasite *Plasmodium yoelii yoelii*. *Nature.* (2002) 419:512–9. doi: 10.1038/nature01099
148. Hall N, Karras M, Raine JD, Carlton JM, Kooij TW, Berriman M, et al. A comprehensive survey of the Plasmodium life cycle by genomic, transcriptomic, and proteomic analyses. *Science.* (2005) 307:82–6. doi: 10.1126/science.1103717
149. Vaughan AM, Mikolajczak SA, Wilson EM, Grompe M, Kaushansky A, Camargo N, et al. Complete *Plasmodium falciparum* liver-stage development in liver-chimeric mice. *J Clin Invest.* (2012) 122:3618–28. doi: 10.1172/JCI62684
150. Krotoski WA, Collins WE, Bray RS, Garnham PC, Cogswell FB, Gwadz RW, et al. Demonstration of hypnozoites in sporozoite-transmitted *Plasmodium vivax* infection. *Am J Trop Med Hyg.* (1982) 31:1291–3. doi: 10.4269/ajtmh.1982.31.1291
151. Landau I, Chabaud AG, Adam JP, Michel JC, Boulard Y. Morphologie et evolution des schizontes hépatiques secondaires dans le paludisme des rongeurs de la Maboké. *Cahiers de la Maboké.* (1968) 6:63–72.
152. Beura LK, Hamilton SE, Bi K, Schenkel JM, Odumade OA, Casey KA, et al. Normalizing the environment recapitulates adult human immune traits in laboratory mice. *Nature.* (2016) 532:512–6. doi: 10.1038/nature17655
153. Beignon AS, Le Grand R, Chapon C. *In vivo* imaging in NHP models of malaria: challenges, progress and outlooks. *Parasitol Int.* (2014) 63:206–15. doi: 10.1016/j.parint.2013.09.001
154. Herrera S, Perlaza BL, Bonelo A, Arevalo-Herrera M. Aotus monkeys: their great value for anti-malaria vaccines and drug testing. *Int J Parasitol.* (2002) 32:1625–35. doi: 10.1016/S0020-7519(02)00191-1
155. Collins WE, Sullivan JS, Williams A, Nace D, Williams T, Galland GG, et al. *Aotus nancymaae* as a potential model for the testing of anti-sporozoite and liver stage vaccines against *Plasmodium falciparum*. *Am J Trop Med Hyg.* (2006) 74:422–4. doi: 10.4269/ajtmh.2006.74.422
156. Joyner C, Barnwell JW, Galinski MR. No more monkeying around: primate malaria model systems are key to understanding *Plasmodium vivax* liver-stage biology, hypnozoites, and relapses. *Front Microbiol.* (2015) 6:145. doi: 10.3389/fmicb.2015.00145
157. Deans JA. Protective antigens of bloodstage *Plasmodium knowlesi* parasites. *Philos Trans R Soc Lond B Biol Sci.* (1984) 307:159–69. doi: 10.1098/rstb.1984.0116
158. Wijayalath WA, Cheesman S, Rajakaruna J, Handunnetti SM, Carter R, Pathirana PP. Evidence for strain-specific protective immunity against blood-stage parasites of *Plasmodium cynomolgi* in toque monkey. *Parasite Immunol.* (2008) 30:630–6. doi: 10.1111/j.1365-3024.2008.01065.x
159. Wijayalath W, Cheesman S, Tanabe K, Handunnetti S, Carter R, Pathirana S. Strain-specific protective effect of the immunity induced by live malarial sporozoites under chloroquine cover. *PLoS ONE.* (2012) 7:e45861. doi: 10.1371/journal.pone.0045861
160. Good MF, Hawkes MT, Yanow SK. Humanized mouse models to study cell-mediated immune responses to liver-stage malaria vaccines. *Trends Parasitol.* (2015) 31:583–94. doi: 10.1016/j.pt.2015.06.008
161. Minkah NK, Schafer C, Kappe SHI. Humanized mouse models for the study of human malaria parasite biology, pathogenesis, and immunity. *Front Immunol.* (2018) 9:807. doi: 10.3389/fimmu.2018.00807
162. Morosan S, Hez-Deroubaix S, Lunel F, Renia L, Giannini C, Van Rooijen N, et al. Liver-stage development of *Plasmodium falciparum*, in a humanized mouse model. *J Infect Dis.* (2006) 193:996–1004. doi: 10.1086/500840
163. Sacci JB Jr, Alam U, Douglas D, Lewis J, Tyrrell DL, Azad AF, et al. *Plasmodium falciparum* infection and exoerythrocytic development in mice with chimeric human livers. *Int J Parasitol.* (2006) 36:353–60. doi: 10.1016/j.ijpara.2005.10.014
164. Mikolajczak SA, Sacci JB Jr, de La Vega P, Camargo N, Vanbuskirk K, Krzych U, et al. Disruption of the *Plasmodium falciparum* liver-stage antigen-1 locus causes a differentiation defect in late liver-stage parasites. *Cell Microbiol.* (2011) 13:1250–60. doi: 10.1111/j.1462-5822.2011.01617.x
165. Brezillon NM, Dasilva L, L'hote D, Bernex F, Piquet J, Binart N, et al. Rescue of fertility in homozygous mice for the urokinase plasminogen activator transgene by the transplantation of mouse hepatocytes. *Cell Transplant.* (2008) 17:803–12. doi: 10.3727/096368908786516800
166. Heckel JL, Sandgren EP, Degen JL, Palmiter RD, Brinster RL. Neonatal bleeding in transgenic mice expressing urokinase-type plasminogen activator. *Cell.* (1990) 62:447–56. doi: 10.1016/0092-8674(90)90010-C
167. Mikolajczak SA, Lakshmanan V, Fishbaugher M, Camargo N, Harupa A, Kaushansky A, et al. A next-generation genetically attenuated *Plasmodium falciparum* parasite created by triple gene deletion. *Mol Ther.* (2014) 22:1707–15. doi: 10.1038/mt.2014.85
168. Hasegawa M, Kawai K, Mitsui T, Taniguchi K, Monnai M, Wakui M, et al. The reconstituted 'humanized liver' in TK-NOG mice is mature and functional. *Biochem Biophys Res Commun.* (2011) 405:405–10. doi: 10.1016/j.bbrc.2011.01.042
169. Soulard V, Bosson-Vanga H, Lorthiois A, Roucher C, Franetich JF, Zanghi G, et al. *Plasmodium falciparum* full life cycle and *Plasmodium ovale* liver stages in humanized mice. *Nat Commun.* (2015) 6:7690. doi: 10.1038/ncomms8690
170. Foquet L, Hermsen CC, Van Gemert GJ, Van Braeckel E, Weening KE, Sauerwein R, et al. Vaccine-induced monoclonal antibodies targeting circumsporozoite protein prevent *Plasmodium falciparum* infection. *J Clin Invest.* (2014) 124:140–4. doi: 10.1172/JCI70349
171. Sack B, Kappe SH, Sather DN. Towards functional antibody-based vaccines to prevent pre-erythrocytic malaria infection. *Expert Rev Vaccines.* (2017) 16:403–14. doi: 10.1080/14760584.2017.1295853
172. Foquet L, Schafer C, Minkah NK, Alanine DGW, Flannery EL, Steel RWJ, et al. *Plasmodium falciparum* liver stage infection and transition to stable blood stage infection in liver-humanized and blood-humanized FRGN KO mice enables testing of blood stage inhibitory antibodies (reticulocyte-binding protein homolog 5) *in vivo*. *Front Immunol.* (2018) 9:524. doi: 10.3389/fimmu.2018.00524
173. Walsh NC, Kenney LL, Jangalwe S, Aryee KE, Greiner DL, Brehm MA, et al. Humanized mouse models of clinical disease. *Annu Rev Pathol.* (2017) 12:187–215. doi: 10.1146/annurev-pathol-052016-100332
174. Huang J, Li X, Coelho-Dos-Reis JG, Wilson JM, Tsuji M. An AAV vector-mediated gene delivery approach facilitates reconstitution of functional human CD8+ T cells in mice. *PLoS ONE.* (2014) 9:e88205. doi: 10.1371/journal.pone.0088205
175. Huang J, Li X, Coelho-Dos-Reis JG, Zhang M, Mitchell R, Nogueira RT, et al. Human immune system mice immunized with Plasmodium falciparum circumsporozoite protein induce protective human humoral immunity against malaria. *J Immunol Methods.* (2015) 427:42–50. doi: 10.1016/j.jim.2015.09.005
176. Dunachie SJ, Walther M, Vuola JM, Webster DP, Keating SM, Berthoud T, et al. A clinical trial of prime-boost immunisation with the candidate malaria vaccines RTS,S/AS02A and MVA-CS. *Vaccine.* (2006) 24:2850–9. doi: 10.1016/j.vaccine.2005.12.041
177. Schofield L, Villaquiran J, Ferreira A, Schellekens H, Nussenzweig R, Nussenzweig V. Gamma interferon, CD8+ T cells and antibodies required for immunity to malaria sporozoites. *Nature.* (1987) 330:664–6. doi: 10.1038/330664a0
178. Weiss WR, Sedegah M, Beaudoin RL, Miller LH, Good MF. CD8+ T cells (cytotoxic/suppressors) are required for protection in mice immunized with malaria sporozoites. *Proc Natl Acad Sci USA.* (1988) 85:573–6. doi: 10.1073/pnas.85.2.573
179. Liehl P, Zuzarte-Luis V, Chan J, Zillinger T, Baptista F, Carapau D, et al. Host-cell sensors for Plasmodium activate innate immunity against liver-stage infection. *Nat Med.* (2014) 20:47–53. doi: 10.1038/nm.3424
180. Nussler AK, Renia L, Pasquetto V, Miltgen F, Matile H, Mazier D. *In vivo* induction of the nitric oxide pathway in hepatocytes after injection with irradiated malaria sporozoites, malaria blood parasites or adjuvants. *Eur J Immunol.* (1993) 23:882–7. doi: 10.1002/eji.1830230417
181. Mellouk S, Hoffman SL, Liu ZZ, De La Vega P, Billiar TR, Nussler AK. Nitric oxide-mediated antiplasmodial activity in human and murine hepatocytes induced by gamma interferon and the parasite itself: enhancement by exogenous tetrahydrobiopterin. *Infect Immun.* (1994) 62:4043–6.
182. Seguin MC, Klotz FW, Schneider I, Weir JP, Goodbary M, Slayter M, et al. Induction of nitric oxide synthase protects against malaria in mice exposed to irradiated *Plasmodium berghei* infected mosquitoes: involvement of interferon gamma and CD8+ T cells. *J Exp Med.* (1994) 180:353–8. doi: 10.1084/jem.180.1.353

183. Muniz-Junqueira MI, Dos Santos-Neto LL, Tosta CE. Influence of tumor necrosis factor-alpha on the ability of monocytes and lymphocytes to destroy intraerythrocytic *Plasmodium falciparum* in vitro. *Cell Immunol.* (2001) 208:73–9. doi: 10.1006/cimm.2001.1770
184. Butler NS, Schmidt NW, Harty JT. Differential effector pathways regulate memory CD8 T cell immunity against *Plasmodium berghei* versus *P. yoelii* sporozoites. *J Immunol.* (2010) 184:2528–38. doi: 10.4049/jimmunol.0903529
185. Roland J, Soulard V, Sellier C, Drapier AM, Di Santo JP, Cazenave PA, et al. NK cell responses to Plasmodium infection and control of intrahepatic parasite development. *J Immunol.* (2006) 177:1229–39. doi: 10.4049/jimmunol.177.2.1229
186. Ing R, Stevenson MM. Dendritic cell and NK cell reciprocal cross talk promotes gamma interferon-dependent immunity to blood-stage *Plasmodium chabaudi* AS infection in mice. *Infect Immun.* (2009) 77:770–82. doi: 10.1128/IAI.00994-08
187. Ryg-Cornejo V, Nie CQ, Bernard NJ, Lundie RJ, Evans KJ, Crabb BS, et al. NK cells and conventional dendritic cells engage in reciprocal activation for the induction of inflammatory responses during *Plasmodium berghei* ANKA infection. *Immunobiology.* (2013) 218:263–71. doi: 10.1016/j.imbio.2012.05.018
188. D'Ombrain MC, Hansen DS, Simpson KM, Schofield L. Gammadelta-T cells expressing NK receptors predominate over NK cells and conventional T cells in the innate IFN-gamma response to *Plasmodium falciparum* malaria. *Eur J Immunol.* (2007) 37:1864–73. doi: 10.1002/eji.2006 36889
189. D'Ombrain MC, Robinson LJ, Stanisic DI, Taraika J, Bernard N, Michon P, et al. Association of early interferon-gamma production with immunity to clinical malaria: a longitudinal study among Papua New Guinean children. *Clin Infect Dis.* (2008) 47:1380–7. doi: 10.1086/592971
190. Tsuji M, Mombaerts P, Lefrancois L, Nussenzweig RS, Zavala F, Tonegawa S. Gamma delta T cells contribute to immunity against the liver stages of malaria in alpha beta T-cell-deficient mice. *Proc Natl Acad Sci USA.* (1994) 91:345–9. doi: 10.1073/pnas.91.1.345
191. McKenna KC, Tsuji M, Sarzotti M, Sacci JB Jr, Witney AA, Azad AF. Gammadelta T cells are a component of early immunity against preerythrocytic malaria parasites. *Infect Immun.* (2000) 68:2224–30. doi: 10.1128/IAI.68.4.2224-2230.2000
192. Brandes M, Willimann K, Moser B. Professional antigen-presentation function by human gammadelta T Cells. *Science.* (2005) 309:264–8. doi: 10.1126/science.1110267
193. Brandes M, Willimann K, Bioley G, Levy N, Eberl M, Luo M, et al. Cross-presenting human gammadelta T cells induce robust CD8+ alphabeta T cell responses. *Proc Natl Acad Sci USA.* (2009) 106:2307–12. doi: 10.1073/pnas.0810059106
194. Zaidi I, Diallo H, Conteh S, Robbins Y, Kolasny J, Orr-Gonzalez S, et al. Gammadelta T cells are required for the induction of sterile immunity during irradiated sporozoite vaccinations. *J Immunol.* (2017) 199:3781–8. doi: 10.4049/jimmunol.1700314
195. Amino R, Thiberge S, Martin B, Celli S, Shorte S, Frischknecht F, et al. Quantitative imaging of Plasmodium transmission from mosquito to mammal. *Nat Med.* (2006) 12:220–4. doi: 10.1038/nm1350
196. Chakravarty S, Cockburn IA, Kuk S, Overstreet MG, Sacci JB, Zavala F. CD8+ T lymphocytes protective against malaria liver stages are primed in skin-draining lymph nodes. *Nat Med.* (2007) 13:1035–41. doi: 10.1038/nm1628
197. Obeid M, Franetich JF, Lorthiois A, Gego A, Gruner AC, Tefit M, et al. Skin-draining lymph node priming is sufficient to induce sterile immunity against pre-erythrocytic malaria. *EMBO Mol Med.* (2013) 5:250–63. doi: 10.1002/emmm.201201677
198. Janeway CAJ, Travers P, Walport M, Shlomcik MJ. *Immunobiology: The Immune System in Health and Disease.* New York, NY: Garland Science (2001).
199. Renia L, Maranon C, Hosmalin A, Gruner AC, Silvie O, Snounou G. Do apoptotic Plasmodium-infected hepatocytes initiate protective immune responses? *J Infect Dis.* (2006) 193:163–4; author reply 164–5. doi: 10.1086/498536
200. Cockburn IA, Amino R, Kelemen RK, Kuo SC, Tse SW, Radtke A, et al. *In vivo* imaging of CD8+ T cell-mediated elimination of malaria liver stages. *Proc Natl Acad Sci USA.* (2013) 110:9090–5. doi: 10.1073/pnas.1303858110
201. Berenzon D, Schwenk RJ, Letellier L, Guebre-Xabier M, Williams J, Krzych U. Protracted protection to *Plasmodium berghei* malaria is linked to functionally and phenotypically heterogeneous liver memory CD8+ T cells. *J Immunol.* (2003) 171:2024–34. doi: 10.4049/jimmunol.171.4.2024
202. Tse SW, Cockburn IA, Zhang H, Scott AL, Zavala F. Unique transcriptional profile of liver-resident memory CD8+ T cells induced by immunization with malaria sporozoites. *Genes Immun.* (2013) 14:302–9. doi: 10.1038/gene.2013.20
203. Patel H, Yadav N, Parmar R, Patel S, Singh AP, Shrivastava N, et al. Frequent inoculations with radiation attenuated sporozoite is essential for inducing sterile protection that correlates with a threshold level of Plasmodia liver-stage specific CD8(+) T cells. *Cell Immunol.* (2017) 317:48–54. doi: 10.1016/j.cellimm.2017.05.001
204. Sacci JBJr, Hollingdale MR, Sedegah M. Cellular immune response to DNA and vaccinia prime-boost immunization kills *Plasmodium yoelii*-infected hepatocytes *in vitro. Pathog Dis.* (2017) 75. doi: 10.1093/femspd/ftx051
205. Carvalho LH, Sano G, Hafalla JC, Morrot A, Curotto De Lafaille MA, Zavala F. IL-4-secreting CD4+ T cells are crucial to the development of CD8+ T-cell responses against malaria liver stages. *Nat Med.* (2002) 8:166–70. doi: 10.1038/nm0202-166
206. Overstreet MG, Chen YC, Cockburn IA, Tse SW, Zavala F. CD4+ T cells modulate expansion and survival but not functional properties of effector and memory CD8+ T cells induced by malaria sporozoites. *PLoS ONE.* (2011) 6:e15948. doi: 10.1371/journal.pone.0015948
207. Vanderberg JP, Frevert U. Intravital microscopy demonstrating antibody-mediated immobilisation of *Plasmodium berghei* sporozoites injected into skin by mosquitoes. *Int J Parasitol.* (2004) 34:991–6. doi: 10.1016/j.ijpara.2004.05.005
208. Aliprandini E, Tavares J, Panatieri RH, Thiberge S, Yamamoto MM, Silvie O, et al. Cytotoxic anti-circumsporozoite antibodies target malaria sporozoites in the host skin. *Nat Microbiol.* (2018) 3:1224–33. doi: 10.1038/s41564-018-0254-z
209. Schwenk R, Lumsden JM, Rein LE, Juompan L, Kester KE, Heppner DG, et al. Immunization with the RTS,S/AS malaria vaccine induces IFN-gamma(+)CD4 T cells that recognize only discrete regions of the circumsporozoite protein and these specificities are maintained following booster immunizations and challenge. *Vaccine.* (2011) 29:8847–54. doi: 10.1016/j.vaccine.2011.09.098
210. Nudelman S, Renia L, Charoenvit Y, Yuan L, Miltgen F, Beaudoin RL, et al. Dual action of anti-sporozoite antibodies *in vitro. J Immunol.* (1989) 143:996–1000.
211. Renia L, Mattei D, Goma J, Pied S, Dubois P, Miltgen F, et al. A malaria heat-shock-like determinant expressed on the infected hepatocyte surface is the target of antibody-dependent cell-mediated cytotoxic mechanisms by nonparenchymal liver cells. *Eur J Immunol.* (1990) 20:1445–9. doi: 10.1002/eji.1830200706
212. Miller JL, Sack BK, Baldwin M, Vaughan AM, Kappe SHI. Interferon-mediated innate immune responses against malaria parasite liver stages. *Cell Rep.* (2014) 7:436–47. doi: 10.1016/j.celrep.2014.03.018
213. Mellouk S, Maheshwari RK, Rhodes-Feuillette A, Beaudoin RL, Berbiguier N, Matile H, et al. Inhibitory activity of interferons and interleukin 1 on the development of *Plasmodium falciparum* in human hepatocyte cultures. *J Immunol.* (1987) 139:4192–5.
214. Ferreira A, Schofield L, Enea V, Schellekens H, Van Der Meide P, Collins WE, et al. Inhibition of development of exoerythrocytic forms of malaria parasites by gamma-interferon. *Science.* (1986) 232:881–4. doi: 10.1126/science.3085218
215. Depinay N, Franetich JF, Gruner AC, Mauduit M, Chavatte JM, Luty AJ, et al. Inhibitory effect of TNF-alpha on malaria pre-erythrocytic stage development: influence of host hepatocyte/parasite combinations. *PLoS ONE.* (2011) 6:e17464. doi: 10.1371/journal.pone.0017464
216. Nussler A, Pied S, Goma J, Renia L, Miltgen F, Grau GE, et al. TNF inhibits malaria hepatic stages *in vitro* via synthesis of IL-6. *Int Immunol.* (1991) 3:317–21. doi: 10.1093/intimm/3.4.317

217. Nussler A, Drapier JC, Renia L, Pied S, Miltgen F, Gentilini M, et al. L-arginine-dependent destruction of intrahepatic malaria parasites in response to tumor necrosis factor and/or interleukin 6 stimulation. *Eur J Immunol.* (1991) 21:227–30. doi: 10.1002/eji.1830210134
218. Pied S, Renia L, Nussler A, Miltgen F, Mazier D. Inhibitory activity of IL-6 on malaria hepatic stages. *Parasite Immunol.* (1991) 13:211–7. doi: 10.1111/j.1365-3024.1991.tb00276.x
219. Liehl P, Meireles P, Albuquerque IS, Pinkevych M, Baptista F, Mota MM, et al. Innate immunity induced by Plasmodium liver infection inhibits malaria reinfections. *Infect Immun.* (2015) 83:1172–80. doi: 10.1128/IAI.02796-14
220. Uldrich AP, Le Nours J, Pellicci DG, Gherardin NA, Mcpherson KG, Lim RT, et al. CD1d-lipid antigen recognition by the gammadelta TCR. *Nat Immunol.* (2013) 14:1137–45. doi: 10.1038/ni.2713
221. Jagannathan P, Kim CC, Greenhouse B, Nankya F, Bowen K, Eccles-James I, et al. Loss and dysfunction of Vdelta2(+) gammadelta T cells are associated with clinical tolerance to malaria. *Sci Transl Med.* (2014) 6:251ra117. doi: 10.1126/scitranslmed.3009793
222. Jagannathan P, Lutwama F, Boyle MJ, Nankya F, Farrington LA, Mcintyre TI, et al. Vdelta2+ T cell response to malaria correlates with protection from infection but is attenuated with repeated exposure. *Sci Rep.* (2017) 7:11487. doi: 10.1038/s41598-017-10624-3
223. Radtke AJ, Kastenmuller W, Espinosa DA, Gerner MY, Tse SW, Sinnis P, et al. Lymph-node resident CD8alpha+ dendritic cells capture antigens from migratory malaria sporozoites and induce CD8+ T cell responses. *PLoS Pathog.* (2015) 11:e1004637. doi: 10.1371/journal.ppat.1004637
224. Jung S, Unutmaz D, Wong P, Sano G, De Los Santos K, Sparwasser T, et al. *In vivo* depletion of CD11c+ dendritic cells abrogates priming of CD8+ T cells by exogenous cell-associated antigens. *Immunity.* (2002) 17:211–20. doi: 10.1016/S1074-7613(02)00365-5
225. Jobe O, Donofrio G, Sun G, Liepinsh D, Schwenk R, Krzych U. Immunization with radiation-attenuated *Plasmodium berghei* sporozoites induces liver cCD8alpha+DC that activate CD8+T cells against liver-stage malaria. *PLoS ONE.* (2009) 4:e5075. doi: 10.1371/journal.pone.0005075
226. Lau LS, Fernandez-Ruiz D, Mollard V, Sturm A, Neller MA, Cozijnsen A, et al. CD8+ T cells from a novel T cell receptor transgenic mouse induce liver-stage immunity that can be boosted by blood-stage infection in rodent malaria. *PLoS Pathog.* (2014) 10:e1004135. doi: 10.1371/journal.ppat.1004135
227. Kurup SP, Anthony SM, Hancox LS, Vijay R, Pewe LL, Moioffer SJ, et al. Monocyte-derived CD11c(+) cells acquire plasmodium from hepatocytes to prime CD8 T cell immunity to liver-stage malaria. *Cell Host Microbe.* (2019) 25:565–77.e6. doi: 10.1016/j.chom.2019.02.014
228. Leiriao P, Mota MM, Rodriguez A. Apoptotic plasmodium-infected hepatocytes provide antigens to liver dendritic cells. *J Infect Dis.* (2005) 191:1576–81. doi: 10.1086/429635
229. Mauduit M, See P, Peng K, Renia L, Ginhoux F. Dendritic cells and the malaria pre-erythrocytic stage. *Immunol Res.* (2012) 53:115–26. doi: 10.1007/s12026-012-8269-7
230. Trimnell A, Takagi A, Gupta M, Richie TL, Kappe SH, Wang R. Genetically attenuated parasite vaccines induce contact-dependent CD8+ T cell killing of *Plasmodium yoelii* liver stage-infected hepatocytes. *J Immunol.* (2009) 183:5870–8. doi: 10.4049/jimmunol.0900302
231. Chakravarty S, Baldeviano GC, Overstreet MG, Zavala F. Effector CD8+ T lymphocytes against liver stages of *Plasmodium yoelii* do not require gamma interferon for antiparasite activity. *Infect Immun.* (2008) 76:3628–31. doi: 10.1128/IAI.00471-08
232. Hill AV, Elvin J, Willis AC, Aidoo M, Allsopp CE, Gotch FM, et al. Molecular analysis of the association of HLA-B53 and resistance to severe malaria. *Nature.* (1992) 360:434–9. doi: 10.1038/360434a0
233. Aidoo M, Lalvani A, Gilbert SC, Hu JT, Daubersies P, Hurt N, et al. Cytotoxic T-lymphocyte epitopes for HLA-B53 and other HLA types in the malaria vaccine candidate liver-stage antigen 3. *Infect Immun.* (2000) 68:227–32. doi: 10.1128/IAI.68.1.227-232.2000
234. Bonelo A, Valmori D, Triponez F, Tiercy JM, Mentha G, Oberholzer J, et al. Generation and characterization of malaria-specific human CD8(+) lymphocyte clones: effect of natural polymorphism on T cell recognition and endogenous cognate antigen presentation by liver cells. *Eur J Immunol.* (2000) 30:3079–88. doi: 10.1002/1521-4141(200011)30:11<3079::AID-IMMU3079>3.0.CO;2-7
235. Doolan DL, Southwood S, Freilich DA, Sidney J, Graber NL, Shatney L, et al. Identification of *Plasmodium falciparum* antigens by antigenic analysis of genomic and proteomic data. *Proc Natl Acad Sci USA.* (2003) 100:9952–7. doi: 10.1073/pnas.1633254100
236. Epstein JE, Tewari K, Lyke KE, Sim BK, Billingsley PF, Laurens MB, et al. Live attenuated malaria vaccine designed to protect through hepatic CD8(+) T cell immunity. *Science.* (2011) 334:475–80. doi: 10.1126/science.1211548
237. Reyes-Sandoval A, Wyllie DH, Bauza K, Milicic A, Forbes EK, Rollier CS, et al. CD8+ T effector memory cells protect against liver-stage malaria. *J Immunol.* (2011) 187:1347–57. doi: 10.4049/jimmunol.1100302
238. Schmidt NW, Podyminogin RL, Butler NS, Badovinac VP, Tucker BJ, Bahjat KS, et al. Memory CD8 T cell responses exceeding a large but definable threshold provide long-term immunity to malaria. *Proc Natl Acad Sci USA.* (2008) 105:14017–22. doi: 10.1073/pnas.0805452105
239. Holz LE, Prier JE, Freestone D, Steiner TM, English K, Johnson DN, et al. CD8(+) T cell activation leads to constitutive formation of liver tissue-resident memory T cells that seed a large and flexible niche in the liver. *Cell Rep.* (2018) 25:68–79 e64. doi: 10.1016/j.celrep.2018.08.094
240. McNamara HA, Cai Y, Wagle MV, Sontani Y, Roots CM, Miosge LA, et al. Up-regulation of LFA-1 allows liver-resident memory T cells to patrol and remain in the hepatic sinusoids. *Sci Immunol.* (2017) 2:eaaj1996. doi: 10.1126/sciimmunol.aaj1996
241. Fernandez-Ruiz D, Ng WY, Holz LE, Ma JZ, Zaid A, Wong YC, et al. Liver-resident memory CD8(+) T cells form a front-line defense against malaria liver-stage infection. *Immunity.* (2016) 45:889–902. doi: 10.1016/j.immuni.2016.08.011
242. Renia L, Marussig MS, Grillot D, Pied S, Corradin G, Miltgen F, et al. *In vitro* activity of CD4+ and CD8+ T lymphocytes from mice immunized with a synthetic malaria peptide. *Proc Natl Acad Sci USA.* (1991) 88:7963–7. doi: 10.1073/pnas.88.18.7963
243. Renia L, Grillot D, Marussig M, Corradin G, Miltgen F, Lambert PH, et al. Effector functions of circumsporozoite peptide-primed CD4+ T cell clones against *Plasmodium yoelii* liver stages. *J Immunol.* (1993) 150:1471–8.
244. Bongfen SE, Torgler R, Romero JF, Renia L, Corradin G. *Plasmodium berghei*-infected primary hepatocytes process and present the circumsporozoite protein to specific CD8+ T cells *in vitro*. *J Immunol.* (2007) 178:7054–63. doi: 10.4049/jimmunol.178.11.7054
245. Pichugin A, Steers N, De La Vega P, Zarling S, Chalom I, Krzych U. TAP-mediated processing of exoerythrocytic antigens is essential for protection induced with radiation-attenuated *Plasmodium sporozoites*. *Eur J Immunol.* (2016) 46:885–96. doi: 10.1002/eji.201545748
246. Takita-Sonoda Y, Tsuji M, Kamboj K, Nussenzweig RS, Clavijo P, Zavala F. *Plasmodium yoelii*: peptide immunization induces protective CD4+ T cells against a previously unrecognized cryptic epitope of the circumsporozoite protein. *Exp Parasitol.* (1996) 84:223–30. doi: 10.1006/expr.1996.0108
247. Weiss WR, Sedegah M, Berzofsky JA, Hoffman SL. The role of CD4+ T cells in immunity to malaria sporozoites. *J Immunol.* (1993) 151:2690–8.
248. Reece WH, Pinder M, Gothard PK, Milligan P, Bojang K, Doherty T, et al. A CD4(+) T-cell immune response to a conserved epitope in the circumsporozoite protein correlates with protection from natural *Plasmodium falciparum* infection and disease. *Nat Med.* (2004) 10:406–10. doi: 10.1038/nm1009
249. Schwenk R, Asher LV, Chalom I, Lanar D, Sun P, White K, et al. Opsonization by antigen-specific antibodies as a mechanism of protective immunity induced by *Plasmodium falciparum* circumsporozoite protein-based vaccine. *Parasite Immunol.* (2003) 25:17–25. doi: 10.1046/j.1365-3024.2003.00495.x
250. Flores-Garcia Y, Nasir G, Hopp CS, Munoz C, Balaban AE, Zavala F, et al. Antibody-mediated protection against *Plasmodium sporozoites* begins at the dermal inoculation site. *MBio.* (2018) 9:e02194-18. doi: 10.1128/mBio.02194-18
251. Sack BK, Keitany GJ, Vaughan AM, Miller JL, Wang R, Kappe SH. Mechanisms of stage-transcending protection following immunization of mice with late liver stage-arresting genetically attenuated malaria parasites. *PLoS Pathog.* (2015) 11:e1004855. doi: 10.1371/journal.ppat.1004855

252. Zenklusen I, Jongo S, Abdulla S, Ramadhani K, Lee Sim BK, Cardamone H, et al. Immunization of malaria-preexposed volunteers with PfSPZ vaccine elicits long-lived IgM invasion-inhibitory and complement-fixing antibodies. *J Infect Dis.* (2018) 217:1569–78. doi: 10.1093/infdis/jiy080
253. Finney OC, Keitany GJ, Smithers H, Kaushansky A, Kappe S, Wang R. Immunization with genetically attenuated *P. falciparum* parasites induces long-lived antibodies that efficiently block hepatocyte invasion by sporozoites. *Vaccine.* (2014) 32:2135–8. doi: 10.1016/j.vaccine.2014.02.055
254. Herrington D, Davis J, Nardin E, Beier M, Cortese J, Eddy H, et al. Successful immunization of humans with irradiated malaria sporozoites: humoral and cellular responses of the protected individuals. *Am J Trop Med Hyg.* (1991) 45:539–47. doi: 10.4269/ajtmh.1991.45.539
255. Edelman R, Hoffman SL, Davis JR, Beier M, Sztein MB, Losonsky G, et al. Long-term persistence of sterile immunity in a volunteer immunized with X-irradiated *Plasmodium falciparum* sporozoites. *J Infect Dis.* (1993) 168:1066–70. doi: 10.1093/infdis/168.4.1066
256. Egan JE, Hoffman SL, Haynes JD, Sadoff JC, Schneider I, Grau GE, et al. Humoral immune responses in volunteers immunized with irradiated *Plasmodium falciparum* sporozoites. *Am J Trop Med Hyg.* (1993) 49:166–73. doi: 10.4269/ajtmh.1993.49.166
257. Campo JJ, Aponte JJ, Skinner J, Nakajima R, Molina DM, Liang L, et al. RTS,S vaccination is associated with serologic evidence of decreased exposure to *Plasmodium falciparum* liver- and blood-stage parasites. *Mol Cell Proteomics.* (2015) 14:519–31. doi: 10.1074/mcp.M114.044677
258. Behet MC, Foquet L, Van Gemert GJ, Bijker EM, Meuleman P, Leroux-Roels G, et al. Sporozoite immunization of human volunteers under chemoprophylaxis induces functional antibodies against pre-erythrocytic stages of *Plasmodium falciparum. Malar J.* (2014) 13:136. doi: 10.1186/1475-2875-13-136
259. Kaushansky A, Rezakhani N, Mann H, Kappe SH. Development of a quantitative flow cytometry-based assay to assess infection by *Plasmodium falciparum* sporozoites. *Mol Biochem Parasitol.* (2012) 183:100–3. doi: 10.1016/j.molbiopara.2012.01.006
260. Zou X, House BL, Zyzak MD, Richie TL, Gerbasi VR. Towards an optimized inhibition of liver stage development assay (ILSDA) for *Plasmodium falciparum. Malar J.* (2013) 12:394. doi: 10.1186/1475-2875-12-394
261. Tan J, Sack BK, Oyen D, Zenklusen I, Piccoli L, Barbieri S, et al. A public antibody lineage that potently inhibits malaria infection through dual binding to the circumsporozoite protein. *Nat Med.* (2018) 24:401–7. doi: 10.1038/nm.4513

6

Induction of Plasmodium-Specific Immune Responses Using Liposome-Based Vaccines

Aloysious Ssemaganda[1], Ashwini Kumar Giddam[1†], Mehfuz Zaman[1], Mariusz Skwarczynski[2], Istvan Toth[2,3,4], Danielle I. Stanisic[1] and Michael F. Good[1*]*

[1] Institute for Glycomics, Griffith University, Southport, QLD, Australia, [2] School of Chemistry and Molecular Biosciences, The University of Queensland, Brisbane, QLD, Australia, [3] School of Pharmacy, The University of Queensland, Brisbane, QLD, Australia, [4] Institute for Molecular Bioscience, The University of Queensland, Brisbane, QLD, Australia

Correspondence:
Danielle I. Stanisic
d.stanisic@griffith.edu.au
Michael F. Good
michael.good@griffith.edu.au

†Present Address:
Ashwini Kumar Giddam, Q-Pharm, Royal Brisbane and Women's Hospital, Herston, QLD, Australia

In the development of vaccines, the ability to initiate both innate and subsequent adaptive immune responses need to be considered. Live attenuated vaccines achieve this naturally, while inactivated and sub-unit vaccines generally require additional help provided through delivery systems and/or adjuvants. Liposomes present an attractive adjuvant/delivery system for antigens. Here, we review the key aspects of immunity against *Plasmodium* parasites, liposome design considerations and their current application in the development of a malaria vaccine.

Keywords: malaria, *Plasmodium*, immunity, adjuvant, liposomes, vaccine

INTRODUCTION

Malaria vaccine development has been a focus of research since the 1940s when inoculation with homologous inactivated sporozoites and/or serum resulted in control of parasitemia amongst immunized domestic fowls (1, 2). Follow-up studies also showed that monkeys and ducks were protected against *Plasmodium (P) knowlesi* and *P. lophurae* following vaccination with killed, adjuvanted parasites (3, 4). Additionally, in 1967, it was demonstrated for the first time, that immunization with irradiated sporozoites protected mice against *P. berghei* (5). Despite these early promising findings, an effective vaccine for malaria still eludes scientists with only one vaccine candidate, RTS, S, receiving a positive scientific opinion from European regulators and it is currently approved for use in pilot implementation trials in 3–5 epidemiologically distinct locations in sub-Saharan Africa (6, 7). The complexity of *Plasmodium* parasites, antigenic polymorphism and failure to maintain long-lived immune responses calls for continued efforts in the search for novel vaccines which can effectively prevent *P. falciparum* and *P. vivax* infections (8).

A major bottleneck in the development of vaccines against infectious diseases is the failure to initiate robust innate immune responses and subsequent potentiation and maintenance of downstream adaptive immune responses. This is achieved naturally with live attenuated vaccines while inactivated and sub-unit vaccines require delivery systems and/or adjuvants for efficient presentation to the immune system and additional stimulation to enhance potency (9). To address this, careful selection of adjuvants and delivery systems needs to be considered early in the vaccine development process. However, only a handful of adjuvants have been licensed or tested for use in human vaccines and these are summarized in **Table 1**.

TABLE 1 | Clinically tested and licensed vaccine adjuvants (10, 11).

Adjuvant	Status of vaccine adjuvant
Aluminum-based salts (Alum)	Licensed for tetanus, diphtheria, pneumococcus vaccines (12).
Mf59 (an oil-in-water emulsion consisting of squalene, Tween 80 and span 85)	Licensed for influenza vaccines (13, 14).
AS01: Liposome-based adjuvant comprised of Monophosphoryl Lipid A (MPLA) and QS-21	Tested in phase III malaria and shingles vaccine trials (15, 16).
AS02: squalene emulsion comprised of MPLA and QS-21	Tested in phase II malaria trials (17).
AS03: An oil-in-water emulsion comprised of squalene, Tween 90 and α-tocopherol	Licensed for influenza vaccines (18, 19).
AS04: comprised of aluminum hydroxide and MPLA	Licensed for Cervarix vaccine against HPV and Fendrix against hepatitis B (20–22).
ISA-51 Montanide: Mineral oil with a Mannide monooleate emulsifier	Licensed for Cimavax vaccine against non-small cell lung cancer (NSCLC) (23).
Virosomes: Comprised of influenza virus envelopes reconstituted in liposomes	Licensed for hepatitis A (Epaxal) (22, 24) and Influenza vaccines (Invivac, Inflexal) (25).
CAF01: Cationic liposomes comprised of dimethyldioctadecylammonium bromide (DDAB) and trehalose 6,6-dibehenate (TDB)	Tested in phase I HIV and tuberculosis vaccine trials (26, 27).
IC31: TLR9 agonist	Tested in phase I tuberculosis vaccine trials (28–30).
Poly I:C: TLR3 agonist comprised of repeating units of double stranded inosine and cytosine	Tested in phase I/II cancer vaccine trials (31).
Imiquimod: TLR7/8 agonist	Tested in phase II therapeutic vaccine trials against vulval intraepithelial neoplasia (32)
SE/SE-GLA: Squalene emulsion co-formulated with TLR4 agonist GLA	Tested in phase I influenza vaccine trials (33–36)
ISCOMS, ISCOMATRIX/ Matrix-M^{TM}: Lipid-based adjuvants formulated with cholesterol and saponins	Tested in a phase I vaccine trials against HCV, HPV and influenza (33–35, 37) (NCT02905019)
Recombinant CTB: B subunit of cholera toxin	Licensed for the cholera vaccine, Dukoral (38)

First proposed by Gregoriadis and Allison in 1974 as immunological adjuvants (39), liposomes are a promising vaccine adjuvant/antigen delivery system. Historically well-known as drug carriers, liposomes are self-assembling phospholipid vesicles capable of incorporating and protecting antigens from degradation, as well as facilitating antigen delivery to professional antigen presenting cells (APCs) (9, 40–43). Liposomes generally act by depot formation resulting in enhanced uptake by APCs and subsequent induction of the desired immune responses. To date, the extensive use of liposomes can be attributed to their safety profile, biocompatibility, biodegradability, versatility, and plasticity and therefore they present an attractive platform for malaria vaccine development.

In a natural malaria infection, the acquisition of clinical immunity is slow, spanning several years of repeated exposure, and it is not sterile (44). An ideal vaccine capable of inducing sterile immunity against the different life-cycle stages of malaria will need to induce a qualitatively and/or quantitatively different immune response to that induced during natural infection immunity (45). Since stage-specific immunity to malaria requires humoral and cell-mediated immune responses, the ideal vaccine-induced responses should preferably be comprised of both forms of responses. However, for rational vaccine development, a clear understanding of the complex nature of immunity to malaria is required and this in turn may help to inform the selection of an appropriate adjuvant/delivery system. This review highlights key aspects of the immune response to malaria, design considerations of liposomes, and their current application in malaria vaccine development.

IMMUNITY TO MALARIA

Plasmodium parasites, the causative agents of malaria, are obligate intracellular organisms which undergo a complex life-cycle in the vertebrate host broadly divided into: the mosquito stage which occurs in the vector; the pre-erythrocytic stage which occurs in the vertebrate host's liver; and the erythrocytic stage which occurs in the blood of the vertebrate host (46). At all life-cycle stages, the immune responses induced following infection differ significantly and a clear understanding of these responses will inform the vaccine development process.

Pre-erythrocytic Stage Immunity to Malaria

The pre-erythrocytic stage of malaria infection is clinically quiescent, probably due to the low number of sporozoites inoculated by the mosquito while taking a blood meal. During this stage, studies in mice have shown that antibodies can control infection through immobilization of sporozoites by inhibiting sporozoite motility and subsequent invasion of hepatocytes (47, 48). Following natural infection, studies demonstrated the existence of pre-erythrocytic antigen-specific antibodies to *P. falciparum*; however, their role remains unclear (49–51). To date, the best model that has enabled the study of pre-erythrocytic immune response mechanisms has utilized irradiated sporozoites in both humans and animals. Radiation-attenuated sporozoites retain the capacity to infect hepatocytes but cannot develop into an erythrocytic infection. Studies in rodent models involving inoculation of radiation-attenuated sporozoites demonstrated that antibodies were involved in the enhanced clearance of sporozoites, reduction in sporozoite motility and inhibition of hepatocyte invasion (52, 53). In clinical studies, induction of antibodies to the circumsporozoite protein (CSP) following immunization with the *P. falciparum* sporozoite (PfSPZ) vaccine has been shown to partially correlate with protection (54–58). Furthermore, following immunization with RTS, S/AS01, high CSP-specific antibody titers are induced and are a surrogate measure of protective efficacy for this vaccine candidate (16, 59–63).

Cell-mediated immunity following inoculation of radiation-attenuated sporozoites has also been shown to contribute to vaccine-induced sterilizing immunity to *Plasmodium* infection in both mice and humans (54–58, 64–72). Studies in rodent models, however, indicate that a network of cellular mechanisms mediates immunity to pre-erythrocytic infection (64–66, 68, 70–72). Initial studies in mice immunized with irradiated *P. yoelii* 17XNL sporozoites reported that cytotoxic CD8^{+} T cells mediated protection against a wild-type challenge of infectious sporozoites (64, 65). Further studies indicated that IL-12 from liver antigen presenting cells (APCs) stimulated CD8^{+} T cells and Natural killer (NK) cells to produce interferon (IFN)-γ. IFN-γ, in turn, induces the infected hepatocytes to produce nitric oxide (NO), which subsequently kills the parasite in the hepatocyte (66, 68, 71). In addition, the balance between IL-2, IL-10, IL-12, and IFN-γ results in an inflammatory response that contributes to pre-erythrocytic immunity (70, 72). In human volunteers, both CD4^{+} and CD8^{+} T cell responses against pre-erythrocytic antigens have been observed following immunization with irradiated sporozoites (54–58, 67, 69).

Controlled infection immunization (CII) studies, involving experimental sporozoite inoculation via infectious mosquito bites with concurrent chemoprophylaxis provides another model for investigating pre-erythrocytic immunity to malaria. These studies have shown that a protective polyfunctional T cell response to pre-erythrocytic antigens predominantly characterized by the production of IFN-γ, tumor necrosis factor (TNF), and IL-2 is induced following CII (73–76). Purified IgG against *P. falciparum* sporozoites, obtained from CII trial participants was also shown to inhibit liver stage infection in a humanized liver-chimeric mouse model (73, 75, 77).

Erythrocytic Stage Immunity to Malaria

During the erythrocytic stage, clinical signs, and symptoms of malaria manifest as the parasites invade and replicate in RBCs. Studies in animal models have demonstrated that the innate immune system is involved in the initial recognition of blood-stage parasites, promotion of inflammation, inhibition of parasite growth and potentiation of the adaptive immune response (78, 79). *Plasmodium falciparum* pathogen-associated molecular patterns (PAMPs) such as glycosylphosphatidylinositol (GPI) anchors (Toll-like receptor 2 [TLR2]), hemozoin (NOD-like receptor containing pyrin domain 3 [NLRP3] inflammasome), CpG-containing DNA motifs bound to hemozoin (TLR9) and AT-rich DNA motifs (unidentified cytosolic receptor) have been shown to trigger an inflammatory cascade by binding pattern recognition receptors (PRRs) on the surface of innate immune cells (79–83). This interaction of PAMPs and PRRs results in the production of pro-inflammatory cytokines (IL-12 [p70], IFN-γ and TNF) by APCs, as well as regulatory cytokines (IL-10 and TGF-β) that have been implicated in immunity and pathogenesis to blood-stage malaria infection (79, 84, 85).

Several innate immune cells such as dendritic cells (DCs), macrophages, mast cells, neutrophils, NK cells, natural killer T (NKT) cells, and γδ T cells have been implicated in this initial immune response (85–88). *Plasmodium* parasites have been shown to modulate DC maturation and function resulting in the induction of regulatory T cells which in turn modulates CD4^{+} T cell responses, suppressing protective immune responses while averting immune-mediated pathology (85). IL-12 production by DCs has also been implicated in the production of IFN-γ by NK cells and CD4^{+} Th1 cells resulting in the control of parasite growth (85). Understanding the balance between protective and immunopathologic responses following DC activation and maturation might have favorable implications in designing vaccines to prevent severe malaria (85). *In vitro*, NK cells have been shown to be an early source of IFN-γ, promoting the destruction of infected red blood cells by activated macrophages (79, 89). γδ T cells and monocytes on the other hand have been associated with elevated levels of TNF, IL- 10, IP-10, IL-6, macrophage inflammatory protein (MIP)-1β and MIP-1α which is linked with severe disease (90). Furthermore, downregulation of γδ T cell responses following repeated exposures to *Plasmodia* has also been implicated with better tolerance to clinical malaria (91, 92). Given their specificity for restricted TCR ligands, γδ T cells present an attractive target for a vaccine to protect against severe disease (45, 90).

Antibodies play a role in naturally acquired immunity to erythrocytic stage malaria, as it has been shown that the passive transfer of immunoglobulin from immune donors resulted in the reduction of parasitaemia and clinical disease among semi-immune recipients from East Africa as well as non-immune Thai patients (93–95). Antibodies may function by inhibiting merozoite invasion of RBCs (96), binding to pRBCs and enhancing clearance by the spleen (97, 98), as well as opsonizing pRBCs, resulting in phagocytosis by macrophages (99, 100).

Cell-mediated immunity against the erythrocytic stage is primarily mediated by CD4^{+} T cells, as demonstrated in both murine and human models. Studies showed that mice depleted of CD4^{+} T cells developed very high parasitaemia and were unable to control the infection compared to mice depleted of CD8^{+} T cells, which developed mild parasitaemia that subsequently resolved; this indicated a clear role of CD4^{+} T cells in erythrocytic stage immunity (101, 102). Additionally, adoptive transfer of CD4^{+} T cells was shown to confer protection and control parasitaemia in immunodeficient mice (103). Further investigation of the role of CD4^{+} T cells demonstrated that during the acute phase of infection, there was a significant upregulation of an IFN-γ-specific CD4^{+} T cell (Th1) response followed by an IL-4-specific CD4^{+} T cell-mediated (Th2) antibody response during the chronic phase (104). These data indicate that early activation of Th1 cells enables control of the infection via effector mechanisms such as macrophages, followed by a Th2 response which activates B cells to clear the parasite in the later stages of the infection in mice (105, 106).

In human studies, the role of CD4$^+$ T cells was demonstrated when volunteers were infected with low doses of blood-stage *P. falciparum* followed by drug cure (107). In this study, volunteers appeared to be protected against a homologous challenge infection with immunity associated with an IFN-γ-specific CD4$^+$ T cell response and nitric oxide synthase (NOS) production in the absence of detectable antibodies (107). However, a follow-up study suggested that residual drug may have contributed to the apparent protection (108). Another study showed that stimulation of T cells obtained from children living in Papua New Guinea resulted in parasite-specific IFN-γ and TNF responses, which were associated with protection against clinical episodes of malaria (109). More recently, studies in African children showed that CD4$^+$ T cells may play an important modulatory role in the development of blood-stage immunity (110, 111). Higher IFN-γ/IL-10+ specific-CD4$^+$ T cell responses were observed amongst children heavily exposed to malaria compared to children with low exposure indicating that CD4$^+$ T cells may play an important immunomodulatory role in the pathogenesis of childhood malaria (110). Additionally, the induction of IL-10-producing CD4$^+$ T cells amongst highly exposed children may interfere with the development of immunity, which may have implications for vaccine development (111).

T follicular helper cells (Tfh) are a subset of CD4$^+$ T cells, capable of providing B cell help as well as activating follicular B-cell responses (112–114). Recent studies in mice showed that Tfh cells play a critical role in controlling *P. chabaudi* blood-stage infection via activation of IL-21 mediated responses (115). Therefore, since humoral responses are critical to the erythrocytic stages of *Plasmodium*, an in-depth understanding of the activation and maintenance of Tfh cells during malaria will be critical in designing blood-stage vaccines (115).

Regulatory T cells (Tregs) are another CD4$^+$ T cell subset implicated in the maintenance of immune homeostasis and control of excessive pathogen-driven inflammatory responses (116, 117). Following *Plasmodium* infection, uncontrolled production of pro-inflammatory cytokines is associated with pathology in both mice and humans (118–121) and anti-inflammatory cytokines (TGF-β and IL-10) are known to be critical in the modulation of this inflammatory response (118, 120, 122, 123). The immunomodulatory function of IL-10 and TGF-β is associated with Tregs whose role in rodent malaria remains unclear. Some studies have shown that Tregs are critical in the control of pro-inflammatory responses associated with pathology (124, 125) while other studies have associated upregulation of Tregs with detrimental outcomes (124, 126, 127). These discrepancies may have been dependent on the rodent parasite strains utilized in the study (128). Tregs may inhibit protective immune responses resulting in enhanced parasite growth if induced early in infection but may also limit immune-mediated pathology (45, 128–130). Clinical studies have shown that acute infection with *Plasmodium* parasites resulted in upregulation of Tregs which positively correlated with augmented parasite load and subsequent disease severity amongst these individuals (131–134). Given this background, a vaccine capable of inducing Tregs with the ability to protect against the immunopathology associated with malaria infection would be desirable if parasite persistence is required for the maintenance of protective immune responses. However, since Tregs are known to inhibit protective immune responses, treatment with antimalaria drugs at the time of vaccination may be necessary to "normalize" the pre-existing immune response and ensure induction of the appropriate vaccine-specific responses (45).

The role of CD8$^+$ T cells in defense against blood-stage parasites remains unclear due to the fact that mature RBCs do not express MHC class I molecules. However, *in vitro* studies have shown that both *P. falciparum* and *P. vivax* are able to invade erythroblasts—immature erythrocytes that possess a nucleus and express MHC class I molecules (135, 136). Additionally, studies in mice demonstrated that blood-stage parasite antigens were cross-presented by CD8-α$^+$ DCs, inducing parasite-specific CD8$^+$ T cell responses capable of lysing APCs (137). These findings indicated the possible relevance of CD8$^+$ T cells in erythrocytic immunity to *Plasmodium*. Indeed, additional studies in mice demonstrated that parasitized erythroblasts activated CD8$^+$ T cells in an antigen-specific manner (138). This contact-dependent Fas—Fas Ligand (FasL) interaction of CD8$^+$ T cells with the parasitized erythroblasts results in the exposure of phosphatidylserine (PS) on the erythroblast surface (139). Cells displaying PS on their surface are rapidly phagocytosed by macrophages. Thus, CD8$^+$ T cells in conjunction with macrophages are able to mediate immunity to a blood-stage malaria infection in mice (139). Earlier studies in a *P. yoelii* infection model demonstrated that professional APCs might cross-present parasite-derived peptides on MHC class I to CD8$^+$ T cells leading to cytotoxicity through the production of IFN-γ, perforin and granzyme B (140). Furthermore, parasite-specific CD8$^+$ T cells have also been shown to clear infected reticulocytes, which express MHC class I molecules, via the secretion of IFN-γ and expression of granzyme B (141).

These data highlighted in the studies above provide an insight into the complex nature of immune responses elicited following infection with malaria parasites. Understanding the balance between protective immunity and immunopathology is critical for the development of an ideal vaccine capable of inducing both humoral and cell-mediated immune responses against different life-cycle stages of the malaria parasite. To achieve this balance, careful selection of antigen delivery systems and adjuvants during the vaccine development process is paramount and the pliability of liposome-based platforms can be utilized for this purpose.

DESIGN CONSIDERATIONS OF LIPOSOMAL VACCINE FORMULATIONS

Based on their design, liposome vaccine formulations can be tailored to achieve desired immune responses and adjuvant properties by modification of vesicle physicochemical factors (summarized in **Figure 1**), such as lipid composition, charge, PEGylation, antigen encapsulation, and addition of immunomodulators (9, 40–43).

The choice of phospholipid has been shown to enhance the adjuvanticity of liposomes. Long chain lipids tend to form

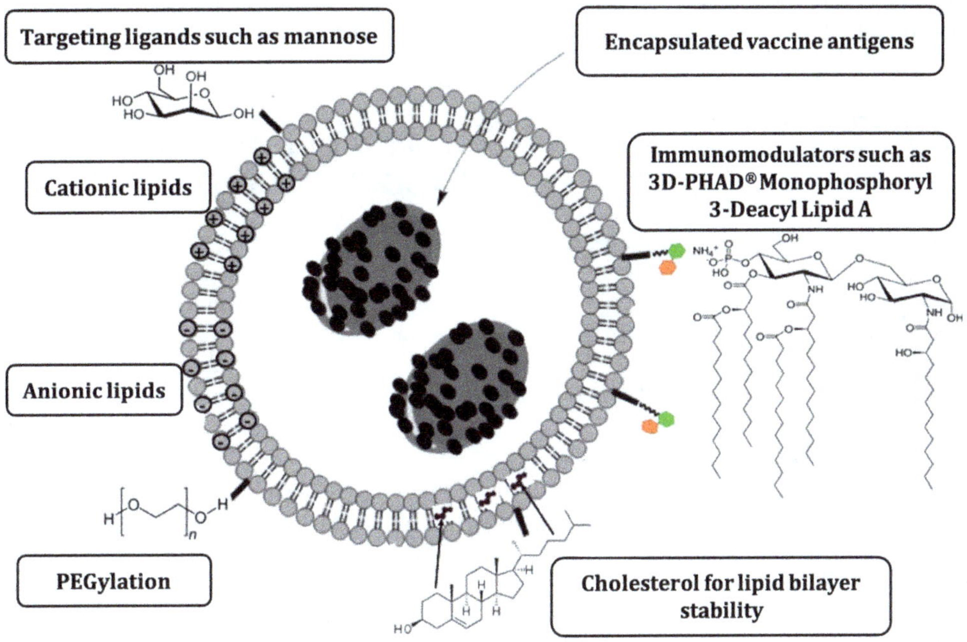

FIGURE 1 | Major liposome physicochemical characteristics that can be modified to direct immune responses elicited following vaccination (9).

rigid ordered bilayer structures while those with shorter tails tend to form fluid and disordered vesicles (9). Immunization of animals with liposomes formulated with long chain lipids such as dimethyldioctadecylammonium bromide (DDAB) and distearyol derivative of L-α-phosphatidyl choline (DSPC) resulted in stronger antigen-specific antibody responses when compared to animals that received liposomes formulated with shorter chain lipids (142). Additionally, the stability of the lipid bilayer can be enhanced further with the addition of cholesterol within the liposome formulation resulting in improved antibody responses compared to formulations without cholesterol (143–145).

Positively charged (cationic) liposomes formulated with saturated acyl chain lipids (with a quaternary ammonium head group) have been shown to promote the binding of antigen at the site of injection stimulating interaction with APCs to elicit a robust Th1 cytokine response (146). In contrast, highly fluid unsaturated acyl chain liposomes that are rapidly cleared from the injection site result in lower activation of APCs as measured by the decreased expression of DC co-stimulatory molecules CD40 and CD86 (146). Additionally, cationic liposomes have been shown to promote retention of higher levels of antigen at the injection site, resulting in a depot-effect allowing continuous attraction of APCs and subsequent induction of robust cell-mediated immune responses comprised of IFN-γ, IL-2, TNF, and IL-17 (147). On the other hand, negatively charged (anionic) and neutral liposomes were rapidly cleared from the injection site resulting in lower activation of APCs and lower Th1 as well as Th17 cytokine responses (9, 147, 148).

The inclusion of polyethylene glycol (PEG), known as PEGylation, has been extensively used for the stabilization of liposomes (149). PEGylation has been shown to mask the charge, due to the hydrophilic chains of PEG extending out from the surface of the liposomes subsequently reducing the electrostatic retention of antigen to the surface of these vesicles (150, 151). Additionally, PEGylation influences lipid packaging reducing the number of bilayers and resulting in reduced vesicle size (151). This modification of liposome size and antigen adsorption properties by PEG was shown to reduce depot formation, resulting in reduced IgG2b antibody and Th1 (IFN-γ) cytokine responses as well as an elevated Th2 (IL-5) cytokine response compared to non- PEGylated liposome formulations (150, 151).

The particle size of liposomes has also been shown to impact adjuvanticity and direct the development of the resulting cell-mediated immune response (42). Studies have shown that the immune response induced following administration of small-sized liposome vesicles (10–100 nm) was skewed toward Th2 whilst larger vesicles (400–2,500 nm) induced a Th1 response characterized by augmented IFN-γ and IgG2a production (152). The differences in the profiles of the induced immune response of large vs. small vesicles could be due to differences in antigen processing and trafficking to lymph nodes. Large-sized vesicles (560 nm) were shown to be more efficiently phagocytosed and processed by macrophages compared to smaller vesicles (155 nm) (153). Additionally, trafficking of liposome particles to lymph nodes has been shown to be size dependent, with small-sized vesicles (20–200 nm) freely draining to and specifically targeting lymph node-resident cells, while large-sized vesicles (500–2,000 nm) require dendritic cells for trafficking from the injection site to lymph nodes (154). More recently, immunization using a formulation containing large-sized cationic liposomes (∼500 nm) resulted in enhanced splenocyte proliferative responses and reduced IL-10 production compared to small sized liposomes (∼100 nm) (155). Interestingly, smaller unilamellar liposomes (70 nm) were reported to stimulate higher IgG titers than larger unilamellar (400 nm) but not large submicron size multilamellar liposomes in mice (156). The potency of multilamellar liposomes can be explained by more efficient antigen protection against degradation in their multiple lipid bilayers.

Liposomes can be modified to incorporate additional lipophilic immunomodulators within or attached to the lipid bilayer to enhance adjuvanticity. Such immunomodulators are crucial in the activation of the cells of the innate immune system via PRRs which recognize PAMPs on the surface of pathogens, subsequently activating the adaptive immune system. The activation of innate immune cells such as dendritic cells and macrophages requires the use of Toll-like receptor (TLR) and NOD-like receptor (NLR) type PRRs to direct a robust immune response (157). Therefore, the use of synthetic PRR agonists has been predicted to be critical in the formulation of liposome-based vaccine adjuvants (9, 158).

Liposome formulations can be customized by incorporating PRR agonists that mediate activation and maturation of APCs which in turn facilitates the uptake and processing of liposome-associated antigens resulting in potent cell-mediated immune responses (9). The most widely used PRR agonist monophosphoryl lipid A (MPLA), a TLR-4 agonist, has been used in licensed vaccine formulations Fendrix (hepatitis B) (159) and Cervarix (human papillomavirus) (160). A synthetic analog of MPLA, 3′-O-desacyl-4′-monophosphoryl lipid A formulated with *Quillaja saponaria* Molina, fraction 21 (QS-21) saponin is included in the liposome-based GSK Adjuvant System 01 (AS01) and has been tested in human studies for the malaria vaccine RTS, S (Mosquirix) (16), as well as a shingles sub-unit vaccine HZ/su which demonstrated over 90% efficacy amongst elderly persons (15). Similarly, liposomes can be tagged with sugars such as mannose to target them to lectin-like molecules on APCs to facilitate phagocytic uptake thereby promoting MHC class II involvement and, via cross presentation, MHC class I. This targeting of liposomes to different uptake pathways may aid in directing the resulting immune response toward a mixed Th1/Th2 response (9, 161).

The route of administration of particulate antigen delivery systems such as liposomes has been shown to affect the type and magnitude of immune response induced. Interestingly liposomes can be even administered orally; however, they need to be extensively modified to improve their stability in the gastrointestinal tract and their mucosa adhesive properties (162). In a cross-sectional study in mice, the intramuscular, intradermal and intralymphatic routes of administration were associated with intermediate to high induction of IgG2a and IFN-γ cytokine production while the subcutaneous route was associated with low elicitation of IgG2a and IFN-γ cytokine production (163). These data indicate that the route of administration is critical in the generation of the desired immune response and should be considered while interpreting immunological data following immunization with liposome-based vaccine formulations. Together, it is evident that the versatility and plasticity of liposomes facilitates the tailoring of the desired immune responses, as well as enhanced adjuvanticity and this can be exploited for the development of a malaria vaccine.

UTILITY OF LIPOSOMES IN MALARIA VACCINE DEVELOPMENT

Liposomes are increasingly becoming used in a number of malaria vaccine candidates targeting the different life-cycle stages. The use of liposomes in the development of sporozoite-stage malaria vaccines dates back to the mid-1980s where tetrapeptide antigens (asparagine-alanine-asparagine-proline) derived from the repetitive region of the circumsporozoite (CS) protein of *P. falciparum* sporozoites were conjugated to carrier proteins and were incorporated into liposomes. These studies demonstrated that liposomes containing carrier protein-conjugated peptide induced a potent humoral immune response which was further enhanced when lipid A was incorporated in the liposome formulation (164–169). The aforementioned studies laid the foundation for the development of RTS, S, the only vaccine against malaria that has received approval for use in pilot implementation trials in sub-Saharan Africa (7). The RTS, S vaccine construct is made of the central repeat region (amino acids 210-398) (R) and the C-terminal region containing the T-cell epitopes of CSP (T), fused to hepatitis B surface antigen (HBsAg) (S), co-expressed in *Saccharomyces cerevisiae* yeast and self-assembled with unfused HBsAg antigen (170, 171). These hybrid virus-like particles (VLPs) were co-formulated with GSK's proprietary liposome-based adjuvant system, AS01, which contains potent immunostimulants, MPLA and QS-21 that was selected over AS02, an oil-in-water emulsion adjuvant following evidence of enhanced antigen-specific antibody and CD4+ T-cell responses as well as improved efficacy in large-scale clinical studies (61, 172–175). The level of and mechanism of immunity induced by RTS, S in endemic settings are topics of much research. Over 4 years of follow up, the level of protection ranged from 18 to 36%, depending on the age of the child and whether the child received 3 or 4 doses of vaccine. Protection was clearly greater in the early months after vaccination, but waned rapidly after that and there was a 'negative efficacy' during the 5th year in some children (176). This is a sub-optimal response and as such the mechanism of immunity came under great scrutiny. Evidence suggests that the level of antibody to the CS protein and serum levels of IFN-γ post vaccination both correlate with protection (177, 178). A major concern, has been the rapid diminution of antibody levels over time, in the face of parasite exposure. The problem is not that RTS,S is not immunogenic. The adjuvant system is one of the most potent there is for human use and is used elsewhere with great effect. It has made Shingrix a highly successful vaccine where even in the elderly there is 90% efficacy. Also, the problem is not with boosting *per se*, as each dose of RTS,S is accompanied by a rapid rise in antibody titer. In our view, the main problem is that even though RTS,S has a powerful adjuvant system, it is still not powerful enough. Titres wane after vaccination and natural infection will not boost. The main reasons for this appear to be: (i) antigenic polymorphism; and (ii) that the dose of sporozoites that individuals are exposed to (and which express the CS protein) are simply too low to boost or maintain antibody levels. T cell epitopes present on the CS protein which are incorporated into the vaccine are polymorphic (179), and this polymorphism does contribute to the low efficacy (180). The T-cell epitopes are known to be non-cross-reactive (181). An additional factor may relate to liposome design *per se*. Indeed, efforts are currently underway to remodel RTS, S such that each HBsAg particle expresses CSP thereby increasing the concentration of parasite antigens (182). Here, CSP-HBsAg fusion proteins were co-expressed in *Pichia pastoris* yeast which in the presence of a tightly regulated inducible alcohol oxidase (AOX1) promoter allows production of a higher density of hybrid VLPs (182, 183). This vaccine construct, co-formulated with Matrix-M ™, a saponin-based liposomal adjuvant is now undergoing clinical testing NCT02905019[1].

In the development of transmission-blocking vaccines, gel core liposomes encapsulating Pfs25, an antigen expressed on zygotes and ookinetes of *P. falciparum* and a leading transmission-blocking vaccine (TBV) candidate, have been tested in mouse models (184). Gel core liposomes are a stabilized form of liposomes bearing a core of biocompatible polymer inside the lipid vesicle which serves to prevent the rapid release of antigen content from liposomes (184, 185). Following 2 intramuscular injections with gel core liposomes, Pfs25-specific antibody responses were observed in immunized mice, and these were maintained for up to 8 weeks. Additionally, strong Th1 cytokine (IL-2 and IFN-γ) responses were elicited and these responses were augmented when the gel core liposomes were formulated with CpG oligodeoxynucleotide (CpG-ODN) (184, 185).

A cationic adjuvant liposome formulation (CAF01) consisting of DDAB, synthetic mycobacterial cordfactor as an immunomodulator, and merozoite surface protein 1 (MSP1) antigen derived from *P. yoelii* genomic DNA, *Py*MSP1, has been tested in pre-clinical studies as a blood-stage malaria vaccine (186). Compared to the Alum adjuvanted vaccine formulation, immunization with CAF01- *Py*-MSP-1 resulted in significantly higher antibody and IFN-γ cytokine responses. Furthermore, following challenge, immunization with CAF01- *Py*MSP1 resulted in significant control of parasite growth (186).

Tyagi et al. (187), utilized a liposome-mediated transdermal immunization approach to deliver *P. falciparum* merozoite surface protein-1 (PfMSP-1) antigens through intact skin to antigen presenting cells in the skin (187). Similar to observations following immunization with CAF01- *Py*MSP1(186), durable and stronger parasite-specific humoral responses were observed up to 10 weeks post-immunization. Additionally, robust cell-mediated responses critical in immunity against blood-stage malaria parasites were induced following transdermal administration of elastic liposomes loaded with PfMSP-1 antigens when compared to Alum based vaccine formulations (187). Collectively, these data underscore the substantial superiority of liposome-based formulations over aluminum-based vaccine adjuvant formulations in the induction of parasite-specific immune responses to malaria.

More recently, our group formulated liposomes with mannosylated lipid core peptides (MLCPs) as targeting ligands for the delivery of whole blood-stage parasite antigens to professional antigen presenting cells (188). Immunization with these mannosylated liposome formulations resulted in the induction of significant $CD8^+$ T cell responses; immunized mice demonstrated better control of parasitemia as well as extended survival following challenge, when compared with control mice, availing an alternative delivery system for inactivated whole parasite antigens (188). Together, the studies above indicate that liposomes are being considerably used in malaria vaccine development for targeting all of the different life-cycle stages and their pliability can be further explored to develop a multi-stage vaccine.

CONCLUDING REMARKS

The quest for a vaccine against malaria continues despite the partial success with RTS, S/AS01, which showed modest efficacy in phase III clinical trials (16). Given the complex network of immune responses elicited following infection with *Plasmodium* parasites, an ideal vaccine should aim to induce the appropriate life-cycle stage-specific-antibody and cell-mediated responses capable of protecting against disease and immunopathology. The versatility of liposomes can be exploited to achieve an optimal formulation via the use of charged lipids to promote antigen retention at the injection site (depot-effect) (186), inclusion of targeting ligands to promote uptake by professional APCs (188), to control their stability, release of antigen, enhance antigen protection, and include immunomodulators (40, 43). Additionally, as the poor efficacy of most malaria vaccines evaluated thus far in field trials has been attributed to antigenic polymorphism, the use of whole parasite antigens (188) in liposome formulations needs to be explored further in malaria vaccine development. In summary, the modification of vesicle physicochemical properties may be further exploited to design an optimal liposome formulation with a high level of efficacy required for complete eradication of malaria by 2030 (8).

AUTHOR CONTRIBUTIONS

AS, DS, and MG drafted and reviewed original manuscript. AG, MZ, MS, and IT critically reviewed original manuscript and provided important intellectual content.

ACKNOWLEDGMENTS

We wish to thank Dr. Leanne M. Low for critically reviewing this manuscript. We acknowledge the generous support from Griffith

[1] A Safety and Efficacy Study of R21 +/- ChAd63/MVA ME-TRAP. https://ClinicalTrials.gov/show/NCT02905019.

University (Griffith University International Postgraduate Research Scholarship and Griffith University Postgraduate Research Scholarship) awarded to AS. We also acknowledge the grant support from a National Health and Medical Research Council Fellowship and Program Grant 1037304 awarded to IT and MG.

REFERENCES

1. Russell PF, Mohan BN. The immunisation of fowls against mosquito-borne *Plasmodium Gallinaceum* by injections of serum and of inactivated homologous sporozoites. *J Exp Med.* (1942) 76:477–95. doi: 10.1084/jem.76.5.477
2. Hill AV. Vaccines against malaria. *Philos Trans R Soc Lond B Biol Sci.* (2011) 366:2806–14. doi: 10.1098/rstb.2011.0091
3. Freund J, Sommer HE, Walter AW. Immunisation against malaria: vaccination of ducks with killed parasites incorporated with adjuvants. *Science* (1945) 102:200–2. doi: 10.1126/science.102.2643.200
4. Freund J, Thomson KJ, Sommer HE, Walter AW, Schenkein EL. Immunisation of rhesus monkeys against malarial infection (*P. knowlesi*) with killed parasites and adjuvants. *Science* (1945) 102:202–4. doi: 10.1126/science.102.2643.202
5. Nussenzweig RS, Vanderberg J, Most H, Orton C. Protective immunity produced by the injection of x-irradiated sporozoites of *Plasmodium berghei. Nature* (1967) 216:160–2. doi: 10.1038/216160a0
6. Kaslow DC, Biernaux S. RTS,S: toward a first landmark on the malaria vaccine technology roadmap. *Vaccine* (2015) 33:7425–32. doi: 10.1016/j.vaccine.2015.09.061
7. World Health Organization. Malaria vaccine: WHO position paper, January 2016-Recommendations. *Vaccine* (2018) 36:3576–7. doi: 10.1016/j.vaccine.2016.10.047
8. Malaria Vaccine Funders Group (2013). *Malaria Vaccine Technology Roadmap.*
9. Perrie Y, Crofts F, Devitt A, Griffiths HR, Kastner E, Nadella, V. Designing liposomal adjuvants for the next generation of vaccines. *Adv Drug Deliv Rev* (2016) 99(Pt A):85–96. doi: 10.1016/j.addr.2015.11.005
10. Brito LA, O'Hagan DT. Designing and building the next generation of improved vaccine adjuvants. *J Control Release* (2014) 190:563–79. doi: 10.1016/j.jconrel.2014.06.027
11. Nevagi RJ, Toth I, Skwarczynski M. Peptide-based vaccines. In: Koutsopoulos S, editor. *Peptide Applications in Biomedicine, Biotechnology and Bioengineering.* Oxford: Elsevier Inc. (2018). p. 327–58.
12. Baylor NW, Egan W, Richman P. Aluminum salts in vaccines–US perspective. *Vaccine* (2002) 20 (Suppl. 3):S18–23. doi: 10.1016/S0264-410X(02)00166-4
13. O'Hagan DT, Ott GS, De Gregorio E, Seubert A. The mechanism of action of MF59 - an innately attractive adjuvant formulation. *Vaccine* (2012) 30:4341–8. doi: 10.1016/j.vaccine.2011.09.061
14. Durando P, Icardi G, Ansaldi F. MF59-adjuvanted vaccine: a safe and useful tool to enhance and broaden protection against seasonal influenza viruses in subjects at risk. *Expert Opin Biol Ther.* (2010) 10:639–51. doi: 10.1517/14712591003724662
15. Lal H, Cunningham AL, Godeaux O, Chlibek R, Diez-Domingo J, Hwang SJ, et al. Efficacy of an adjuvanted herpes zoster subunit vaccine in older adults. *N Engl J Med.* (2015) 372:2087–96. doi: 10.1056/NEJMoa1501184
16. RTSS Clinical Trials Partnership (2015). Efficacy and safety of RTS,S/AS01 malaria vaccine with or without a booster dose in infants and children in Africa: final results of a phase 3, individually randomised, controlled trial. *Lancet* 386:31–45. doi: 10.1016/S0140-6736(15)60721-8
17. Regules JA, Cummings JF, Ockenhouse CF. The RTS,S vaccine candidate for malaria. *Expert Rev Vaccines* (2011) 10:589–99. doi: 10.1586/erv.11.57
18. Nohynek H, Jokinen J, Partinen M, Vaarala O, Kirjavainen T, Sundman J, et al. AS03 adjuvanted AH1N1 vaccine associated with an abrupt increase in the incidence of childhood narcolepsy in Finland. *PLoS ONE* (2012) 7:e33536. doi: 10.1371/journal.pone.0033536
19. Morel S, Didierlaurent A, Bourguignon P, Delhaye S, Baras B, Jacob V, et al. Adjuvant System AS03 containing alpha-tocopherol modulates innate immune response and leads to improved adaptive immunity. *Vaccine* (2011) 29:2461–73. doi: 10.1016/j.vaccine.2011.01.011
20. Kundi M, Kundi M. New hepatitis B vaccine formulated with an improved adjuvant system. *Expert Rev Vaccines* (2007) 6:133–40. doi: 10.1586/14760584.6.2.133
21. Paavonen J, Jenkins D, Bosch FX, Naud P, Salmerón J, Wheeler CM, et al. Efficacy of a prophylactic adjuvanted bivalent L1 virus-like-particle vaccine against infection with human papillomavirus types 16 and 18 in young women: an interim analysis of a phase III double-blind, randomised controlled trial. *Lancet* (2007) 369:2161–70. doi: 10.1016/S0140-6736(07)60946-5
22. Garçon N, Chomez P, Van Mechelen M. GlaxoSmithKline adjuvant systems in vaccines: concepts, achievements and perspectives. *Expert Rev Vaccines* (2007) 6:723–39. doi: 10.1586/14760584.6.5.723
23. Rodríguez PC, Rodríguez G, González G, Lage A. Clinical development and perspectives of CIMAvax EGF, Cuban vaccine for non-small-cell lung cancer therapy. *MEDICC Rev.* (2010) 12:17–23.
24. Bovier PA. Recent advances with a virosomal hepatitis A vaccine. *Expert Opin Biol Ther.* (2008) 8:1177–85. doi: 10.1517/14712598.8.8.1177
25. Mischler R, Metcalfe IC. Inflexal V a trivalent virosome subunit influenza vaccine: production. *Vaccine* (2002) 20 (Suppl. 5):B17–23 doi: 10.1016/S0264-410X(02)00512-1
26. Román VR, Jensen KJ, Jensen SS, Leo-Hansen C, Jespersen S, da Silva Te. D, et al. Therapeutic vaccination using cationic liposome-adjuvanted HIV type 1 peptides representing HLA-supertype-restricted subdominant T cell epitopes: safety, immunogenicity, and feasibility in Guinea-Bissau. *AIDS Res Hum Retroviruses* (2013) 29:1504–12. doi: 10.1089/AID.2013.0076
27. van Dissel JT, Joosten SA, Hoff ST, Soonawala D, Prins C, Hokey DA, et al. A novel liposomal adjuvant system, CAF01, promotes long-lived *Mycobacterium tuberculosis*-specific T-cell responses in human. *Vaccine* (2014) 32:7098–107. doi: 10.1016/j.vaccine.2014.10.036
28. Luabeya AK, Kagina BM, Tameris MD, Geldenhuys H, Hoff ST, Shi Z, et al. First-in-human trial of the post-exposure tuberculosis vaccine H56:IC31 in *Mycobacterium tuberculosis* infected and non-infected healthy adults. *Vaccine* (2015) 33:4130–40. doi: 10.1016/j.vaccine.2015.06.051
29. Norrby M, Vesikari T, Lindqvist L, Maeurer M, Ahmed R, Mahdavifar S, et al. Safety and immunogenicity of the novel H4:IC31 tuberculosis vaccine candidate in BCG-vaccinated adults: Two phase I dose escalation trials. *Vaccine* (2017) 35:1652–61. doi: 10.1016/j.vaccine.2017.01.055
30. Hussein J, Zewdie M, Yamuah L, Bedru A, Abebe M, Dagnew AF, et al. A phase I, open-label trial on the safety and immunogenicity of the adjuvanted tuberculosis subunit vaccine H1/IC31(R) in people living in a TB-endemic area. *Trials* (2018) 19:24. doi: 10.1186/s13063-017-2354-0
31. Levine AS, Levy HB. Phase I-II trials of poly IC stabilized with poly-L-lysine. *Cancer Treat Rep.* (1978) 62:1907–12.
32. Daayana S, Elkord E, Winters U, Pawlita M, Roden R, Stern PL, et al. Phase II trial of imiquimod and HPV therapeutic vaccination in patients with vulval intraepithelial neoplasia. *Br J Cancer* (2010) 102:1129–36. doi: 10.1038/sj.bjc.6605611
33. Drane D, Gittleson C, Boyle J, Maraskovsky E. ISCOMATRIX adjuvant for prophylactic and therapeutic vaccines. *Expert Rev Vaccines* (2007) 6:761–72. doi: 10.1586/14760584.6.5.761
34. Maraskovsky E, Schnurr M, Wilson NS, Robson NC, Boyle J, Drane D. Development of prophylactic and therapeutic vaccines using the ISCOMATRIX adjuvant. *Immunol Cell Biol.* (2009) 87:371–6. doi: 10.1038/icb.2009.21
35. Morelli AB, Becher D, Koernig S, Silva A, Drane D, Maraskovsky E. ISCOMATRIX: a novel adjuvant for use in prophylactic and therapeutic vaccines against infectious diseases. *J Med Microbiol.* (2012) 61 (Pt 7):935–43. doi: 10.1099/jmm.0.040857-0

36. Behzad H, Huckriede AL, Haynes L, Gentleman B, Coyle K, Wilschut JC, et al. GLA-SE, a synthetic toll-like receptor 4 agonist, enhances T-cell responses to influenza vaccine in older adults. *J Infect Dis.* (2012) 205:466–73. doi: 10.1093/infdis/jir769
37. McKenzie A, Watt M, Gittleson C. ISCOMATRIX() vaccines: safety in human clinical studies. *Hum Vaccin* (2010) 6:237–46. doi: 10.4161/hv.6.3.10754
38. Stratmann T. Cholera Toxin Subunit B as adjuvant–an accelerator in protective immunity and a break in autoimmunity. *Vaccines* (2015) 3:579–96. doi: 10.3390/vaccines3030579
39. Allison AG, Gregoriadis G. Liposomes as immunological adjuvants. *Nature* (1974) 252:252. doi: 10.1038/252252a0
40. Schwendener RA. Liposomes as vaccine delivery systems: a review of the recent advances. *Ther Adv Vaccines* (2014) 2:159–82. doi: 10.1177/2051013614541440
41. Marasini N, Ghaffar KA, Skwarczynski M, Toth I. Liposomes as a vaccine delivery system. In: Skwarczynski M, Toth I, editors. *Micro and Nanotechnologies for Vaccine Development.* Oxford, UK: Elsevier Inc. (2017). p. 221–39. doi: 10.1016/B978-0-323-39981-4.00012-9
42. Ghaffar KA, Giddam AK, Zaman M, Skwarczynski M, Toth I. Liposomes as nanovaccine delivery systems. *Curr Top Med Chem.* (2014) 14:1194–208. doi: 10.2174/1568026614666140329232757
43. Giddam AK, Zaman M, Skwarczynski M, Toth I. Liposome-based delivery system for vaccine candidates: constructing an effective formulation. *Nanomedicine* (2012) 7:1877–93. doi: 10.2217/nnm.12.157
44. Tran TM, Li S, Doumbo S, Doumtabe D, Huang CY, Dia S, et al. An intensive longitudinal cohort study of Malian children and adults reveals no evidence of acquired immunity to *Plasmodium falciparum* infection. *Clin Infect Dis.* (2013) 57:40–7. doi: 10.1093/cid/cit174
45. Stanisic DI, Good MF. Examining cellular immune responses to inform development of a blood-stage malaria vaccine. *Parasitology* (2016) 143:208–23. doi: 10.1017/S0031182015001092
46. Fujioka H, Aikawa M. The malaria parasite and its life-cycle. In: editors M. Wahlgren and P. Perlmann, *Malaria Molecular and Clinical Aspects.* Amsterdam: Harwood Academic Publishers (1999). p. 19–53.
47. Chatterjee S, Wery M, Sharma P, Chauhan VS. A conserved peptide sequence of the *Plasmodium falciparum* circumsporozoite protein and antipeptide antibodies inhibit *Plasmodium berghei* sporozoite invasion of Hep-G2 cells and protect immunized mice against *P. berghei* sporozoite challenge. *Infect Immun.* (1995) 63:4375–81.
48. Sultan AA, Thathy V, Frevert U, Robson KJ, Crisanti A, Nussenzweig V, et al. TRAP is necessary for gliding motility and infectivity of *Plasmodium* sporozoites. *Cell* (1997) 90:511–22. doi: 10.1016/S0092-8674(00)80511-5
49. John CC, Zickafoose JS, Sumba PO, King CL, Kazura JW. Antibodies to the *Plasmodium falciparum* antigens circumsporozoite protein, thrombospondin-related adhesive protein, and liver-stage antigen 1 vary by ages of subjects and by season in a highland area of Kenya. *Infect Immun.* (2003) 71:4320–5. doi: 10.1128/IAI.71.8.4320-4325.2003
50. John CC, Moormann AM, Pregibon DC, Sumba PO, McHugh MM, Narum DL, et al. Correlation of high levels of antibodies to multiple pre-erythrocytic *Plasmodium falciparum* antigens and protection from infection. *Am J Trop Med Hyg.* (2005) 73:222–8. doi: 10.4269/ajtmh.2005.73.222
51. Offeddu V, Thathy V, Marsh K, Matuschewski K. Naturally acquired immune responses against *Plasmodium falciparum* sporozoites and liver infection. *Int J Parasitol.* (2012) 42:535–48. doi: 10.1016/j.ijpara.2012.03.011
52. Vanderberg JP, Frevert U. Intravital microscopy demonstrating antibody-mediated immobilisation of *Plasmodium berghei* sporozoites injected into skin by mosquitoes. *Int J Parasitol.* (2004) 34:991–6. doi: 10.1016/j.ijpara.2004.05.005
53. Sinnis P, Coppi A. A long and winding road: the *Plasmodium* sporozoite's journey in the mammalian host. *Parasitol Int.* (2007) 56:171–8. doi: 10.1016/j.parint.2007.04.002
54. Seder RA, Chang LJ, Enama ME, Zephir KL, Sarwar UN, Gordon IJ, et al. Protection against malaria by intravenous immunisation with a nonreplicating sporozoite vaccine (PfSPZ). *Science* (2013) 341:1359–65. doi: 10.1126/science.1241800
55. Ishizuka AS, Lyke KE, DeZure A, Berry AA, Richie TL, Mendoza FH, et al. Protection against malaria at 1 year and immune correlates following PfSPZ vaccination. *Nat Med.* (2016) 22:614–23. doi: 10.1038/nm.4110
56. Epstein JE, Paolino KM, Richie TL, Sedegah M, Singer A, Ruben AJ, et al. Protection against *Plasmodium falciparum* malaria by PfSPZ vaccine. *JCI Insight* (2017) 2:e89154. doi: 10.1172/jci.insight.89154
57. Lyke KE, Ishizuka AS, Berry AA, Chakravarty S, DeZure A, Enama ME, et al. Attenuated PfSPZ Vaccine induces strain-transcending T cells and durable protection against heterologous controlled human malaria infection. *Proc Natl Acad Sci USA.* (2017) 114:2711–6. doi: 10.1073/pnas.1615324114
58. Sissoko MS, Healy SA, Katile A, Omaswa F, Zaidi I, Gabriel EE, et al. Safety and efficacy of PfSPZ Vaccine against *Plasmodium falciparum* via direct venous inoculation in healthy malaria-exposed adults in Mali: a randomised, double-blind phase 1 trial. *Lancet Infect Dis.* (2017) 17:498–509. doi: 10.1016/S1473-3099(17)30104-4
59. Cohen J, Nussenzweig V, Nussenzweig R, Vekemans J, Leach A. From the circumsporozoite protein to the RTS, S/AS01 candidate vaccine. *Hum Vaccine* (2010) 6:90–6. doi: 10.4161/hv.6.1.9677
60. Agnandji ST, Lell B, Soulanoudjingar SS, Fernandes JF, Abossolo BP, et al. First results of phase 3 trial of RTS,S/AS01 malaria vaccine in African children. *N Engl J Med.* (2011) 365:1863–75. doi: 10.1056/NEJMoa1102287
61. Olotu A, Moris P, Mwacharo J, Vekemans J, Kimani D, Janssens M, et al. Circumsporozoite-specific T cell responses in children vaccinated with RTS,S/AS01E and protection against *P. falciparum* clinical malaria. *PLoS ONE* (2011) 6:e25786. doi: 10.1371/journal.pone.0025786
62. White MT, Verity R, Griffin JT, Asante KP, Owusu-Agyei S, Greenwood B, et al. Immunogenicity of the RTS,S/AS01 malaria vaccine and implications for duration of vaccine efficacy: secondary analysis of data from a phase 3 randomised controlled trial. *Lancet Infect Dis.* (2015) 15:1450–8. doi: 10.1016/S1473-3099(15)00239-X
63. Agnandji ST, Lell B, Fernandes JF, Abossolo BP, Methogo BG, et al. A phase 3 trial of RTS,S/AS01 malaria vaccine in African infants. *N Engl J Med.* (2012) 367:2284–95. doi: 10.1056/NEJMoa1208394
64. Schofield L, Villaquiran J, Ferreira A, Schellekens H, Nussenzweig R, Nussenzweig V. Gamma interferon, CD8+ T cells and antibodies required for immunity to malaria sporozoites. *Nature* (1987) 330:664–6. doi: 10.1038/330664a0
65. Weiss WR, Sedegah M, Beaudoin RL, Miller LH, Good MF. CD8+ T cells (cytotoxic/suppressors) are required for protection in mice immunized with malaria sporozoites. *Proc Natl Acad Sci USA.* (1988) 85:573–6. doi: 10.1073/pnas.85.2.573
66. Seguin MC, Klotz FW, Schneider I, Weir JP, Goodbary M, Slayter M, et al. Induction of nitric oxide synthase protects against malaria in mice exposed to irradiated *Plasmodium berghei* infected mosquitoes: involvement of interferon gamma and CD8+ T cells. *J Exp Med.* (1994) 180:353–8. doi: 10.1084/jem.180.1.353
67. Krzych U, Lyon JA, Jareed T, Schneider I, Hollingdale MR, Gordon DM, et al. T-lymphocytes from volunteers immunized with irradiated *Plasmodium falciparum* sporozoites recognize liver and blood-stage malaria antigens. *J Immunol.* (1995) 155:4072–7.
68. Doolan DL, Hoffman SL. IL-12 and NK cells are required for antigen-specific adaptive immunity against malaria initiated by CD8+ T cells in the *Plasmodium yoelii* model. *J Immunol.* (1999) 163:884–92.
69. Hoffman SL, Goh LM, Luke TC, Schneider I, Le TP, Doolan D, et al. Protection of humans against malaria by immunisation with radiation-attenuated *Plasmodium falciparum* sporozoites. *J Infect Dis.* (2002) 185:1155–64. doi: 10.1086/339409
70. Hollingdale MR, Krzych U. Immune responses to liver-stage parasites: implications for vaccine development. In: Perlmann P, Troye-Blomberg M, editors. *Malaria Immunology.* Basel: Karger (2002). p. 27.
71. Sinnis P, Nardin E. Sporozoite antigens: biology and immunology of the circumsporozoite protein and thrombospondin-related anonymous protein. In: Perlmann P, Troye-Blomberg M, editors. *Malaria Immunology* Basel: Karger (2002). p. 26.
72. Steers N, Schwenk R, Bacon DJ, Berenzon D, Williams J, Krzych U. The immune status of Kupffer cells profoundly influences their responses to infectious *Plasmodium berghei* sporozoites. *Eur J Immunol.* (2005) 35:2335–46. doi: 10.1002/eji.200425680

73. Roestenberg M, McCall M, Hopman J, Wiersma J, Luty AJ, van Gemert GJ, et al. Protection against a malaria challenge by sporozoite inoculation. *N Engl J Med.* (2009) 361:468–77. doi: 10.1056/NEJMoa0805832
74. Roestenberg M, Teirlinck AC, McCall MB, Teelen K, Makamdop KN, Wiersma J, et al. Long-term protection against malaria after experimental sporozoite inoculation: an open-label follow-up study. *Lancet* (2011) 377:1770–6. doi: 10.1016/S0140-6736(11)60360-7
75. Bijker EM, Bastiaens GJ, Teirlinck AC, van Gemert GJ, Graumans W, van de Vegte-Bolmer M, et al. Protection against malaria after immunisation by chloroquine prophylaxis and sporozoites is mediated by preerythrocytic immunity. *Proc Natl Acad Sci USA.* (2013) 110:7862–7. doi: 10.1073/pnas.1220360110
76. Mordmüller B, Surat G, Lagler H, Chakravarty S, Ishizuka AS, Lalremruata A, et al. Sterile protection against human malaria by chemoattenuated PfSPZ vaccine. *Nature* (2017) 542:445–9. doi: 10.1038/nature21060
77. Behet MC, Foquetm L, van Gemert GJ, Bijker EM, Meuleman P, Leroux-Roels G. Sporozoite immunisation of human volunteers under chemoprophylaxis induces functional antibodies against pre-erythrocytic stages of *Plasmodium falciparum. Malar J.* (2014) 13:136. doi: 10.1186/1475-2875-13-136
78. Stevenson MM, Riley EM. Innate immunity to malaria. *Nat Rev Immunol.* (2004) 4:169–80. doi: 10.1038/nri1311
79. Crompton PD, Moebius J, Portugal S, Waisberg M, Hart G, Garver LS, et al. Malaria immunity in man and mosquito: insights into unsolved mysteries of a deadly infectious disease. *Annu Rev Immunol.* (2014) 32:157–87. doi: 10.1146/annurev-immunol-032713-120220
80. Krishnegowda G, Hajjar AM, Zhu J, Douglass EJ, Uematsu S, Akira S, et al. Induction of proinflammatory responses in macrophages by the glycosylphosphatidylinositols of *Plasmodium falciparum*: cell signaling receptors, glycosylphosphatidylinositol (GPI) structural requirement, and regulation of GPI activity. *J Biol Chem.* (2005) 280:8606–16. doi: 10.1074/jbc.M413541200
81. Parroche P, Lauw FN, Goutagny N, Latz E, Monks BG, Visintin A, et al. Malaria hemozoin is immunologically inert but radically enhances innate responses by presenting malaria DNA to Toll-like receptor 9. *Proc Natl Acad Sci USA.* (2007) 104:1919–24. doi: 10.1073/pnas.0608745104
82. Shio MT, Eisenbarth SC, Savaria M, Vinet AF, Bellemare MJ, Harder KW, et al. Malarial hemozoin activates the NLRP3 inflammasome through Lyn and Syk kinases. *PLoS Pathog.* (2009) 5:e1000559. doi: 10.1371/annotation/abca067d-b82b-4de6-93c5-0fcc38e3df05
83. Sharma S, DeOliveira RB, Kalantari P, Parroche P, Goutagny N, Jiang, Z, et al. Innate immune recognition of an AT-rich stem-loop DNA motif in the *Plasmodium falciparum* genome. *Immunity* (2011) 35:194–207. doi: 10.1016/j.immuni.2011.05.016
84. Ing R, Stevenson MM. Dendritic cell and NK cell reciprocal cross talk promotes gamma interferon-dependent immunity to blood-stage *Plasmodium chabaudi* AS infection in mice. *Infect Immun.* (2009) 77:770–82. doi: 10.1128/IAI.00994-08
85. Stevenson MM, Ing R, Berretta F, Miu J. Regulating the adaptive immune response to blood-stage malaria: role of dendritic cells and CD4(+)Foxp3(+) regulatory T cells. *Int J Biol Sci.* (2011) 7:1311–22. doi: 10.7150/ijbs.7.1311
86. Urban BC, Ing R, Stevenson MM. Early interactions between blood-stage *Plasmodium* parasites and the immune system. *Curr Top Microbiol Immunol.* (2005) 297:25–70. doi: 10.1007/3-540-29967-X_2
87. Hansen DS, D'Ombrain MC, Schofield L. The role of leukocytes bearing natural killer complex receptors and killer immunoglobulin-like receptors in the immunology of malaria. *Curr Opin Immunol.* (2007) 19:416–23. doi: 10.1016/j.coi.2007.07.011
88. Porcherie A, Mathieu C, Peronet R, Schneider E, Claver J, Commere PH, et al. Critical role of the neutrophil-associated high-affinity receptor for IgE in the pathogenesis of experimental cerebral malaria. *J Exp Med.* (2011) 208:2225–36. doi: 10.1084/jem.20110845
89. Horowitz A, Newman KC, Evans JH, Korbel DS, Davis DM, Riley EM. Cross-talk between T cells and NK cells generates rapid effector responses to *Plasmodium falciparum*-infected erythrocytes. *J Immunol.* (2010) 184:6043–52. doi: 10.4049/jimmunol.1000106
90. Stanisic DI, Cutts J, Eriksson E, Fowkes FJ, Rosanas-Urgell A, Siba P, et al. γδ T cells and CD14+ monocytes are predominant cellular sources of cytokines and chemokines associated with severe malaria. *J Infect Dis.* 210:295–305. (2014). doi: 10.1093/infdis/jiu083
91. Jagannathan P, Kim CC, Greenhouse B, Nankya F, Bowen K, Eccles-James I, et al.. Loss and dysfunction of Vdelta2(+) gammadelta T cells are associated with clinical tolerance to malaria. *Sci Transl Med.* (2014) 6:251ra117. doi: 10.1126/scitranslmed.3009793
92. Kurup SP, Harty JT. γδ T cells and immunity to human malaria in endemic regions. *Ann Transl Med.* (2015) 3(Suppl. 1):S22. doi: 10.3978/j.issn.2305-5839.2015.02.22
93. Cohen S, Mc Gregor IA, Carrington S. Gamma-globulin and acquired immunity to human malaria. *Nature* (1961) 192:733–7. doi: 10.1038/192733a0
94. McGregor IA, Carrington SP, Cohen S. Treatment of East African *P. falciparum* malaria with West African human γ-globulin. *Trans R Soc Trop Med Hyg.* (1963) 57:170–5. doi: 10.1016/0035-9203(63)90058-0
95. Sabchareon A, Burnouf T, Ouattara D, Attanath P, Bouharoun-Tayoun H, Chantavanich P, et al. Parasitologic and clinical human response to immunoglobulin administration in falciparum malaria. *Am J Trop Med Hyg.* (1991) 45:297–308. doi: 10.4269/ajtmh.1991.45.297
96. Wåhlin B, Wahlgren M, Perlmann H, Berzins K, Björkman A, Patarroyo ME, et al. Human antibodies to a Mr 155,000 *Plasmodium falciparum* antigen efficiently inhibit merozoite invasion. *Proc Natl Acad Sci USA.* (1984) 81:7912–6.
97. Udeinya IJ, Schmidt JA, Aikawa M, Miller LH, Green I. *Falciparum* malaria-infected erythrocytes specifically bind to cultured human endothelial cells. *Science* (1981) 213:555–7. doi: 10.1126/science.7017935
98. Treutiger CJ, Hedlund I, Helmby H, Carlson J, Jepson A, Twumasi P, et al. Rosette formation in *Plasmodium falciparum* isolates and anti-rosette activity of sera from Gambians with cerebral or uncomplicated malaria. *Am J Trop Med Hyg.* (1992) 46:503–10. doi: 10.4269/ajtmh.1992.46.503
99. Bouharoun-Tayoun H, Oeuvray C, Lunel F, Druilhe P. Mechanisms underlying the monocyte-mediated antibody-dependent killing of *Plasmodium falciparum* asexual blood stages. *J Exp Med.* (1995) 182:409–18. doi: 10.1084/jem.182.2.409
100. Perlmann P, Troye-Blomberg M. Malaria and the immune system in humans. In: Perlmann P, Troye-Blomberg M, editors. *Malaria Immunology.* Basel: Kager (2002). p. 229–242. doi: 10.1159/000058846
101. Süss G, Eichmann K, Kury E, Linke A, Langhorne J. Roles of CD4- and CD8-bearing T lymphocytes in the immune response to the erythrocytic stages of *Plasmodium chabaudi. Infect Immun.* (1988) 56:3081–8.
102. Podoba JE, Stevenson MM. CD4+ and CD8+ T lymphocytes both contribute to acquired immunity to blood-stage *Plasmodium chabaudi* AS. *Infect Immun.* (1991) 59:51–8.
103. Amante FH, Good MF. Prolonged Th1-like response generated by a *Plasmodium yoelii*-specific T cell clone allows complete clearance of infection in reconstituted mice. *Parasite Immunol.* (1997) 19:16. doi: 10.1046/j.1365-3024.1997.d01-187.x
104. Langhorne J, Gillard S, Simon B, Slade S, Eichmann K. Frequencies of CD4+ T cells reactive with *Plasmodium chabaudi chabaudi*: distinct response kinetics for cells with Th1 and Th2 characteristics during infection. *Int Immunol.* (1989) 1:416–24. doi: 10.1093/intimm/1.4.416
105. Langhorne J, Meding SJ, Eichmann K, Gillard SS. The response of CD4+ T cells to *Plasmodium chabaudi chabaudi. Immunol Rev.* (1989) 112:71–94. doi: 10.1111/j.1600-065X.1989.tb00553.x
106. Perez-Mazliah D, Langhorne J. CD4 T-cell subsets in malaria: TH1/TH2 revisited. *Front Immunol.* (2015) 5:671. doi: 10.3389/fimmu.2014.00671
107. Pombo DJ, Lawrence G, Hirunpetcharat C, Rzepczyk C, Bryden M, Cloonan N, et al. Immunity to malaria after administration of ultra-low doses of red cells infected with *Plasmodium falciparum. Lancet* (2002) 360:610–7. doi: 10.1016/S0140-6736(02)09784-2
108. Edstein MD, Kotecka BM, Anderson KL, Pombo DJ, Kyle DE, Rieckmann KH, et al. Lengthy antimalarial activity of atovaquone in human plasma following atovaquone-proguanil administration. *Antimicrob Agents Chemother.* (2005) 49:4421–2. doi: 10.1128/AAC.49.10.4421-44 22.2005
109. Robinson LJ, D'Ombrain MC, Stanisic DI, Taraika J, Bernard N, Richards JS, et al. Cellular tumor necrosis factor, gamma interferon, and interleukin-6 responses as correlates of immunity and risk of clinical *Plasmodium*

falciparum malaria in children from Papua New Guinea. *Infect Immun.* (2009) 77:3033–43. doi: 10.1128/IAI.00211-09
110. Jagannathan P, Eccles-James I, Bowen K, Nankya F, Auma A, Wamala S, et al. IFNγ/IL-10 co-producing cells dominate the CD4 response to malaria in highly exposed children. *PLoS Pathog.* (2014) 10:e1003864. doi: 10.1371/journal.ppat.1003864
111. Boyle MJ, Jagannathan P, Bowen K, McIntyre TI, Vance HM, Farrington LA, et al. Effector phenotype of *Plasmodium falciparum*-specific CD4(+) T cells is influenced by both age and transmission intensity in naturally exposed populations. *J Infect Dis.* (2015) 212:416–25. doi: 10.1093/infdis/jiv054
112. Breitfeld D, Ohl L, Kremmer E, Ellwart J, Sallusto F, Lipp M, et al. Follicular B helper T cells express CXC chemokine receptor 5, localize to B cell follicles, and support immunoglobulin production. *J Exp Med.* (2000) 192:1545–52. doi: 10.1084/jem.192.11.1545
113. Schaerli P, Willimann K, Lang AB, Lipp M, Loetscher P, Moser B. CXC chemokine receptor 5 expression defines follicular homing T cells with B cell helper function. *J Exp Med.* (2000) 192:1553–62. doi: 10.1084/jem.192.11.1553
114. Kim CH, Rott LS, Clark-Lewis I, Campbell DJ, Wu L, Butcher EC. Subspecialization of CXCR5(+) T cells: B helper activity is focused in a germinal center-localized subset of CXCR5(+) T cells. *J Exp Med.* (2001) 193:1373–81. doi: 10.1084/jem.193.12.1373
115. Pérez-Mazliah D, Nguyen MP, Hosking C, McLaughlin S, Lewis MD, Tumwine I, et al. Follicular helper T cells are essential for the elimination of *Plasmodium* infection. *EBio Med.* (2017) 24:216–30. doi: 10.1016/j.ebiom.2017.08.030
116. Stockinger B, Kassiotis G, Bourgeois C. Homeostasis and T cell regulation. *Curr Opin Immunol.* (2004) 16:775–9. doi: 10.1016/j.coi.2004.09.003
117. Tang Q, Bluestone JA. The Foxp3+ regulatory T cell: a jack of all trades, master of regulation. *Nat Immunol.* (2008) 9:239–44. doi: 10.1038/ni1572
118. Omer FM, Riley EM. Transforming growth factor beta production is inversely correlated with severity of murine malaria infection. *J Exp Med.* (1998) 188:39–48. doi: 10.1084/jem.188.1.39
119. Day NP, Hien TT, Schollaardt T, Loc PP, Chuong LV, Chau TT, et al. The prognostic and pathophysiologic role of pro- and antiinflammatory cytokines in severe malaria. *J Infect Dis.* (1999) 180:1288–97. doi: 10.1086/315016
120. Li C, Corraliza I, Langhorne J. A defect in interleukin-10 leads to enhanced malarial disease in *Plasmodium chabaudi chabaudi* infection in mice. *Infect Immun.* (1999) 67:4435–42.
121. Dodoo D, Omer FM, Todd J, Akanmori BD, Koram KA, Riley EM. Absolute levels and ratios of proinflammatory and anti-inflammatory cytokine production *in vitro* predict clinical immunity to *Plasmodium falciparum* malaria. *J Infect Dis.* (2002) 185:971–9. doi: 10.1086/339408
122. Couper KN, Blount DG, Wilson MS, Hafalla JC, Belkaid Y, Kamanaka M, et al. IL-10 from CD4CD25Foxp3CD127 adaptive regulatory T cells modulates parasite clearance and pathology during malaria infection. *PLoS Pathog.* (2008) 4:e1000004. doi: 10.1371/journal.ppat.1000004
123. Scholzen A, Mittag D, Rogerson SJ, Cooke BM, Plebanski M. *Plasmodium falciparum*-mediated induction of human CD25Foxp3 CD4T cells is independent of direct TCR stimulation and requires IL-2, IL-10 and TGFbeta. *PLoS Pathog.* (2009) 5:e1000543. doi: 10.1371/journal.ppat.1000543
124. Nie CQ, Bernard NJ, Schofield L, Hansen DS. CD4+ CD25+ regulatory T cells suppress CD4+ T-cell function and inhibit the development of *Plasmodium berghei-specific* TH1 responses involved in cerebral malaria pathogenesis. *Infect Immun.* (2007) 75:2275–82. doi: 10.1128/IAI.01783-06
125. Cambos M, Bélanger B, Jacques A, Roulet A, Scorza T. Natural regulatory (CD4+CD25+FOXP+) T cells control the production of pro-inflammatory cytokines during *Plasmodium chabaudi adami* infection and do not contribute to immune evasion. *Int J Parasitol.* (2008) 38:229–38. doi: 10.1016/j.ijpara.2007.07.006
126. Hisaeda H, Maekawa Y, Iwakawa D, Okada H, Himeno K, Kishihara K, et al. Escape of malaria parasites from host immunity requires CD4+ CD25+ regulatory T cells. *Nat Med.* (2004) 10:29–30. doi: 10.1038/nm975
127. Amante FH, Stanley AC, Randall LM, Zhou Y, Haque A, McSweeney K, et al. A role for natural regulatory T cells in the pathogenesis of experimental cerebral malaria. *Am J Pathol.* (2007) 171:548–59. doi: 10.2353/ajpath.2007.061033
128. Finney OC, Riley EM, Walther M. Regulatory T cells in malaria - friend or foe? *Trends Immunol.* (2010) 31:63–70. doi: 10.1016/j.it.2009.12.002
129. Hansen DS, Schofield L. Natural regulatory T cells in malaria: host or parasite allies? *PLoS Pathog* (2010) 6:e1000771. doi: 10.1371/journal.ppat.1000771
130. Scholzen A, Minigo G, Plebanski M. Heroes or villains? T regulatory cells in malaria infection. *Trends Parasitol.* (2010) 26:16–25. doi: 10.1016/j.pt.2009.10.004
131. Walther M, Tongren JE, Andrews L, Korbel D, King E, Fletcher H, et al. Upregulation of TGF-beta, FOXP3, and CD4+CD25+ regulatory T cells correlates with more rapid parasite growth in human malaria infection. *Immunity* (2005) 23:287–96. doi: 10.1016/j.immuni.2005.08.006
132. Jangpatarapongsa K, Chootong P, Sattabongkot J, Chotivanich K, Sirichaisinthop J, Tungpradabkul S, et al. *Plasmodium vivax* parasites alter the balance of myeloid and plasmacytoid dendritic cells and the induction of regulatory T cells. *Eur J Immunol.* (2008) 38:2697–705. doi: 10.1002/eji.200838186
133. Minigo G, Woodberry T, Piera KA, Salwati E, Tjitra E, Kenangalem E, et al. Parasite-dependent expansion of TNF receptor II-positive regulatory T cells with enhanced suppressive activity in adults with severe malaria. *PLoS Pathog.* (2009) 5:e1000402. doi: 10.1371/journal.ppat.1000402
134. Bueno LL, Morais CG, Araújo FF, Gomes JA, Corrêa-Oliveira R, Soares IS, et al. *Plasmodium vivax*: induction of CD4+CD25+FoxP3+ regulatory T cells during infection are directly associated with level of circulating parasites. *PLoS ONE* (2010) 5:e9623. doi: 10.1371/journal.pone.0009623
135. Panichakul T, Sattabongkot J, Chotivanich K, Sirichaisinthop J, Cui L, Udomsangpetch R. Production of erythropoietic cells *in vitro* for continuous culture of *Plasmodium vivax*. *Int J Parasitol.* (2007) 37:1551–7. doi: 10.1016/j.ijpara.2007.05.009
136. Tamez PA, Liu H, Fernandez-Pol S, Haldar K, Wickrema A. Stage-specific susceptibility of human erythroblasts to *Plasmodium falciparum* malaria infection. *Blood* (2009) 114:3652–5. doi: 10.1182/blood-2009-07-231894
137. Lundie RJ, de Koning-Ward TF, Davey GM, Nie CQ, Hansen DS, Lau LS, et al. Blood-stage *Plasmodium* infection induces CD8+ T lymphocytes to parasite-expressed antigens, largely regulated by CD8alpha+ dendritic cells. *Proc Natl Acad Sci USA.* (2008) 105:14509–14. doi: 10.1073/pnas.0806727105
138. Imai T, Ishida H, Suzue K, Hirai M, Taniguchi T, Okada H, et al. CD8(+) T cell activation by murine erythroblasts infected with malaria parasites. *Sci Rep.* (2013) 3:1572. doi: 10.1038/srep01572
139. Imai T, Ishida H, Suzue K, Taniguchi T, Okada H, Shimokawa C, et al. Cytotoxic activities of CD8(+) T cells collaborate with macrophages to protect against blood-stage murine malaria. *Elife* (2015) 4:e04232. doi: 10.7554/eLife.04232
140. Imai T, Shen J, Chou B, Duan X, Tu L, Tetsutani K, et al. Involvement of CD8+ T cells in protective immunity against murine blood-stage infection with *Plasmodium yoelii* 17XL strain. *Eur J Immunol.* (2010) 40:1053–61. doi: 10.1002/eji.200939525
141. Horne-Debets JM, Faleiro R, Karunarathne DS, Liu XQ, Lineburg KE, Poh CM, et al. PD-1 dependent exhaustion of CD8+ T cells drives chronic malaria. *Cell Rep.* (2013) 5:1204–13. doi: 10.1016/j.celrep.2013.11.002
142. Mazumdar T, Anam K, Ali N. Influence of phospholipid composition on the adjuvanticity and protective efficacy of liposome-encapsulated Leishmania donovani antigens. *J Parasitol.* (2005) 91:269–74. doi: 10.1645/GE-356R1
143. van Houte AJ, Snippe H, Schmitz MG, Willers JM. Characterization of immunogenic properties of haptenated liposomal model membranes in mice. V Effect of membrane composition on humoral and cellular immunogenicity. *Immunology* (1981) 44:561–8.
144. Bakouche O, Gerlier D. Enhancement of immunogenicity of tumour virus antigen by liposomes: the effect of lipid composition. *Immunology* (1986) 58:507–13.
145. Mannock DA, Lee MY, Lewis RN, McElhaney RN. Comparative calorimetric and spectroscopic studies of the effects of cholesterol and epicholesterol on the thermotropic phase behaviour of dipalmitoylphosphatidylcholine bilayer membranes. *Biochim Biophys Acta* (2008) 1778:2191–202. doi: 10.1016/j.bbamem.2008.05.004
146. Christensen D, Henriksen-Lacey M, Kamath AT, Lindenstrøm T, Korsholm KS, Christensen JP, et al. A cationic vaccine adjuvant based

on a saturated quaternary ammonium lipid have different *in vivo* distribution kinetics and display a distinct CD4 T cell-inducing capacity compared to its unsaturated analog. *J Control Release* (2012) 160:468–76. doi: 10.1016/j.jconrel,.2012.03.016
147. Henriksen-Lacey M, Christensen D, Bramwell VW, Lindenstrøm T, Agger EM, Andersen P, et al. Liposomal cationic charge and antigen adsorption are important properties for the efficient deposition of antigen at the injection site and ability of the vaccine to induce a CMI response. *J Control Release* (2010) 145:102–8. doi: 10.1016/j.jconrel.2010.03.027
148. Henriksen-Lacey M, Bramwell VW, Christensen D, Agger EM, Andersen P, Perrie Y, et al. Liposomes based on dimethyldioctadecylammonium promote a depot effect and enhance immunogenicity of soluble antigen. *J Control Release* (2010) 142:180–6. doi: 10.1016/j.jconrel.2009.10.022
149. Basile L, Passirani C, Huynh NT, Béjaud J, Benoit JP, Puglisi G, et al. Serum-stable, long-circulating paclitaxel-loaded colloidal carriers decorated with a new amphiphilic PEG derivative. *Int J Pharm.* (2012) 426:231–8. doi: 10.1016/j.ijpharm.2012.01.038
150. Levchenko TS, Rammohan R, Lukyanov AN, Whiteman KR, Torchilin VP. Liposome clearance in mice: the effect of a separate and combined presence of surface charge and polymer coating. *Int J Pharm.* (2002) 240:95–102. doi: 10.1016/S0378-5173(02)00129-1
151. Kaur R, Bramwell VW, Kirby DJ, Perrie Y. Pegylation of DDA:TDB liposomal adjuvants reduces the vaccine depot effect and alters the Th1/Th2 immune responses. *J Control Release* (2012) 158:72–7. doi: 10.1016/j.jconrel.2011.10.012
152. Mann JF, Shakir E, Carter KC, Mullen AB, Alexander J, Ferro VA. Lipid vesicle size of an oral influenza vaccine delivery vehicle influences the Th1/Th2 bias in the immune response and protection against infection. *Vaccine* (2009) 27:3643–9. doi: 10.1016/j.vaccine.2009.03.040
153. Brewer JM, Pollock KG, Tetley L, Russell DG. Vesicle size influences the trafficking, processing, and presentation of antigens in lipid vesicles. *J Immunol* (2004) 173:6143–50. doi: 10.4049/jimmunol.173.10.6143
154. Manolova V, Flace A, Bauer M, Schwarz K, Saudan P, Bachmann MF. Nanoparticles target distinct dendritic cell populations according to their size. *Eur J Immunol.* (2008) 38:1404–13. doi: 10.1002/eji.200737984
155. Henriksen-Lacey M, Devitt A, Perrie Y. The vesicle size of DDA:TDB liposomal adjuvants plays a role in the cell-mediated immune response but has no significant effect on antibody production. *J Control Release* (2011) 154:131–7. doi: 10.1016/j.jconrel.2011.05.019
156. Ghaffar KA, Marasini N, Giddam AK, Batzloff MR, Good MF, Skwarczynski M, et al. The role of size in development of mucosal liposome-lipopeptide vaccine candidates against group A Streptococcus. *Med Chem.* (2016) 13:22–7. doi: 10.2174/1573406412666160720093138
157. Janeway CA. How the immune system works to protect the host from infection: a personal view. *Proc Natl Acad Sci USA.* (2001) 98:7461–8. doi: 10.1073/pnas.131202998
158. Gnjatic S, Sawhney NB, Bhardwaj N. Toll-like receptor agonists: are they good adjuvants? *Cancer J.* (2010) 16:382–91. doi: 10.1097/PPO.0b013e3181eaca65
159. Tong NK, Beran J, Kee SA, Miguel JL, Sánchez C, Bayas JM, et al. Immunogenicity and safety of an adjuvanted hepatitis B vaccine in pre-hemodialysis and hemodialysis patients. *Kidney Int.* (2005) 68:2298–303. doi: 10.1111/j.1523-1755.2005.00689.x
160. Monie A, Hung CF, Roden R, Wu TC. Cervarix: a vaccine for the prevention of HPV 16, 18-associated cervical cancer. *Biologics* (2008) 2:97–105.
161. Vyas SP, Goyal AK, Khatri K. Mannosylated liposomes for targeted vaccines delivery. *Methods Mol Biol.* (2010) 605:177–88. doi: 10.1007/978-1-60327-360-2_12
162. Marasini N, Giddam AK, Ghaffar KA, Batzloff MR, Good MF, Skwarczynski M, et al. Multilayer engineered nanoliposomes as a novel tool for oral delivery of lipopeptide-based vaccines against group A Streptococcus. *Nanomedicine* (2016) 11:1223–36. doi: 10.2217/nnm.16.36
163. Mohanan D, Slütter B, Henriksen-Lacey M, Jiskoot W, Bouwstra JA, Perrie Y, et al. Administration routes affect the quality of immune responses: a cross-sectional evaluation of particulate antigen-delivery systems. *J Control Release* (2010) 147:342–9.
164. Ballou WR, Rothbard J, Wirtz R, Gordon D, Williams J, Gore R, et al. Immunogenicity of synthetic peptides from circumsporozoite protein of *Plasmodium falciparum*. *Science* (1985) 228:996–9. doi: 10.1126/science.2988126
165. Alving CR, Richards RL, Moss J, Alving LI, Clements JD, Shiba T, et al. Effectiveness of liposomes as potential carriers of vaccines: applications to cholera toxin and human malaria sporozoite antigen. *Vaccine* (1986) 4:166–72. doi: 10.1016/0264-410X(86)90005-8
166. Richards RL, Hayre MD, Hockmeyer WT, Alving CR. Liposomes, lipid A, and aluminum hydroxide enhance the immune response to a synthetic malaria sporozoite antigen. *Infect Immun.* (1988) 56:682–6.
167. Alving CR, Richards RL, Hayre MD, Hockmeyer WT, Wirtz RA. Liposomes as carriers of vaccines: development of a liposomal malaria vaccine. In: Gregoriadis G, Allison AC, Poste G, editors. *Immunological Adjuvants and Vaccines.* Boston, MA: Springer (1989). p. 123–31. doi: 10.1007/978-1-4757-0283-5_13
168. Fries LF, Gordon DM, Richards RL, Egan JE, Hollingdale MR, Gross M, et al. Liposomal malaria vaccine in humans: a safe and potent adjuvant strategy. *Proc Natl Acad Sci USA.* (1992) 89:358–62. doi: 10.1073/pnas.89.1.358
169. Richards RL, Swartz GM, Schultz C, Hayre MD, Ward GS, Ballou WR, et al. Immunogenicity of liposomal malaria sporozoite antigen in monkeys: adjuvant effects of aluminium hydroxide and non-pyrogenic liposomal lipid A. *Vaccine* (1989) 7:506–12. doi: 10.1016/0264-410X(89)90274-0
170. Rutgers T, Gordon D, Gathoye AM, Hollingdale M, Hockmeyer W, Rosenberg M, et al. Hepatitis B surface antigen as carrier matrix for the repetitive epitope of the circumsporozoite protein of *Plasmodium Falciparum*. *Nat Biotechnol.* (1988) 6:1065–70. doi: 10.1038/nbt0988-1065
171. Gordon DM, McGovern TW, Krzych U, Cohen JC, Schneider I, LaChance R, et al. Safety, immunogenicity, and efficacy of a recombinantly produced *Plasmodium falciparum* circumsporozoite protein-hepatitis B surface antigen subunit vaccine. *J Infect Dis.* (1995) 171:1576–85. doi: 10.1093/infdis/171.6.1576
172. Ansong D, Asante KP, Vekemans J, Owusu SK, Owusu R, Brobby NA, et al. T cell responses to the RTS,S/AS01(E) and RTS,S/AS02(D) malaria candidate vaccines administered according to different schedules to Ghanaian children. *PLoS ONE* (2011) 6:e18891. doi: 10.1371/journal.pone.0018891
173. Owusu-Agyei S, Ansong D, Asante K, Kwarteng Owusu S, Owusu R, Wireko Brobby NA, et al. Randomized controlled trial of RTS,S/AS02D and RTS,S/AS01E malaria candidate vaccines given according to different schedules in Ghanaian children. *PLoS ONE* (2009) 4:e7302. doi: 10.1371/journal.pone.0007302
174. Kester KE, Cummings JF, Ofori-Anyinam O, Ockenhouse CF, Krzych U, Moris P, et al. Randomized, double-blind, phase 2a trial of *falciparum* malaria vaccines RTS,S/AS01B and RTS,S/AS02A in malaria-naive adults: safety, efficacy, and immunologic associates of protection. *J Infect Dis.* (2009) 200:337–46. doi: 10.1086/600120
175. Leroux-Roels G, Leroux-Roels I, Clement F, Ofori-Anyinam O, Lievens M, Jongert E, et al. Evaluation of the immune response to RTS,S/AS01 and RTS,S/AS02 adjuvanted vaccines: randomized, double-blind study in malaria-naive adults. *Hum Vaccin Immunother* (2014) 10:2211–9. doi: 10.4161/hv.29375
176. Olotu A, Fegan G, Wambua J, Nyangweso G, Leach A, Lievens M, et al. Seven-year efficacy of RTS,S/AS01 malaria vaccine among young african children. *N Engl J Med.* (2016) 374:2519–29. doi: 10.1056/NEJMoa1515257
177. Kazmin D, Nakaya HI, Lee EK, Johnson MJ, van der Most R., van den Berg RA, et al. Systems analysis of protective immune responses to RTS,S malaria vaccination in humans. *Proc Natl Acad Sci USA.* (2017) 114:2425–30. doi: 10.1073/pnas.1621489114
178. van den Berg RA, Coccia M, Ballou WR, Kester KE, Ockenhouse CF, Vekemans J, et al. Predicting RTS,S vaccine-mediated protection from transcriptomes in a malaria-challenge clinical trial. *Front Immunol.* (2017) 8:557. doi: 10.3389/fimmu.2017.00557
179. Good MF, Pombo D, Quakyi IA, Riley EM, Houghten RA, Menon A, et al. Human T-cell recognition of the circumsporozoite protein of *Plasmodium falciparum*: immunodominant T-cell domains map to the polymorphic regions of the molecule. *Proc Natl Acad Sci USA.* (1988) 85:1199–203. doi: 10.1073/pnas.85.4.1199
180. Neafsey DE, Juraska M, Bedford T, Benkeser D, Valim C, Griggs A, et al. Genetic Diversity and protective efficacy of the RTS,S/AS01 malaria vaccine. *N Engl J Med.* (2015) 373:2025–37. doi: 10.1056/NEJMoa1505819

181. Zevering Y, Khamboonruang C, Good MF. Natural amino acid polymorphisms of the circumsporozoite protein of *Plasmodium falciparum* abrogate specific human CD4+ T cell responsiveness. *Eur J Immunol.* (1994) 24:1418–25. doi: 10.1002/eji.1830240627
182. Collins KA, Snaith R, Cottingham MG, Gilbert SC, Hill AVS. Enhancing protective immunity to malaria with a highly immunogenic virus-like particle vaccine. *Sci Rep.* (2017) 7:46621. doi: 10.1038/srep46621
183. Ahmad M, Hirz M, Pichler H, Schwab H. Protein expression in *Pichia pastoris*: recent achievements and perspectives for heterologous protein production. *Appl Microbiol Biotechnol.* (2014) 98:5301–17. doi: 10.1007/s00253-014-5732-5
184. Tiwari S, Goyal AK, Mishra N, Khatri K, Vaidya B, Mehta A, et al. Development and characterization of novel carrier gel core liposomes based transmission blocking malaria vaccine. *J Control Release* (2009) 140:157–65. doi: 10.1016/j.jconrel.2009.08.004
185. Tiwari S, Goyal AK, Khatri K, Mishra N, Vyas SP. Gel core liposomes: an advanced carrier for improved vaccine delivery. *J Microencapsul* (2009) 26:75–82. doi: 10.1080/02652040802170897
186. Agger EM, Rosenkrands I, Hansen J, Brahimi K, Vandahl BS, Aagaard C, et al. Cationic liposomes formulated with synthetic mycobacterial cordfactor (CAF01): a versatile adjuvant for vaccines with different immunological requirements. *PLoS ONE* (2008) 3:e3116. doi: 10.1371/journal.pone.0003116
187. Tyagi RK, Garg NK, Jadon R, Sahu T, Katare OP, Dalai SK, et al. XElastic liposome-mediated transdermal immunisation enhanced the immunogenicity of *P. falciparum* surface antigen, MSP-119. *Vaccine* (2017) 33:4630–8. doi: 10.1016/j.vaccine.2015.06.054
188. Giddam AK, Reiman JM, Zaman M, Skwarczynski M, Toth I, Good MF. A semi-synthetic whole parasite vaccine designed to protect against blood stage malaria. *Acta Biomater.* (2016). doi: 10.1016/j.actbio.2016.08.020

7

The Role of IL-10 in Malaria: A Double Edged Sword

Rajiv Kumar[1,2]**, *Susanna Ng*[3] *and Christian Engwerda*[3]*

[1] *Department of Biochemistry, Institute of Science, Banaras Hindu University, Varanasi, India,* [2] *Centre of Experimental Medicine and Surgery, Institute of Medical Sciences, Banaras Hindu University, Varanasi, India,* [3] *Immunology and Infection Lab, QIMR Berghofer Medical Research Institute, Brisbane, QLD, Australia*

Correspondence:
Rajiv Kumar
rajiv082@yahoo.com
Christian Engwerda
christian.engwerda@qimr.edu.au

IL-10 produced by $CD4^+$ T cells suppresses inflammation by inhibiting T cell functions and the upstream activities of antigen presenting cells (APCs). IL-10 was first identified in Th2 cells, but has since been described in IFNγ-producing $Tbet^+$ Th1, $FoxP3^+$ $CD4^+$ regulatory T (Treg) and IL-17-producing $CD4^+$ T (Th17) cells, as well as many innate and innate-like immune cell populations. IL-10 production by Th1 cells has emerged as an important mechanism to dampen inflammation in the face of intractable infection, including in African children with malaria. However, although these type I regulatory T (Tr1) cells protect tissue from inflammation, they may also promote disease by suppressing Th1 cell-mediated immunity, thereby allowing infection to persist. IL-10 produced by other immune cells during malaria can also influence disease outcome, but the full impact of this IL-10 production is still unclear. Together, the actions of this potent anti-inflammatory cytokine along with other immunoregulatory mechanisms that emerge following *Plasmodium* infection represent a potential hurdle for the development of immunity against malaria, whether naturally acquired or vaccine-induced. Recent advances in understanding how IL-10 production is initiated and regulated have revealed new opportunities for manipulating IL-10 for therapeutic advantage. In this review, we will summarize our current knowledge about IL-10 production during malaria and discuss its impact on disease outcome. We will highlight recent advances in our understanding about how IL-10 production by specific immune cell subsets is regulated and consider how this knowledge may be used in drug delivery and vaccination strategies to help eliminate malaria.

Keywords: IL-10, malaria, protozoan, T cells, Inflammation

INTRODUCTION

Malaria remains a major public health problem in tropical and sub-tropical regions of the world despite substantial efforts to reduce associated morbidity and mortality. There are still around 250 million cases and 500,000 deaths annually, with young children in sub-Saharan Africa being most affected (1). A major unmet medical need for malaria is an effective vaccine. No vaccine tested to date in malaria endemic areas has performed as well as when tested in healthy volunteers, including RTS,S/AS01 (2–4).

$CD4^+$ T cells play critical roles in coordinating immune responses during infection by differentiating into functional subsets best suited to control pathogen growth (5). Diseases caused by intracellular protozoan parasites, such as *Plasmodium* species, require the generation of IFNγ-producing, $Tbet^+$ $CD4^+$ (Th1) cells to promote antigen capture and presentation by dendritic cells (DCs) and macrophages, as well as stimulate phagocytic cells to kill captured or resident pathogens (6). However, the inflammatory cytokines produced by Th1 cells can also damage tissues. In addition, recent data suggests that Th1 cell development may also influence the development of T follicular helper (Tfh) cells, another important $CD4^+$ T cell subset in malaria needed for the expansion of antigen-specific B cell populations and the production anti-parasitic antibody (7, 8). Hence, a better understanding about the development of $CD4^+$ T cell responses during malaria is needed to improve strategies aimed at improving anti-parasitic immunity.

The development of a robust host immune response is essential to eliminate parasites that cause malaria and protect against re-infection. Concurrently, these responses need to be tightly regulated to avoid immune-mediated damage to host tissue. This requires the establishment of immunoregulatory networks which ultimately determine the magnitude of immune response following infection. However, if these networks over-power anti-parasitic immunity too early, parasites can persist and cause associated disease. Many molecules and cell types contribute to these immunoregulatory networks, including anti-inflammatory cytokines such as interleukine-10 (IL-10) and transforming growth factor (TGF)β, immune check point molecules such as PD-1, CTLA-4, and LAG-3, as well as $CD4^+$ $FoxP3^+$ regulatory T (Treg) cells. However, our understanding about how immunoregulatory networks develop following *Plasmodium* infection and are maintained after resolution of infection is still incomplete.

One possible explanation for the failure of RTS,S/AS01 vaccine is the early imprinting of potent, pathogen-specific immunoregulatory networks in children following first exposure to malaria that prevents the generation of robust, vaccine-induced anti-parasitic immunity (9). Hence, targeting these networks may be critical step needed for malaria vaccines to stimulate long-lasting, anti-parasitic immunity in disease-endemic areas.

IL-10 has emerged as an important regulatory molecule in malaria that protects tissues by preventing excessive inflammation (10). It suppresses inflammation not only by directly dampening pro-inflammatory cytokine and/or chemokine production, but also by down-regulating the expression of MHC-II and co-stimulatory molecules on antigen presenting cells (APCs) and increasing expression of immune checkpoint molecules (11–13). IL-10 is secreted by many different cells, including B cells, Th1, Th2, Th17, and Treg cells, as well as innate immune cells such as macrophages and DCs (14). More recently, IL-10-producing Th1 (type 1 regulatory; Tr1) cells were found to develop relatively quickly in healthy volunteers participating in controlled human malaria infection (CHMI) studies and children living in malaria-endemic areas (15–18). Results from both pre-clinical malaria models and human studies show that IL-10 not only protects against severe disease, but also inhibits protective anti-parasitic immunity. In this review, we will discuss the role of IL-10 during the blood stage of experimental and human malaria, as well as describe the cellular sources of IL-10 and how the production of this potent anti-inflammatory cytokine is regulated. We will also examine how IL-10 mediated immune response may be manipulated to improve vaccine efficacy and/or current drug treatment regimes.

IL-10 AND MALARIA

The balance between host pro- and anti-inflammatory immune responses plays a critical role in determining the outcome of *Plasmodium* infection. A weak pro-inflammatory response may result in uncontrolled replication of parasites, while an excessive pro-inflammatory response may cause tissue damage, such as occurs in severe malaria syndromes, including cerebral malaria and multi-organ failure. Studies from mice have identified a clear role of IL-10 in controlling inflammatory responses and preventing tissue damage (14). IL-10-deficient mice infected with *P. chaubadi chaubadi* AS displayed exacerbated disease pathology, including hypoglycemia, hypothermia, and a loss in body weight, along with enhanced pro-inflammatory cytokine (IFN-γ, TNF-α, and IL-12) production (19). The excessive pro-inflammatory conditions in *P. chabaudi* AS-infected IL-10-deficient mice were also thought to cause parasite sequestration to the brain, associated with cerebral edema and hemorrhages (20). IL-10 has also been reported to play a protective role in experimental cerebral malaria (ECM) caused by *P. berghei* ANKA (21). In this model, decreased expression of IL-10 mRNA in spleen and brain tissue was associated with susceptibility to ECM. Sequestration of parasitized RBC (pRBC) in brain was mediated by ICAM-1 expressed by endothelial cells, and IL-10 inhibited expression of ICAM-I on these cells, thus providing a potential mechanism for the prevention of pathology associated with ECM. In a lethal *P. yoelii* infection in mice, production of IL-10 and TGF-β were thought to inhibit pro-inflammatory responses, and this was correlated with high parasitemia and severe anemia (22, 23). IL-10 has also been reported to promote hyper-parasitemia in mice infected with *P. chabaudi adami* (24). Therefore, data from mouse models of malaria indicates that IL-10 is required to protect host tissue from inflammation, but by doing so, can also promote growth of parasites and associated disease manifestations.

In a prospective longitudinal study conducted in a malaria endemic area, *IL10* gene polymorphisms associated with high IL-10 production were found to increase the risk of developing clinical malaria in young children (25). High levels of circulating IL-10 have been reported in patients with mild, severe and cerebral malaria (26, 27). Similar to studies in pre-clinical models, African children with severe anemia had lower plasma IL-10 levels than patients with moderate anemia or cerebral malaria, suggesting that IL-10 plays an important role in preventing severe anemia (28). However, a case control study in an African population with mild or severe malaria showed that both IL-10 and TNF-α were elevated in severe malaria and positively correlated with parasitemia (29). In another study with children living in a holo-endemic area of Western Kenya, higher ratios of plasma IL-10 to TNF levels were strongly associated with protection against severe malaria anemia, providing evidence that IL-10 may be protective by inhibiting TNF activity (30). This was supported by data from pre-clinical malaria models that have shown over-expression of TNF can suppress haematopoiesis in the bone marrow and promote RBC destruction (31), while IL-10 is thought to enhance hematopoietic activity (32). High levels of plasma TNF have also been associated with anemia and high-density *P. falciparum* infection in Zairian children (33), as well as being associated with other severe malaria complications such as renal failure (34). Thus, IL-10 appears to play a critical role in regulating the pathogenic effects of TNF during malaria, but in performing this important role, IL-10 may promote high-density infections that can result in other complications of malaria, including accumulation of pRBC in tissue that can cause hypoxia and direct damage to the vasculature.

IL-10 suppressed IL-12 production by monocytes (35), which was required for the development of protective immunity against malaria and skewing the cytokine production pattern toward a pro-inflammatory response (36, 37). A study in patients with severe malaria anemia living in a holo-endemic region of western Kenya showed that ingestion of *Plasmodium*-derived pigment (hemozoin; [PfHz]) by monocytes, suppressed IL-12 production in an IL-10-dependent manner (38). IFNγ signaling is critical for the development of hematopoietic progenitor subsets during acute experimental malaria (39), and given the important role for IL-12 in IFNγ production, reduced levels of IL-12 would likely impact hematopoiesis during malaria.

IL-10 can also augment antibody production and B cell maturation (37, 40). In experimental malaria caused by *P. yoelli* infection of C57BL/6 mice, B cell intrinsic IL-10 signaling enhanced germinal center (GC) B cell responses by limiting IFNγ activity and subsequent Tbet expression by these cells, thereby promoting antibody production and parasite clearance (41). Hence, IL-10 may be beneficial for the development of humoral immunity, but detrimental for cell-mediated immune responses during malaria.

CELLULAR SOURCES OF IL-10 DURING PLASMODIUM INFECTION

IL-10 production was initially identified in Th2 cells (42), but has since been shown to be produced by many immune cells, including Th1 cells (43, 44), Treg cells (45), IL-17-producing $CD4^+$ T (Th17) cells (46), Tfh cells (47), $CD8^+$ T cells (48), B cells (49), including regulatory B cells (50), NK cells (51), and γδ T cells (52, 53). Additionally, innate immune cells such as macrophages and DCs (12) have also been shown to produce IL-10. In both lethal and non-lethal mouse models caused by *P. yoelii* infection, the major source of IL-10 were FoxP3-negative $CD4^+$ T cells that didn't produce Th1, Th2, or Th17-associated cytokines, and these cells not only prevented hepatic immunopathology but also suppressed the effector T cell response, preventing parasite clearance (54). These regulatory cells are amongst several specialized $CD4^+$ T cell sub-populations which emerge from the thymus as conventional $CD4^+$ T cells and acquire regulatory functions in the periphery following exposure to inflammatory conditions (55–57). The most well-studied of these subsets are IL-10-producing Th1 (Tr1) cells that have been identified in many infectious diseases, including visceral leishmaniasis (58), tuberculosis (59), and human immunodeficiency virus (60). Importantly, they have also be identified as an important immunoregulatory cell population in African children with *P. falciparum* malaria (16–18, 61), as well as in healthy volunteers participating in CHMI studies (15). A high frequency of antigen-specific Tr1 cells were also found in neonates whose mothers had active placental malaria during pregnancy, suggesting that these cells might be able to influence anti-parasitic immunity from very early in life (62). Hence, the rapid generation of Tr1 cells during malaria may play a critical role in determining the outcome of infection. Furthermore, because these cells are likely to be generated prior to vaccination in malaria endemic areas, they are also likely to impact the efficacy of malaria vaccines, and their presence and function may be an important factor contributing to the failure of these vaccines to date.

γδ T cells play several different roles in host defense against *Plasmodium* infection (63), including their rapid expansion upon exposure to *P. falciparum* antigen in malaria naïve individuals (64). However, studies in children with chronic malaria exposure showed that the $V\delta2^+$ subset of γδ T cells declined in number and switched from a predominant pro-inflammatory response to an anti-inflammatory response that was postulated to contribute to clinical tolerance during malaria (52). Another recent study in a malaria endemic area found a subset of γδ T cells from uncomplicated malaria patients expressing Vδ9 T cell receptor that expanded and produced IFNγ and IL-10 when cultured in presence of *P. falciparum* antigen (53). Given that these γδ T cells produce IL-10 and can provide help to B cells for antibody production (65), they may play a role in the acquisition of natural immunity against malaria.

NK cells have also been reported to produce IL-10 during many systemic infections (66, 67). A recent study in mice infected with *P. berghei ANKA* showed that systemic inflammation during ECM stimulated NK cell IL-10 production but was induced too late to prevent inflammation-mediated disease pathology (51). However, in the same study, treatment of mice with recombinant IL-15 complexed with antibody to extend cytokine half-life and target NK cell induced IL-10 production which protected against disease without affecting the parasite burden.

REGULATION OF IL-10 BY CYTOKINES

Tr1 cells are an important immunoregulatory $CD4^+$ T cell subset that not only prevent immune pathology during *Plasmodium* infection but can also promote establishment of infection by suppressing Th1 cell-mediated anti-parasitic immunity. The manipulation of this regulatory T cell subset is being considered for a wide range of immunotherapeutic applications, including in organ transplantation, rheumatoid arthritis, colitis, and cancer (68–71). Therefore, a better understanding about how IL-10 production is initiated and maintained by Tr1 cells is required for the development of new therapeutic approaches targeting this cell population. Tr1 cells are $Tbet^+$ $Foxp3^-$ $CD4^+$ T cells that are most likely derived from Th1 cells, and acquire an ability to co-produce IL-10 and IFNγ under inflammatory conditions

(72). IL-27 has been identified as a critical regulator of T cell IL-10 production in humans and mice (46, 73–76). Generally, IL-27 produced by APC's, such as DC's and macrophages, can induce expression of the transcription factors c-Maf and aryl hydrocarbon receptor (Ahr) via STAT1 and STAT3-dependent mechanisms, which in turn, stimulated IL-21 production by CD4+ T cells which acted in an autocrine manner to expand IL-10-producing Tr1 cells (77–79) (**Figure 1**). In mouse models of malaria, a critical role for IL-27 signaling in the regulation of pro-inflammatory Th1 cell responses and suppression of immune-mediated pathology has been reported (80–83). A study with *P. chaubadi* AS infection showed that although Treg cells produced IL-10 during infection, Tr1 cells were the important source of IL-10 for protection against severe immune-mediated pathology, and that although the generation of these Tr1 cells was dependent on IL-27 signaling, it was independent of IL-21 (84). Similarly, another study with mice infected with *P. yoelli* confirmed that Tr1 cell generation was dependent on IL-27 receptor signaling during blood stage malaria (85). Thus, IL-27 is a critical regulator of IL-10 producing Tr1 cells in mouse models of malaria. The involvement of IL-27 in Tr1 cell generation in human malaria has not been fully established, although patients with severe malaria were reported to have reduced IL-27 plasma levels, compared to uncomplicated malaria patients and endemic controls, suggesting a potential role in controlling pathology (86). Additionally, many of the intracellular signaling

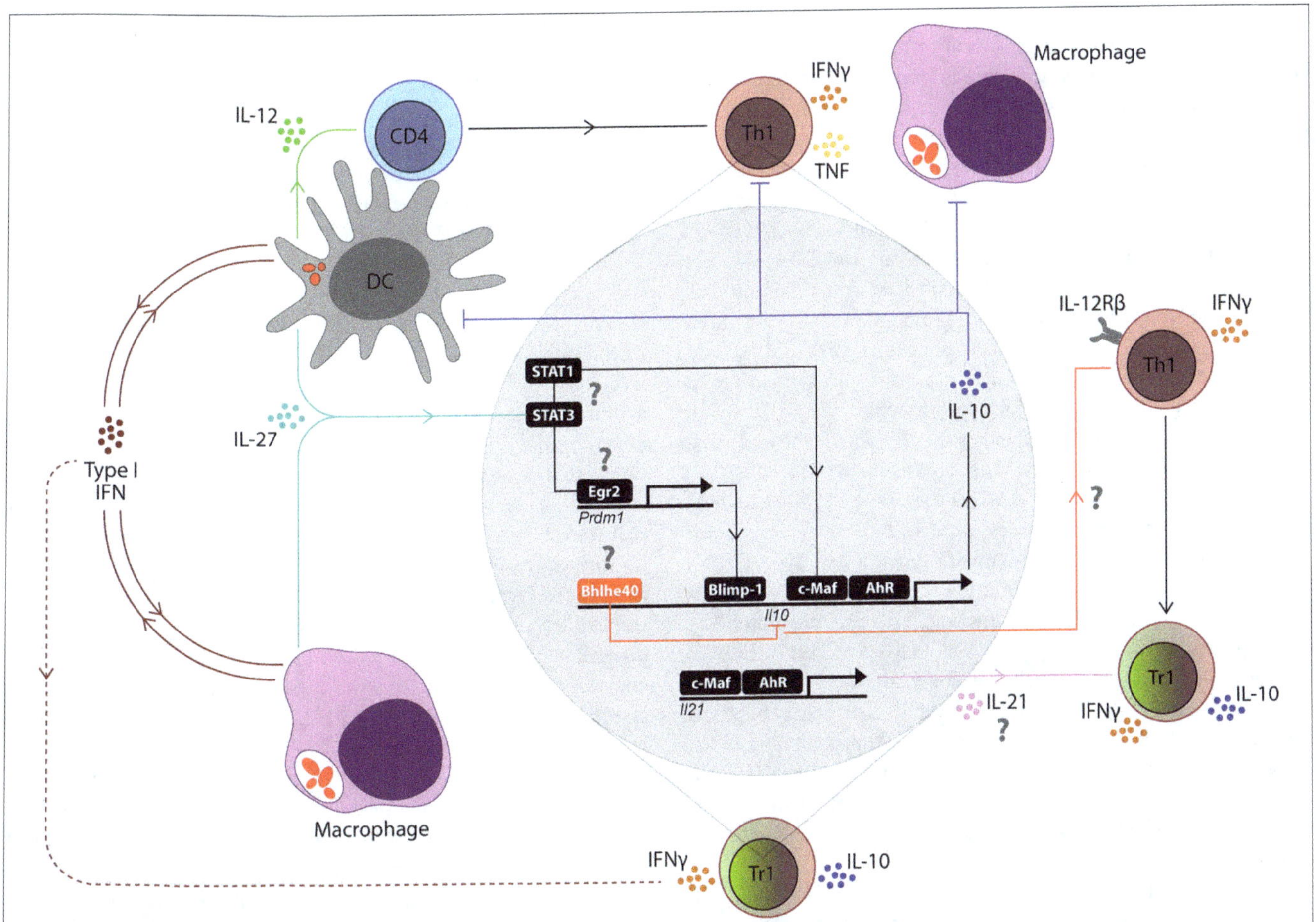

FIGURE 1 | Key regulators of the Th1/Tr1 cell axis in mouse malaria models. Following blood-stage infection with *Plasmodium* parasites, dendritic cells (DC's) recognize parasite molecules and produce IL-12 to drive the expansion of antigen-specific CD4+ T cells into IFNγ-producing Th1 cells. Soon after, type I interferon (IFN) and IL-27 production is initiated by macrophages and DC's, presumably in response to activation of pattern recognition receptors by parasite molecules. Type I IFNs promote the development of IL-10-producing Th1 (Tr1) cells by T cell-independent and T cell-dependent activities (dashed red line), depending on the *Plasmodium* species. IL-27 stimulates STAT1 and STAT3-dependent transcription of c-Maf and aryl hydrocarbon receptor (AhR) in Th1 cells, which then drive *IL-10* and *IL-21* gene transcription. T cell receptor signaling of Th1 cells promotes expression of the transcription factor Erg2, which in turn, induces *Prdm1* (encoding Blimp1) transcription and IL-10-production by Th1 cells in a STAT3-dependent manner. IL-21 acts as an autocrine growth factor for IL-10-producing Th1 (Tr1) cells. IL-10 produced by these cells can suppress the activity of Th1 cells and phagocytes, as well as the antigen presenting capacity of DC's and macrophages. However, the Bhlhe40 transcription factor can also be upregulated in Th1 cells to block *IL-10* gene transcription and promote IFNγ production and IL-12 receptor β (IL-12Rβ) chain expression, which both re-enforce Th1 cell development and activity. Thus, Bhlhe40 has an important role in determining the balance between Th1 and Tr1 cell development. The small red ellipsoids in DC's and macrophages represent captured parasites and associated antigens. The question marks (?) indicate pathways not yet validated in *Plasmodium* infections.

pathways described above and below (**Figure 1**) have yet to be confirmed in samples from experimental malaria or malaria patients. This is clearly an important gap in our knowledge. It should also be noted that Tr1 cells are likely to represent a heterogenous cell population (87), and cytokine production and responsiveness may be regulated distinctly, depending on local immune conditions.

More recently, type I interferons (IFNs) have emerged as important regulators of IL-10 production by Tr1 cells. Type I IFNs comprise a large family of cytokines that includes several types of IFNα and two types of IFNβ proteins which all signal through the common IFNα receptor (IFNAR) that consists of IFNAR1 and IFNAR2 chains which signal via STAT-1 and STAT-2 (88, 89) to mediate diverse functions during many infections (90). Polymorphisms in the *IFNAR1* gene have been associated with increased risk of severe malaria in The Gambia (91, 92), while a whole-brain transcriptional analysis in genetically resistant and susceptible inbred mice infected with *P. berghei* ANKA identified type I IFN-dependent transcriptional program associated with the pathogenesis of severe malaria ECM (93). Type I IFNs suppress $CD4^+$ T cell-dependent parasite control during experimental blood-stage malaria by modulating the function of $CD8\alpha^-$ cDC following *P. berghei* ANKA infection, rather than acting directly on $CD4^+$ T cells (94, 95). Another study in mice infected with *P. yoelli* YM showed that type I IFNs produced by plasmacytoid DCs (pDCs) activated conventional DCs (cDCs) and macrophages for generating B and T cell responses which are required for controlling parasitemia and mortality during late phase of infection (96). However, another study in mice infected with *P. yoelli* showed that type I IFNs directly promoted the expansion of Tr1 cells (97) (**Figure 1**). Significantly, in CHMI studies, type I IFNs produced by several different cell sources were found to be important regulators of developing anti-parasitic immunity. Type I IFNs not only suppressed innate immune cell function and parasitic-specific $CD4^+$ T cell IFNγ production, but also promoted the development of parasitic-specific Tr1 cells (9). Thus, IL-27 is a major mediator of Tr1 cell development in mouse models of malaria, but to date, the main driver of Tr1 cell generation identified in humans infected with *P. falciparum* are type I IFNs. Whether these results point to separate pathways for Tr1 cell generation in humans and mice is still not clear, but if so, this has significant ramifications for developing strategies to modulate Tr1 cells for clinical advantage.

TNF is a potent pro-inflammatory cytokine that has been implicated in malaria pathogenesis. As mentioned above, the ratio of plasma IL-10 to TNF plays an important role in determining whether children with malaria develop anemia. It is often assumed that the relationship between these two cytokines is characterized by IL-10 dampening the pro-inflammatory activity of TNF. However, TNF can also promote IL-10 production, as demonstrated by TNF playing a major role in lipopolysaccharide-induced IL-10 secretion by human monocytes (98). Similarly, TGFβ was reported to play a protective role against severe malaria in mice (99), and TGFβ can drive IL-10 production by several different $CD4^+$ T cell subsets, including Treg, Th17 and other FoxP3-negative cells (100). Therefore, modulation of IL-10 production in malaria may be achieved by targeting the activities of upstream activating cytokines, such as IL-27, IL-21, type I IFNs, TNF, or TGFβ. However, as indicated previously, the precise roles for these cytokines in clinical malaria still needs to be fully elucidated before these strategies can be developed and implemented.

TRANSCRIPTIONAL REGULATION OF IL-10

As discussed earlier, IL-10 can be produced by most $CD4^+$ T cell subsets in various inflammatory settings, but whether IL-10 production is mediated by common transcription factors or cell lineage-specific transcription factors is unclear. Many transcription factors, including c-Maf, have been shown to modulate *IL10* gene expression *in vitro* (77, 101, 102). The ligand-activated transcription factor Aryl hydrocarbon Receptor (AhR) has also been shown to promote the development of Tr1 cells in humans (102). During IL-27-mediated Tr1 cell differentiation, AhR physically associates with c-Maf and trans-activates the *IL10* and *IL21* promoters (78) (**Figure 1**). A recent study in mice infected with *P. chabaudi* AS showed that c-Maf regulates T cell IL-10 production and T cell-specific c-Maf-deficiency was associated with greater acute-phase pathology, compared to control mice, but had little effect on blood parasitemia, similar to the phenotype observed in IL-10-deficient mice (103). Thus, although c-Maf-dependent T cell IL-10 production protected against the detrimental impact of inflammation, it had a minimal effect of the development of anti-parasitic immunity in this non-lethal, mouse malaria model.

Another transcriptional regulator, B lymphocyte induced maturation protein (BLIMP)1, has been shown to play an important role in IL-10 production by Treg cells (104). BLIMP1 is induced by IL-12 in a STAT4-dependent manner and was shown to control IL-10 expression by Tr1 cells in mice infected with *Toxoplasma gondii* (105). In chronic lymphocytic choriomeningitis viral infection, as well as in central nervous system-related autoimmunity, BLIMP1 was identified as a critical regulator of IL-10 production by Tr1 cells (106, 107). IL-27-dependent production of the early growth response gene 2 (Egr2), a transcription factor required for T cell anergy induction, was also required for IL-10 production by Tr1 cells in a BLIMP1-dependent manner (108, 109). BLIMP1-mediated IL-10 production by Tr1 cells was recently reported in experimental malaria (97), and BLIMP1-dependent IL-10 production by Tr1 cells protected against IFNγ-dependent, TNF-mediated splenic tissue damage, but also limited the control of *P. chabaudi* AS blood parasitemia (110).

More recently, basic helix-loop-helix family member e40 (Bhlhe40) has been identified as a negative transcriptional regulator of IL-10 production during *Mycobacterium tuberculosis* (111) and *T. gondii* infection (112). Interestingly, Bhlhe40 regulated IL-10 production in both T cells and DCs during *M. tuberculosis* infection by binding directly to the *Il10* gene promoter in both cell populations (111). In the case of *T. gondii* infection, Bhlhe40 promoted Tbet-dependent IFNγ production by CD4+ T cells, while also suppressing IL-10 production in this cell population (112). Given the many similar mechanisms of T cell IL-10 generation between these two infectious diseases and malaria, it will be important to establish the role of this transcription factor in IL-10 production during *Plasmodium* infections. Another basic helix-loop-helix family member Twist-1 also regulates IL-10 production (113), although little is currently known about its role in infectious diseases settings.

Therefore, key transcriptional regulators of IL-10 production have been identified with potentially important roles in malaria (**Figure 1**), although as mentioned previously, many still need to be validated with samples from pre-clinical models of malaria or malaria patients. However, this area of research is still at an early stage and it will be necessary to carefully elucidate the specific cell populations in which these transcription factors operate, the range of genes they regulate and whether their modulation can change IL-10 activity to improve anti-parasitic immunity without causing tissue damage.

THERAPEUTIC MANIPULATION OF IL-10

IL-10 plays a critical role in the immunoregulatory networks that protect tissue from infection-mediated inflammation during malaria, and there is convincing mechanistic evidence form pre-clinical malaria models and associative data from malaria patient samples showing key roles for IL-10 is preventing several severe manifestations of malaria, including the development of anemia and damage to organs. These actions of IL-10 are like a double-edged sword, cutting both ways, as they can both suppress important anti-parasitic immune responses, and in particular, the functions of Th1 cell responses, but also protect the host from tissue damage. Furthermore, as mentioned above, IL-10 may also promote anti-parasitic antibody production by B cells. Therefore, given these beneficial and detrimental roles for IL-10 during malaria, it is critically important that we improve our understanding about how IL-10 production is regulated and the specific roles for IL-10 produced by different cell populations. We know that parasite-specific Tr1 cells develop early in children living in malaria endemic areas, as well as in healthy volunteers participating in CHMI studies with *P. falciparum*. However, given the important roles these cells play in preventing disease pathology, as outlined above, modulation of their activity to improve vaccine efficacy or the development of immunity after anti-parasitic drug treatment may be dangerous. However, if modulation of IL-10 production by specific cell populations or subsets can be achieved, leaving in place mechanisms to protect tissue from inflammatory mediators, then clinical benefits may be achieved. This will require the identification of unique cellular signaling pathways that regulate IL-10 production in different cell populations. In addition, strategies to target specific cell signaling pathways will need to be developed.

CONCLUDING REMARKS

IL-10 is a critical immunoregulatory molecule with both positive and negative roles during malaria. Blocking IL-10 activity may promote anti-parasitic immunity by enhancing APC functions and associated T cell activity. However, this will likely result in concomitant tissue pathology and related disease. Therefore, a more selective strategy for IL-10 modulation will be needed. As we identify the cell subsets producing this cytokine, and learn more about upstream regulators, the cell signaling pathways, transcription factors and post-translational modifications controlling IL-10 production, we may be able to manipulate IL-10 activity to improve anti-parasitic immunity in response to vaccination or drug treatment. Although IL-10 is a promising target for immune modulation, it is not the only such target for trying to improve outcomes in malaria. Immune checkpoint molecules, other anti-inflammatory cytokines and alternative host-directed therapies have also been identified (9, 57, 114). Ideally, different approaches should be tested in parallel to establish the safest and best approach to take. However, robust pre-clinical and clinical models will be required, as well as appropriate resourcing. The development of effective, long-lasting immunity to malaria through vaccination or drug-mediated strategies is an important priority, and our increasing knowledge should help make this possible.

AUTHOR CONTRIBUTIONS

RK and CE researched the work and wrote the paper. SN prepared the figure. All authors reviewed and edited the manuscript.

FUNDING

This work was made possible through Queensland State Government funding. It was supported by grants and fellowships from the National Health and Medical Research Council of Australia, as well as an Australian Post-graduate Awards through Griffith University and an INSPIRE Fellowship to RK provided by the Indian government Department of Science and Technology (DST).

ACKNOWLEDGMENTS

We thank staff in the QIMR Berghofer Infection and Immunity laboratory for helpful discussions and comments on the manuscript.

REFERENCES

1. *World Malaria Report Geneva*. World Health Organization (WHO) (2017) p. 1–186.
2. Polhemus ME, Remich SA, Ogutu BR, Waitumbi JN, Otieno L, Apollo S, et al. Evaluation of RTS, S/AS02A and RTS, S/AS01B in adults in a high malaria transmission area. *PLoS ONE* (2009) 4:e6465. doi: 10.1371/journal.pone.0006465

3. Ockenhouse CF, Regules J, Tosh D, Cowden J, Kathcart A, Cummings J, et al. Ad35. CS. 01-RTS, S/AS01 heterologous prime boost vaccine efficacy against sporozoite challenge in healthy malaria-naive adults. *PLoS ONE* (2015) 10:e0131571. doi: 10.1371/journal.pone.0131571
4. Kester KE, Cummings JF, Ofori-Anyinam O, Ockenhouse CF, Krzych U, Moris P, et al. Randomized, double-blind, phase 2a trial of falciparum malaria vaccines RTS, S/AS01B and RTS, S/AS02A in malaria-naive adults: safety, efficacy, and immunologic associates of protection. *J Infect Dis.* (2009) 200:337–46. doi: 10.1086/600120
5. Sallusto F. Heterogeneity of human CD4+ T cells against microbes. *Ann Rev Immunol.* (2016) 34:317–34. doi: 10.1146/annurev-immunol-032414-112056
6. Tubo NJ, Jenkins MK. CD4+ T cells: guardians of the phagosome. *Clin Microbiol Rev.* (2014) 27:200–13. doi: 10.1128/CMR.00097-13
7. Obeng-Adjei N, Portugal S, Tran TM, Yazew TB, Skinner J, Li S, et al. Circulating Th1-cell-type Tfh cells that exhibit impaired B cell help are preferentially activated during acute malaria in children. *Cell Rep.* (2015) 13:425–39. doi: 10.1016/j.celrep.2015.09.004
8. Ryg-Cornejo V, Ioannidis LJ, Ly A, Chiu CY, Tellier J, Hill DL, et al. Severe malaria infections impair germinal center responses by inhibiting T follicular helper cell differentiation. *Cell Rep.* (2016)14:68–81. doi: 10.1016/j.celrep.2015.12.006
9. Montes De Oca M, Good MF, McCarthy JS, Engwerda CR. The impact of established immunoregulatory networks on vaccine efficacy and the development of immunity to malaria. *J Immunol.* (2016) 197:4518–26. doi: 10.4049/jimmunol.1600619
10. Couper KN, Blount DG, Riley EM. IL-10: the master regulator of immunity to infection. *J Immunol.* (2008) 180:5771–7. doi: 10.4049/jimmunol.180.9.5771
11. Fiorentino DF, Zlotnik A, Vieira P, Mosmann TR, Howard M, Moore KW, O'Garra A. IL-10 acts on the antigen-presenting cell to inhibit cytokine production by Th1 cells. *J Immunol.* (1991) 146:3444–51.
12. Moore KW, de Waal Malefyt R, Coffman RL, O'Garra A. Interleukin-10 and the interleukin-10 receptor. *Ann Rev Immunol.* (2001) 19:683–765. doi: 10.1146/annurev.immunol.19.1.683
13. Mege L-J, Meghari S, Honstettre A, Capo C, Raoult D. The two faces of interleukin 10 in human infectious diseases. *Lancet Infect Dis.* (2006) 6:557–69. doi: 10.1016/S1473-3099(06)70577-1
14. A.do Rosario PF, Langhorne J. T cell-derived IL-10 and its impact on the regulation of host responses during malaria. *Int J Parasitol.* (2012) 42:549–55. doi: 10.1016/j.ijpara.2012.03.010
15. Montes de Oca, M, Kumar R, Rivera F, Amante F, Sheel M, Faleiro R, et al. Type I interferons regulate immune responses in humans with blood-stage *Plasmodium falciparum* infection. *Cell Rep.* (2016) 17:399–412. doi: 10.1016/j.celrep.2016.09.015
16. Walther M, Jeffries D, Finney OC, Njie M, Ebonyi A, Deininger S, et al. Distinct roles for FOXP3+ and FOXP3− CD4+ T cells in regulating cellular immunity to uncomplicated and severe *Plasmodium falciparum* malaria. *PLoS Pathog.* (2009) 5:e1000364. doi: 10.1371/journal.ppat.1000364
17. Jagannathan P, Eccles-James I, Bowen K, Nankya F, Auma A, Wamala S, et al. IFNγ/IL-10 co-producing cells dominate the CD4 response to malaria in highly exposed children. *PLoS Pathog.* (2014) 10:e1003864. doi: 10.1371/journal.ppat.1003864
18. Portugal S, Moebius J, Skinner J, Doumbo S, Doumtabe D, Kone Y, et al. Exposure-dependent control of malaria-induced inflammation in children. *PLoS Pathog.* (2014) 10:e1004079. doi: 10.1371/journal.ppat.1004079
19. Li C, Corraliza I, Langhorne J. A defect in interleukin-10 leads to enhanced malarial disease in *Plasmodium chabaudi chabaudi* infection in mice. *Infection Immunity* (1999) 67:4435–42.
20. Sanni LA, Jarra W, Li C, Langhorne J. Cerebral edema and cerebral hemorrhages in interleukin-10-deficient mice infected with *Plasmodium chabaudi*. *Infect Immun.* (2004) 72:3054–8. doi: 10.1128/IAI.72.5.3054-3058.2004
21. Kossodo S, Monso C, Juillard P, Velu T, Goldman M, Grau GE. Interleukin-10 modulates susceptibility in experimental cerebral malaria. *Immunology* (1997) 91:536–40. doi: 10.1046/j.1365-2567.1997.00290.x
22. Omer FM, de Souza JB, Riley EM. Differential induction of TGF-β regulates proinflammatory cytokine production and determines the outcome of lethal and nonlethal *Plasmodium yoelii* infections. *J Immunol.* (2003) 171:5430–36. doi: 10.4049/jimmunol.171.10.5430
23. Kobayashi F, Ishida H, Matsui T, Tsuji M. Effects of *in vivo* administration of anti-IL-10 or anti-IFN-γ monoclonal antibody on the host defense mechanism against *Plasmodium yoelii* yoelii infection. *J Vet Med Sci.* (2000) 62:583–7. doi: 10.1292/jvms.62.583
24. Weidanz WP, Batchelder JM, Flaherty P, LaFleur G, Wong C, Van der Heyde H. *Plasmodium chabaudi* adami: use of the B-cell-deficient mouse to define possible mechanisms modulating parasitemia of chronic malaria. *Exp Parasitol.* (2005) 111:97–104. doi: 10.1016/j.exppara.2005.06.006
25. Zhang G, Manaca MN, McNamara-Smith M, Mayor A, Nhabomba A, Berthoud TK, et al. IL-10 polymorphisms are associated with IL-10 production and clinical malaria in young children. *Infect Immun.* (2012) IAI:00261-12. doi: 10.1128/IAI.00261-12.
26. Peyron F, Burdin N, Ringwald P, Vuillez J, Rousset F, Banchereau J. High levels of circulating IL-10 in human malaria. *Clin Exp Immunol.* (1994) 95:300–3. doi: 10.1111/j.1365-2249.1994.tb06527.x
27. Lyke K, Burges R, Cissoko Y, Sangare L, Dao M, Diarra I, et al. Serum levels of the proinflammatory cytokines interleukin-1 beta (IL-1β), IL-6, IL-8, IL-10, tumor necrosis factor alpha, and IL-12 (p70) in Malian children with severe *Plasmodium falciparum* malaria and matched uncomplicated malaria or healthy controls. *Infect Immun.* (2004) 72:5630–7. doi: 10.1128/IAI.72.10.5630-5637.2004
28. Kurtzhals JA, Adabayeri V, Goka BQ, Akanmori BD, Oliver-Commey JO, Nkrumah FK, et al. Low plasma concentrations of interleukin 10 in severe malarial anaemia compared with cerebral and uncomplicated malaria. *Lancet* (1998) 351:1768–72. doi: 10.1016/S0140-6736(97)09439-7
29. Luty AJ, Perkins DJ, Lell B, Schmidt-Ott R, Lehman LG, Luckner D, et al. Low interleukin-12 activity in severe *Plasmodium falciparum* malaria. *Infect Immun.* (2000) 68:3909–15. doi: 10.1128/IAI.68.7.3909-3915.2000
30. Othoro C, Lal AA, Nahlen B, Koech D, Orago AS, Udhayakumar V. A low interleukin-10 tumor necrosis factor-α ratio is associated with malaria anemia in children residing in a holoendemic malaria region in western Kenya. *J Infect Dis.* (1999) 179:279–82. doi: 10.1086/314548
31. Taverne J, Sheikh N, De Souza J, Playfair J, Probert L, Kollias G. Anaemia and resistance to malaria in transgenic mice expressing human tumour necrosis factor. *Immunology* (1994) 82:397.
32. Van PV, Falla N, R.Van DH, Dasch J. Interleukin-10 stimulates hematopoiesis in murine osteogenic stroma. *Clin Orthop Related Res.* (1995) 313:103–14.
33. Shaffer N, Grau GE, Hedberg K, Davachi F, Lyamba B, Hightower AW, et al. Tumor necrosis factor and severe malaria. *J Infect Dis.* (1991) 163:96–101. doi: 10.1093/infdis/163.1.96
34. Day NP, Hien TT, Schollaardt T, Loc PP, Chuong LV, Chau TT, et al. The prognostic and pathophysiologic role of pro- and antiinflammatory cytokines in severe malaria. *J Infect Dis.* (1999) 180:1288–97. doi: 10.1086/315016
35. D'Andrea A, Rengaraju M, Valiante NM, Chehimi J, Kubin M, Aste M, et al. Production of natural killer cell stimulatory factor (interleukin 12) by peripheral blood mononuclear cells. *J Exp Med.* (1992) 176:1387–98. doi: 10.1084/jem.176.5.1387
36. Crutcher JM, Stevenson MM, Sedegah M, Hoffman SL. Interleukin-12 and malaria. *Res Immunol.* (1995) 146:552–9. doi: 10.1016/0923-2494(96)83031-8
37. Xu X, Sumita K, Feng C, Xiong X, Shen H, Maruyama S, et al. Down-regulation of IL-12 p40 gene in *Plasmodium berghei*-infected mice. *J Immunol.* (2001) 167:235–41. doi: 10.4049/jimmunol.167.1.235
38. Keller CC, Yamo O, Ouma C, Ong'echa JM, Ounah D, Hittner JB, et al. Acquisition of hemozoin by monocytes down-regulates interleukin-12 p40 (IL-12p40) transcripts and circulating IL-12p70 through an IL-10-dependent mechanism: *in vivo* and *in vitro* findings in severe malarial anemia. *Infect Immun.* (2006) 74:5249–60. doi: 10.1128/IAI.00843-06
39. Belyaev NN, Brown DE, Diaz AI, Rae A, Jarra W, Thompson J, et al. Induction of an IL7-R(+)c-Kit(hi) myelolymphoid progenitor critically dependent on IFN-gamma signaling during acute malaria. *Nat Immunol.* (2010) 11:477–85. doi: 10.1038/ni.1869
40. Heine G, Drozdenko G, Grun JR, Chang HD, Radbruch A, Worm M. Autocrine IL-10 promotes human B-cell differentiation into IgM-

or IgG-secreting plasmablasts. *Eur J Immunol.* (2014) 44:1615–21. doi: 10.1002/eji.201343822

41. Guthmiller JJ, Graham AC, Zander RA, Pope RL, Butler NS. Cutting edge: IL-10 is essential for the generation of germinal center B cell responses and anti-plasmodium humoral immunity. *J Immunol.* (2017) 198:617–22. doi: 10.4049/jimmunol.1601762
42. Fiorentino DF, Bond MW, Mosmann T. Two types of mouse T helper cell. IV. Th2 clones secrete a factor that inhibits cytokine production by Th1 clones. *J Exp Med.* (1989) 170:2081–95.
43. Meyaard L, Hovenkamp E, Otto SA, Miedema F. IL-12-induced IL-10 production by human T cells as a negative feedback for IL-12-induced immune responses. *J Immunol.* (1996) 156:2776–82.
44. Groux H, O'garra A, Bigler M, Rouleau M, Antonenko S, De Vries JE, et al. A CD4+ T-cell subset inhibits antigen-specific T-cell responses and prevents colitis. *Nature* (1997) 389:737. doi: 10.1038/39614
45. Rubtsov YP, Rasmussen JP, Chi EY, Fontenot J, Castelli L, Ye X, et al. Regulatory T cell-derived interleukin-10 limits inflammation at environmental interfaces. *Immunity* (2008) 28:546–58. doi: 10.1016/j.immuni.2008.02.017
46. Stumhofer JS, Silver JS, Laurence A, Porrett PM, Harris TH, Turka LA, et al. Interleukins 27 and 6 induce STAT3-mediated T cell production of interleukin 10. *Nat Immunol.* (2007) 8:1363. doi: 10.1038/ni1537
47. Laidlaw BJ, Lu Y, Amezquita RA, Weinstein JS, Vander Heiden JA, Gupta NT, et al. Interleukin-10 from CD4+ follicular regulatory T cells promotes the germinal center response. *Sci Immunol.* (2017) 2:eaan4767. doi: 10.1126/sciimmunol.aan4767
48. Sun J, Madan R, Karp CL, Braciale TJ. Effector T cells control lung inflammation during acute influenza virus infection by producing IL-10. *Nat Med.* (2009) 15:277. doi: 10.1038/nm.1929
49. Madan R, Demircik F, Surianarayanan S, Allen JL, Divanovic S, Trompette A, et al. Nonredundant roles for B cell-derived IL-10 in immune counter-regulation. *J Immunol.* (2009) 183:2312–20. doi: 10.4049/jimmunol.0900185
50. Liu Y, Chen Y, Li Z, Han Y, Sun Y, Wang Q, et al. Role of IL-10-producing regulatory B cells in control of cerebral malaria in *Plasmodium berghei* infected mice. *Eur J Immunol.* (2013) 43:2907–18. doi: 10.1002/eji.201343512
51. Burrack KS, Huggins MA, Taras E, Dougherty P, Henzler CM, Yang R, et al. Interleukin-15 complex treatment protects mice from cerebral malaria by inducing interleukin-10-producing natural killer cells. *Immunity* (2018) 48:760–72 e4. doi: 10.1016/j.immuni.2018.03.012
52. Jagannathan P, Kim CC, Greenhouse B, Nankya F, Bowen K, Eccles-James I, et al. Loss and dysfunction of Vdelta2(+) gammadelta T cells are associated with clinical tolerance to malaria. *Sci Transl Med.* (2014) 6:251ra117. doi: 10.1126/scitranslmed.3009793
53. Taniguchi T, Md Mannoor K, Nonaka D, Toma H, Li C, Narita M, etal. A unique subset of gammadelta T cells expands and produces IL-10 in patients with naturally acquired immunity against *Falciparum malaria*. *Front Microbiol.* (2017) 8:1288. doi: 10.3389/fmicb.2017.01288
54. Couper KN, Blount DG, Wilson MS, Hafalla JC, Belkaid Y, Kamanaka M, et al. IL-10 from CD4+ CD25- Foxp3- CD127- adaptive regulatory T cells modulates parasite clearance and pathology during malaria infection. *PLoS Pathog.* (2008) 4:e1000004. doi: 10.1371/journal.ppat.1000004
55. O'Garra A, Vieira PL, Vieira P, Goldfeld AE. IL-10–producing and naturally occurring CD4+ Tregs: limiting collateral damage. *J Clin Invest.* (2004) 114:1372–8. doi: 10.1172/JCI23215
56. Belkaid Y, Rouse BT. Natural regulatory T cells in infectious disease. *Nat Immunol.* (2005) 6:353. doi: 10.1038/ni1181
57. Engwerda CR, Ng SS, Bunn PT. The regulation of CD4+ T cell responses during protozoan infections. *Front Immunol.* (2014) 5:498. doi: 10.3389/fimmu.2014.00498
58. Nylen S, Maurya R, Eidsmo L, Manandhar KD, Sundar S, Sacks D. Splenic accumulation of IL-10 mRNA in T cells distinct from CD4+CD25+ (Foxp3) regulatory T cells in human visceral leishmaniasis. *J Exp Med.* (2007) 204:805–17. doi: 10.1084/jem.20061141
59. Kumar NP, Moideen K, Banurekha VV, Nair D, Sridhar R, Nutman TB, et al. IL-27 and TGFbeta mediated expansion of Th1 and adaptive regulatory T cells expressing IL-10 correlates with bacterial burden and disease severity in pulmonary tuberculosis. *Immun Inflamm Dis.* (2015) 3:289–99. doi: 10.1002/iid3.68
60. Chevalier MF, Didier C, Petitjean G, Karmochkine M, Girard PM, Barre-Sinoussi F, et al. Phenotype alterations in regulatory T-cell subsets in primary HIV infection and identification of Tr1-like cells as the main interleukin 10-producing CD4+ T cells. *J Infect Dis.* (2015) 211:769–79. doi: 10.1093/infdis/jiu549
61. Boyle MJ, Jagannathan P, Bowen K, McIntyre TI, Vance HM, Farrington LA, et al. The development of *Plasmodium falciparum*-specific il10 cD4 T cells and protection from malaria in children in an area of high malaria transmission. *Front Immunol.* (2017) 8:1329. doi: 10.3389/fimmu.2017.01329
62. Brustoski K, Möller U, Kramer M, Petelski A, Brenner S, Palmer DR, et al. IFN-γ and IL-10 mediate parasite-specific immune responses of cord blood cells induced by pregnancy-associated *Plasmodium falciparum* malaria. *J Immunol.* (2005) 174:1738–45. doi: 10.4049/jimmunol.174.3.1738
63. Deroost K, Langhorne J. Gamma/delta T cells and their role in protection against malaria. *Front Immunol.* (2018) 9:2973. doi: 10.3389/fimmu.2018.02973
64. Behr C, Dubois P. Preferential expansion of V gamma 9 V delta 2 T cells following stimulation of peripheral blood lymphocytes with extracts of *Plasmodium falciparum*. *Int Immunol.* (1992) 4:361–6.
65. Caccamo N, Todaro M, La Manna MP, Sireci G, Stassi G, Dieli F. IL-21 regulates the differentiation of a human gammadelta T cell subset equipped with B cell helper activity. *PLoS ONE* (2012) 7:e41940. doi: 10.1371/journal.pone.0041940
66. Maroof A, Beattie L, Zubairi S, Svensson M, Stager S, Kaye PM. Posttranscriptional regulation of Il10 gene expression allows natural killer cells to express immunoregulatory function. *Immunity* (2008) 29:295–305. doi: 10.1016/j.immuni.2008.06.012
67. Tarrio ML, Lee SH, Fragoso MF, Sun HW, Kanno Y, O'Shea JJ, et al. Proliferation conditions promote intrinsic changes in NK cells for an IL-10 response. *J Immunol.* (2014) 193:354–63. doi: 10.4049/jimmunol.1302999
68. Mfarrej B, Tresoldi E, Stabilini A, Paganelli A, Caldara R, Secchi A, et al. Generation of donor-specific Tr1 cells to be used after kidney transplantation and definition of the timing of their in vivo infusion in the presence of immunosuppression. *J Transl Med.* (2017) 15:40. doi: 10.1186/s12967-017-1133-8
69. Roncarolo MG, Gregori S, Bacchetta R, Battaglia M. Tr1 cells and the counter-regulation of immunity: natural mechanisms and therapeutic applications. *Curr Top Microbiol Immunol.* (2014) 380:39–68. doi: 10.1007/978-3-662-43492-5_3
70. Bacchetta R, Lucarelli B, Sartirana C, Gregori S, Stanghellini L, Teresa M, et al. Immunological outcome in haploidentical-HSC transplanted patients treated with IL-10-anergized donor T cells. *Front Immunol.* (2014) 5:16. doi: 10.3389/fimmu.2014.00016
71. Desreumaux P, Foussat A, Allez M, Beaugerie L, Hébuterne X, Bouhnik Y, et al. Safety and efficacy of antigen-specific regulatory T-cell therapy for patients with refractory Crohn's disease. *Gastroenterology* (2012) 143:1207–17. e2. doi: 10.1053/j.gastro.2012.07.116
72. Jankovic D, Kullberg MC, Feng CG, Goldszmid RS, Collazo CM, Wilson M, et al. Conventional T-bet+ Foxp3- Th1 cells are the major source of host-protective regulatory IL-10 during intracellular protozoan infection. *J Exp Med.* (2007) 204:273–83. doi: 10.1084/jem.20062175
73. Murugaiyan G, Mittal A, Lopez-Diego R, Maier LM, Anderson DE, Weiner HL. IL-27 is a key regulator of IL-10 and IL-17 production by human CD4+ T cells. *J Immunol.* (2009)183:2435–43. doi: 10.4049/jimmunol.0900568
74. Awasthi A, Carrier Y, Peron JP, Bettelli E, Kamanaka M, Flavell RA, et al. A dominant function for interleukin 27 in generating interleukin 10–producing anti-inflammatory T cells. *Nat Immunol.* (2007) 8:1380. doi: 10.1038/ni1541
75. Ansari NA, Kumar R, Gautam S, Nylén S, Singh OP, Sundar S, et al. IL-27 and IL-21 are associated with T cell IL-10 responses in human visceral leishmaniasis. *J Immunol.* (2011) 186:3977–85. doi: 10.4049/jimmunol.1003588
76. Anderson CF, Stumhofer JS, Hunter CA, Sacks D. IL-27 regulates IL-10 and IL-17 from CD4+ cells in nonhealing Leishmania major infection. *J Immunol.* (2009) 183:4619–27. doi: 10.4049/jimmunol.0804024
77. Pot C, Jin H, Awasthi A, Liu SM, Lai CY, Madan R, et al. Cutting edge: IL-27 induces the transcription factor c-Maf, cytokine IL-21, and the costimulatory receptor ICOS that coordinately act together to promote

differentiation of IL-10-producing Tr1 cells. *J Immunol.* (2009) 183:797–801. doi: 10.4049/jimmunol.0901233
78. Apetoh L, Quintana FJ, Pot C, Joller N, Xiao S, Kumar D, et al. The aryl hydrocarbon receptor interacts with c-Maf to promote the differentiation of type 1 regulatory T cells induced by IL-27. *Nat Immunol.* (2010) 11:854. doi: 10.1038/ni.1912
79. Spolski R, Kim H-P, Zhu W, Levy DE, Leonard WJ. IL-21 mediates suppressive effects via its induction of IL-10. *J Immunol.* (2009) 182:2859–67. doi: 10.4049/jimmunol.0802978
80. Villegas-Mendez A, de Souza JB, Lavelle SW, Findlay EG, Shaw TN, van Rooijen N, et al. IL-27 receptor signalling restricts the formation of pathogenic, terminally differentiated Th1 cells during malaria infection by repressing IL-12 dependent signals. *PLoS Pathog.* (2013) 9:e1003293. doi: 10.1371/journal.ppat.1003293
81. Findlay EG, Villegas-Mendez A, O'Regan N, de Souza JB, Grady LM, Saris CJ, et al. IL-27R signalling regulates memory CD4+ T cell populations and suppresses rapid inflammatory responses during secondary malaria infection. *Infect Immun.* (2013) IAI:01091-13. doi: 10.1128/IAI.01091-13
82. Kimura D, Miyakoda M, Kimura K, Honma K, Hara H, Yoshida H, et al. Interleukin-27-producing CD4+ T cells regulate protective immunity during malaria parasite infection. *Immunity* (2016) 44:672–82. doi: 10.1016/j.immuni.2016.02.011
83. Findlay EG, Greig R, Stumhofer JS, Hafalla JC, de Souza JB, Saris CJ, et al. Essential role for IL-27 receptor signaling in prevention of Th1-mediated immunopathology during malaria infection. *J Immunol.* (2010) 185:2482–92 doi: 10.4049/jimmunol.0904019
84. do Rosário APF, Lamb T, Spence P, Stephens R, Lang A, Roers A, et al. IL-27 promotes IL-10 production by effector Th1 CD4+ T cells: a critical mechanism for protection from severe immunopathology during malaria infection. *J Immunol.* (2011) 188:1178–90. doi: 10.4049/jimmunol.1102755
85. Villegas-Mendez A, Shaw TN, Inkson CA, Strangward P, de Souza JB, Couper KN. Parasite-specific CD4+ IFN-γ+ IL-10+ T cells distribute within both lymphoid and non-lymphoid compartments and are controlled systemically by IL-27 and ICOS during blood-stage malaria infection. *Infect Immun.* (2015) IAI:01100–15. doi: 10.1128/IAI.01100-15
86. Ayimba E, Hegewald J, Segbena A, Gantin R, Lechner C, Agosssou A, et al. Proinflammatory and regulatory cytokines and chemokines in infants with uncomplicated and severe *Plasmodium falciparum* malaria. *Clin Exp Immunol.* (2011) 166:218–26. doi: 10.1111/j.1365-2249.2011.04474.x
87. Brockmann L, Soukou S, Steglich B, Czarnewski P, Zhao L, Wende S, et al. Molecular and functional heterogeneity of IL-10-producing CD4(+) T cells. *Nat Commun.* (2018) 9:5457. doi: 10.1038/s41467-018-07581-4
88. Ivashkiv LB, Donlin LT. Regulation of type I interferon responses. *Nat Rev Immunol.* (2014) 14:36–49. doi: 10.1038/nri3581
89. Pestka S, Krause CD, Walter MR. Interferons, interferon-like cytokines, and their receptors. *Immunol. Rev.* (2004) 202:8–32. doi: 10.1111/j.0105-2896.2004.00204.x
90. McNab F, Mayer-Barber K, Sher A, Wack A, O'garra A. Type I interferons in infectious disease. *Nat Rev Immunol.* (2015) 15:87. doi: 10.1038/nri3787
91. Aucan C, Walley A, Hennig B, Fitness J, Frodsham A, Zhang L, et al. Interferon-alpha receptor-1 (IFNAR1) variants are associated with protection against cerebral malaria in the Gambia. *Genes Immun.* (2003) 4:275. doi: 10.1038/sj.gene.6363962
92. Khor CC, Vannberg FO, Chapman SJ, Walley A, Aucan C, Loke H, et al. Positive replication and linkage disequilibrium mapping of the chromosome 21q22. 1 malaria susceptibility locus. *Genes Immun.* (2007) 8:570. doi: 10.1038/sj.gene.6364417
93. Lovegrove FE, Gharib SA, Patel SN, Hawkes CA, Kain KC, Liles WC. Expression microarray analysis implicates apoptosis and interferon-responsive mechanisms in susceptibility to experimental cerebral malaria. *Am J Pathol.* (2007) 171:1894–903. doi: 10.2353/ajpath.2007.070630
94. Haque A, Best SE, De Oca MM, James KR, Ammerdorffer A, Edwards CL, et al. Type I IFN signaling in CD8–DCs impairs Th1-dependent malaria immunity. *J Clin Invest.* (2014) 124:2483–96. doi: 10.1172/JCI70698
95. Haque A, Best SE, Ammerdorffer A, Desbarrieres L, de Oca MM, Amante FH, et al. Type I interferons suppress CD4+ T-cell-dependent parasite control during blood-stage Plasmodium infection. *Eur J Immunol.* (2011) 41:2688–98. doi: 10.1002/eji.201141539
96. Yu X, Cai B, Wang M, Tan P, Ding X, Wu J, et al. Cross-regulation of two type I interferon signaling pathways in plasmacytoid dendritic cells controls anti-malaria immunity and host mortality. *Immunity* (2016) 45:1093–107. doi: 10.1016/j.immuni.2016.10.001
97. Zander RA, Guthmiller JJ, Graham AC, Pope RL, Burke BE, Carr DJ, Butler NS. Type I interferons induce T regulatory 1 responses and restrict humoral immunity during experimental malaria. *PLoS Pathog.* (2016) 12:e1005945. doi: 10.1371/journal.ppat.1005945
98. Wanidworanun C, Strober W. Predominant role of tumor necrosis factor-alpha in human monocyte IL-10 synthesis. *J Immunol.* (1993) 151:6853–61.
99. Omer FM, Riley EM. Transforming growth factor β production is inversely correlated with severity of murine malaria infection. *J Exp Med.* (1998) 188:39–48.
100. Saraiva M, O'garra A. The regulation of IL-10 production by immune cells. *Nat Rev Immunol.* (2010) 10:170. doi: 10.1038/nri2711
101. Xu J, Yang Y, Qiu G, Lal G, Wu Z, Levy DE, et al. c-Maf regulates IL-10 expression during Th17 polarization. *J Immunol.* (2009) 182:6226–36. doi: 10.4049/jimmunol.0900123
102. Gandhi R, Kumar D, Burns EJ, Nadeau M, Dake B, Laroni A, et al. Activation of the aryl hydrocarbon receptor induces human type 1 regulatory T cell–like and Foxp3+ regulatory T cells. *Nature Immunol.* (2010) 11:846. doi: 10.1038/ni.1915
103. Gabryšová L, Alvarez-Martinez M, Luisier R, Cox LS, Sodenkamp J, Hosking C, et al. c-Maf controls immune responses by regulating disease-specific gene networks and repressing IL-2 in CD4+ T cells. *Nat Immunol.* (2018) 19:497. doi: 10.1038/s41590-018-0083-5
104. Cretney E, Xin A, Shi W, Minnich M, Masson F, Miasari M, et al. The transcription factors Blimp-1 and IRF4 jointly control the differentiation and function of effector regulatory T cells. *Nat Immunol.* (2011) 12:304. doi: 10.1038/ni.2006
105. Neumann C, Heinrich F, Neumann K, Junghans V, Mashreghi MF, Ahlers J, et al. Role of Blimp-1 in programing Th effector cells into IL-10 producers. *J Exp Med.* (2014) 211:1807–19. doi: 10.1084/jem.20131548
106. Heinemann C, Heink S, Petermann F, Vasanthakumar A, Rothhammer V, Doorduijn E, et al. IL-27 and IL-12 oppose pro-inflammatory IL-23 in CD4+ T cells by inducing Blimp1. *Nat Commun.* (2014) 5:3770. doi: 10.1038/ncomms4770
107. Parish IA, Marshall HD, Staron MM, Lang PA, Brüstle A, Chen JH, et al. Chronic viral infection promotes sustained Th1-derived immunoregulatory IL-10 via BLIMP-1. *J Clin Invest.* (2014) 124:3455–468. doi: 10.1172/JCI66108
108. Iwasaki Y, Fujio K, Okamura T, Yanai A, Sumitomo S, Shoda H, et al. Egr-2 transcription factor is required for Blimp-1-mediated IL-10 production in IL-27-stimulated CD4+ T cells. *Eur J Immunol.* (2013) 43:1063–73. doi: 10.1002/eji.201242942
109. Okamura T, Fujio K, Shibuya M, Sumitomo S, Shoda H, Sakaguchi S, et al. CD4+ CD25– LAG3+ regulatory T cells controlled by the transcription factor Egr-2. *Proc Nat Acad Sci USA.* 106 (2009) 13974–79. doi: 10.1073/pnas.0906872106
110. Montes de Oca M, Kumar R, de Labastida Rivera F, Amante FH, Sheel M, Faleiro RJ, et al. Blimp-1-dependent IL-10 production by Tr1 cells regulates TNF-mediated tissue pathology. *PLoS Pathog.* (2016) 12:e1005398. doi: 10.1371/journal.ppat.1005398
111. Huynh JP, Lin CC, Kimmey JM, Jarjour NN, Schwarzkopf EA, Bradstreet TR, et al. Bhlhe40 is an essential repressor of IL-10 during *Mycobacterium tuberculosis* infection. *J Exp Med.* (2018) 215:1823–38 doi: 10.1084/jem.20171704

112. Yu F, Sharma S, Jankovic D, Gurram RK, Su P, Hu G, et al. The transcription factor Bhlhe40 is a switch of inflammatory versus antiinflammatory Th1 cell fate determination. *J Exp Med.* (2018) 215:1813–21. doi: 10.1084/jem.20170155
113. Zheng S, Hedl M, Abraham C. Twist1 and Twist2 contribute to cytokine downregulation following chronic NOD2 stimulation of human macrophages through the coordinated regulation of transcriptional repressors and activators. *J Immunol.* (2015) 195:217–26. doi: 10.4049/jimmunol.1402808
114. Wykes MN, Lewin SR. Immune checkpoint blockade in infectious diseases. *Nat Rev Immunol.* (2018) 18:91–104. doi: 10.1038/nri.2017.112

8

Novel Strategies for Malaria Vaccine Design

Augustina Frimpong [1,2,3], Kwadwo Asamoah Kusi [1,2], Michael Fokuo Ofori [1,2] and Wilfred Ndifon [3,4*]*

[1] Department of Biochemistry, Cell and Molecular Biology, West African Centre for Cell Biology of Infectious Pathogens, College of Basic and Applied Sciences, University of Ghana, Accra, Ghana, [2] Immunology Department, College of Health Sciences, Noguchi Memorial Institute for Medical Research, University of Ghana, Accra, Ghana, [3] African Institute for Mathematical Sciences, Cape Coast, Ghana, [4] African Institute for Mathematical Sciences, University of Stellenbosch, Cape Town, South Africa

***Correspondence:**
Augustina Frimpong
tinafrimp@gmail.com
Wilfred Ndifon
wndifon@aims.ac.za

The quest for a licensed effective vaccine against malaria remains a global priority. Even though classical vaccine design strategies have been successful for some viral and bacterial pathogens, little success has been achieved for *Plasmodium falciparum,* which causes the deadliest form of malaria due to its diversity and ability to evade host immune responses. Nevertheless, recent advances in vaccinology through high throughput discovery of immune correlates of protection, lymphocyte repertoire sequencing and structural design of immunogens, provide a comprehensive approach to identifying and designing a highly efficacious vaccine for malaria. In this review, we discuss novel vaccine approaches that can be employed in malaria vaccine design.

Keywords: *Plasmodium falciparum,* malaria, vaccine, immunoinformatics, structure-based, lymphocyte repertoire sequencing

THE GLOBAL MALARIA SITUATION

Malaria caused by *Plasmodium* parasites remains a major infectious disease of public health importance. The disease is caused by five protozoan species, namely *Plasmodium falciparum, P. vivax, P. malariae, P. ovale,* and *P. knowlesi.* The deadliest of these is *P. falciparum* which is predominant in sub-Saharan Africa (SSA). In 2016, approximately $2.7 billion was invested globally in control and elimination programs (1). Meanwhile, it was estimated in 2016 that nearly half of the world's population was at risk of infection, with 91% of the estimated deaths being in Africa and 70% of the mortality occurring in children under 5 years (1). Notwithstanding, preventive control and intervention measures have helped decrease the burden between 2000 and 2015. For instance, the incidence of new malaria cases was down by 37% world wide and 42% for the WHO African region. In addition, the incidence of mortality over the same period decreased by about 60% globally and 66% for the African region (2). Yet, malaria imposes huge economic losses for people in the African Region and there is a need to upscale the available interventions and introduce new ones such as a licensed cost-effective vaccine (3).

CHALLENGES TO THE ERADICATION OF MALARIA

Malaria eradication faces many challenges including insecticide resistance, emerging anti-malarial drug resistance and the presence of asymptomatic and submicroscopic infections.

Indoor residual spraying (IRS) and long-lasting insecticidal nets (LLINs), have been among the most effective tools for malaria control and elimination (4). So far, pyrethroids are the only recommended class of insecticides for LLINs. However, more than 30 countries have reported resistance to pyrethroids, which has the potential to spread to new areas (5–9).

The rapid development of pyrethroid resistance suggests that alternative classes of insecticides need to be identified. As a result, WHO has cautioned against the use of pyrethroids (8), raising the need for alternative measures of control. The development of resistance to malaria drugs by *P. falciparum* remains a major threat to malaria elimination. The WHO-recommended first line treatment for uncomplicated malaria caused by *Plasmodium falciparum* is the artemisinin-based combination therapies (ACTs). Historically, *P. falciparum* has been able to develop resistance to almost all previous first-line antimalarial drugs (10, 11). The development of resistance to these drugs almost always begins from South-East Asia, where mutant parasites resistant to antimalarial drugs are more likely to survive due to lower levels of acquired immunity, poor adherence to administered drugs and higher parasite burdens (11–14). *P. falciparum* resistance to artemisinin-based drugs seems to have emerged sporadically (15), with mutations for resistance found within the kelch 13 propeller gene (15, 16). An inevitable fact is that artemisinin resistance may be imminent and other intervention avenues such as the development of highly effective vaccines need to be rapidly explored.

Also, the presence of asymptomatic and submicroscopic infections poses a major threat to malaria eradication and control. Continuous exposure to infectious mosquito bites leads to the development of anti-disease and anti-parasite immunity. The level of this immunity is determined by the transmission intensity and epidemiology of the disease (17, 18). It has been shown that the microscopic prevalence of malaria is almost half of that detected by nucleic acid amplification techniques and lower in low transmission areas (19, 20). The prevalence of submicroscopic infections has been found to be high in low transmission areas and common in children, probably as a result of a less robust immune response, leading to insufficient time for the development of protective immunity. In addition, asymptomatic infections may persist for several months and serve as a major threat to malaria eradication (21) as they sustain disease transmission (22–25).

CURRENT APPROACHES TO DEVELOPING A MALARIA VACCINE

Malaria Vaccines

The acquisition of partial immunity and the successful treatment of clinical symptoms of malaria in children with purified immunoglobulins from semi-immune adults (26) are positive indications of the feasibility of a vaccine against malaria. This is also supported by the induction of sterile immunity in both animal models and controlled human malaria infection (CHMI) through immunization with either live or attenuated sporozoites and merozoite-infected red cells (27–29). Attenuated sporozoites, even though they still maintain their natural hepatocyte invasion ability, do not fully mature in the liver and hence do not form merozoites that are responsible for the clinical symptoms of malaria (30).

Vaccine Targets

There are three stages to target for a potential malaria vaccine candidate. The first target of vaccine development is the pre-erythrocytic stage. This is the period where sporozoites travel through blood and infect hepatocytes to undergo schizogony, the vigorous multiplication stage that precedes the invasion of red blood cells (RBCs). The main purpose of developing a vaccine against this stage is to inhibit hepatocyte infections and hepatic parasite development, thus limiting RBC invasion (27, 30). The mechanisms of protection for this stage may involve antibody responses that prevent sporozoites from invading hepatocytes or cytotoxic T cells that destroy infected liver cells. So far, the licensed RTS,S, subunit vaccine remains the most advanced malaria vaccine to be developed. Other candidate vaccines include the whole-parasite vaccine candidates such as *Pf* sporozoite (PfSPZ), PfSPZ vaccination with chemoprophylaxis (PfSPZ-CVac) and the genetically attenuated parasite (PfSPZ-GAP).

The second target for malaria vaccine candidate design is the blood-stage of the parasite. The motivation for developing such vaccine candidates comes from evidence that people with repeated malaria infections in endemic areas develop some level of protective immunity, a state in which there is immune-controlled RBC invasion, resulting in fewer disease symptoms or asymptomatic infections (26, 31). Accordingly, vaccine candidates have been designed to elicit immune responses that will block/limit merozoite invasion of RBCs and stop the rapid replication of merozoites by targeting parasite surface proteins such merozoite surface proteins, apical membrane antigen 1 (AMA1), and the reticulocyte homolog (Rh) proteins (32–35). Other blood-stage vaccines target parasite antigens embedded in infected RBC membranes, such as *P. falciparum* Erythrocyte Membrane Protein-1 (PfEMP1) (36).

Despite being highly immunogenic and showing good promise as vaccine candidates, most of these antigens are also highly polymorphic and hence elicit antigen and parasite strain-specific responses (32, 33). Conversely, antigens such as the Rh proteins that show a high level of conservation (34, 35) tend to be less immunogenic (37).

The third malaria vaccine candidate target is the sexual parasite forms or gametocytes. Malaria transmission-blocking vaccines (TBVs) are designed to interrupt parasite transmission between humans and the mosquito vector through host immunological response to parasite targeted proteins such as Pfs230, Pfs45, Pfs48 (pre-fertilization antigens) and Pfs25, Pfs28 (post-fertilization antigens). Successful malaria transmission depends on the availability of infectious gametocytes in human

Abbreviations: ACTs, artemisinin-based combination therapies; PfEMP1, *P. falciparum* Erythrocyte Membrane Protein-1; MSP1, Merozoite Surface Protein; AMA1, Apical Membrane Antigen 1; Rh, Reticulocyte homolog (Rh); MHC, Major histocompatibility complex; HLA, Human leukocyte antigen; PfSPZ, *Pf* sporozoite; PfCVac, *Pf* chemoprophylaxis vaccination; PfGAP, *Pf* genetically attenuated parasite; TBV, transmission-blocking vaccines; BCR, B cell receptor; bnMAb, broadly neutralizing monoclonal antibody; TCR, T cell receptor; VIMT, Vaccine that interrupt malaria transmission; SSM-VIMT, Sexual, sporogenic or mosquito stage VIMT; PE-VIMT, pre-erythrocytic VIMT.

peripheral blood that can be taken up by mosquitoes during a blood meal. Studies have reported that the degree of infectivity of gametocytes to mosquitoes is based on the gametocyte density, drug stress, clonality of infection and immune defenses of the mosquito (38–42). However, according to Churcher et al. (38), even at very low densities, gametocytes remain infectious to mosquitoes. Also, it has been reported that in the human host, transmission can be stable at very low densities and is not directly proportional to the gametocyte density in peripheral blood (43, 44). Basically, a TBV exploits the fact that there is a functional immunological activity against the sexual stage parasite proteins which is able to reduce the infectivity of the parasite, thereby decreasing malaria transmission (45, 46). Vaccine candidates that seek to interrupt malaria transmission (VIMT) are of two main types: (1) sexual, sporogenic or mosquito stage VIMT (SSM-VIMT) candidates which are expected to interrupt human-to-mosquito transmission; and (2) the pre-erythrocytic VIMT (PE-VIMT) candidates, which are expected to interrupt mosquito-to-human transmission (47). Among the TBV candidates, only Pfs25 and Pfs230 have undergone clinical trials in human (48–51). Unfortunately, a major challenge with these candidate vaccines is the inability to elicit higher antibody titers. In regards, there are considerations to conjugate these candidate vaccines (50, 52).

Current Status of Malaria Vaccine Development

After decades of extensive research, the pre-erythrocytic stage vaccine, RTS,S has been licensed and is expected to undergo further testing in malaria endemic areas before possible approval for immunization. Currently, together with RTS,S, only 20 candidate vaccines are undergoing clinical trials (**Table 1**). For RTS,S, a recent evaluation on the safety and immunogenicity of the vaccine co-administered with the recommended expanded programme on immunization showed the vaccine to be safe and immunogenic with no related adverse events (58). The RTS,S/AS01 consists of a recombinant protein of the *P. falciparum* circumsporozoite protein (CSP) conjugated to a hepatitis B virus surface antigen. During clinical trials, the efficacy of the vaccine after 4 doses was observed to be 43.9% in children aged 5–17 months and 27.8% in children 6–12 weeks old (59). However, vaccine efficacy wanes with time and fails to meet the target set by the Malaria Vaccine Technology Roadmap (60). Consequently, other vaccination regimens such as the number of doses, time of immunization, and alternative approaches for vaccination are being evaluated (61).

Also, the R21, a virus-like particle vaccine which is a biosimilar of RTS,S consists of the CSP conjugated to a single hepatitis B surface antigen. The RTS,S-like vaccine has been shown to provide sterile protection in mice at very low doses. In addition, it was observed that most of the immune responses elicited against the candidate vaccine targeted the CSP in contrast to the hepatitis B surface antigen which is often targeted in the RTS,S vaccinated individuals (53). Importantly, this candidate vaccine is designed such that more epitopes of the CSP may be exposed to host immune system to enhance the efficacy of R21.

Furthermore, the whole sporozoite vaccine has been reported to provide significant protection against falciparum malaria. The whole organism candidate vaccine design approaches include the radiation-attenuated sporozoites (PfSPZ), whole PfSPZ with chemoprophylaxis (PfCVac) and the genetically modified sporozoites (PfGAP). Even though PfCVac showed complete protection to homologous *P. falciparum strain,* moderate protection has been observed with heterologous strains in non-exposed vaccines (62). Clinical trials with PfSPZ in endemic areas have been shown to be safe and well tolerated, however, inducing low level of immune responses compared to naïve individuals (63, 64). These may suggest that the breadth of immune responses to PfSPZ vaccines need to be increased by considering other vaccination regimens.

PROMISING APPROACHES TO MALARIA VACCINE DEVELOPMENT

Recent technological advances have greatly improved the prospects for designing an effective malaria vaccine through advances in high-throughput biology and computation. These alternative approaches may be focused on the parasite- or host immune system.

The Parasite-Focused Approach

The technologies involved in this approach center on the identification of immunogenic antigens from the pathogen by interrogating the parasite's genome, transcriptome or proteome. It may modify the structure of the antigenic component(s) identified with the aim of targeting various strains of the pathogen. The parasite-focused approach further tests the immunogenicity and safety of the candidate antigens to design novel and improved vaccines. This approach may involve the application of reverse vaccinology, structural vaccinology, and immunoinformatics.

Reverse Vaccinology

Reverse vaccinology, developed by Rappouli et al. is a technology first used in *Meningococcus* serogroup B bacteria to identify novel vaccine antigens (**Figure 1**). Here, the pathogen's genome is sequenced and analyzed to have access to the entire repertoire of proteins and enable comparison of conserved sequences shared among pathogens of the same species (65). Genomic data is analyzed using bioinformatics tools, taking into consideration all open reading frames. Also, with the use of computational tools, genomic sequences that are homologous to those of humans are eliminated from the vaccine candidates identified. The remaining genes are isolated and inserted into a suitable vector to obtain proteins for testing in animal models. Responses to the vaccine antigens are analyzed in immunized mice to validate their immunogenicity and efficacy levels. Importantly, molecular epidemiology studies are undertaken using various strains of the pathogen to ascertain whether the selected antigens are conserved or highly variable in a given population (66). This approach has been used to develop vaccines against serogroup B *Neisseria meningitidis* (67); and identify vaccine candidates for, *S. agalactia* and *S. pyogenes* (68, 69). This vaccine design approach

TABLE 1 | Current malaria vaccines in clinical trials.

Vaccine candidate	Clinical trial registration number	Clinical trial stage
PRE-ERYTHROCYTIC		
RTS,S/AS01	NCT01345240	Phase 3
R21/AS01B	NCT02600975	Phase 1
R21/ME-TRAP	NCT02905019 (53)	Phase 2
ChAd63/MVA ME-TRAP	NCT01635647 (54–56)	Phase 2
R21/Matrix-M1	NCT02572388/NCT02925403	Phase 1/2
PfSPZ Vaccine	NCT03510481	Phase 1
PfSPZ-CVac (PfSPZ Challenge + chloroquine or + chloroquine/pyrimethamine	NCT03083847	Phase 1
GAP 3KO (52-/36-/sap1-)	NCT02313376	Phase 1
BLOOD-STAGE		
pfAMA1-DiCo	NCT02014727 (57)	Phase 1
P27A	NCT01949909	Phase 2
PAMVAC	NCT02647489	Phase 1
PRIMVAC	NCT02658253	Phase 1
SEXUAL-STAGE		
ChAd63 Pfs25-IMX313/MVA Pfs25-IMX313	NCT02532049	Phase 1
Pfs25-EPA/Alhydrogel	NCT01867463, 51	Phase 1
Pfs230D1M-EPA/Alhydrogel and/or Pfs25-EPA/Alhydrogel	NCT02334462	Phase 1
Pfs25M-EPA/AS01 and/or Pfs230D1M-EPA/ASOI	NCT02942277	Phase 1
Pfs25 VLP-FhCMB	NCT02013687	Phase 1
Pfs25-Pfs25	NCT00977899	Phase 1
Pfs25 & Pvs/Monatide ISA 51	NCT00295581	Phase 1

Adapted from WHO. 9/28/2018. Malaria Vaccine Rainbow Tables. http://www.who.int/vaccine_research/links/Rainbow/en/index.html.

has greatly enhanced the discovery and characterization of several pathogen antigens.

Reverse vaccinology has been applied in malaria to identify parasite proteins either secreted or involved in signaling for consideration as possible vaccine candidates. The genomic sequence of *P. falciparum* has been available since 2002 (70). In addition, the sequence of other diverse *Plasmodium spp* including primate (71, 72) and rodent (73) parasites have been published. Comparative analysis of these sequences has shown similar homologs between species with possibly similar functions. For instance, the conserved Pf48/45 and PfHAP2 genes, both of which are transmission blocking vaccine candidates, functions were determined based on the role of their homologs in other *Plasmodium* spp. The functional analysis of the P48/45 and PHAP2 genes in *P. berghei* established their significant role in reducing the fertility of male gametes during fertilization, promoting these genes as vaccine candidates (74, 75), which are currently in the preclinical stage (76–78).

Despite the success of reverse vaccinology, it cannot be used to identify non-peptide antigens but can identify operons that code for synthesis of such molecules (79). For pathogens with complex genomes such as malaria parasites, no successful vaccine has as yet been developed via this approach. Further progress requires, among other things, improved predictive algorithms to identify the T and B cell epitopes as well as accurate quantitative assessments before inclusion in vaccines.

Structural Vaccinology

An improved understanding of the native structures of biological macromolecules such as proteins and how changes in their structure affect their functions can assist the identification of suitable epitopes (80, 81). Such epitopes can be designed into accessible forms for easy uptake by immune cells. These structural considerations make it possible to improve vaccine immunogenicity and safety and mitigate the effects of sequence variability within different strains of a pathogen (82). For instance, the bacterium *Meningococcus* is able to evade the host's immune system with the aid of a factor H binding protein (Hbp), which inactivates the host complement pathway by blocking factor H. Structural considerations allowed immunodominant epitopes of Hbp from various meningococcal strains to be identified and grafted into a single variant molecule to form a single antigen. This antigen was used in the MenB vaccine, responses against which are able to neutralize all the targeted strains (83).

Also, in an earlier study, short conserved α-helical coiled coil structural domains were identified from the asexual blood stage of the *P. falciparum* by examining the *Plasmodium* genome (84). Upon further screening, an unstructured peptide (P27A) that unfolds in native confirmation was selected. The peptide was the target of human antibodies which were able to restrict parasite replication (85). The vaccine candidate P27A has been considered immunogenic and safe with mild adverse events after PhaseI clinical trials (86).

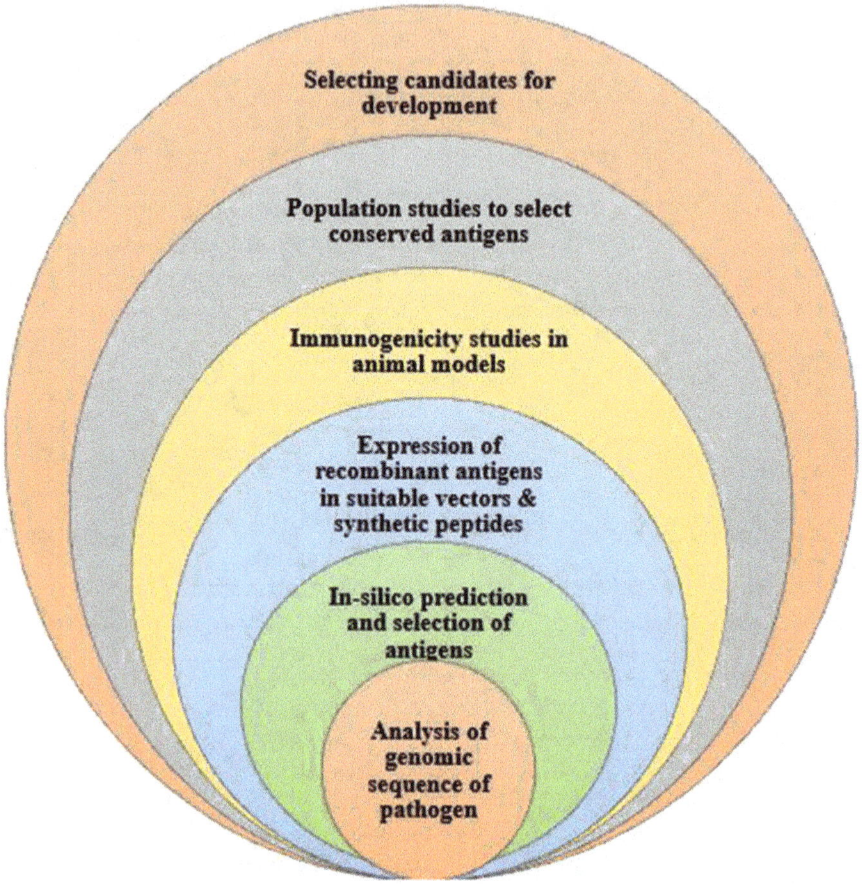

FIGURE 1 | The process of developing a vaccine using reverse vaccinology. Reverse vaccinology starts with obtaining the genomic sequence of the pathogen and using bioinformatics tools to identify all open reading frames to predict protein antigens. The predicted antigens are subsequently expressed in suitable vectors to produce the recombinant proteins which are tested to evaluate the immunogenicity in animal models. Expressed antigens that yield high immunogenicity are selected as vaccine candidates, further tested in population studies to determine and identify conserved antigens for further vaccine development.

For pathogens like *P. falciparum*, structural vaccinology may also help overcome antigenic variation. For instance, the application of structural vaccinology enabled the characterization of the less polymorphic DBL4ε domain of VAR2CSA to identify novel properties in the motif that affects the functional features of the antigen (87); identification and confirmation of the three-dimensional structure of the invasion ligand Cysteine-Rich Protective Antigen (CyRPA) (88). For example, the CyRPA was identified as a protective epitope providing an additive effect with the Reticulocyte binding-like Homologous protein 5 (*Pf*RH5) such that antibodies against *Pf*RH5 and CyRPA can inhibit parasite replication in host RBCs (88). Hopefully malaria vaccines incorporating these epitopes may elicit strong protective immune responses. Combining these protective antigens to create hybrid protein vaccines with enhanced efficacy may be a viable option for malaria.

A key challenge with this approach is the identification of suitable B and T cell epitopes for incorporation into vaccine candidates.

Immunoinformatics Based Approach to Vaccine Design

Immunoinformatics integrates both computational approaches and experimental immunology to develop machine learning algorithms that attempt to predict the immunogenicity of antigens. These approaches can be either pattern- or theory-based and may operate at either the amino acid sequence or the protein structure level. The pattern-based approaches conceive the prediction problem as one of finding sequence/structural patterns associated with immunogenicity. In contrast, the theory-based approaches attempt to model the basis for immunogenicity, for example, by using physical principles. Examples of algorithmic tools employed by pattern-based approaches include quantitative structure-activity relationship analysis, support vector machines, and artificial neural networks (89, 90). Theory-based approaches often employ Markovian and/or Bayesian models as well as models based on statistical mechanics (91).

Immunoinformatic approaches have already been applied to *P. falciparum* to predict possible cytotoxic T cell epitopes coupled with HLA A/B molecules for malaria peptide vaccine design (92). For example, the PfEMP1 gene, a member of the var gene family has been associated with parasite evasion from host immune mechanisms due to its multiple variation and ability to bind to different host receptors (36). In a recent study, both *in-silico* and experimental approaches were used to identify antigenic epitopes from CIDR-1 and DBL-3γ conserved domains of PfEMP1. These epitopes were predicted to have good binding affinity to HLA molecules as well as the capability to induce IFN-γ, IL-4 secretion and T cell proliferation in exposed individuals (93).

Classically, HLA class I molecules optimally require peptides that are 8-10 amino acids long for presentation to CD8 T cells while HLA Class II molecules optimally require 12-25 amino acids long peptides for presentation to CD4 T cells. Of note high predictive accuracies have been achieved for bioinformatics methods for predicting peptide binding to HLA I molecules; whereas those for predicting binding to HLA II molecules require further improvement. An even greater challenge is prediction of peptide binding to B cell receptors for effective antibody responses. On-going work by us and other groups is aimed at addressing some of these challenges (91, 94). However, not all HLA binders are good epitopes for T cells and this poses a major challenge for approaches that predict HLA binders without considering the global picture of HLA-peptide-TCR interactions. Nonetheless, these computational approaches, which are quite cost-effective and are important down-selection tools in instances where there are too many peptides to evaluate experimentally, have the potential to aid in the development of effective vaccines against malaria.

Immune-Focused Approach

Due to the sophisticated immune-evasion mechanisms of *P. falciparum* that allow it to coexist with the host, vaccinologists require new paradigms in vaccine development. One such new paradigm that has been developed to target these pathogens is the immune-focused approach (**Figure 2**). In contrast to the parasite-focused approach, which centers on the pathogen of interest, this new approach seeks to harness the host immune system to more rapidly design effective vaccines. It focuses on studying the host immune system to discover protective immune signatures. It is expected that these protective signatures can be induced *de novo* in susceptible hosts to protect them against infection and/or disease. Compared to the pathogen-focused approach, the immune-focused approach has, in principle, a greater potential for success against pathogens like malaria parasites, which have highly variable genomes. In particular, it may be able to identify and design immune cells with broadly neutralizing antibodies (95) and enhanced cellular immune responses, which has proved difficult to accomplish by using conventional approaches. To provide context for the discussion of opportunities for vaccine development, we begin with a brief overview of human immunity to malaria.

Immunity to Malaria

In contrast to many pathogens against which highly potent, long-lived immunity is achieved, human immunity to malarial parasites is less potent and relatively short-lived (17). In malaria, acquired immunity to infection is rare; rather, what develops naturally, generally over a long period, is acquired immunity to disease (96). Such clinical immunity generally targets the disease-causing asexual blood stage of malarial parasites. It tends to be acquired faster in moderate-to-high transmission settings compared to low transmission areas, and with a higher number of clinical episodes (97–99). As with other infectious diseases, the development of clinical immunity to malaria is dependent on the adaptive arm of the immune system, and the principal mediators consist of specific subsets of B and T cells. Some progress has been made to elucidate the underlying mechanisms, although the key immune determinants remain unclear.

In addition, the ability to predict the beginning and end of transmission seasons have made it possible to study host responses to infection and some immune dynamics that occur before, during and after infection as well as, drug interventions (100) and how they may affect the immunity acquired (101, 102).

In natural infections, acquisition of immunity to sporozoite stage infections is limited, probably due to the low number of sporozoites that are inoculated as well as the limited time that sporozoites have extracellular, prior to hepatocyte invasion. In addition, it has been reported that *Plasmodium* sporozoites are able to modulate the cytokine environment by downregulating Th1 responses and antigen presentation to T cells (103). Recently, it was reported that continuous exposure to *P. falciparum* leads to the induction and expression of immunoregulatory cytokines such as IL-10 and affects the function of dendritic cells (104). These, coupled with frequent infection and immune activation, may profoundly impact on the tolerogenic environment leading to the escape of sporozoites from immune cells. Nevertheless, functional properties of antibodies to sporozoite-stage infections have been associated with natural protection from clinical disease. It has been reported that these antibodies kill sporozoites through complement fixation and inhibit hepatocyte invasion. However, the response to sporozoite antigens was age-dependent and acquired slowly compared to blood-stage antigens (105).

The blood-stage parasite is associated with the clinical symptoms of the disease as it causes an upregulation of pro-inflammatory cytokines, regulatory T cells and parasite sequestration in small blood vessels in host organs. Antibodies have been reported to play functional roles in preventing parasite invasion of red blood cells (106, 107). Antibodies to parasite antigens are associated with clinical immunity in endemic areas (108–110). The mechanisms of antibody activity may include blocking invasion of erythrocytes (111); opsonizing parasites to facilitate their clearance (110, 112) enhancing the killing of infected cells by monocytes (113); complement-mediated lysis of infected cells (114); and inhibiting adherence of infected erythrocytes to vascular endothelium (115). However, the generation of atypical memory B cells which have reduced effector functions has been observed under chronic conditions (116, 117).

T cells have also been shown to play protective roles during blood-stage infection. For instance, protection from the disease has been associated with $FOXP3^{-}$ Th1 cells which are self-regulatory and produce IFNγ, TNF and IL-10 (101, 118, 119). These cells are believed to prevent the production of pyrogenic

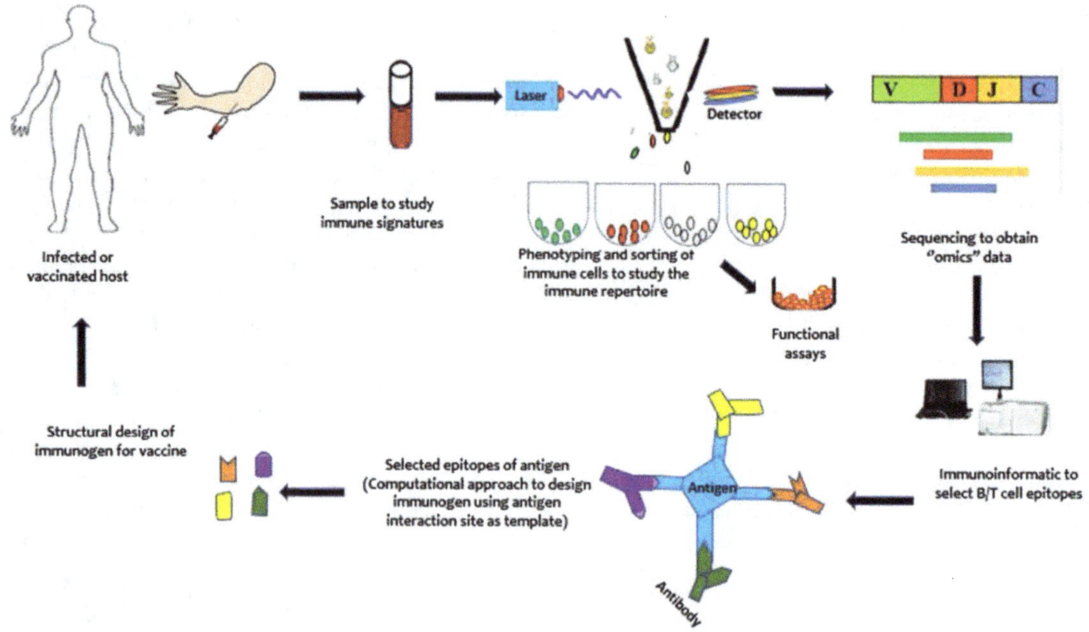

FIGURE 2 | An illustration of the immune-focused approach to vaccine development**.** Briefly, from top left, samples are obtained from an infected but protected or a vaccinated host. Immune cells are phenotyped and sorted using single cell sorting technologies such as the flow cytometry. The sorted cells may be sequenced directly or proliferated for functional studies before sequencing to study the immune repertoires (B/T cell receptor repertoire). With the use of computational approaches, the immunogen is designed and taken through further stages of development to yield a vaccine. After vaccination, mechanisms underlying vaccine efficacy and safety can be studied to further enhance the developed vaccine to achieve maximum protection against the targeted pathogen.

factors that may lead to the manifestation of clinical disease. However, these immune responses are not long-lasting and easily decay after infection has waned. T cell responses are hampered by the upregulation of negative immune regulatory receptors which may blunt or cause anergic responses (116, 120, 121). Our recent study found higher levels of T regulatory cells to be associated with higher blood levels of *P. falciparum* in children (118), suggesting less effective control of the parasite. Indeed, trying to understand these various aspects of the immune responses is a quite complex task (122).

Compared to natural infections, inducing sterile immunity in naïve individuals has been achieved through whole sporozoite immunization (29, 123) although similar outcomes have not been seen in individuals from malaria endemic areas (63, 64). Vaccination of volunteers with radiation-attenuated sporozoites has shown that both T cells and antibody responses play a significant role in protecting vaccinated cohorts against clinical challenge. It was observed that T cells from the periphery of these individuals, when stimulated with *P. falciparum* sporozoites *in vitro*, produced effector cytokines in a dose-dependent manner whereas antibody levels increased and prevented hepatocyte invasion (124–127).

The challenges of inducing immunity to malaria by natural or artificial means are compounded by the sophisticated immune-evasion strategies of the parasite. The parasite has a large genome consisting of about 5,300–5,500 possible antigenic targets (70). This extensive gene repertoire coupled with the parasite's high mutation rate allows for extensive variation of antigens that can be potential vaccine targets. Moreover, the epitopes targeted by the immune system exhibit a hierarchy of immunogenicity, with immunodominant epitopes that induce large amounts of antibodies, not all of which are neutralizing and may mask sub-dominant epitopes bound by neutralizing antibodies (73). In addition, the parasite switches off antigenic phenotypes, associated with the variant antigens resulting in functional diversity. Consequently, infections are mostly characterized by successive parasitemia waves caused by different parasite variants, making the development of long-lived immunity to the parasite very challenging (36, 128). Furthermore, key antigens such as CSP contain tandem repeats that have been implicated in immune evasion by suppressing antibody responses against adjacent antigens (129).

High Throughput Identification of Immune Correlates of Protection

The age and genetics of a person may modulate the immune responses elicited during infections and vaccinations (130, 131). Nonetheless, these responses that modulate infection may help to systematically define factors associated with protection from disease. Conventional approaches to understanding immune correlates of protection against *P. falciparum* includes, but is not limited to, ELISA, Elispot and Western blots. However, recent advances in high throughput assays have allowed in-depth analysis of immune correlates of protection to multiple *falciparum* antigens. Individuals in malaria-endemic areas generate antibodies to different *P. falciparum* proteins which may be protective or serve as a serological marker for exposure.

High throughput assays that probe the genomic, proteomic and transcriptomic data of immune responses are useful means of determining correlates of protection in exposed and vaccine trial cohorts. Independent studies using library expression and protein microarray has characterized host immune reactivity to different *P. falciparum* antigens. Using these approaches, Doolan et al. (132) were able to identify stage-specific *P. falciparum* antigens associated with protection in naturally exposed individuals, vaccine protected and non-protected individuals using a protein microarray chip with 250 proteins. They observed distinctive antibody profiles in the various groups to these antigens. Also, in an independent study, involving a large cohort of children naturally exposed to malaria (≤10 years old) in Kenya, it was observed that responses to fewer proteins from the 39 *P. falciparum* antigens analyzed were significantly associated with protection, and these included AMA1 and MSP2. Also, antibodies to the top 10 proteins provided an additive effect whereas most antibody responses to the other antigens were markers of malaria exposure (133).

A similar study conducted in Mali probed sera from malaria-exposed children and adults against 1204 proteins. Among these proteins, 91 were associated with sexual stage-specific immunity with specific-IgG responses culminating during the transmission season. It was further observed that immunity to these sexual stage vaccine candidates (Pfs48/45 and Pfs230 but not Pfs25) can be boosted in natural infections (134). These studies showed evidence that the breadth and magnitude of the antibody response is a better correlate of immune protection. Furthermore, in analyzing PBMCs for non-humoral immune responses associated with protection using DNA microarrays, qRT-PCR and flow cytometry, it was observed that repeated exposure to malaria in children was associated with the upregulation of genes involved in immune regulation (such as IL-10 secretion from CD4+Foxp3-), phagocytosis and activation of adaptive immune system. In contrast, gene expression levels of chemokines and cytokines associated with fever and inflammation (such as IL-1β, TNF, CXCL2 and IL-8) were downregulated (101).

Interestingly, the application of next-generation sequencing techniques such as lymphocyte immune repertoire sequencing, including T cell receptor (TCR), membrane-bound B cell receptor (BCR) or secreted BCR can allow an in-depth analysis of host factors associated with pathogen recognition, identification and protection from disease. The TCR structure is heterodimeric with two protein subunits; an alpha and beta chain or gamma and delta chain with both a constant and variable region. Similarly, the BCR consists of two heavy and light chains which are joined together by disulphide bonds to form a Y shaped immunoglobulin together with a variable and a constant region. The lymphocyte receptors (TCR/BCR) have similar structures including a variable, diversity and joining regions that enable diversification in identifying different host pathogens. In the generation of receptor diversity, there is a recombination of a V, D, and J segment of a beta or heavy chain, and a V and J segment for the alpha or light chain. For the BCR, this process helps expose very potent neutralizing antibodies that may be public in protecting against clinical disease. The generation of the variable regions may help guarantee higher levels of somatic mutation at the antigen binding site which may be shared or unique to an individual(s).

Despite the documented importance of lymphocyte receptors for antigen recognition and, hence, for the initiation of adaptive immune responses, the specific TCRs/BCRs that determine immunity to particular pathogens remain poorly understood. To our knowledge, no previous study has comprehensively mapped these receptors and analyzed how their expression profiles may correlate with individual variations in immune protection against malaria. In addition, the application of machine learning algorithms such as random forests, support vector machines may allow the identification of patterns on immune correlates that may predict protection against disease (118, 135).

Moreover, these approaches generate huge amounts of data that can be computationally analyzed to generate new, experimentally testable hypotheses. These may yield novel insights into the mechanisms underlying vaccine safety and efficacy. Importantly, data from such studies will inform pathways to which vaccine strategies should focus.

The B Cell Response and Vaccine Design

Effective vaccines are supposed to elicit and provide long-term protection as well as require both B and T cells to produce effective antibodies to neutralize surface-expressed antigens. B cell lineage vaccine design is an immune-focused approach that combines human immunology, structural biology, and computational protein design to develop a vaccine. The aim is to identify in both naïve and memory B cell receptors, paratopes (antigen binding sites) that interact with immunogens of interest. For a vaccine to be designed through this approach, memory B cell clones from the same lineage (or clone) are first identified and isolated from patients that produce broadly neutralizing antibodies or protective antibodies. These clones are then sequenced to obtain the V(D)J and VJ gene pairs that make up the B cell receptors in order to identify the paratope. Computational approaches are used to design an immunogen that interacts with the identified paratope (95). For *P. falciparum*, neutralizing antibodies produced by activated B cells are required to prevent the infection of new RBCs. By isolating such protective B cells from malaria patients and sequencing and analyzing their antigen receptors, it might be possible to identify immunogens able to induce protective immunity in susceptible individuals.

In malaria, the identification of broadly neutralizing antibodies remained elusive partly due to the high polymorphic nature of *P. falciparum* antigens. In addition, malaria vaccine candidates tend to induce antibodies with weak neutralizing ability, low breadth and strain-specific. However, Tan et al. (136) have recently identified monoclonal antibodies that can recognize *P. falciparum*-infected RBCs (iRBCs) from different strains of parasites. These antibodies recognize and bind to iRBCs through the RIFIN proteins, a group of variant antigens that are extracellularly expressed on the surface of iRBCs and have been associated with immune evasion (128) to initialize opsonization.

Another remarkable example is the identification of the novel antigenic target NPDP (part of the sequence in the N-terminal junction peptide) that is found between genes for the CSP and NANP and NVDP tandem repeats (137, 138). Independent studies in 2018 by Tan et al. (137) and Kisalu et al. (138) identified and isolated neutralizing antibodies from memory B cells and plasmablasts that could inhibit hepatocyte infection by PfSPZ. Through structural information, they were able to identify that these antibodies bind to conserved epitopes in the N-terminus of the CSP that is not found within the RTS,S vaccine.

Furthermore, mAbs that can inhibit parasite replication to about 97% have been isolated from CHMI donors immunized with RTS,S. Deciphering the structure and functionality of these antibodies have provided an informed overview on the structure of the CSP *in vivo*. Thus provides positive implications in the design of CSP immunogens against *P. falciparum* (139). However, there are still unsolved questions on the antibody responses to the PfCSP which have been described to be protective (139) and non-protective (129) as well as more structural information is needed to induce such potent neutralizing antibodies during vaccination Nonetheless, it is very interesting since they have implications in designing immunogens that can target specific immune responses and probably improve the efficacy of the RTS,S vaccine.

T Cell Response and Vaccine Design

Protective immunity to malaria liver-stage infection has been attributed to T cells in both human and rodent models. In studying immune responses to malaria such as cerebral malaria, murine models have provided significant understanding of various immunological properties that have impacted our understanding of the immune activity in humans.

For instance, Lau et al. (140) characterize MHC-restricted TCR that have potential in enhancing antigen presentation to T cells to enhance T cell immunity. They developed a novel CD8+ T cell receptor to *P. berghei* termed PbT-I from transgenic mouse with immune specificity for liver-stage and blood-stage infections. Isolated TCR genes from Vα8.3 and Vβ10 were isolated from a restricted hybridoma T cell line generated from *Plasmodium berghei* ANKA (PbA) blood-stage infection. Despite been developed for PbA, this transgenic MHC-I restricted T cell line was cross-reactive to *P. chabaudi* and *P. yoelli*. This implies that they may recognize conserved regions in rodent *Plasmodium spp.* Functional analysis revealed that the PbT-I cells produced effector cytokines (IFNγ, TNFα) and was positive for the degranulation marker (CD107a) showing their involvement in immune activity during the PbA infection. Using PbT-I CD8+ T cells, the peptides responsible for their activation were elucidated.

In a subsequent research, they identified and developed PbT-II CD4+ T cells from mouse transgenic line using the TCRα (Vα2.7, Jα12, Cα) and TCRβ gene (Vβ12, Dβ2, Jβ2.4) segments to blood-stage PbA infection (141). These cells were cross-reactive to rodent parasites (*P. berghei, yoelli and chabaudi*) and to *P. falciparum*. These MHC-II restricted PbT CD4+ T cells enhanced both humoral activity of B cells and cytotoxic activity of CD8+ T cells. In addition, the study confirmed that immunity to antigens in both blood stage and liver-stage development can restrict parasite replication in the hepatic stage and characterize the impact of blood stage antigen presentation to T cells that can enhance such T-cell immunity during infection. The uses of these target antigens may delineate protective immune responses and possibly circumvent pathologic outcomes. More importantly, further work should be focused on identifying and understanding such broadly reactive *Plasmodium*-specific T cells in host infections.

Structure-Based Immunogen Vaccine Design

The structure-based vaccine approach can be employed in both the parasite and immune-focused approach. However, in the immune-focused approach, the principle is based on understanding the structural properties of the immune cell providing the desired response. Here, the properties of the antigenic binding site on the immune cell is studied at the atomic level (80, 81). By understanding these properties, the approach seeks to design and develop immunogens to target the protective response or develop these immune cells for use as interventions.

Structural-based vaccine design has aided in unmasking immunodominant epitopes in the haemagglutinin-stem of the influenza virus (142), the fusion protein in the respiratory syncytial virus (143) and CD4 binding site in HIV-1 virus. For example, identifying conserved immunogenic epitopes in HIV has been quite challenging. However, elucidating the structure of broadly neutralizing antibodies (bNAbs) has been very useful. Using NAb, subdominant epitopes in the CD4 binding site by the gp120 viral protein were identified. Probing the structure of the antigenic binding site on CD4, the structural properties helped in the development of a recombinant protein (RSC3) with specificity to the NAb. The RSC3 was further used to identify and isolate B cells that expressed broadly neutralizing antibodies with increased breadth. VRC01 and 3BNC117, highly potent monoclonal bnMAb with reactivity to about 91% to HIV-1 isolates were developed (144). Phase I clinical trials of the VRC01 were reported as safe with no allergenicity (145, 146). It is currently being evaluated in a Phase IIB trials with a projected overall efficacy of 53 and 82% (147). These observations indicate that using structural properties, subdominant epitopes can be uncovered to design immunogens to target a specific immune response.

Currently, there are few examples of the successful use of these approaches in malaria vaccine design. For instance, using invasion-inhibitory monoclonal antibodies, the novel structure of PfRh5 in complex with basigin was characterized, together with novel protective epitopes found in the complex (148). Similarly, for *P. vivax* infections, bNAbs that confer strain-specific immune responses (149) were isolated. These bNAbs, enabled the characterization of protective epitopes in the duffy binding protein that can be included in the design of a potent *P. vivax* vaccine (150).

CONCLUSION

The development of a highly efficacious malaria vaccine faces many challenges, both technical and biological. Partly because the parasite is equipped with a variety of evasion mechanisms allow it to co-exist with the host. With the recent advent of high throughput approaches such as lymphocyte repertoire sequencing and structural design of immunogens, the breadth of protection of previous and current vaccine candidates may be enhanced as well as the identification of new candidate vaccines. In addition, vaccinologist may be able to design vaccines that drive the immune system through unusual yet protective pathways. Likewise, the application of mathematical modeling and computational approaches to the data thus obtained will open new pathways toward designing highly effective vaccines against malaria and aid in achieving the targets set by the malaria vaccine technology roadmap for 2030.

AUTHOR CONTRIBUTIONS

All authors listed have made a substantial, direct and intellectual contribution to the work, and approved it for publication.

FUNDING

Augustina Frimpong is supported by a Ph.D. fellowship from a World Bank African Centers of Excellence Grant (ACE02-WACCBIP: Awandare) and the International Development Research Center grant from the African Institute for Mathematical Sciences, Ghana, the Carnegie Corporation of New York and the University of Ghana BanGA Ph.D. Research Grant. WN is supported by the AIMS Global Secretariat.

REFERENCES

1. WHO. *World Malaria Report 2017.* Geneva: World Health Organization (2017).
2. World Health Organization. *World Malaria Report 2015*: World Health Organization (2015).
3. Alonso PL, Brown G, Arevalo-Herrera M, Binka F, Chitnis C, Collins F, et al. A Research Agenda to Underpin Malaria Eradication. *PLoS Med.* (2011) 8:e1000406. doi: 10.1371/journal.pmed.1000406
4. Bhatt S, Weiss DJ, Cameron E, Bisanzio D, Mappin B, Dalrymple U, et al. The effect of malaria control on Plasmodium falciparum in Africa between 2000 and 2015. *Nature* (2015) 526:207.doi: 10.1038/nature 15535
5. WHO. *Global Plan for Insecticide Resistance Management in Malaria Vectors (GPIRM).* Geneva: World Health Organization (2012).
6. Müller P, Donnelly MJ, Ranson H. Transcription profiling of a recently colonised pyrethroid resistant Anopheles gambiae strain from Ghana. *BMC Genomics* (2007) 8:36. doi: 10.1186/1471-2164-8-36
7. Toé KH, N'Falé S, Dabiré RK, Ranson H, Jones CM. The recent escalation in strength of pyrethroid resistance in Anopheles coluzzi in West Africa is linked to increased expression of multiple gene families. *BMC Genomics* (2015) 16:146. doi: 10.1186/s12864-015-1342-6
8. Ranson H, Lissenden N. Insecticide resistance in African Anopheles mosquitoes: a worsening situation that needs urgent action to maintain malaria control. *Trends Parasitol.* (2016) 32:187–96. doi: 10.1016/j.pt.2015.11.010
9. Choi KS, Christian R, Nardini L, Wood OR, Agubuzo E, Muleba M, et al. Insecticide resistance and role in malaria transmission of Anopheles funestus populations from Zambia and Zimbabwe. *Parasit Vectors* (2014) 7:464. doi: 10.1186/s13071-014-0464-z
10. Moore DV, Lanier JE. Observations on two Plasmodium falciparum infections with an abnormal response to chloroquine. *Am J Trop Med Hyg.* (1961) 10:5–9. doi: 10.4269/ajtmh.1961.10.5
11. Roper C, Pearce R, Nair S, Sharp B, Nosten F, Anderson T. Intercontinental spread of pyrimethamine-resistant malaria. *Science* (2004) 305:1124. doi: 10.1126/science.1098876
12. Hanboonkunupakarn B, White NJ. The threat of antimalarial drug resistance. *Trop Dis Travel Med Vaccin.* (2016) 2:10. doi: 10.1186/s40794-016-0027-8
13. Ataíde R, Powell R, Moore K, McLean A, Phyo AP, Nair S, et al. Declining transmission and immunity to malaria and emerging artemisinin resistance in Thailand: a longitudinal study. *J Infect Dis.* (2017) 216:723–31. doi: 10.1093/infdis/jix371
14. Ataide R, Ashley EA, Powell R, Chan J-A, Malloy MJ, O'Flaherty K, et al. Host immunity to Plasmodium falciparum and the assessment of emerging artemisinin resistance in a multinational cohort. *Proc Natl. Acad. Sci.* (2017) 114:3515–20. doi: 10.1073/pnas.16158 75114
15. Ashley EA, Dhorda M, Fairhurst RM, Amaratunga C, Lim P, Suon S, et al. Spread of artemisinin resistance in *Plasmodium falciparum* malaria. *N Engl J Med.* (2014) 371:411–23. doi: 10.1056/NEJMoa1314981
16. Imwong M, Suwannasin K, Kunasol C, Sutawong K, Mayxay M, Rekol H, et al. The spread of artemisinin-resistant Plasmodium falciparum in the Greater Mekong subregion: a molecular epidemiology observational study. *Lancet Infect Dis.* (2017) 17:491–7. doi: 10.1016/S1473-3099(17)30048-8
17. Doolan DL, Dobaño C, Baird JK. Acquired immunity to malaria. *Clin Microbiol Rev.* (2009) 22:13–36. doi: 10.1128/CMR.00025-08
18. Tran TM, Li S, Doumbo S, Doumtabe D, Huang C-Y, Dia S, et al. An intensive longitudinal cohort study of malian children and adults reveals no evidence of acquired immunity to *Plasmodium falciparum* infection. *Clin Infect Dis* (2013) 57:40-7. doi: 10.1093/cid/cit17
19. Okell LC, Ghani AC, Lyons E, Drakeley CJ. Submicroscopic infection in Plasmodium falciparum-endemic populations: a systematic review and meta-analysis. *J Infect Dis.* (2009) 200:1509–17. doi: 10.1086/644781
20. Idris ZM, Chan CW, Kongere J, Gitaka J, Logedi J, Omar A, et al. High and heterogeneous prevalence of asymptomatic and sub-microscopic malaria infections on islands in Lake Victoria, Kenya. *Sci Reports* (2016) 6:36958. doi: 10.1038/srep36958
21. Roucher C, Rogier C, Dieye-Ba F, Sokhna C, Tall A, Trape J-F. Changing Malaria Epidemiology and Diagnostic Criteria for *Plasmodium falciparum* Clinical Malaria. *PLoS ONE* (2012) 7:e46188. doi: 10.1371/journal.pone.0046188
22. Baum E, Sattabongkot J, Sirichaisinthop J, Kiattibutr K, Jain A, Taghavian O, et al. Common asymptomatic and submicroscopic malaria infections in Western Thailand revealed in longitudinal molecular and serological studies: a challenge to malaria elimination. *Malaria J.* (2016) 15:333. doi: 10.1186/s12936-016-1393-4
23. Lindblade KA, Steinhardt L, Samuels A, Kachur SP, Slutsker L. The silent threat: asymptomatic parasitemia and malaria transmission. *Expert Rev Anti Infect Ther.* (2013) 11:623–39. doi: 10.1586/eri.13.45
24. Bousema JT, Gouagna LC, Drakeley CJ, Meutstege AM, Okech BA, Akim IN, et al. Plasmodium falciparum gametocyte carriage in asymptomatic children in western Kenya. *Mal J.* (2004) 3:18. doi: 10.1186/1475-2875-3-18
25. Coleman RE, Kumpitak C, Ponlawat A, Maneechai N, Phunkitchar V, Rachapaew N, et al. Infectivity of asymptomatic Plasmodium-infected human populations to Anopheles dirus mosquitoes in western Thailand. *J Med Entomol.* (2004) 41:201–8. doi: 10.1603/0022-2585-41.2.201
26. Cohen S, McGregor I, Carrington S. Gamma-globulin and acquired immunity to human malaria. *Nature* 1961:733–7. doi: 10.1038/192733a0
27. Roestenberg M, McCall M, Hopman J, Wiersma J, Luty AJ, van Gemert GJ, et al. Protection against a malaria challenge by sporozoite inoculation. *N Engl J Med.* (2009) 361:468–77. doi: 10.1056/NEJMoa0805832
28. Pombo DJ, Lawrence G, Hirunpetcharat C, Rzepczyk C, Bryden M, Cloonan N, et al. Immunity to malaria after administration of ultra-low doses of red cells infected with *Plasmodium falciparum*. *Lancet* (2002) 360:610–7. doi: 10.1016/S0140-6736(02)09784-2

29. Hoffman SL, Goh LM, Luke TC, Schneider I, Le TP, Doolan DL, et al. Protection of humans against malaria by immunization with radiation-attenuated Plasmodium falciparum sporozoites. *J Infect Dis* (2002) 185:1155–64. doi: 10.1086/339409
30. Nussenzweig V, Nussenzweig RS. Rationale for the development of an engineered sporozoite malaria vaccine. *Adv Immunol.* (1989) 45:283–334. doi: 10.1016/S0065-2776(08)60695-1
31. Baruch D, Gormely J, Ma C, Howard R, Pasloske B. *Plasmodium falciparum* erythrocyte membrane protein 1 is a parasitized erythrocyte receptor for adherence to CD36, thrombospondin, and intercellular adhesion molecule 1. *Proc Natl Acad Sci USA.* (1996) 93:3497–502. doi: 10.1073/pnas.93.8.3497
32. Hill DL, Wilson DW, Sampaio NG, Eriksson EM, Ryg-Cornejo V, Harrison GLA, et al. Merozoite Antigens of *Plasmodium falciparum* elicit strain-transcending opsonizing immunity. *Infect Immun* (2016) 84:2175–84. doi: 10.1128/IAI.00145-16
33. Kusi KA, Dodoo D, Bosomprah S, van der Eijk M, Faber BW, Kocken CHM, et al. Measurement of the plasma levels of antibodies against the polymorphic vaccine candidate apical membrane antigen 1 in a malaria-exposed population. *BMC Infect Dis.* (2012) 12:32. doi: 10.1186/1471-2334-12-32
34. Baum J, Chen L, Healer J, Lopaticki S, Boyle M, Triglia T, et al. Reticulocyte-binding protein homologue 5–an essential adhesin involved in invasion of human erythrocytes by *Plasmodium falciparum. Int J Parasitol.* (2009) 39:371–80. doi: 10.1016/j.ijpara.2008.10.006
35. Rodriguez M, Lustigman S, Montero E, Oksov Y, Lobo CA. PfRH5: a novel reticulocyte-binding family homolog of *Plasmodium falciparum* that binds to the erythrocyte, and an investigation of its receptor. *PLoS ONE* (2008) 3:e3300. doi: 10.1371/journal.pone.0003300
36. Mkumbaye SI, Wang CW, Lyimo E, Jespersen JS, Manjurano A, Mosha J, et al. The severity of Plasmodium falciparum infection is associated with transcript levels of var genes encoding EPCR-binding PfEMP1. *Infect Immun.* (2017) 85:e00841-16. doi: 10.1128/IAI.00841-16
37. Partey FD, Castberg FC, Sarbah EW, Silk SE, Awandare GA, Draper SJ, et al. Kinetics of antibody responses to PfRH5-complex antigens in Ghanaian children with *Plasmodium falciparum* malaria. *PLoS ONE* (2018) 13:e0198371. doi: 10.1371/journal.pone.0198371
38. Churcher TS, Bousema T, Walker M, Drakeley C, Schneider P, Ouédraogo AL, et al. Predicting mosquito infection from Plasmodium falciparum gametocyte density and estimating the reservoir of infection. *Elife* (2013) 2:e00626. doi: 10.7554/eLife.00626
39. Bousema T, Okell L, Shekalaghe S, Griffin JT, Omar S, Sawa P, et al. Revisiting the circulation time of *Plasmodium falciparum* gametocytes: molecular detection methods to estimate the duration of gametocyte carriage and the effect of gametocytocidal drugs. *Mal J.* (2010) 9:136. doi: 10.1186/1475-2875-9-136
40. Nsango SE, Abate L, Thoma M, Pompon J, Fraiture M, Rademacher A, et al. Genetic clonality of *Plasmodium falciparum* affects the outcome of infection in Anopheles gambiae. *Int J Parasitol.* (2012) 42:589–95. doi: 10.1016/j.ijpara.2012.03.008
41. Lefèvre T, Vantaux A, Dabiré KR, Mouline K, Cohuet A. Non-Genetic Determinants of Mosquito Competence for Malaria Parasites. *PLoS Pathogens* (2013) 9:e1003365. doi: 10.1371/journal.ppat.1003365
42. Dong Y, Manfredini F, Dimopoulos G. Implication of the mosquito midgut microbiota in the defense against malaria parasites. *PLoS Pathogens* (2009) 5:e1000423. doi: 10.1371/journal.ppat.1000423
43. Schneider P, Bousema JT, Gouagna LC, Otieno S, Van de Vegte-Bolmer M, Omar SA, et al. Submicroscopic *Plasmodium falciparum* gametocyte densities frequently result in mosquito infection. *Am J Tropic Med Hygiene* (2007) 76:470–4. doi: 10.4269/ajtmh.2007.76.470
44. Hallett RL, Dunyo S, Ord R, Jawara M, Pinder M, Randall A, et al. Chloroquine/sulphadoxine-pyrimethamine for gambian children with malaria: transmission to mosquitoes of multidrug-resistant *Plasmodium falciparum. PLoS Clin Trials* (2006) 1:e15. doi: 10.1371/journal.pctr.0010015
45. Saul A. Efficacy model for mosquito stage transmission blocking vaccines for malaria. *Parasitology* (2008) 135:1497–506. doi: 10.1017/S0031182008000280
46. Carter R, Mendis KN, Miller LH, Molineaux L, Saul A. Malaria transmission-blocking vaccines—how can their development be supported? (2000) 6:241–4. doi: 10.1038/73062
47. Jones S, Grignard L, Nebie I, Chilongola J, Dodoo D, Sauerwein R, Theisen M, Roeffen W, Singh SK, Singh RK: Naturally acquired antibody responses to recombinant Pfs230 and Pfs48/45 transmission blocking vaccine candidates. *J Infect* (2015) 71:117–27. doi: 10.1016/j.jinf.2015.03.007
48. Doumbo OK, Niaré K, Healy SA, Sagara I, Duffy PE. Malaria transmission-blocking vaccines: present status and future perspectives. In: *Towards Malaria Elimination-A Leap Forward.* IntechOpen. (2018). doi: 10.5772/intechopen.77241
49. MacDonald NJ, Nguyen V, Shimp R, Reiter K, Herrera R, Burkhardt M, et al. Structural and immunological characterization of recombinant 6-cysteine domains of the *Plasmodium falciparum* sexual stage protein Pfs230. *J Bioll Chem.* (2016) 291:19913–22. doi: 10.1074/jbc.M116.732305
50. Talaat KR, Ellis RD, Hurd J, Hentrich A, Gabriel E, Hynes NA, et al. Safety and immunogenicity of Pfs25-EPA/Alhydrogel®, a transmission blocking vaccine against *Plasmodium falciparum*: an open label study in malaria naïve adults. *PLoS ONE* (2016) 11:e0163144. doi: 10.1371/journal.pone.0163144
51. Wu Y, Ellis RD, Shaffer D, Fontes E, Malkin EM, Mahanty S, et al. Phase 1 trial of malaria transmission blocking vaccine candidates Pfs25 and Pvs25 formulated with montanide ISA 51. *PLoS ONE* (2008) 3:e2636. doi: 10.1371/journal.pone.0002636
52. Sagara I, Healy SA, Assadou MH, Gabriel EE, Kone M, Sissoko K, et al. Safety and immunogenicity of Pfs25H-EPA/Alhydrogel, a transmission-blocking vaccine against Plasmodium falciparum: a randomised, double-blind, comparator-controlled, dose-escalation study in healthy Malian adults. *Lancet Infect Dis* (2018) 18:969–82. doi: 10.1016/S1473-3099(18)30344-X
53. Collins KA, Snaith R, Cottingham MG, Gilbert SC, Hill AVS. Enhancing protective immunity to malaria with a highly immunogenic virus-like particle vaccine. *Sci Reports* (2017) 7:46621. doi: 10.1038/srep46621
54. Ogwang C, Kimani D, Edwards NJ, Roberts R, Mwacharo J, Bowyer G, et al. Prime-boost vaccination with chimpanzee adenovirus and modified vaccinia Ankara encoding TRAP provides partial protection against *Plasmodium falciparum* infection in Kenyan adults. *Sci Transl Med.* (2015) 7:286re285. doi: 10.1126/scitranslmed.aaa2373
55. Bliss CM, Drammeh A, Bowyer G, Sanou GS, Jagne YJ, Ouedraogo O, et al. Viral vector malaria vaccines induce high-level T cell and antibody responses in West African children and infants. *Mol Ther.* (2017) 25:547–59. doi: 10.1016/j.ymthe.2016.11.003
56. Mensah VA, Roetynck S, Kanteh EK, Bowyer G, Ndaw A, Oko F, et al. Safety and immunogenicity of malaria vectored vaccines given with routine expanded program on immunization vaccines in gambian infants and neonates: a randomized controlled trial. *Front Immunol.* (2017) 8:1551. doi: 10.3389/fimmu.2017.01551
57. Sirima S, Durier C, Kara L, Houard S, Gansane A, Loulergue P, et al. Safety and immunogenicity of a recombinant Plasmodium falciparum AMA1-DiCo malaria vaccine adjuvanted with GLA-SE or Alhydrogel® in European and African adults: a phase 1a/1b, randomized, double-blind multi-centre trial. *Vaccine* (2017) 35:6218–27. doi: 10.1016/j.vaccine.2017.09.027
58. Valéa I, Adjei S, Usuf E, Traore O, Ansong D, Tinto H, et al. Immune response to the hepatitis B antigen in the RTS, S/AS01 malaria vaccine, and co-administration with pneumococcal conjugate and rotavirus vaccines in African children: a randomized controlled trial. *Hum Vaccin Immunotherapeut.* (2018) 14: 1489–1500. doi: 10.1080/21645515.2018.1442996
59. Rts S. Efficacy and safety of RTS, S/AS01 malaria vaccine with or without a booster dose in infants and children in Africa: final results of a phase 3, individually randomised, controlled trial. *Lancet* (2015) 386:31–45. doi: 10.1016/S0140-6736(15)60721-8
60. Gosling R, von Seidlein L. The future of the RTS, S/AS01 malaria vaccine: an alternative development plan. *PLoS Med.* (2016) 13:e1001994. doi: 10.1371/journal.pmed.1001994
61. Chaudhury S, Regules JA, Darko CA, Dutta S, Wallqvist A, Waters NC, et al. Delayed fractional dose regimen of the RTS, S/AS01 malaria vaccine candidate enhances an IgG4 response that inhibits serum opsonophagocytosis. *Sci Reports* (2017) 7:7998. doi: 10.1038/s41598-017-08526-5

62. Walk J, Reuling IJ, Behet MC, Meerstein-Kessel L, Graumans W, van Gemert G-J, et al. Modest heterologous protection after *Plasmodium falciparum* sporozoite immunization: a double-blind randomized controlled clinical trial. *BMC Med.* (2017) 15:168. doi: 10.1186/s12916-017-0923-4
63. Sissoko MS, Healy SA, Katile A, Omaswa F, Zaidi I, Gabriel EE, et al. Safety and efficacy of PfSPZ Vaccine against *Plasmodium falciparum* via direct venous inoculation in healthy malaria-exposed adults in Mali: a randomised, double-blind phase 1 trial. *Lancet Infect Dis.* (2017) 17:498–509. doi: 10.1016/S1473-3099(17)30104-4
64. Olotu A, Urbano V, Hamad A, Eka M, Chemba M, Nyakarungu E, et al. Advancing global health through development and clinical trials partnerships: a randomized, placebo-controlled, double-blind assessment of safety, tolerability, and immunogenicity of PfSPZ vaccine for malaria in healthy equatoguinean men. *Am J Tropic Med Hyg.* (2018) 98:308–18. doi: 10.4269/ajtmh.17-0449
65. Seib KL, Zhao X, Rappuoli R. Developing vaccines in the era of genomics: a decade of reverse vaccinology. *Clin. Microbiol. Infect* (2012) 18:109–116. doi: 10.1111/j.1469-0691.2012.03939.x
66. Rappuoli R. Reverse vaccinology. *Curr Opin Microbiol.* (2000) 3:445–50. doi: 10.1016/S1369-5274(00)00119-3
67. Watson PS, Turner DP. Clinical experience with the meningococcal B vaccine, Bexsero®: Prospects for reducing the burden of meningococcal serogroup B disease. *Vaccine* (2016) 34:875–80. doi: 10.1016/j.vaccine.2015.11.057
68. Vesikari T, Esposito S, Prymula R, Ypma E, Kohl I, Toneatto D, et al. Immunogenicity and safety of an investigational multicomponent, recombinant, meningococcal serogroup B vaccine (4CMenB) administered concomitantly with routine infant and child vaccinations: results of two randomised trials. *Lancet* (2013) 381:825–35. doi: 10.1016/S0140-6736(12)61961-8
69. Maione D, Margarit I, Rinaudo CD, Masignani V, Mora M, Scarselli M, et al. Identification of a Universal Group B Streptococcus Vaccine by Multiple Genome Screen. *Science* (2005) 309:148–50. doi: 10.1126/science.1109869
70. Gardner MJ, Hall N, Fung E, White O, Berriman M, Hyman RW, et al. Genome sequence of the human malaria parasite *Plasmodium falciparum*. *Nature* (2002) 419:498. doi: 10.1038/nature01097
71. Sundararaman SA, Plenderleith LJ, Liu W, Loy DE, Learn GH, Li Y, et al. Genomes of cryptic chimpanzee *Plasmodium* species reveal key evolutionary events leading to human malaria. *Nat Commun.* (2016) 7:11078. doi: 10.1038/ncomms11078
72. Otto TD, Rayner JC, Böhme U, Pain A, Spottiswoode N, Sanders M, et al. Genome sequencing of chimpanzee malaria parasites reveals possible pathways of adaptation to human hosts. *Nature Commun.* (2014) 5:4754. doi: 10.1038/ncomms5754
73. Hall N, Karras M, Raine JD, Carlton JM, Kooij TW, Berriman M, et al. A comprehensive survey of the Plasmodium life cycle by genomic, transcriptomic, and proteomic analyses. *Science* (2005) 307:82–6. doi: 10.1126/science.1103717
74. van Dijk MR, Janse CJ, Thompson J, Waters AP, Braks JA, Dodemont HJ, et al. A central role for P48/45 in malaria parasite male gamete fertility. *Cell* (2001) 104:153–64. doi: 10.1016/S0092-8674(01)00199-4
75. Blagborough AM, Sinden RE. *Plasmodium berghei* HAP2 induces strong malaria transmission-blocking immunity *in vivo* and *in vitro*. *Vaccine* (2009) 27:5187–94. doi: 10.1016/j.vaccine.2009.06.069
76. Pritsch M, Ben-Khaled N, Chaloupka M, Kobold S, Berens-Riha N, Peter A, et al. Comparison of intranasal outer membrane vesicles with cholera toxin and injected MF59C. 1 as adjuvants for malaria transmission blocking antigens AnAPN1 and Pfs48/45. *J Immunol Res.* (2016) 2016:3576028. doi: 10.1155/2016/3576028
77. Merino KM, Bansal GP, Kumar N. Reduced immunogenicity of *Plasmodium falciparum* gamete surface antigen (Pfs48/45) in mice after disruption of disulphide bonds–evaluating effect of interferon-γ-inducible lysosomal thiol reductase. *Immunology* (2016) 148:433–47. doi: 10.1111/imm.12621
78. Miura K, Takashima E, Deng B, Tullo G, Diouf A, Moretz SE, et al. Functional comparison of *Plasmodium falciparum* transmission-blocking vaccine candidates by the standard membrane-feeding assay. *Infect Immun.* (2013) 81:4377–82. doi: 10.1128/IAI.01056-13
79. Sette A, Rappuoli R. Reverse vaccinology: developing vaccines in the era of genomics. *Immunity* (2010) 33:530–41. doi: 10.1016/j.immuni.2010.09.017
80. Delany I, Rappuoli R, De Gregorio E. Vaccines for the 21st century. *EMBO Molr Med.* (2014) 6:708–20. doi: 10.1002/emmm.201403876
81. Thomas S, Luxon BA. Vaccines based on structure-based design provide protection against infectious diseases. *Expert Rev Vaccin.* (2013) 12:1301–11. doi: 10.1586/14760584.2013.840092
82. Nuccitelli A, Cozzi R, Gourlay LJ, Donnarumma D, Necchi F, Norais N, et al. Structure-based approach to rationally design a chimeric protein for an effective vaccine against Group B Streptococcus infections. *Proc Natl Acad Sci. USA.* (2011) 108:10278–83. doi: 10.1073/pnas.1106590108
83. Scarselli M, Aricò B, Brunelli B, Savino S, Di Marcello F, Palumbo E, et al. Rational design of a meningococcal antigen inducing broad protective immunity. *Sci Transl Med.* (2011) 3:91ra62. doi: 10.1126/scitranslmed.3002234
84. Villard V, Agak GW, Frank G, Jafarshad A, Servis C, Nébié I, et al. Rapid identification of malaria vaccine candidates based on α-helical coiled coil protein motif. *PLoS ONE* (2007) 2:e645. doi: 10.1371/journal.pone.0000645
85. Olugbile S, Kulangara C, Bang G, Bertholet S, Suzarte E, Villard V, et al. Vaccine potentials of an intrinsically unstructured fragment derived from the blood stage-associated *Plasmodium falciparum* protein PFF0165c. *Infect immun.* (2009) 77:5701–9. doi: 10.1128/IAI.00652-09
86. Steiner-Monard V, Kamaka K, Karoui O, Roethlisberger S, Audran R, Daubenberger C, et al. The candidate blood stage malaria vaccine P27A induces a robust humoral response in a fast track to the field phase I trial in exposed and non exposed volunteers. *Clin Infect Dis.* (2018) ciy514. doi: 10.1093/cid/ciy514
87. Gangnard S, Lewit-Bentley A, Dechavanne S, Srivastava A, Amirat F, Bentley GA, et al. Structure of the DBL3X-DBL4ε region of the VAR2CSA placental malaria vaccine candidate: insight into DBL domain interactions. *Sci Reports* (2015) 5:14868. doi: 10.1038/srep14868
88. Favuzza P, Guffart E, Tamborrini M, Scherer B, Dreyer AM, Rufer AC, et al. Structure of the malaria vaccine candidate antigen CyRPA and its complex with a parasite invasion inhibitory antibody. *Elife* (2017) 6:e20383. doi: 10.7554/eLife.20383
89. Wan J, Liu W, Xu Q, Ren Y, Flower DR, Li T. SVRMHC prediction server for MHC-binding peptides. *BMC Bioinformat.* (2006) 7:463. doi: 10.1186/1471-2105-7-463
90. Liu W, Meng X, Xu Q, Flower DR, Li T. Quantitative prediction of mouse class I MHC peptide binding affinity using support vector machine regression (SVR) models. *BMC Bioinformat.* (2006) 7:182. doi: 10.1186/1471-2105-7-182
91. Degoot AM, Chirove F, Ndifon W. Trans-Allelic Model for Prediction of Peptide:MHC-II Interactions. *Front Immunol.* (2018) 9:1410. doi: 10.3389/fimmu.2018.01410
92. Doolan DL. Plasmodium immunomics. *Int J Parasitol.* (2011) 41:3–20. doi: 10.1016/j.ijpara.2010.08.002
93. Khan N, Kumar R, Chauhan S, Farooq U. An immunoinformatics approach to promiscuous peptide design for the Plasmodium falciparum erythrocyte membrane protein-1. *Mol BioSyst.* (2017) 13:2160–7. doi: 10.1039/C7MB00332C
94. Jensen KK, Andreatta M, Marcatili P, Buus S, Greenbaum JA, Yan Z, et al. Improved methods for predicting peptide binding affinity to MHC class II molecules. *Immunology* (2018) 154:394–406. doi: 10.1111/imm.12889
95. Haynes BF, Kelsoe G, Harrison SC, Kepler TB. B-cell-lineage immunogen design in vaccine development with HIV-1 as a case study. *Nature Biotechnol.* (2012) 30:423–33. doi: 10.1038/nbt.2197
96. Stanisic DI, Good MF. Examining cellular immune responses to inform development of a blood-stage malaria vaccine. *Parasitology* (2016) 143:208–23. doi: 10.1017/S0031182015001092
97. Rodriguez-Barraquer I, Arinaitwe E, Jagannathan P, Kamya MR, Rosenthal PJ, Rek J, et al. Quantification of anti-parasite and anti-disease immunity to malaria as a function of age and exposure. *eLife* (2018) 7:e35832. doi: 10.7554/eLife.35832
98. Rodriguez-Barraquer I, Arinaitwe E, Jagannathan P, Boyle MJ, Tappero J, Muhindo M, et al. Quantifying heterogeneous malaria exposure and clinical protection in a cohort of Ugandan children. *J Infect Dis.* (2016) 214:1072–80. doi: 10.1093/infdis/jiw301

99. Baird JK, Basri H, Bangs MJ, Andersen EM, Jones TR, Masbar S, et al. Age-specific prevalence of Plasmodium falciparum among six populations with limited histories of exposure to endemic malaria. *Am J Tropic Med Hyg.* (1993) 49:707–19. doi: 10.4269/ajtmh.1993.49.707
100. Portugal S, Tran TM, Ongoiba A, Bathily A, Li S, Doumbo S, et al. Treatment of chronic asymptomatic *Plasmodium falciparum* infection does not increase the risk of clinical malaria upon reinfection. *Clin Infect Dis.* (2016) 64:645–53. doi: 10.1093/cid/ciw849
101. Portugal S, Moebius J, Skinner J, Doumbo S, Doumtabe D, Kone Y, et al. Exposure-dependent control of malaria-induced inflammation in children. *PLoS Pathog.* (2014) 10:e1004079. doi: 10.1371/journal.ppat.1004079
102. Boyle MJ, Jagannathan P, Farrington LA, Eccles-James I, Wamala S, McIntyre TI, et al. Decline of FoxP3+ Regulatory CD4 T cells in peripheral blood of children heavily exposed to malaria. *PLoS Pathog.* (2015) 11:e1005041. doi: 10.1371/journal.ppat.1005041
103. Guilbride DL, Gawlinski P, Guilbride PD. Why functional pre-erythrocytic and bloodstage malaria vaccines fail: a meta-analysis of fully protective immunizations and novel immunological model. *PLoS ONE* (2010) 5:e10685. doi: 10.1371/journal.pone.0010685
104. Loughland JR, Woodberry T, Boyle MJ, Tipping PE, Piera KA, Amante FH, et al. *Plasmodium falciparum* activates CD16+ dendritic cells to produce TNF and IL-10 in subpatent malaria. *J Infect Dis.* (2018) jiy555. doi: 10.1093/infdis/jiy555. [Epub ahead of print].
105. Kurtovic L, Behet MC, Feng G, Reiling L, Chelimo K, Dent AE, et al. Human antibodies activate complement against *Plasmodium falciparum* sporozoites, and are associated with protection against malaria in children. *BMC Med.* (2018) 16:61. doi: 10.1186/s12916-018-1054-2
106. Teo A, Feng G, Brown GV, Beeson JG, Rogerson SJ. Functional antibodies and protection against blood-stage malaria. *Trends Parasitol.* (2016) 32:887–898. doi: 10.1016/j.pt.2016.07.003
107. Hart GT, Tran T, Theorell J, Arora G, Crompton P, Bryceson Y, et al. A new malaria killer: Fc receptor gamma chain and PLZF identify NK cell subsets that correlate with reduced *Plasmodium falciparum* parasitemia and increased antibody dependent cellular cytotoxicity against opsonized infected RBCs. *Am Assoc Immnol.* (2018).
108. Jäschke A, Coulibaly B, Remarque EJ, Bujard H, Epp C. Merozoite surface protein-1 from *P. falciparum* is a major target of opsonizing antibodies in individuals with acquired immunity against malaria. *Clin Vaccine Immunol.* (2017).
109. Laurens MB, Kouriba B, Bergmann-Leitner E, Angov E, Coulibaly D, Diarra I, et al. Strain-specific Plasmodium falciparum growth inhibition among Malian children immunized with a blood-stage malaria vaccine. *PLoS One (2017)* 12:e0173294. doi: 10.1371/journal.pone.0173294
110. Chiu CYH, Hodder AN, Lin CS, Hill DL, Li Wai Suen CSN, Schofield L, et al. Antibodies to the Plasmodium falciparum Proteins MSPDBL1 and MSPDBL2 Opsonize Merozoites, Inhibit Parasite Growth, and Predict Protection From Clinical Malaria. *J Infect Dis.* (2015) 212:406–15. doi: 10.1093/infdis/jiv057
111. Persson KEM, Fowkes FJI, McCallum FJ, Gicheru N, Reiling L, Richards JS, et al. Erythrocyte-binding antigens of *Plasmodium falciparum* are targets of human inhibitory antibodies and function to evade naturally acquired immunity. *J Immunol.* (2013) 191:785–94. doi: 10.4049/jimmunol.1300444
112. Osier FH, Feng G, Boyle MJ, Langer C, Zhou J, Richards JS, et al. Opsonic phagocytosis of *Plasmodium falciparum* merozoites: mechanism in human immunity and a correlate of protection against malaria. *BMC Med.* (2014) 12:108. doi: 10.1186/1741-7015-12-108
113. Hill DL, Schofield L, Wilson DW. IgG opsonization of merozoites: multiple immune mechanisms for malaria vaccine development. *Int J Parasitol.* (2017) 47:585–95. doi: 10.1016/j.ijpara.2017.05.004
114. Boyle Michelle J, Reiling L, Feng G, Langer C, Osier Faith H, Aspeling-Jones H, et al. Human antibodies fix complement to inhibit *Plasmodium falciparum* invasion of erythrocytes and are associated with protection against malaria. *Immunity* (2015) 42:580–90. doi: 10.1016/j.immuni.2015.02.012
115. Olsen RW, Ecklu-Mensah G, Bengtsson A, Ofori MF, Lusingu JPA, Castberg FC, et al. Natural and Vaccine-Induced Acquisition of Cross-Reactive IgG-Inhibiting ICAM-1-Specific Binding of a <span class="named-content genus-species" id="named-content-1">*Plasmodium falciparum*</span> PfEMP1 Subtype Associated Specifically with Cerebral Malaria. *Infect Immun.* (2018) 86:e00622-17. doi: 10.1128/IAI.00622-17
116. Illingworth J, Butler NS, Roetynck S, Mwacharo J, Pierce SK, Bejon P, et al. Chronic exposure to *Plasmodium falciparum* is associated with phenotypic evidence of B and T cell exhaustion. *J Immunol* (2013) 190:1038–47. doi: 10.4049/jimmunol.1202438
117. Portugal S, Tipton CM, Sohn H, Kone Y, Wang J, Li S, et al. Malaria-associated atypical memory B cells exhibit markedly reduced B cell receptor signaling and effector function. *Elife* (2015) 4:e07218. doi: 10.7554/eLife.07218
118. Frimpong A, Kusi KA, Tornyigah B, Ofori MF, Ndifon W. Characterization of T cell activation and regulation in children with asymptomatic Plasmodium falciparum infection. *Mal J.* (2018) 17:263. doi: 10.1186/s12936-018-2410-6
119. Walther M, Jeffries D, Finney OC, Njie M, Ebonyi A, Deininger S, et al. Distinct roles for FOXP3+ and FOXP3− CD4+ T cells in regulating cellular immunity to uncomplicated and severe Plasmodium falciparum malaria. *PLoS Pathog.* (2009) 5:e1000364. doi: 10.1371/journal.ppat.1000364
120. Kurup SP, Obeng-Adjei N, Anthony SM, Traore B, Doumbo OK, Butler NS, et al. Regulatory T cells impede acute and long-term immunity to blood-stage malaria through CTLA-4. *Nature Med.* (2017) 23:1220. doi: 10.1038/nm.4395
121. Abel A, Steeg C, Aminkiah F, Addai-Mensah O, Addo M, Gagliani N, et al. Differential expression pattern of co-inhibitory molecules on CD4+ T cells in uncomplicated versus complicated malaria. *Sci Reports* (2018) 8:4789. doi: 10.1038/s41598-018-22659-1
122. Valletta JJ, Recker M. Identification of immune signatures predictive of clinical protection from malaria. *PLoS Comput Biol.* (2017) 13:e1005812. doi: 10.1371/journal.pcbi.1005812
123. Mordmüller B, Surat G, Lagler H, Chakravarty S, Ishizuka AS, Lalremruata A, et al. Sterile protection against human malaria by chemoattenuated PfSPZ vaccine. *Nature* (2017) 542:445. doi: 10.1038/nature21060
124. Lyke KE, Ishizuka AS, Berry AA, Chakravarty S, DeZure A, Enama ME, et al. Attenuated PfSPZ Vaccine induces strain-transcending T cells and durable protection against heterologous controlled human malaria infection. *Proc Natl Acad Sci USA.* (2017) 114:2711–16. doi: 10.1073/pnas.1615324114
125. Ishizuka AS, Lyke KE, DeZure A, Berry AA, Richie TL, Mendoza FH, et al. Protection against malaria at 1 year and immune correlates following PfSPZ vaccination. *Nat Med.* (2016) 22:614. doi: 10.1038/nm.4110
126. Seder RA, Chang L-J, Enama ME, Zephir KL, Sarwar UN, Gordon IJ, et al. Protection against malaria by intravenous immunization with a nonreplicating sporozoite vaccine. *Science* (2013) 341:1359–65. doi: 10.1126/science.1241800
127. Epstein JE, Tewari K, Lyke K, Sim B, Billingsley P, Laurens M, et al. Live attenuated malaria vaccine designed to protect through hepatic CD8+ T cell immunity. *Science* 2011:1211548. doi: 10.1126/science.1211548
128. Saito F, Hirayasu K, Satoh T, Wang CW, Lusingu J, Arimori T, et al. Immune evasion of Plasmodium falciparum by RIFIN via inhibitory receptors. *Nature* (2017) 552:101. doi: 10.1038/nature24994
129. Scally SW, Murugan R, Bosch A, Triller G, Costa G, Mordmüller B, et al. Rare PfCSP C-terminal antibodies induced by live sporozoite vaccination are ineffective against malaria infection. *J Exp Med.* (2018) 215:63–75. doi: 10.1084/jem.20170869
130. Pulendran B. Systems vaccinology: probing humanity's diverse immune systems with vaccines. *Proc Natl Acad Sci USA.* (2014) 111:12300–6. doi: 10.1073/pnas.1400476111
131. Pulendran B, Li S, Nakaya HI. Systems vaccinology. *Immunity* (2010) 33:516–29. doi: 10.1016/j.immuni.2010.10.006
132. Doolan DL, Mu Y, Unal B, Sundaresh S, Hirst S, Valdez C, et al. Profiling humoral immune responses to *P. falciparum* infection with protein microarrays. *Proteomics* (2008) 8:4680–94. doi: 10.1002/pmic.200800194
133. Osier FH, Mackinnon MJ, Crosnier C, Fegan G, Kamuyu G, Wanaguru M, et al. New antigens for a multicomponent blood-stage malaria vaccine. *Sci Transl Med.* (2014) 6:247ra102. doi: 10.1126/scitranslmed.3008705.

134. Skinner J, Huang C-Y, Waisberg M, Felgner PL, Doumbo OK, Ongoiba A, et al. *Plasmodium falciparum* gametocyte-specific antibody profiling reveals boosting through natural infection and identifies potential markers of gametocyte exposure. *Infect Immun.* (2015) 83:4229–36. doi: 10.1128/IAI.00644-15
135. Arevalillo JM, Sztein MB, Kotloff KL, Levine MM, Simon JK. Identification of immune correlates of protection in Shigella infection by application of machine learning. *J Biomed Informat.* (2017) 74:1–9. doi: 10.1016/j.jbi.2017.08.005
136. Tan J, Pieper K, Piccoli L, Abdi A, Foglierini M, Geiger R, et al. A LAIR1 insertion generates broadly reactive antibodies against malaria variant antigens. *Nature* (2016) 529:105. doi: 10.1038/nature16450
137. Tan J, Sack BK, Oyen D, Zenklusen I, Piccoli L, Barbieri S, et al. A public antibody lineage that potently inhibits malaria infection through dual binding to the circumsporozoite protein. *Nature Med.* (2018) 24:401. doi: 10.1038/nm.4513
138. Kisalu NK, Idris AH, Weidle C, Flores-Garcia Y, Flynn BJ, Sack BK, et al. A human monoclonal antibody prevents malaria infection by targeting a new site of vulnerability on the parasite. *Nature Med.* (2018) 24:408. doi: 10.1038/nm.4512
139. Oyen D, Torres JL, Wille-Reece U, Ockenhouse CF, Emerling D, Glanville J, et al. Structural basis for antibody recognition of the NANP repeats in Plasmodium falciparum circumsporozoite protein. *Proc Natl Acad Sci USA.* (2017) 114:E10438-445. doi: 10.1073/pnas.1715812114
140. Lau LS, Fernandez-Ruiz D, Mollard V, Sturm A, Neller MA, Cozijnsen A, et al. CD8+ T Cells from a Novel T cell receptor transgenic mouse induce liver-stage immunity that can be boosted by blood-stage infection in rodent malaria. *PLoS Pathog.* (2014) 10:e1004135. doi: 10.1371/journal.ppat.1004135
141. Fernandez-Ruiz D, Lau LS, Ghazanfari N, Jones CM, Ng WY, Davey GM, et al. Development of a Novel $CD4^+$ TCR transgenic line that reveals a dominant role for $CD8^+$ dendritic cells and CD40 signaling in the generation of helper and CTL responses to blood-stage malaria. *J Immunol.* (2017) 199:4165–79. doi: 10.4049/jimmunol.1700186
142. Impagliazzo A, Milder F, Kuipers H, Wagner MV, Zhu X, Hoffman RM, et al. A stable trimeric influenza hemagglutinin stem as a broadly protective immunogen. *Science* (2015) 349:1301–6. doi: 10.1126/science.aac7263
143. Ngwuta JO, Chen M, Modjarrad K, Joyce MG, Kanekiyo M, Kumar A, et al. Prefusion F-specific antibodies determine the magnitude of RSV neutralizing activity in human sera. *Science Transl Med.* (2015) 7:309ra162. doi: 10.1126/scitranslmed.aac4241
144. Wu X, Yang Z-Y, Li Y, Hogerkorp C-M, Schief WR, Seaman MS, et al. Rational design of envelope identifies broadly neutralizing human monoclonal antibodies to HIV-1. *Science* (2010) 329:856–61. doi: 10.1126/science.1187659
145. Lynch RM, Boritz E, Coates EE, DeZure A, Madden P, Costner P, et al. Virologic effects of broadly neutralizing antibody VRC01 administration during chronic HIV-1 infection. *Science Transl Med.* (2015) 7:319ra206. doi: 10.1126/scitranslmed.aad5752
146. Ledgerwood J, Coates E, Yamshchikov G, Saunders J, Holman L, Enama M, et al. Safety, pharmacokinetics and neutralization of the broadly neutralizing HIV-1 human monoclonal antibody VRC01 in healthy adults. *Clin Exper Immunol.* (2015) 182:289–301. doi: 10.1111/cei.12692
147. Huang Y, Karuna S, Carpp LN, Reeves D, Pegu A, Seaton K, et al. Modeling cumulative overall prevention efficacy for the VRC01 phase 2b efficacy trials. *Hum Vaccin Immunother.* (2018) 14:2116–27. doi: 10.1080/21645515.2018.1462640
148. Wright KE, Hjerrild KA, Bartlett J, Douglas AD, Jin J, Brown RE, et al. Structure of malaria invasion protein RH5 with erythrocyte basigin and blocking antibodies. *Nature* (2014) 515:427. doi: 10.1038/nature13715
149. Payne RO, Silk SE, Elias SC, Milne KH, Rawlinson TA, Llewellyn D, et al. Human vaccination against Plasmodium vivax Duffy-binding protein induces strain-transcending antibodies. *JCI Insight* (2017) 2:e93683. doi: 10.1172/jci.insight.93683
150. Chen E, Salinas ND, Huang Y, Ntumngia F, Plasencia MD, Gross ML, et al. Broadly neutralizing epitopes in the *Plasmodium vivax* vaccine candidate Duffy Binding Protein. *Proc Natl Acad Sci USA.* (2016) 113:6277–82. doi: 10.1073/pnas.1600488113

9

CXCR3+ T Follicular Helper Cells Induced by Co-Administration of RTS,S/AS01B and Viral-Vectored Vaccines are Associated with Reduced Immunogenicity and Efficacy Against Malaria

Georgina Bowyer[1], Amy Grobbelaar[1], Tommy Rampling[1], Navin Venkatraman[1], Danielle Morelle[2], Ripley W. Ballou[2], Adrian V. S. Hill[1] and Katie J. Ewer[1]*

[1] *The Jenner Institute, University of Oxford, Oxford, United Kingdom,* [2] *GSK Vaccines, Rixensart, Belgium*

***Correspondence:**
Georgina Bowyer
georgina.bowyer@ndm.ox.ac.uk

A malaria vaccine strategy targeting multiple lifecycle stages may be required to achieve a high level of efficacy. In two Phase IIa clinical trials, we tested immunogenicity and efficacy of RTS,S/AS01B administered alone, in a staggered regimen with viral-vectored vaccines or co-administered with viral-vectored vaccines. RTS,S/AS01B induces high titers of antibody against sporozoites and viral-vectored vaccines ChAd63 ME-TRAP and MVA ME-TRAP induce potent T cell responses against infected hepatocytes. By combining these two strategies, we aimed to improve efficacy by inducing immune responses targeting multiple parasite antigens. Vaccination with RTS,S/AS01B alone or in a staggered regimen with viral vectors produced strong immune responses and demonstrated high levels of protection against controlled human malaria infection. However, concomitant administration of these vaccines significantly reduced humoral immunogenicity and protective efficacy. Strong Th1-biased cytokine responses induced by MVA ME-TRAP were associated with a skew in circulating T follicular helper cells toward a CXCR3+ phenotype and a reduction in antibody quantity and quality. This study illustrates that while a multistage-targeting vaccine strategy could provide high-level efficacy, the regimen design will require careful optimization.

Keywords: malaria, vaccine, T follicular helper cell, antibody, efficacy, CXCR3, RTSS viral-vectored vaccines

INTRODUCTION

Despite years of remarkable success in reducing malaria morbidity and mortality, progress appears to have stalled with 216 million new cases in 2016, 5 million more than 2015 (1). An efficacious vaccine could be an essential tool to enable any further reduction in morbidity and mortality, and for the ultimate goal of eradication (2). The most advanced vaccine candidate, RTS,S, has shown significant short-term protective efficacy and has completed testing in a large Phase III trial (3–7).

Abbreviations: ChAd, chimpanzee adenovirus; CHMI, controlled human malaria infection; CSP, circumsporozoite protein; cTfh, circulating T follicular helper cell; GC, germinal center; ISI, inhibition of sporozoite invasion; ME, multi-epitope; MVA, modified vaccinia virus Ankara; PBMCs, peripheral blood mononucleocytes; pfu, plaque-forming units; TRAP, thrombospondin-related adhesive protein; VE, vaccine efficacy; VP, viral particles.

However, there remains a need to improve efficacy to achieve the goals laid out in the Malaria Vaccine Technology Roadmap (8). To improve efficacy, it may be necessary to develop a vaccine regimen targeting multiple stages of the parasite lifecycle (9). In addition to RTS,S, which targets the pre-liver stage, vaccines are being developed to target liver- and blood-stage parasites, or block parasite transmission and these could be combined into a multistage malaria vaccine program (9–12). It is likely that for a multistage vaccine regimen to provide high-level efficacy, it will need to induce both potent T cell and antibody responses (9).

The primary mechanism by which RTS,S induces protection appears to be antibody responses against the NANP repeat region of the circumsporozoite protein (CSP) on the sporozoite surface (13–16). The viral-vectored vaccines used in this study were chimpanzee adenovirus serotype 63 (ChAd63) and modified vaccinia virus Ankara (MVA), both expressing a multi-epitope (ME) string fused to the *Plasmodium falciparum* protein thrombospondin-related adhesive protein (TRAP). The ME string contains 17 epitopes from potentially protective *P. falciparum* and bacille Calmette–Guérin antigens in addition to epitopes from tetanus toxoid. TRAP is expressed on the surface of sporozoites and contains a thrombospondin domain that binds to heparin sulfate proteoglycans to facilitate sporozoite entry into host hepatocytes. ChAd63 ME-TRAP and MVA ME-TRAP provide protection by inducing $CD8^+$ T cell responses against infected hepatocytes (17). When RTS,S/AS01B and viral-vectored vaccines were tested in a combination regimen, efficacy against controlled human malaria infection (CHMI) was higher for volunteers receiving the combination of vaccines (14/17 subjects protected; vaccine efficacy (VE) 82.4% [95% CI 64–100]) than for those receiving RTS,S/AS01B alone (12/16 subjects protected; VE 75% [95% CI 54–96]), suggesting that TRAP-specific T cell responses could add to the protective effect of RTS,S-induced antibody responses (18). In that study, NANP IgG titers in the combination group were comparable to those in the group given RTS,S/AS01B alone and were significantly higher in protected individuals. Titers of IgG against NANP were negatively correlated with parasitemia at day 7.5, indicating a reduced liver to blood inoculum. However, as viral-vectored vaccinations were given at staggered time points, a minimum of 2 weeks after RTS,S/AS01B, this regimen required five separate clinic visits over a period of 10 weeks. For a vaccine regimen to be logistically and economically feasible for deployment in malaria-endemic regions, the number of clinic visits should be reduced. For this reason, we conducted a further Phase I/IIa clinical trial to assess concomitant administration of RTS,S/AS01B with viral-vectored vaccines (Rampling et al. manuscript under review). On the basis of high efficacy in two previous trials, additional groups were included to test a reduced third dose of RTS,S/AS01B (1/5th, 10 μg) (14, 19). In this study, co-administration of these two vaccine platforms resulted in a significant reduction in humoral immunogenicity and efficacy with only 11/19 volunteers protected (VE 57.9% 95% CI [33.2–76.3]), compared with 14/17 (82.4% 95% CI [54.7–93.9]) in the group receiving RTS,S/AS01B alone.

Durable, high-affinity IgG is generated in germinal center (GC) reactions in secondary lymphoid organs, during which B cells undergo class-switching, somatic hypermutation, and differentiation into memory B cells and plasma cells. T follicular helper cells (Tfh) expressing CD4 and CXCR5 and the transcription factor Bcl-6 provide essential help to B cells for this process in the form of cytokine production (IL-21) and the expression of costimulatory molecules (CD40L, ICOS) (20, 21). Circulating $PD1^+CXCR5^+CD45RA^-$ $CD4^+$ T cells appear to be a peripheral counterpart of conventional lymphoid resident Tfh, may represent GC responses, and are a useful tool for clinical trials in which lymphoid tissue is rarely available for analysis (22–24). Circulating T follicular helper cells (cTfh) can be further defined by differential expression of chemokine receptors CXCR3 and CCR6: Th17-like (cTfh17) $CXCR3^-CCR6^+$, double-positive $CXCR3^+CCR6^+$, Th1-like (cTfh1) $CXCR3^+CCR6^-$, and Th2-like (cTfh2) $CXCR3^-CCR6^-$. These subsets have been associated with varying degrees of helper activity in different contexts (25). In particular, $CXCR3^-$ Tfh have been associated with the production of broadly neutralizing antibodies against HIV and Tfh17 induced by rVSV-ZEBOV vaccination were associated with antibody responses against Ebola (26, 27). Therefore, the type of cTfh induced by vaccination may be an indicator of the quality of the GC reaction and the resulting antibodies produced.

To investigate the mechanisms underlying the reduction in humoral immunogenicity after co-administration of ChAd63-MVA ME-TRAP and RTS,S, we conducted a thorough analysis of the differences in antibody quality and cTfh responses in volunteers receiving RTS,S/AS01B alone (R), RTS,S/AS01B given with viral vectors in a staggered regimen (R2V) or co-administered (R + V). Trial regimens are summarized in **Table 1**. This is the first study to assess the impact of vaccine co-administration on the cTfh response in humans and also defines a functional antibody quality that may explain the improved efficacy observed in RTS,S regimens with a reduced third dose.

MATERIALS AND METHODS

Samples and Study Details

Full details of these studies are available in the clinical trial reports [(18), Rampling et al. manuscript under review]. Healthy adult volunteers were recruited and vaccinated at four UK sites, in Oxford, Southampton, London, and Surrey. The CHMI procedure was performed as previously described using five infectious bites from *P. falciparum* 3D7-strain infected *Anopheles stephensi* mosquitoes at Imperial College, London (28). All subjects were infected with a single batch of infected mosquitoes for each trial, supplied by the Department of Entomology, Walter Reed Army Institute of Research, Washington DC, USA. All vaccinations were administered intramuscularly into the deltoid region of the arm. For participants who received concomitant vaccinations, RTS,S/AS01B was administered first followed by the viral-vectored vaccine in the same site no longer than 5 min later.

Ethics Statement

All volunteers gave written informed consent prior to participation, and the studies were conducted according to the principles of the Declaration of Helsinki and in accordance with Good

TABLE 1 | Vaccination schedules.

	Co-administration study (VAC59)					Staggered study (VAC55)		
	RTS,S/AS01B (R)		RTS,S/AS01B co-administered with viral vectors (R + V)			RTS,S/AS01B and viral vectors staggered (R2V)	RTS,S/AS01B (R)	
Group	G1 R-R-R	G2 R-R-r	G3 RA-RM-RM	G4 RA-RM-rM	Controls	R-A-R-R-M	R-R-R	Controls
No. volunteers enrolled	10	10	10	11	4	20	17	6
No. volunteers at C-1	9	10	10	9	4	17	16	6
No. volunteers challenged	8	9	10	9	4	17	16	6
Week 0	R	R	RA	RA		R	R	
Week 2						A		
Week 4	R	R	RM	RM		R	R	
Week 8	R	r	RM	rM		R	R	
Week 10						M		
Week 11	CHMI	CHMI	CHMI	CHMI	CHMI			
Week 12						CHMI	CHMI	CHMI
Efficacy: sterilely protected volunteers	6/8 (75%)	8/9 (89%)	6/10 (60%)	5/9 (56%)	0/4	(14/17) 82%	(12/16) 75%	0/6

R, 50 µg RTS,S/AS01B; r, 10 µg RTS,S/AS01B; A, 5 × 10^{10} viral particles (vp) ChAd63 ME-TRAP; M, 2 × 10^{8} plaque-forming units (pfu) MVA ME-TRAP; CHMI, controlled human malaria infection; (R), RTS,S/AS01B groups; (R2V), RTS,S/AS01B and viral-vectored vaccinations staggered by 2 weeks; (R + V), RTS,S/AS01B and viral vectors co-administered.

Clinical Practice. The trials were registered with ClinicalTrials.gov (Ref: NCT01883609 and NCT02252640). The study protocols were approved by the UK National Research Ethics Service, Committee South Central—Oxford A (Refs: 13/SC/0208 and 14/SC/0227), the Western Institution Review Board (Ref: 20130698), and the UK Medicines and Healthcare products Regulatory Agency (Refs: 21584/0317/001-0001 and 21584/0333/001-0001). The Local Safety Committee provided safety oversight for both trials and GCP compliance was monitored by the Clinical Trials and Research Governance Team (CTRG) of the University of Oxford.

Total IgG ELISA

ELISA 96-well plates were coated with a synthetic peptide (Eurogentec, Liège, Belgium) based on the PfCSP repeat region ($(NANP)_6C$) diluted to 0.2 µg/mL in 100 µL dPBS per well and incubated overnight at room temperature (RT). Plates were washed six times with PBS containing 0.5% Tween-20 (PBS/T) and blocked with casein for 1 h at RT. Plates were washed again and serum samples diluted in casein at 1:100, 1:500, 1:1,000, or 1:5,000, were added for 2 h at RT. After washing again, secondary antibody (goat anti-human IgG conjugated to alkaline phosphatase, Sigma) was added at 1:1,000 in casein for 1 h at RT. Plates were washed a final time and developed using 4-nitrophenyl phosphate in diethanolamine buffer (Pierce, Rockford, IL, USA). Optical density (OD) was read at 405 nm using an ELx800 microplate reader (Bio-Rad, Hercules, CA, USA). A reference pool of positive serum formed a standard curve on each plate and was used to calculate ELISA units for each sample. An internal control was included on each plate to standardize between assays. All samples were tested in triplicate.

Isotype ELISA

Isotype ELISAs were conducted as described above, except that all serum samples were diluted to 1:100 and added to the plate in duplicate wells on each of six plates. One of six secondary antibodies against IgG1, IgG2, IgG3, IgG4, IgM, or IgA was added to each plate at 1:1,000 in casein before developing as above. Blank wells and internal development controls were included on each plate. A "seropositive cut-off" value was calculated for each isotype or subclass using the mean plus 3 SDs of 36 UK malaria-naïve serum samples.

Indirect Immunofluorescence Assay (IFA)

Chambered microscope slides coated with *P. falciparum* sporozoites were stored at −80°C until use. Slides were brought to RT and then fixed for 15 min in 4% paraformaldehyde. After washing twice in PBS for 5 min, slides were blocked for 1 h in casein. Slides were washed as before and 10 µL of serum sample diluted 1:100 in casein was added to each well. Slides were incubated for 30 min at RT in a humidity chamber then wells were individually washed with PBS three times for 5 min. Secondary antibody (anti-IgG-AlexaFluor488) was diluted 1:800 in casein and 15 µL was added to each well for 30–45 min in a humidity chamber at RT protected from the light. Slides were washed a final time, rinsed in distilled water and left to dry before mounting with DAPI-containing media. Slides were left to set overnight at 4°C before being examined under a Leica DMI3000 B microscope. Images were captured in QCapturePro software using brightfield illumination, GFP and DAPI filters at set exposure levels. ImageJ software was used to measure the median fluorescence intensity (MFI) for five sporozoites in each well and an average was taken.

Inhibition of Sporozoite Invasion (ISI) Assay

The ISI assay was carried out as previously described (29). Human hepatoma cells (HC04) cultured in R10 medium (RPMI 1640 with 10% FCS, 1% penicillin/streptomycin, and 1% L-glutamine) were added to 96-well culture plates at 30,000 cells/well and left to settle overnight at 37°C, 5% CO_2. Viable GFP-labeled *Plasmodium berghei* sporozoites expressing *P. falciparum* CSP at the *P. berghei* CSP locus (*P. berghei* PfCSP@CSP) were obtained by dissecting infected *A. stephensi* mosquitoes. Salivary glands were pooled into RPMI 1640 medium and homogenized. Sporozoites were counted and diluted to 100,000/mL in RPMI 1640. Culture medium was aspirated from the hepatoma cells then 100 μL of serum diluted 1:5 in R10 and 100 μL of sporozoite dilution (10,000 sporozoites, 10% final serum concentration) were added to each well. Samples were tested in duplicate and an average calculated. "Hepatoma only" wells and infectivity control wells that contained hepatoma cells and sporozoites but no serum were included. Pre-vaccination and C-1 samples were run for each volunteer. After incubation for 20–26 h at 37°C, medium was aspirated, and plates were washed with 90 μL/well dPBS. Cells were trypsinized, re-suspended in 65 μL dPBS with 1% bovine serum albumin (BSA), and acquired immediately using a BD LSRII. DAPI stain was added to each sample just before acquisition. Data were analyzed in Flow Jo software v10.6 (Tree Star Inc., Ashland, OR, USA) according to a predefined gating strategy. The percentage of sporozoite inhibition was calculated for each sample (average of duplicate wells) based on the reduction in the percentage of infected cells compared with the infectivity controls (average of 4–6 wells).

Ex Vivo IFNγ ELISpot

Ex vivo ELISpot assays were performed for TRAP-specific T cell responses as previously described (10). Average responses were taken across triplicate wells, background subtracted and then responses in individual pools were summed.

cTfh Phenotyping and ICS

Surface phenotyping of cTfh was carried out using cryopreserved peripheral blood mononucleocytes (PBMCs). Thawing was performed rapidly in a water bath and cells were rested for 2 h at 37°C with 5% CO_2 and Benzonase at 25U/10^6 PBMC (Novagen, Madison, WI, USA) before staining. For surface phenotyping 1–2 million PBMC were stained. Cells were washed in FACS buffer (PBS containing 0.1% BSA and 0.01% sodium azide) and stained with LIVE/DEAD aqua amine reactive dye (Life Technologies Ltd., Carlsbad, CA, USA) for 20 min at RT in the dark. Cells were washed in FACS buffer and a cocktail of antibodies for Tfh surface staining (**Table 2**) was added for 30 min at RT. Cells were washed again in FACS Buffer and re-suspended in PBS containing 1% paraformaldehyde, prior to acquisition on a BD LSR II using FACSDiva v6.2 (BD Biosciences, Franklin Lakes, NJ, USA) on the day of staining. Compensation control beads (OneComp Beads, eBioscience, San Diego, CA, USA, ArC Amine Reactive Beads, Invitrogen, Carlsbad, CA, USA) were stained according to the manufacturer's instructions for compensation between parameters. A median of 100,000 live $CD4^+$ cells were acquired [inter-quartile range (IQR) 25% = 68,406, 75% = 143,000] per sample. Data analysis was performed using Flow Jo v9.6.2 (Tree Star Inc.). IFNγ production was measured after overnight stimulation with 2 μg/mL of a pool of 31 peptides spanning the CSP antigen (15mers overlapping by 11 amino acids, at 2 μg/mL, all volunteers) or 10 μg/mL superantigen *Staphylococcus* enterotoxin B (SEB). Brefeldin A and monensin were added at 10 μg/mL after 2 h. The staining protocol was the same as for cTfh phenotyping, except that after surface staining, cells were permeabilized with fix/perm buffer (BD biosciences)

TABLE 2 | Circulating T follicular helper cell phenotyping panel.

Marker	Fluorophore	Supplier	Clone	Dilution	Volume (μL)
CD3	Alexa Fluor 700	eBioscience	UCHT1	1:33	1.5
CD4	APC-eFluor 780	eBioscience	SK3 (SK-3)	1:50	1
CD45RA	eFluor450	BioLegend	HI101	1:50	1
CXCR5	PerCP-eFluor 710	BioLegend	MU5UBEE	1:16	3
CXCR3	APC	BioLegend	1C6/CXCR3	1:16	3
CCR6	PE	BioLegend	G034E3	1:16	3
PD-1	BV650	BioLegend	EH12.2H7	1:100	0.5
Live/dead	AmCyan	Invitrogen	N/A	1:500	0.1
IFNγ (in ICS assay)	FITC	eBioscience	4S.B3	1:250	0.2

then stained intracellularly at RT for 30 min with IFNγ-FITC (1:250, eBioscience), washed and fixed in 1% paraformaldehyde. Acquisition and analysis was performed as for cTfh phenotyping.

Multiplex Cytokine Assay

Between 1 and 2 million PBMC from the C-1 time point were plated per well in a 96-well plate and stimulated for 21 h at 37°C. Cells were stimulated either with a pool of 31 peptides spanning the CSP antigen (15mers overlapping by 11 amino acids, at 2 μg/mL, all volunteers) or 10^6 pfu of MVA. Supernatants were taken and stored at −20°C in 96-well U-bottom polypropylene plates until use. Cytokine concentrations in the supernatants were measured using the LEGENDplex human Th cytokine panel 13-plex assay (BioLegend, San Diego, CA, USA) according to the manufacturer's instructions. The samples were read on the same day on a BD LSR II using FACSDiva v6.2 (BD Biosciences) with 5,000 beads acquired per sample. Data analysis was conducted using the LEGENDplex data analysis software.

Statistical Analysis

Data tested negative for a normal distribution by D'Agostina–Pearson omnibus normality test; therefore, non-parametric tests were used and medians with IQRs are presented. Mann–Whitney analysis was used to compare differences between two groups. Kruskal–Wallis with Dunn's multiple comparisons post-test was used to compare responses across multiple groups at a given time point. Wilcoxon matched-pairs analysis was used to compare responses at two time points within a group. Spearman's rank was calculated for correlations. $P < 0.05$ was considered significant and all P values are two-tailed. Analyses were performed in GraphPad Prism, version 7.

RESULTS

Reduced Quantity and Quality of Antibody Responses When RTS,S/AS01B Is Co-Administered With Viral-Vectored Vaccines

Antibody responses against the NANP repeat region of CSP were measured in each of the clinical trials and reported separately (18) (Rampling et al. manuscript under review). Total

NANP-specific IgG was measured by ELISA at baseline (day 0, D0), D28, D42, D56, D76 (the day before CHMI, C-1, in the co-administration trial) and 35 and 90 days after CHMI (C + 35, C + 90). In the staggered regimen trial, anti-NANP-specific IgG was also measured at D83 (C-1 for that trial) as the CHMI was 1 week later to accommodate the additional vaccinations (**Figure 1A**). Titers were comparable in all regimens after the first two vaccinations but failed to re-boost after the third vaccination

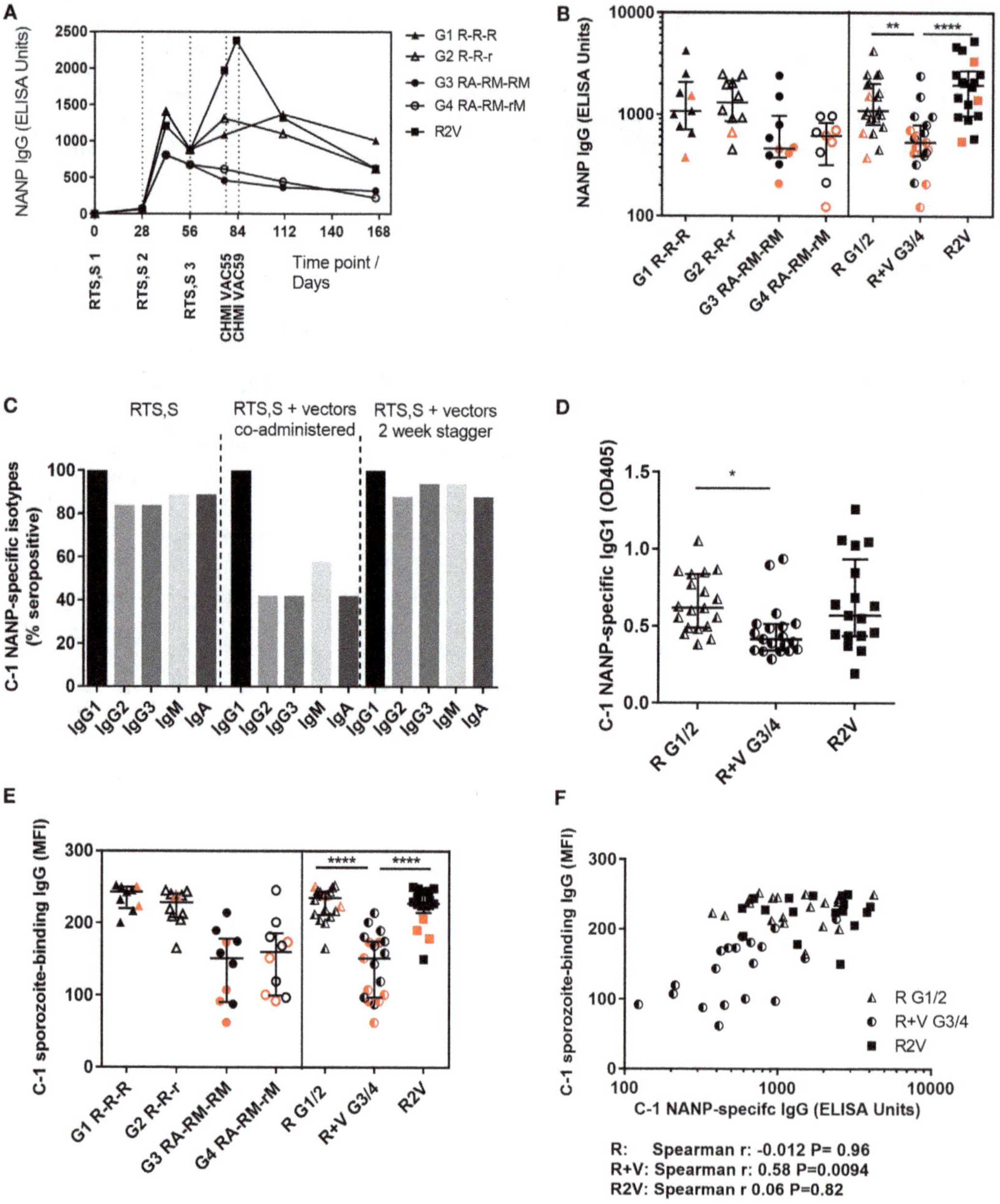

FIGURE 1 | Antibody quantity and quality. **(A)** Median NANP-specific IgG time courses. **(B)** Total IgG titers against the CSP repeat region NANP in each group at D76 (2 weeks after third dose of RTS,S/AS01B), in G1/2 combined (R) and G3/4 combined (R + V) or in the staggered regimen (R2V), Kruskal–Wallis with Dunn's post-test $P < 0.0001$. **(C)** NANP-specific isotype and IgG subclass responses at C-1. **(D)** NANP-specific IgG1 at C-1, Kruskal–Wallis $P = 0.0062$. **(E)** MFI of sporozoite-binding IgG at C-1 measured by IFA, Kruskal–Wallis $P < 0.0001$. **(F)** Relationship between NANP IgG titer and level of sporozoite-binding at C-1. Volunteers receiving RTS,S/AS01B alone (G1/2, R) Spearman r: –0.012, $P = 0.96$, RTS,S/AS01B co-administered with vectors (G3/4, R + V) Spearman r: 0.58, $P = 0.0094$ or RTS,S/AS01B and viral vectors given in a staggered regimen Spearman r: 0.06, $P = 0.82$. Medians + IQRs shown and non-protected volunteers highlighted in red for all column graphs. Abbreviations: R G1/2, RTS,S/AS01B vaccinated; R + V G3/4, RTS,S/AS01B and viral-vectored vaccines co-administered; R2V, RTS,S/AS01B and viral-vectored vaccines at a 2-week stagger; A, ChAd63 ME-TRAP; M, MVA ME-TRAP; R, 50 µg third dose of RTS,S/AS01B; r, 10 µg third dose of RTS,S/AS01B; CHMI, controlled human malaria infection; C-1, day before CHMI; CSP, circumsporozoite protein; TRAP, thrombospondin-related adhesive protein; IQRs, inter-quartile ranges; IFA, immunofluorescence assay; MFI, median fluorescence intensity.

in the co-administration regimen, resulting in significantly lower titers in these groups at D76 (**Figure 1B**, median ELISA units, R: 1,102 IQR [757–2,035], R + V: 533 IQR [394–790], R2V: 1,969 IQR [983–2,724] Kruskal–Wallis $P < 0.0001$). There were no significant differences in NANP IgG titers between groups receiving a full or reduced third dose of RTS,S/AS01B either alone or co-administered with viral-vectored vaccines. The highest titers were seen in the staggered regimen at D83 (4 weeks after the third dose of RTS,S/AS01B), although there was no comparable time point in the co-administration study.

Isotype and subclass responses were measured by ELISA against the NANP repeat region at C-1 in both trials (**Figure 1C**). Titers were measured for IgG1-4, IgM, and IgA. No NANP-specific IgG4 was detected in any volunteers (data not shown). Over 80% of volunteers given RTS,S/AS01B alone were seropositive for NANP-specific IgG2, IgG3, IgM, and IgA. There were significant reductions in seroconversion for these isotypes/subclasses in groups that received concomitant viral-vectored vaccinations, but not in the staggered regimen. All volunteers were positive for NANP IgG1 and titers were comparable in the RTS,S/AS01B only groups (R) and the staggered administration group (R2V), but were significantly reduced in the co-administration regimen (R + V) (**Figure 1D**, median OD, R: 0.617 IQR [0.488–0.835], R + V: 0.415 [0.343–0.514], R2V: 0.570 [0.438–0.935] Kruskal–Wallis $P = 0.0062$). There were no significant differences in IgG1 titers between groups receiving full or reduced third doses of RTS,S/AS01B (G1 R-R-R vs G2 R-R-r and G3 RA-RM-RM vs G4 RA-RM-rM, data not shown).

Antibody binding to fixed whole sporozoites was measured for all volunteers at C-1 using an indirect IFA. Sporozoite-binding IgG was significantly lower in the co-administration regimen but the staggered regimen was comparable to RTS,S/AS01B alone (**Figure 1E**, MFI, R: 238 IQR [213–245] R + V: 151 [98–175], R2V: 228 [215–245] Kruskal–Wallis $P < 0.0001$). There were no differences between groups receiving full or reduced third doses of RTS,S/AS01B. Sporozoite-binding was significantly associated with NANP IgG titers in the co-administration groups (**Figure 1F**, Spearman r: 0.58, $P = 0.0094$). There was no association in the RTS,S/AS01B alone or staggered regimens (Spearman r: −0.012, $P = 0.96$ and r: 0.058, $P = 0.83$, respectively), in which sporozoite-binding was higher for a given NANP IgG titer than in the co-administration regimen.

ISI Is Associated With Protection From CHMI

The functional quality of vaccine-induced antibodies was assessed using an *in vitro* assay measuring the ability of serum to block sporozoite infection of hepatoma cells (29). A defined gating strategy was used to identify infected hepatoma cells (**Figure 2**).

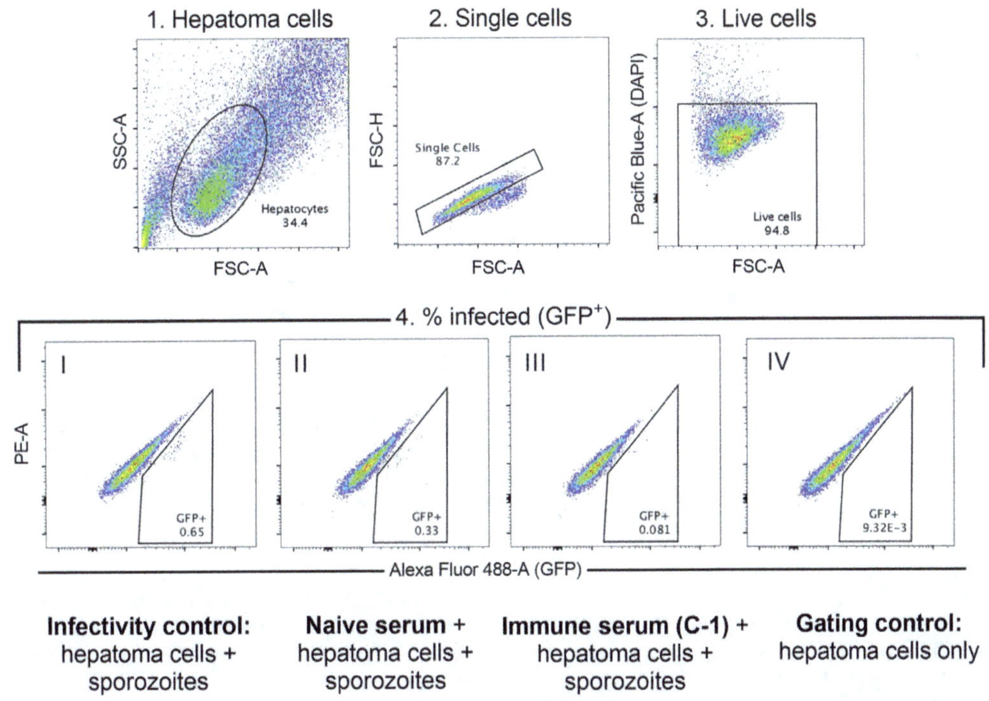

FIGURE 2 | Inhibition of sporozoite invasion assay. Hierarchical gating strategy used to determine the percentage of hepatoma cells infected with GFP-expressing sporozoites. 1. Hepatoma cells are gated based on size to exclude debris and large cell clumps. 2. Singlets are gated to exclude smaller cell clumps. 3. Live cells (DAPI-negative) are gated to exclude dead cells. 4. Cells infected with the GFP-expressing sporozoites are GFP^{+}. Cells are gated against both GFP (Alexa Fluor-AF488 channel, GFP^{+}) and the adjacent channel (PE^{-}) to exclude signal that is caused by autofluorescence. Representative populations in each of the conditions are shown: I. Infectivity control—sporozoite infection of hepatoma cells in the absence of any serum; II. Sporozoite infection of hepatoma cells in the presence of naïve serum (D0); III. Sporozoite infection of hepatoma cells in the presence of immune serum (C-1); IV. Gating control—hepatoma cells only, no sporozoites or serum added.

The percentage of infection blocked by vaccine-induced antibody was significantly lower in the co-administration regimen compared with RTS,S/AS01B alone (**Figure 3A**, median percentage infection blocked R, 90% IQR [76–98], R + V 80% [52–89], Mann–Whitney $P = 0.016$). However, blocking ability was significantly higher in groups receiving a reduced third dose of RTS,S/AS01B than those receiving three standard doses, even when this dose was co-administered with viral-vectored vaccines (**Figure 3A**, medians + IQRs G1 R-R-R: 80% [71.5–91.5], G2 R-R-r: 96% [89.3–98], G3 RA-RM-RM: 55% [50–73.5], G4 RA-RM-rM: 89% [85–95], Mann–Whitney analyses G1 R-R-R vs G2 R-R-r $P = 0.014$, G3 RA-RM-RM vs G4 RA-RM-rM $P < 0.0001$, G1 R-R-R and G3 RA-RM-RM vs G2 R-R-r and G4 RA-RM-rM $P < 0.0001$). ISI was significantly associated with C-1 NANP IgG titer for groups receiving three standard doses of RTS,S/AS01B (**Figure 3B**, G1 R-R-R and G3

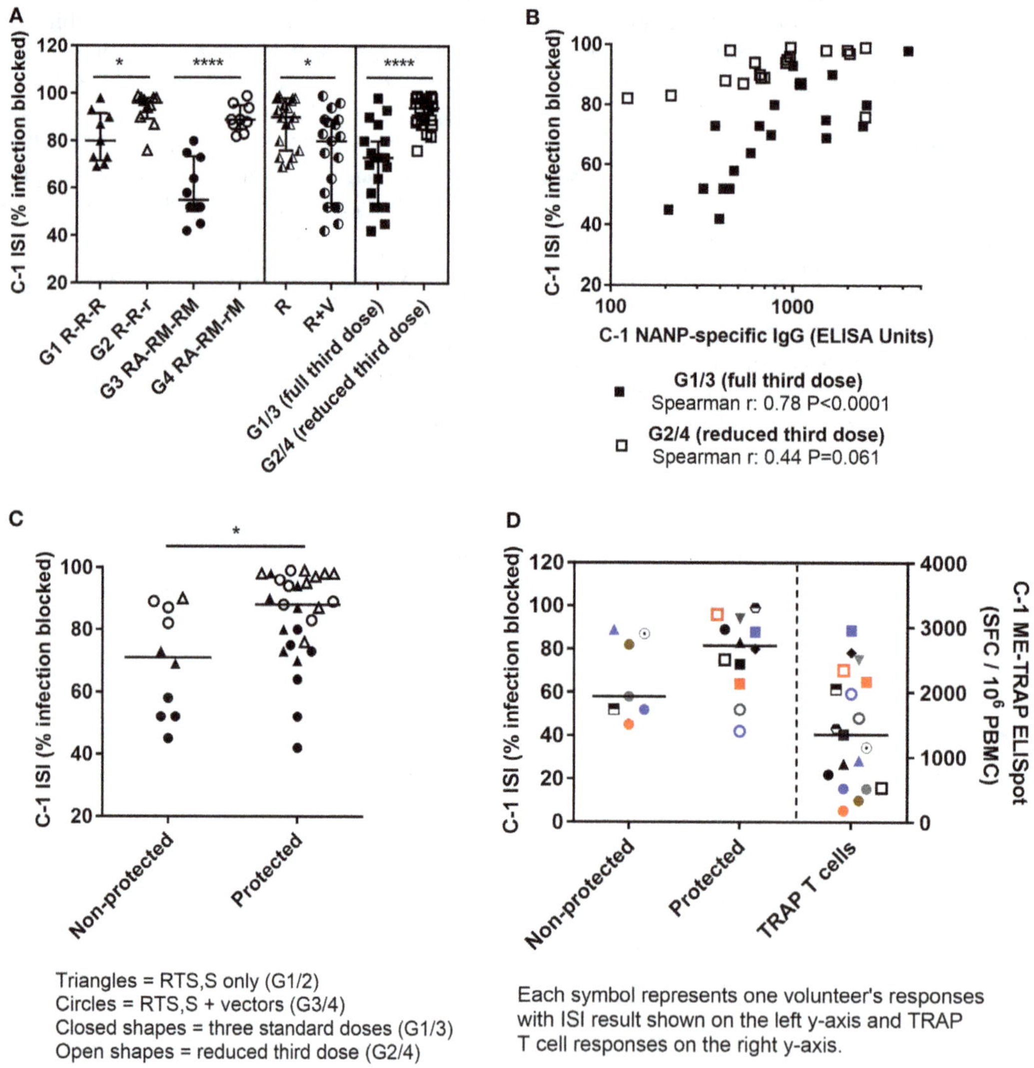

FIGURE 3 | ISI results. **(A)** Percentage of sporozoite invasion into hepatoma cells that was blocked by serum at C-1. Comparison of groups given three standard doses of RTS,S/AS01B or a reduced (1/5th) third dose of RTS,S/AS01B. Mann–Whitney analyses G1 R-R-R vs G2 R-R-r $P = 0.014$, G3 RA-RM-RM vs G4 RA-RM-rM $P < 0.0001$, G1/2 (R) vs G3/4 (R + V) $P = 0.016$, G1/3 (full third dose of RTS,S/AS01B) vs G2/4 (reduced third dose of RTS,S/AS01B) $P < 0.0001$, medians + IQRs. **(B)** Relationship between C-1 NANP IgG titers and sporozoite-blocking ability in individuals who received three full doses of RTS,S/AS01B with or without vectored vaccines (G1 and G3, closed squares, Spearman r: 0.78, $P < 0.0001$) or a reduced third dose of RTS,S/AS01B with, or without vectored vaccines (G2 and G4, open squares, Spearman r: 0.44, $P = 0.061$). **(C)** Percentage of sporozoite invasion blocked by C-1 serum protected and non-protected individuals, Mann–Whitney $P = 0.017$. Closed triangles: G1, open triangles: G2, closed circles: G3, open circles: G4. **(D)** Percentage of sporozoite invasion blocked by serum at C-1 in protected and non-protected volunteers in G3/4, R + V (left Y-axis) and corresponding TRAP T cell responses (right Y-axis) at C-1 for each volunteer measured by IFNγ ELISpot, summed responses from T9/96 TRAP pools + ME, spot-forming cells per million PBMC (SFC/10^6 PBMC), lines at medians. Abbreviations: R G1/2, RTS,S/AS01B vaccinated; R + V G3/4, RTS,S/AS01B and viral-vectored vaccines co-administered; R2V, RTS,S/AS01B and viral-vectored vaccines at a 2-week stagger; A, ChAd63 ME-TRAP; M, MVA ME-TRAP; R, 50 µg third dose of RTS,S/AS01B; r, 10 µg third dose of RTS,S/AS01B; CHMI, controlled human malaria infection; C-1: day before CHMI; ISI, inhibition of sporozoite invasion; PBMCs, peripheral blood mononucleocytes; TRAP, thrombospondin-related adhesive protein; IQRs, inter-quartile ranges.

RA-RM-RM Spearman r: 0.78, $P < 0.0001$) but not in groups receiving a reduced third dose, in which blocking ability was higher even at lower NANP titers (G2 R-R-r and G4 RA-RM-rM Spearman r: 0.44, $P = 0.061$). The relationship between blocking ability and the NANP-specific isotype/subclass titers was also assessed (Figure S1 in Supplementary Material). Relationships between all subclasses and isotypes tested and blocking ability demonstrated a similar pattern to total IgG, with a positive correlation in G1/3 and high blocking regardless of titer in G2/4. However, IgG1 was the only isotype that showed an association with blocking ability in the data set as a whole (G1–4, Spearman r: 0.42, $P = 0.009$).

Blocking ability was associated with protection from malaria after CHMI, with significantly higher percentages of infection blocked in protected than non-protected volunteers (**Figure 3C**, medians + IQRs protected: 88% [75–97], non-protected: 71% [52–87.5] Mann–Whitney $P = 0.019$). TRAP-specific T cell responses elicited by the viral-vectored vaccines were measured by IFNγ ELISpot and previously reported (Rampling et al. manuscript under review). T cell responses (IFNγ responses against summed T9/96 TRAP pools + the multi-epitope, ME) were not reduced by co-administration and responses were significantly higher in protected than non-protected individuals in these groups (Rampling et al. manuscript under review). Volunteers in the co-administration groups that were protected despite having low levels of sporozoite-blocking antibody had high TRAP-specific T cell responses (**Figure 3D**).

Proportion of CXCR3$^+$ cTfh Increases When RTS,S/AS01B Is Co-Administered With Viral-Vectored Vaccines and Negatively Correlates With Antibody Responses

To determine whether cellular differences associated with the reduction in antibody responses in the co-administration regimen could be detected in the blood, cTfh were phenotyped at C-1 by surface staining and flow cytometry using a defined gating strategy (**Figure 4A**). Total cTfh were analyzed for all volunteers in the co-administration study (except 1 volunteer in G4 for which there were no cryopreserved cells remaining) and 10 volunteers in the staggered administration study with enough cryopreserved cells remaining for the experiment (**Figure 4B**). The proportion of cTfh (PD1$^+$CXCR5$^+$) within memory CD4$^+$ T cells ranged from 0.1 to 4.8%, was comparable across groups and did not correlate with CSP- or TRAP-specific antibody responses. Subsets within cTfh were identified using CXCR3 and CCR6: cTfh17 (CXCR3$^-$CCR6$^+$), CXCR3$^+$ [including double-positive (CXCR3$^+$CCR6$^+$) and cTfh1 (CXCR3$^+$CCR6$^-$)] and cTfh2 (CXCR3$^-$CCR6$^-$). Volunteers who received RTS,S/AS01B co-administered with viral-vectored vaccines had significantly higher frequencies of CXCR3$^+$ cTfh and significantly lower frequencies of cTfh2 than those who received RTS,S/AS01B alone, while the staggered administration group had an intermediate phenotype which was not significantly different to either of the other regimens (**Figure 4C**). There were no significant differences in frequencies of any population between G1 R-R-R and G2 R-R-r or G3 RA-RM-RM and G4 RA-RM-rM (data not shown). In the co-administration regimen, the percentage of CXCR3$^+$ cTfh was negatively correlated with antibody responses to both vaccines (**Figure 4D**, NANP Spearman r: −0.78, $P = 0.0001$, TRAP Spearman r: −0.50, $P = 0.036$). For groups that received RTS,S/AS01B alone, the frequency of CXCR3$^+$ cTfh was lower, and there was no association with antibody responses (**Figure 4E**, Spearman r: 0.32, $P = 0.18$). Although in the staggered regimen the proportion of CXCR3$^+$ cTfh was comparable to that in the co-administration regimen, they were not associated with a reduction in antibody responses in this regimen (Spearman r: 0.26, $P = 0.47$). The proportion of CXCR3$^+$ in CXCR5$^-$ memory CD4$^+$ T cells was not associated with antibody responses in any regimen (data not shown).

Co-Administration of Viral-Vectored Vaccines With RTS,S/AS01B Drives Th1-Biased Cytokine Responses Which Are Associated With the Increase in CXCR3$^+$ cTfh and Reduction in Antibody Responses

Concentrations of a range of T-helper cytokines in the supernatant of C-1 PBMC from the co-administration study were measured using a cytometric bead array (LEGENDplex, BioLegend). PBMCs were stimulated with CSP (all groups) or MVA (G3&4) and concentrations of IL-5, IL-13, IL-2, IL-6, IL-9, IL-10, IFNγ, TNFα, IL-17A, IL17-F, IL-4, IL-21, and IL-22 were measured (**Figure 5A**). High concentrations of IL-2, IFNγ, TNFα, IL-6, and IL-22 were detected. The concentration of IFNγ was particularly high in the supernatant from MVA-stimulated PBMCs where all samples produced >3,000 pg/mL. In comparison, IFNγ responses were significantly lower after CSP stimulation, with no detectable IFNγ in 9/34 samples and less than 1,000 pg/mL in most where responses were detected. However, PBMCs from volunteers in the co-administration groups produced more IFNγ in response to CSP stimulation than those from volunteers who received RTS,S/AS01B alone (**Figure 5B**, median pg/mL + IQR, R CSP: 114 [1–348], R + V CSP: 311 [96–610], R + V MVA: 16,796 [11,409–20,462], Kruskal-Wallis $P < 0.0001$). In addition, IFNγ was a greater proportion of the cytokine response to CSP stimulation in PBMC from G3/4 (R + V) volunteers who were not sterilely protected after CHMI than those who were protected (**Figure 5C**).

The concentration of IFNγ in the CSP supernatant was positively associated with the proportion of CXCR3$^+$ cTfh (**Figure 6A**, Spearman r: 0.41, $P = 0.01$) and negatively with the proportion of cTfh17 within cTfh (**Figure 6B**, Spearman r: −0.63, $P < 0.0001$). In addition, there was a negative association between the concentration of IFNγ in the CSP supernatant and the ability of antibody to block sporozoite entry into hepatocytes (**Figure 6C**, Spearman r: −0.79, $P = 0.0001$). Analysis of IFNγ production by ICS of cTfh after stimulation with CSP or the superantigen SEB showed very low frequencies of these cells expressing IFNγ [**Figure 6D**, less than 2% in G1/2 (R) and less than 3% in G3/4 (R + V) after CSP stimulation].

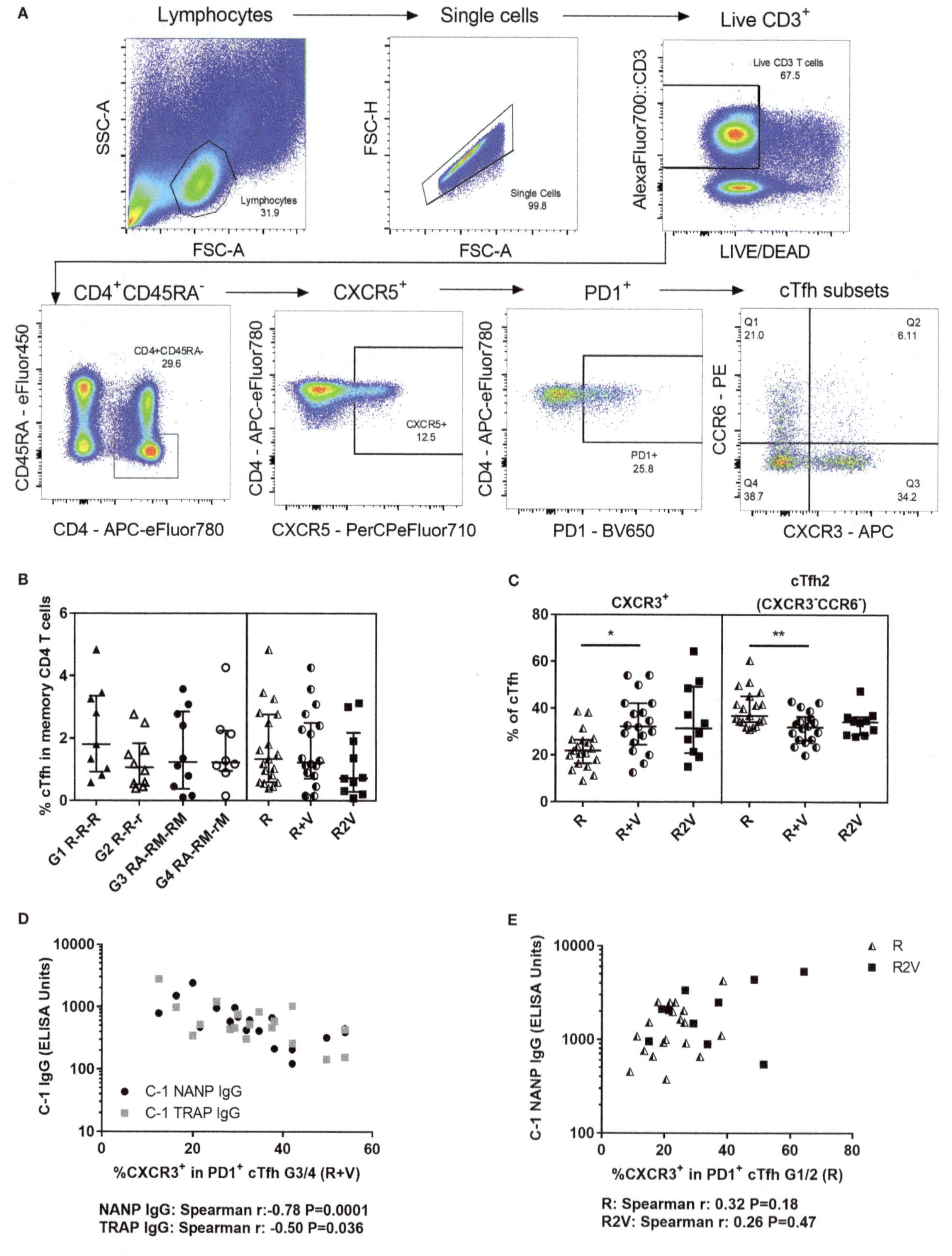

FIGURE 4 | Continued

FIGURE 4 | Total cTfhs. **(A)** Gating strategy for cTfh phenotyping using cell surface staining and flow cytometry. **(B)** Percentage of cTfh ($PD1^+CXCR5^+$) within memory CD4 T cells ($CD45RA^-$) at C-1. **(C)** Subsets within cTfh (at C-1) defined by chemokine receptor expression: cTfh2 ($CXCR3^-CCR6^-$), or $CXCR3^+$; including double-positive, dp ($CXCR3^+CCR6^+$), and cTfh1 ($CXCR3^+CCR6^-$). Kruskal–Wallis analyses; cTfh2 $P = 0.009$, $CXCR3^+$ $P = 0.01$. **(D)** Relationship between percentage of $CXCR3^+$ cTfh and antibody responses at C-1 in individuals who received RTS,S/AS01B co-administered with viral-vectored vaccines (G3/4). NANP IgG (Spearman *r*: −0.78, $P = 0.0001$), TRAP IgG (Spearman *r*: −0.50, $P = 0.036$). **(E)** Relationship between percentage of $CXCR3^+$ cTfh and C-1 NANP IgG in individuals vaccinated with RTS,S/AS01B alone (R, G1/2, Spearman *r*: 0.32, $P = 0.18$) or RTS,S/AS01B and viral-vectored vaccines in a staggered regimen (R2V, Spearman *r*: 0.26, $P = 0.47$). Abbreviations: R G1/2, RTS,S/AS01B vaccinated; R + V G3/4, RTS,S/AS01B and viral-vectored vaccines co-administered; R2V, RTS,S/AS01B and viral-vectored vaccines at a 2-week stagger; A, ChAd63 ME-TRAP; M, MVA ME-TRAP; R, 50 µg third dose of RTS,S/AS01B; r, 10 µg third dose of RTS,S/AS01B; CHMI, controlled human malaria infection; C-1, day before CHMI; cTfh, circulating T follicular helper cell; TRAP, thrombospondin-related adhesive protein.

DISCUSSION

Viral-vectored vaccines ChAd63 ME-TRAP and MVA ME-TRAP given with RTS,S/AS01B in a staggered regimen induced high titers of antibodies against sporozoites and potent T cell responses against infected liver cells (18). This regimen required five separate vaccinations and would likely be impractical and uneconomical for deployment in malaria-endemic regions. One way to overcome this obstacle would be to co-administer the RTS,S/AS01B and viral-vectored vaccines. Co-administration of vaccines can lead to interactions between the immune responses, which may be beneficial, enhancing the response as seen after co-administration of the live and attenuated polio vaccines or may result in a reduction of immunogenicity as is the case for multivalent inactivated or live viral vaccines (30, 31).

We examined the immune responses induced by both vaccines when co-administered to assess the extent of the immunological interaction between RTS,S/AS01B and viral-vectored vaccines. An *in vitro* assay measuring the ability of vaccine-induced antibody to block sporozoite invasion of hepatocytes was used to assess the functional quality of antibody. Infection-blocking ability was associated with protection. However, some volunteers who received viral-vectored vaccines were protected despite having antibodies with only low levels of infection-blocking activity. These volunteers had some of the highest TRAP-specific T cell responses, suggesting that cellular responses may provide protection by killing infected hepatocytes in volunteers who do not produce sufficient anti-NANP titers to block sporozoite entry. This demonstrates the potential of a multistage targeting regimen to provide high-level efficacy if each vaccine can be given without interfering with the immunogenicity of the other. However, co-administration of viral-vectored vaccines with RTS,S/AS01B in this study induced a strong Th1 cytokine response and increased proportions of $CXCR3^+$ cTfh, which were associated with reduced antibody quantity and quality and lower efficacy in these groups.

In addition, we observed qualitative differences in RTS,S-induced antibody responses when a reduced third (1/5th, 10 µg) dose was given compared with three standard doses (50 µg). Although NANP IgG titers were comparable, administration of a reduced third dose of RTS,S/AS01B-induced antibodies that were capable of blocking a significantly higher level of sporozoite infection *in vitro*—a measure which was associated with protection from CHMI. Previously, a reduced third dose of RTS,S/AS01B was shown to provide higher levels of protection (14, 19) and in a more recent study, a fractional third dose boost induced antibody with increased somatic hypermutation and higher avidity (19). However, it was unclear whether this effect was due to the delayed boost (0, 1, and 7-month regimen) or the fractional dose. Our study is the first to demonstrate a functional difference in the antibodies induced by the reduced third dose regimen that is associated with protection. However, it is unclear whether the quality of the antibody response is enhanced by a reduced third dose in particular or whether this could be achieved with a reduction of all three doses, which would also have economical and practical advantages. Lower vaccine doses decrease the availability of antigen and therefore could result in greater affinity maturation through increased competition between B cells for T cell help and preferential expansion of B cell clones with the highest affinity B cell receptors (32, 33). Lower doses of antigen at priming also preferentially drive the induction of memory, while higher antigen doses drive differentiation of plasma cells (34). The preferential induction of memory by reducing the priming dose could enhance responses to the subsequent vaccinations and also potentially generate more durable protection. This suggests that the dosing regimen should also be carefully tested to ensure the optimal type of immune response is achieved.

Previous studies have demonstrated that cTfh may be useful biomarkers for GC responses in the absence of lymphoid tissue (35). However, cTfh are a heterogeneous population composed of a number of different subsets, some of which appear to more closely resemble *bona fide* GC Tfh than others (22, 36). The proportions of these subsets have been associated with different diseases: increases in cTfh2/cTfh17 subsets are associated with the production of autoantibodies and disease severity in various autoimmune diseases (22, 37, 38), the development of allergy (39, 40) and the production of broadly neutralizing antibody in HIV^+ individuals (26, 41). By contrast, increases in $CXCR3^+$ cTfh have been implicated in the poor development of humoral immunity against malaria (42, 43) and are proportionally increased in patients with primary immunodeficiencies (44). In addition, a study that observed $CXCR3^+$ cTfh to positively correlate with antibody responses after influenza vaccination also showed that $CXCR3^+$ Tfh that were localized to tonsillar GCs, expressed Fas-L, secreted IFNγ, lacked CD154 expression, and suppressed the activity of GC B cells. Therefore, although this subset was correlated with antibody responses, they were not optimal for their induction (45). In our study, co-administration of RTS,S/AS01B with viral-vectored vaccines led to an increased frequency of $CXCR3^+$ total cTfh compared with RTS,S/AS01B administered alone, and this phenotype was associated with the observed reduction in antibody quantity and quality. Although the observed association was for total cTfh, it would be useful

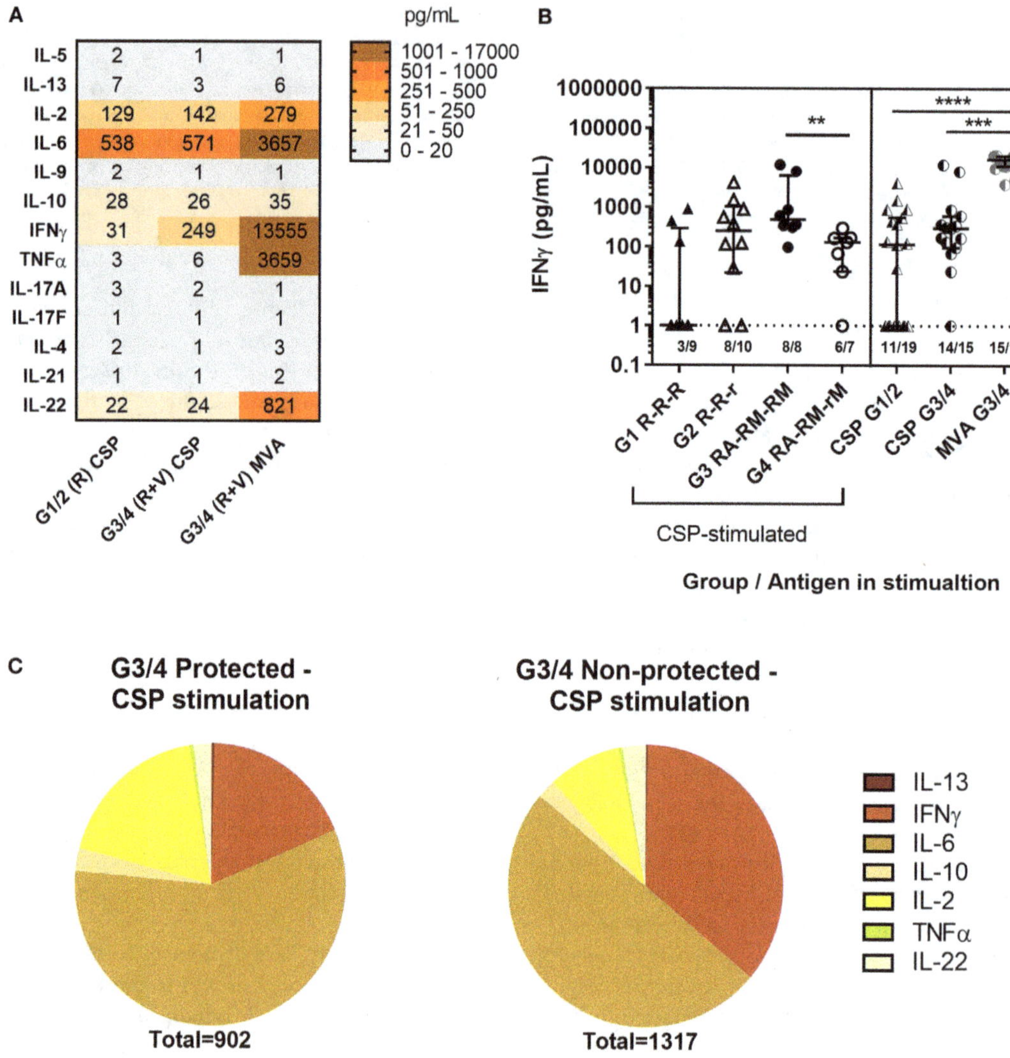

Percentage of column total	G3/4 CSP Protected	G3/4 CSP Not protected
IL-13	0.33%	0.23%
IFNγ	18.29%	35.84%
IL-6	57.87%	49.89%
IL-10	2.66%	2.20%
IL-2	18.18%	8.58%
TNFα	0.55%	0.53%
IL-22	2.11%	2.73%

FIGURE 5 | Cytokine responses to CSP and MVA. Cytokine responses measured in supernatant after stimulation of 1–2 × 10^6 PBMC at C-1 with CSP or MVA. A multiplex cytokine bead assay (Legendplex, BioLegend) was used to measure a panel of T-helper cytokines. Responses were measured for 19 G1/2 samples stimulated with CSP and 15 G3/4 samples for which there were enough cells to run both CSP and MVA stimulations. **(A)** Heatmap of geomean cytokine concentrations in pg/mL in supernatant of PBMC from G1/2 stimulated with CSP and G3/4 stimulated with CSP or MVA. **(B)** Concentration of IFNγ in supernatant of PBMC stimulated with CSP or MVA, Kruskal–Wallis with Dunn's multiple comparisons $P < 0.0001$. Mann–Whitney analysis between G3 RA-RM-RM and G4 RA-RM-rM $P = 0.0037$. Lower limit of detection for all cytokines in this assay was 1 pg/mL (indicated by the dashed line). **(C)** Proportions of cytokines produced in response to CSP stimulation (geomeans) in G3/4 (R + V) volunteers who were protected compared with those who were not. Table shows the level of each cytokine produced as a percentage of the total cytokine response to CSP in each group. Abbreviations: R G1/2, RTS,S/AS01B vaccinated; R + V G3/4, RTS,S/AS01B and viral-vectored vaccines co-administered; R2V, RTS,S/AS01B and viral-vectored vaccines at a 2-week stagger; A, ChAd63 ME-TRAP; M, MVA ME-TRAP; R, 50 µg third dose of RTS,S/AS01B; r, 10 µg third dose of RTS,S/AS01B; CHMI, controlled human malaria infection; C-1, day before CHMI; CSP, circumsporozoite protein; PBMCs, peripheral blood mononucleocytes; TRAP, thrombospondin-related adhesive protein.

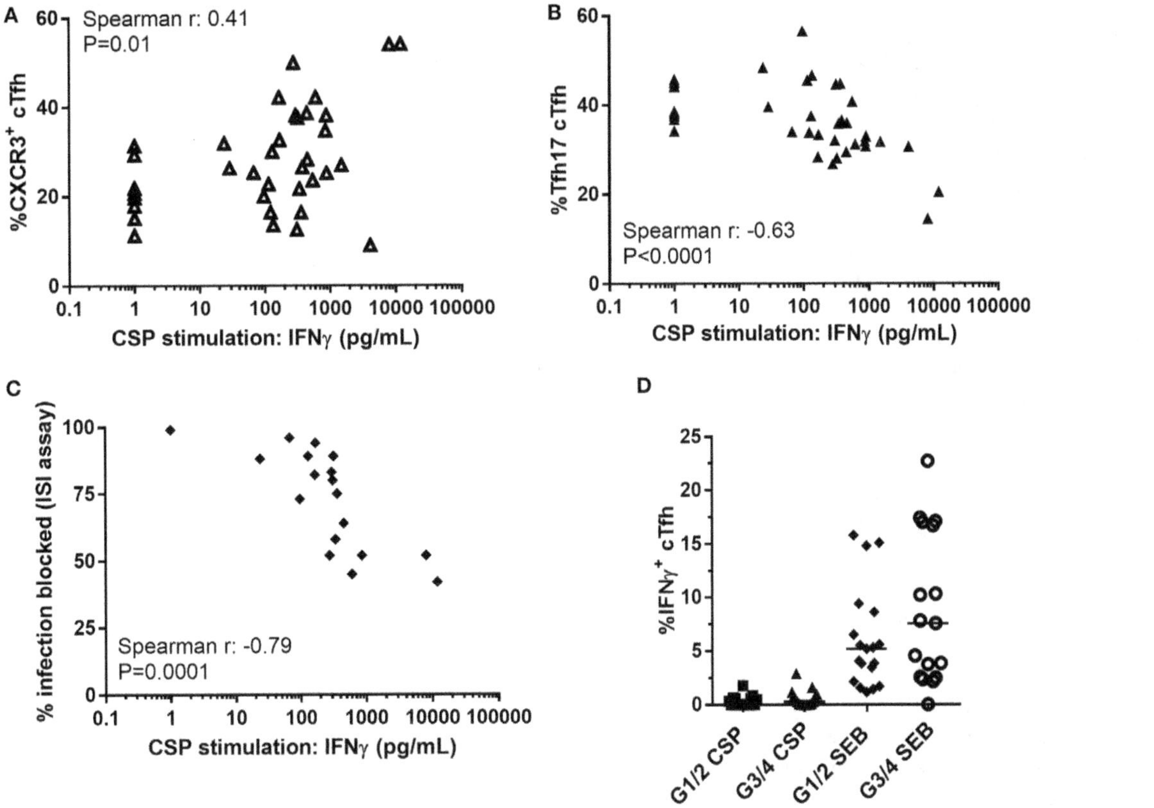

FIGURE 6 | Association between Th1-biased cytokine responses and suppressed humoral immunity. Relationship between concentration of IFNγ in supernatant of PBMCs stimulated with CSP in co-administration trial (G1–4, R, and R + V combined) and: **(A)** Proportion of CXCR3⁺ cTfh (Spearman *r*: 0.41, $P = 0.01$); **(B)** Proportion of cTfh17 (CXCR3⁺CCR6⁻) within cTfh (Spearman *r*: -0.63, $P < 0.0001$); **(C)** Percentage of infection blocked in the ISI assay (Spearman *r*: -0.79, $P = 0.0001$). **(D)** Proportion of IFNγ⁺ cTfh after stimulation with CSP or SEB, Mann–Whitney analyses between G1/2 (R) and G3/4 (R + V) $P = 0.14$ and $P = 0.26$ for CSP and SEB stimulations, respectively. Abbreviations: R G1/2, RTS,S/AS01B vaccinated; R + V G3/4, RTS,S/AS01B and viral-vectored vaccines co-administered; R2V, RTS,S/AS01B and viral-vectored vaccines at a 2-week stagger; A, ChAd63 ME-TRAP; M, MVA ME-TRAP; R, 50 μg third dose of RTS,S/AS01B; r, 10 μg third dose of RTS,S/AS01B; CHMI, controlled human malaria infection; C-1, day before CHMI; CSP, circumsporozoite protein; cTfh, circulating T follicular helper cell; ISI, inhibition of sporozoite invasion; PBMCs, peripheral blood mononucleocytes; TRAP, thrombospondin-related adhesive protein; SEB, *Staphylococcus* enterotoxin B.

to profile the antigen-specificity of these cells to determine if the increase in CXCR3⁺ cTfh was due to the induction of cTfh specific for the vector or whether this was a change in the phenotype of the CSP-specific cTfh. There are several methods used to look at antigen-specific cTfh, including cytokine production or CD154 expression after overnight antigen stimulation or the use of antigen-induced markers (45–48). Unfortunately, we found that staining for the chemokine receptors CXCR3 and CCR6 could not reliably be incorporated into these assays (unpublished data). Therefore, we were unable to determine the specificity of the CXCR3⁺ cTfh.

Circulating Tfh have been shown to produce cytokines, with CXCR3⁺ cTfh in particular producing IFNγ (49). However, the association we saw between IFNγ in the supernatant and CXCR3⁺ cTfh was not likely due to production of IFNγ by the CXCR3⁺ cTfh themselves as only very low percentages of cTfh were observed to produce IFNγ after CSP or SEB stimulation. This suggests that exogenous sources of IFNγ are associated with the polarization of cTfh toward a CXCR3⁺ phenotype, although vector-specific CXCR3⁺ cTfh could be a source IFNγ in G3/4 volunteers. MVA has previously been shown to drive a strong IFNγ response, particularly in CD8⁺ T cells and IFNγ enhances CXCR3 expression on T cells through STAT1 signaling (50–53). It is perhaps therefore unsurprising that MVA induced a CXCR3-skewed cTfh response. However, the impact of this skew on the antibody responses was less predictable, given that CXCR3⁺ cTfh have in some contexts been positively associated with antibody responses (45, 54) while in other studies they have been associated with suboptimal GC responses and poor humoral immunity (42, 55). In our study when the two different vaccine platforms were co-administered, the IFNγ-dominated cytokine responses driven by viral-vectored vaccines were associated with an increase in CXCR3⁺ cTfh and a reduction in humoral immunity and protective efficacy. However, if given 2 weeks after RTS,S/AS01B the extent of this CXCR3⁺ cTfh skew, although only slightly reduced, is no longer associated with a reduction in humoral immunogenicity.

IFNγ induces the production of chemokines CXCL9 (MIG, monokine induced by gamma-interferon), CXCL10 (IP-10, interferon-induced protein of 10 kDa), and CXCL11 (I-TAC, interferon inducible T cell alpha chemoattractant), which all bind CXCR3. This chemokine system mediates the migration of Th1 CD4+ T cells and cytotoxic T lymphocytes to sites of Th1 inflammation in the periphery (56). MVA has been shown to induce high systemic levels of IP-10 (57). The systemic induction of CXCR3 ligands, in combination with the CXCR3+ cTfh polarization, may result in the reduction of antibody responses by causing an egress of these cTfh from the draining lymph node, preventing them from providing help to B cells in the GC response. A staggered regimen may reduce this effect by allowing time for the RTS,S/AS01B-induced GC response to occur before MVA-induced inflammation begins. Alternative strategies to reduce or avoid the observed immune interference without increasing the number of clinic visits could be to reduce the dose of MVA or to exclude the additional MVA vaccination at week 4, which was included for practical reasons to simplify the vaccination protocol and is not required to induce potent T cell responses (17, 18).

Producing an effective vaccine against malaria will likely depend on a combination of vaccines targeting multiple stages of the parasite lifecycle. In resource-poor settings, mixing, or co-administering, the vaccines will be necessary to reduce the number of clinic visits required, particularly in infants to fit in with the established Expanded Program on Immunisation vaccine schedule. However, the effects of co-administration on immunogenicity and protective efficacy of each vaccine must be carefully examined. Ideally, a combination regimen could be designed to elicit antibody and T cell responses with an additive protective effect and without the immune interference observed here. Examining the cellular mechanisms underlying these differences in antibody responses will be critical for determining how effective, long-lived antibody responses can be induced by vaccination and for informing rational design of vaccine regimens.

ETHICS STATEMENT

All volunteers gave written informed consent prior to participation, and the studies were conducted according to the principles of the Declaration of Helsinki and in accordance with Good Clinical Practice. The trials were registered with ClinicalTrials.gov (Ref: NCT01883609 and NCT02252640). The study protocols were approved by the UK National Research Ethics Service, Committee South Central—Oxford A (Refs: 13/SC/0208 and 14/SC/0227), the Western Institution Review Board (Ref: 20130698) and the UK Medicines and Healthcare products Regulatory Agency (Refs: 21584/0317/001-0001 and 21584/0333/001-0001). The Local Safety Committee provided safety oversight for both trials and GCP compliance was monitored by the Clinical Trials and Research Governance Team (CTRG) of the University of Oxford.

AUTHOR CONTRIBUTIONS

GB designed laboratory study, interpreted data, and wrote the manuscript. GB and AG acquired and analyzed data. DM, RB, AH, and KE conceived clinical studies and provided project over-sight. TR, NV, AH, and KE designed clinical studies. TR and NV conducted clinical work. All the authors revised the manuscript.

ACKNOWLEDGMENTS

We thank the VAC55/59 clinical and laboratory team — N. Edwards, D. Wright, S. Sridhar, R. Payne, J. Powlson, C. Bliss, N. Venkatraman, I. Poulton, R. Roberts, B. Angus, A. Lawrie, R. Lopez-Ramon, O. Griffiths, N. Lella, and C. Tyson for logistical support; the study volunteers; J. Furze for laboratory assistance; J. Illingworth and A. Douglas for production of recombinant TRAP protein; the staff at the NIHR Wellcome Trust Clinical Research Facilities at the Southampton, Guildford and Hammersmith Hospital sites; S. Davidson and colleagues at the WRAIR Ento-mology laboratories for supply of infected mosquitoes for CHMI; GSK for supply of RTS,S/AS01B vaccine and scientific input; A. Spencer, M. Ulaszewska and the Jenner insectary for *A. stephensi* mosquitoes; A. Salman for *P. berghei* PfCSP@CSP sporozoites; K. Collins and F. Halstead for preparation of IFA slides; N. Obeng-Adjei and P. Crompton for their advice and training on the Tfh phenotyping flow cytometry; PATH for funding.

FUNDING

This work was supported by the PATH Malaria Vaccine Initiative and by the United Kingdom NIHR, through the NIHR Oxford Biomedical Research Centre, the Southampton NIHR Wellcome Trust Clinical Research Facility, and the Imperial College NIHR Wellcome Trust Clinical Research Facility. Support was also received from the UK National Institute for Health Research Oxford Biomedical Research Centre (Vaccines Theme). AVS Hill is supported by a Wellcome Trust Senior Investigator Award (104750/Z/14).

REFERENCES

1. World Health Organization. *World Malaria Report* [Online]. (2016). Available from: http://www.who.int/malaria/publications/world-malaria-report-2016/report/en/ [Accessed: July 15, 2018].
2. malERA Consultative Group on Vaccines. A research agenda for malaria eradication: vaccines. *PLoS Med* (2011) 8:e1000398. doi:10.1371/journal.pmed.1000398
3. RTS,S Clinical Trials Partnership, Agnandji ST, Lell B, Soulanoudjingar SS, Fernandes JF, Abossolo BP, et al. First results of phase 3 trial of RTS,S/AS01 malaria vaccine in African children. *N Engl J Med* (2011) 365:1863–75. doi:10.1056/NEJMoa1102287
4. RTS,S Clinical Trials Partnership, Agnandji ST, Lell B, Fernandes JF, Abossolo BP, Methogo BG, et al. A phase 3 trial of RTS,S/AS01 malaria vaccine in African infants. *N Engl J Med* (2012) 367:2284–95. doi:10.1056/NEJMoa1208394

5. Olotu A, Fegan G, Wambua J, Nyangweso G, Leach A, Lievens M, et al. Seven-year efficacy of RTS,S/AS01 malaria vaccine among young African children. *N Engl J Med* (2016) 374:2519–29. doi:10.1056/NEJMoa1515257
6. RTS,S Clinical Trials Partnership. Efficacy and safety of the RTS,S/AS01 malaria vaccine during 18 months after vaccination: a phase 3 randomized, controlled trial in children and young infants at 11 African sites. *PLoS Med* (2014) 11:e1001685. doi:10.1371/journal.pmed.1001685
7. RTS,S Clinical Trials Partnership. Efficacy and safety of RTS,S/AS01 malaria vaccine with or without a booster dose in infants and children in Africa: final results of a phase 3, individually randomised, controlled trial. *Lancet* (2015) 386:31–45. doi:10.1016/S0140-6736(15)60721-8
8. Malaria Vaccine Funders Group. *Malaria, Vaccine Technology Roadmap* [Online]. (2013). Available from: http://www.who.int/immunization/topics/malaria/vaccine_roadmap/TRM_update_nov13.pdf [Accessed: July 15, 2018].
9. Ewer KJ, Sierra-Davidson K, Salman AM, Illingworth JJ, Draper SJ, Biswas S, et al. Progress with viral vectored malaria vaccines: a multi-stage approach involving "unnatural immunity". *Vaccine* (2015) 33:7444–51. doi:10.1016/j.vaccine.2015.09.094
10. Ogwang C, Kimani D, Edwards NJ, Roberts R, Mwacharo J, Bowyer G, et al. Prime-boost vaccination with chimpanzee adenovirus and modified vaccinia Ankara encoding TRAP provides partial protection against *Plasmodium falciparum* infection in Kenyan adults. *Sci Transl Med* (2015) 7:286re285. doi:10.1126/scitranslmed.aaa2373
11. Hodgson SH, Choudhary P, Elias SC, Milne KH, Rampling TW, Biswas S, et al. Combining viral vectored and protein-in-adjuvant vaccines against the blood-stage malaria antigen AMA1: report on a phase 1a clinical trial. *Mol Ther* (2014) 22:2142–54. doi:10.1038/mt.2014.157
12. Kapulu MC, Da DF, Miura K, Li Y, Blagborough AM, Churcher TS, et al. Comparative assessment of transmission-blocking vaccine candidates against *Plasmodium falciparum*. *Sci Rep* (2015) 5:11193. doi:10.1038/srep11193
13. Moorthy VS, Ballou WR. Immunological mechanisms underlying protection mediated by RTS,S: a review of the available data. *Malar J* (2009) 8:312–312. doi:10.1186/1475-2875-8-312
14. Stoute JA, Slaoui M, Heppner DG, Momin P, Kester KE, Desmons P, et al. A preliminary evaluation of a recombinant circumsporozoite protein vaccine against *Plasmodium falciparum* malaria. RTS,S Malaria Vaccine Evaluation Group. *N Engl J Med* (1997) 336:86–91. doi:10.1056/NEJM199701093360202
15. White MT, Bejon P, Olotu A, Griffin JT, Riley EM, Kester KE, et al. The relationship between RTS,S vaccine-induced antibodies, $CD4^+$ T cell responses and protection against *Plasmodium falciparum* infection. *PLoS One* (2013) 8:e61395. doi:10.1371/journal.pone.0061395
16. White MT, Verity R, Griffin JT, Asante KP, Owusu-Agyei S, Greenwood B, et al. Immunogenicity of the RTS,S/AS01 malaria vaccine and implications for duration of vaccine efficacy: secondary analysis of data from a phase 3 randomised controlled trial. *Lancet Infect Dis* (2015) 15:1450–8. doi:10.1016/S1473-3099(15)00239-X
17. Ewer KJ, O'Hara GA, Duncan CJ, Collins KA, Sheehy SH, Reyes-Sandoval A, et al. Protective CD8+ T-cell immunity to human malaria induced by chimpanzee adenovirus-MVA immunisation. *Nat Commun* (2013) 4:2836. doi:10.1038/ncomms3836
18. Rampling T, Ewer KJ, Bowyer G, Bliss CM, Edwards NJ, Wright D, et al. Safety and high level efficacy of the combination malaria vaccine regimen of RTS,S/AS01B with chimpanzee adenovirus 63 and modified vaccinia Ankara vectored vaccines expressing ME-TRAP. *J Infect Dis* (2016) 214:772–81. doi:10.1093/infdis/jiw244
19. Regules JA, Cicatelli SB, Bennett JW, Paolino KM, Twomey PS, Moon JE, et al. Fractional third and fourth dose of RTS,S/AS01 malaria candidate vaccine: a phase 2a controlled human malaria parasite infection and immunogenicity study. *J Infect Dis* (2016) 214:762–71. doi:10.1093/infdis/jiw237
20. Breitfeld D, Ohl L, Kremmer E, Ellwart J, Sallusto F, Lipp M, et al. Follicular B helper T cells express CXC chemokine receptor 5, localize to B cell follicles, and support immunoglobulin production. *J Exp Med* (2000) 192:1545–52. doi:10.1084/jem.192.11.1545
21. Ma CS, Deenick EK, Batten M, Tangye SG. The origins, function, and regulation of T follicular helper cells. *J Exp Med* (2012) 209:1241–53. doi:10.1084/jem.20120994
22. Morita R, Schmitt N, Bentebibel SE, Ranganathan R, Bourdery L, Zurawski G, et al. Human blood CXCR5(+)CD4(+) T cells are counterparts of T follicular cells and contain specific subsets that differentially support antibody secretion. *Immunity* (2011) 34:108–21. doi:10.1016/j.immuni.2010.12.012
23. Chevalier N, Jarrossay D, Ho E, Avery DT, Ma CS, Yu D, et al. CXCR5 expressing human central memory CD4 T cells and their relevance for humoral immune responses. *J Immunol* (2011) 186:5556–68. doi:10.4049/jimmunol.1002828
24. Vinuesa CG, Cook MC. Blood relatives of follicular helper T cells. *Immunity* (2011) 34:10–2. doi:10.1016/j.immuni.2011.01.006
25. Schmitt N, Bentebibel S-E, Ueno H. Phenotype and functions of memory Tfh cells in human blood. *Trends Immunol* (2014) 35:436–42. doi:10.1016/j.it.2014.06.002
26. Locci M, Havenar-Daughton C, Landais E, Wu J, Kroenke MA, Arlehamn CL, et al. Human circulating PD-1+CXCR3-CXCR5+ memory Tfh cells are highly functional and correlate with broadly neutralizing HIV antibody responses. *Immunity* (2013) 39:758–69. doi:10.1016/j.immuni.2013.08.031
27. Farooq F, Beck K, Paolino KM, Phillips R, Waters NC, Regules JA, et al. Circulating follicular T helper cells and cytokine profile in humans following vaccination with the rVSV-ZEBOV Ebola vaccine. *Sci Rep* (2016) 6:27944. doi:10.1038/srep27944
28. Thompson FM, Porter DW, Okitsu SL, Westerfeld N, Vogel D, Todryk S, et al. Evidence of blood stage efficacy with a virosomal malaria vaccine in a phase IIa clinical trial. *PLoS One* (2008) 3:e1493. doi:10.1371/journal.pone.0001493
29. Rodríguez-Galán A, Salman AM, Bowyer G, Collins KA, Longley RJ, Brod F, et al. An in vitro assay to measure antibody-mediated inhibition of *P. berghei* sporozoite invasion against *P. falciparum* antigens. *Sci Rep* (2017) 7:17011. doi:10.1038/s41598-017-17274-5
30. WHO collaborative Study Group on Oral and Inactivated Poliovirus Vaccines. Combined immunization of infants with oral and inactivated poliovirus vaccines: results of a randomized trial in The Gambia, Oman, and Thailand/WHO Collaborative Study Group on oral and inactivated poliovirus vaccines. *Bull World Health Organ* (1996) 74:253–68.
31. Migasena S, Simasathien S, Samakoses R, Pitisuttitham P, Sangaroon P, van Steenis G, et al. Simultaneous administration of oral rhesus-human reassortant tetravalent (RRV-TV) rotavirus vaccine and oral poliovirus vaccine (OPV) in Thai infants. *Vaccine* (1995) 13:168–74. doi:10.1016/0264-410X(95)93131-R
32. Eisen HN, Siskind GW. Variations in affinities of antibodies during the immune response. *Biochemistry* (1964) 3:996–1008.
33. González-Fernández A, Milstein C. Low antigen dose favours selection of somatic mutants with hallmarks of antibody affinity maturation. *Immunology* (1998) 93:149–53. doi:10.1046/j.1365-2567.1998.00423.x
34. Ahman H, Käyhty H, Vuorela A, Leroy O, Eskola J. Dose dependency of antibody response in infants and children to pneumococcal polysaccharides conjugated to tetanus toxoid. *Vaccine* (1999) 17:2726–32.
35. He J, Tsai LM, Leong YA, Hu X, Ma CS, Chevalier N, et al. Circulating precursor CCR7(lo)PD-1(hi) $CXCR5^+$ $CD4^+$ T cells indicate Tfh cell activity and promote antibody responses upon antigen reexposure. *Immunity* (2013) 39:770–81. doi:10.1016/j.immuni.2013.09.007
36. Heit A, Schmitz F, Gerdts S, Flach B, Moore MS, Perkins JA, et al. Vaccination establishes clonal relatives of germinal center T cells in the blood of humans. *J Exp Med* (2017) 214:2139–52. doi:10.1084/jem.20161794
37. Li XY, Wu ZB, Ding J, Zheng ZH, Li XY, Chen LN, et al. Role of the frequency of blood CD4(+) CXCR5(+) CCR6(+) T cells in autoimmunity in patients with Sjögren's syndrome. *Biochem Biophys Res Commun* (2012) 422:238–44. doi:10.1016/j.bbrc.2012.04.133
38. Romme Christensen J, Börnsen L, Ratzer R, Piehl F, Khademi M, Olsson T, et al. Systemic inflammation in progressive multiple sclerosis involves follicular T-helper, Th17- and activated B-cells and correlates with progression. *PLoS One* (2013) 8:e57820. doi:10.1371/journal.pone.0057820
39. Gong F, Qian C, Zhu H, Zhu J, Pan Y, Dong Q, et al. Circulating follicular T-helper cell subset distribution in patients with asthma. *Allergy Asthma Proc* (2016) 37:154–61. doi:10.2500/aap.2016.37.3982
40. Kamekura R, Shigehara K, Miyajima S, Jitsukawa S, Kawata K, Yamashita K, et al. Alteration of circulating type 2 follicular helper T cells and regulatory B cells underlies the comorbid association of allergic rhinitis with bronchial asthma. *Clin Immunol* (2015) 158:204–11. doi:10.1016/j.clim.2015.02.016

41. Schmitt N, Ueno H. Human T follicular helper cells: development and subsets. *Adv Exp Med Biol* (2013) 785:87–94. doi:10.1007/978-1-4614-6217-0_10
42. Obeng-Adjei N, Portugal S, Tran TM, Yazew TB, Skinner J, Li S, et al. Circulating Th1-cell-type Tfh cells that exhibit impaired B cell help are preferentially activated during acute malaria in children. *Cell Rep* (2015) 13:425–39. doi:10.1016/j.celrep.2015.09.004
43. Ryg-Cornejo V, Ioannidis LJ, Ly A, Chiu CY, Tellier J, Hill DL, et al. Severe malaria infections impair germinal center responses by inhibiting T follicular helper cell differentiation. *Cell Rep* (2016) 14:68–81. doi:10.1016/j.celrep.2015.12.006
44. Cunill V, Clemente A, Lanio N, Barceló C, Andreu V, Pons J, et al. Follicular T cells from smB(-) common variable immunodeficiency patients are skewed toward a Th1 phenotype. *Front Immunol* (2017) 8:174. doi:10.3389/fimmu.2017.00174
45. Bentebibel SE, Lopez S, Obermoser G, Schmitt N, Mueller C, Harrod C, et al. Induction of ICOS+CXCR3+CXCR5+ TH cells correlates with antibody responses to influenza vaccination. *Sci Transl Med* (2013) 5:176ra132. doi:10.1126/scitranslmed.3005191
46. Chattopadhyay PK, Yu J, Roederer M. Live-cell assay to detect antigen-specific CD4+ T-cell responses by CD154 expression. *Nat Protoc* (2006) 1:1–6. doi:10.1038/nprot.2006.1
47. Dan JM, Lindestam Arlehamn CS, Weiskopf D, da Silva Antunes R, Havenar-Daughton C, Reiss SM, et al. A cytokine-independent approach to identify antigen-specific human germinal center t follicular helper cells and rare antigen-specific CD4+ T cells in blood. *J Immunol* (2016) 197:983–93. doi:10.4049/jimmunol.1601321
48. Havenar-Daughton C, Reiss SM, Carnathan DG, Wu JE, Kendric K, Torrents de la Peña A, et al. Cytokine-independent detection of antigen-specific germinal center T follicular helper cells in immunized nonhuman primates using a live cell activation-induced marker technique. *J Immunol* (2016) 197:994–1002. doi:10.4049/jimmunol.1600320
49. Ma CS, Wong N, Rao G, Avery DT, Torpy J, Hambridge T, et al. Monogenic mutations differentially affect the quantity and quality of T follicular helper cells in patients with human primary immunodeficiencies. *J Allergy ClinImmunol* (2015) 136:993–1006.e1. doi:10.1016/j.jaci.2015.05.036
50. Remy-Ziller C, Germain C, Spindler A, Hoffmann C, Silvestre N, Rooke R, et al. Immunological characterization of a modified vaccinia virus Ankara vector expressing the human papillomavirus 16 E1 protein. *Clin Vaccine Immunol* (2014) 21:147–55. doi:10.1128/CVI.00678-13
51. Kimani D, Jagne YJ, Cox M, Kimani E, Bliss CM, Gitau E, et al. Translating the immunogenicity of prime-boost immunization with ChAd63 and MVA ME-TRAP from malaria naive to malaria-endemic populations. *Mol Ther* (2014) 22:1992–2003. doi:10.1038/mt.2014.109
52. Reyes-Sandoval A, Berthoud T, Alder N, Siani L, Gilbert SC, Nicosia A, et al. Prime-boost immunization with adenoviral and modified vaccinia virus Ankara vectors enhances the durability and polyfunctionality of protective malaria CD8+ T-cell responses. *Infect Immun* (2010) 78:145–53. doi:10.1128/IAI.00740-09
53. Nakajima C, Mukai T, Yamaguchi N, Morimoto Y, Park WR, Iwasaki M, et al. Induction of the chemokine receptor CXCR3 on TCR-stimulated T cells: dependence on the release from persistent TCR-triggering and requirement for IFN-gamma stimulation. *Eur J Immunol* (2002) 32:1792–801. doi:10.1002/1521-4141(200206)32:6<1792::AID-IMMU1792>3.0.CO;2-0
54. Bentebibel SE, Khurana S, Schmitt N, Kurup P, Mueller C, Obermoser G, et al. ICOS(+)PD-1(+)CXCR3(+) T follicular helper cells contribute to the generation of high-avidity antibodies following influenza vaccination. *Sci Rep* (2016) 6:26494. doi:10.1038/srep26494
55. Keitany GJ, Kim KS, Krishnamurty AT, Hondowicz BD, Hahn WO, Dambrauskas N, et al. Blood stage malaria disrupts humoral immunity to the pre-erythrocytic stage circumsporozoite protein. *Cell Rep* (2016) 17:3193–205. doi:10.1016/j.celrep.2016.11.060
56. Groom JR, Luster AD. CXCR3 in T cell function. *Exp Cell Res* (2011) 317:620–31. doi:10.1016/j.yexcr.2010.12.017
57. Teigler JE, Phogat S, Franchini G, Hirsch VM, Michael NL, Barouch DH. The canarypox virus vector ALVAC induces distinct cytokine responses compared to the vaccinia virus-based vectors MVA and NYVAC in rhesus monkeys. *J Virol* (2014) 88:1809–14. doi:10.1128/JVI.02386-13

10

Different Life Cycle Stages of *Plasmodium falciparum* Induce Contrasting Responses in Dendritic Cells

Xi Zen Yap [1,2†], Rachel J. Lundie [3†], Gaoqian Feng [1,2], Joanne Pooley [3], James G. Beeson [1,2,4,5] and Meredith O'Keeffe [1,3*]*

[1] Burnet Institute, Melbourne, VIC, Australia, [2] Department of Medicine, The University of Melbourne, Parkville, VIC, Australia, [3] Department of Biochemistry and Molecular Biology and Biomedicine Discovery Institute, Monash University, Clayton, VIC, Australia, [4] Department of Microbiology, Monash University, Clayton, VIC, Australia, [5] Central Clinical School, Monash University, Melbourne, VIC, Australia

***Correspondence:**
James G. Beeson
james.beeson@burnet.edu.au
Meredith O'Keeffe
meredith.okeeffe@monash.edu

†Present Address:
Xi Zen Yap,
Radboud University Medical Centre, Nijmegen, Netherlands
Rachel J. Lundie,
The Walter and Eliza Hall Institute of Medical Research, Parkville, VIC, Australia

Dendritic cells are key linkers of innate and adaptive immunity. Efficient dendritic cell activation is central to the acquisition of immunity and the efficacy of vaccines. Understanding how dendritic cells are affected by *Plasmodium falciparum* blood-stage parasites will help to understand how immunity is acquired and maintained, and how vaccine responses may be impacted by malaria infection or exposure. This study investigates the response of dendritic cells to two different life stages of the malaria parasite, parasitized red blood cells and merozoites, using a murine model. We demonstrate that the dendritic cell responses to merozoites are robust whereas dendritic cell activation, particularly CD40 and pro-inflammatory cytokine expression, is compromised in the presence of freshly isolated parasitized red blood cells. The mechanism of dendritic cell suppression by parasitized red blood cells is host red cell membrane-independent. Furthermore, we show that cryopreserved parasitized red blood cells have a substantially reduced capacity for dendritic cell activation.

Keywords: dendritic cell (DC), malaria, malaria vaccines, parasite-host interactions, innate immunity

INTRODUCTION

Dendritic cells (DCs) are key linkers of innate and adaptive immunity and their activation is essential to vaccination. Ablating DCs in murine models leads to vaccination failure and subsequent loss of antigen-specific T cells (1). Immunization of individuals living in malaria-infested regions has been notoriously difficult, with even the most promising vaccines failing to provide high levels of efficacy. A failure to activate DCs in people infected with *Plasmodium falciparum* blood-stage parasites may provide some explanation to the low efficacy of malaria vaccines [reviewed in (2)]. It may also explain the slow acquisition of natural anti-malarial immunity in individuals residing in malaria-endemic settings.

Activation of DCs is required for their subsequent efficient activation of T cells. Activated DCs increase surface expression of the co-stimulatory markers MHCII, CD40, CD80, and CD86, which are all involved in T cell co-stimulation. In particular, the interaction between CD40 on DC and its ligand CD40L on T cells is integral to enhance both T cell and DC responses for effective adaptive immune responses (3).

There remains an unresolved question of whether exposure to *P. falciparum* inhibits DC activation, leading to DC "suppression." Literature from *ex vivo* studies has suggested that DCs from infected individuals are inhibited in core DC functions, namely: expression of co-stimulatory markers, cytokine secretion, antigen uptake, and the ability to induce primary and secondary T cell responses (4–7). However, there is a lack of consensus among *in vitro* studies as to what effect *P. falciparum* has directly upon DCs. To date the majority of literature has examined DC responses to parasitized erythrocytes (pRBCs), the intracellular stage of the asexual parasite. In this life stage *P. falciparum* is concealed from host immunity by the host erythrocyte membrane, though parasite proteins such as the adhesion ligand *PfEMP1* are exported to the erythrocyte surface. Very little research into cellular responses to the infectious extracellular stage, known as the merozoite, has been carried out. Furthermore, it is important to note that the majority of *in vitro* studies have been carried out in monocyte-derived (mo) DCs (8), which are phenotypically and functionally different from *bona fide* DCs (8, 9).

The murine Flt3 ligand-induced DCs (FL-DCs) closely recapitulate the DCs of the blood, similar to spleen DC, but slightly less mature conventional (cDC) and plasmacytoid (pDC) DC subsets (10–13). Therefore, the FL-DC model was used here for its ease and its capacity to generate large volumes of *bona fide* DCs, enabling us to test a broad variety of parameters.

The FL-DC cDCs can be divided into two subsets by expression of CD24 and CD11b. The FL-DC $CD24^+$ cDCs ($CD24^+CD11b^-$) are immature cDC1. The cDC1 subset is specialized in cross-presentation and has a superior ability to prime naive cytotoxic $CD8^+$ T cells, and polarize T cells toward the T_H1 pathway via IL-12 production. Meanwhile, the FL-DC $CD11b^+$ subset ($CD24^-CD11b^+$) is equivalent to immature cDC2 (11). These FL-DC cDC1 and cDC2 populations share many pattern recognition receptors with their human blood DC counterparts and the core surface phenotypes and functions of cross-presentation (cDC1) and bacterial recognition and $CD4^+$ T cell stimulation (cDC2) are conserved [reviewed in Macri et al. (14)].

In contrast, pDCs are overall poor stimulators of T cell responses and do not upregulate co-stimulatory markers. Their defining characteristic is the secretion of Type I and III interferons (IFNs) in response to viral infection and/or the ligation of endosomal TLRs (15–17). In humans, pDCs are also the only subset to express TLR9, which is a known receptor for malarial DNA (18, 19).

Previous literature has described pDC production of IFN-α in response to *P. falciparum* merozoites *in vitro* (19) and during natural infection in humans (20), where pDCs appear suppressed in the presence of malaria parasites (21). Further studies hinted at pDC as a source of replicating malaria parasites (22), but this subset has, overall, been poorly studied in malaria.

This study aimed to identify how DC responses to the pRBC and the merozoite differ, with findings indicating that merozoites induce DC activation whereas pRBCs induce low co-stimulatory marker expression but high production of cytokines, with greater suppression at increasing doses of pRBCs. We reveal that the mechanism of suppression of DC activation occurs independently of the host RBC membrane, is not seen with pRBCs that have undergone a freeze-thaw cycle, and cannot be rescued by merozoites nor an exogenous TLR9 stimulus.

METHODS

Culture, Purification, and Freeze-Thawing of *P. falciparum* Blood-Stage Parasites

Plasmodium falciparum 3D7 parasites were cultured as per standard protocols. Briefly, parasites were maintained in RPMI1640 (Gibco) enriched with 5% Albumax (Gibco) and 5% AB^+ human serum obtained from the Red Cross, Melbourne, Australia. Parasites were cultured at 3–5% haematocrit using type-O negative blood (Red Cross) and incubated in medical gas (1% O_2 and 5% CO_2 in nitrogen gas) at 37°C as per standard protocols. Parasite growth was assessed daily by thin smear (23) stained with Giemsa's azur eosin methylene blue solution (Merck Millipore). Parasites were sorbitol synchronized (24) and selected for knob expression by gelatin flotation (25). All parasites were initially treated with *Mycoplasma* removal agent (MP Biomedicals) for 2 weeks as per the manufacturer's instructions. Subsequently, parasites were tested at 1-monthly intervals for *Mycoplasma* contamination using the MycoAlert test kit (Lonza).

Trophozoite Preparation

Trophozoites at 24–28 h post-invasion were isolated by magnetic selection with the VarioMACS (Miltenyi Biotech) system. Purity was assessed by counting 200 cells via Giemsa thin smear. Preparations varied from 70 to 99% parasite purity and preparations with purity of <90% were re-purified by repeating magnet selection. Purified preparations were counted using a haemocytometer and resuspended to the appropriate cell concentration in complete medium (CM): RPMI1640 containing GlutaMAX (Gibco) supplemented with 10% heat-inactivated FCS, 0.1 mM 2-beta-mercaptoethanol, 100 U/mL penicillin and 100 μg/mL streptomycin. Aliquots of purified trophozoites with >95% purity were also frozen in glycerolyte 57 (Baxter Healthcare Corporation) and stored at −80°C to compare efficacy of DC stimulation with same-day isolated cultures.

Merozoite Preparation

Merozoites were purified as per Boyle et al. (26). Briefly, late-stage (30–34 h) trophozoites were purified and returned to culture without uninfected RBCs (uRBCs). When trophozoites had matured into schizonts (40 h), 10 μM of protease inhibitor E64 (Sigma) was added to culture medium to inhibit merozoite egress. Upon maturation into late-stage schizonts (46–48 h), pRBCs were resuspended in 20 mL of RPMI-HEPES and schizont rupture was induced by pushing through a 1.2 μM syringe filter (Pall), resulting in purified merozoites. Merozoites were stained with ethidium bromide (EtBr) and counted by flow cytometry. For storage, late-stage segmented schizonts derived by this method were frozen in PBS at a concentration of 150 × 10^7/mL after arrest with E64 but prior to filter lysis and stored at −80°C until use in assays.

Saponin Lysis to Remove Host RBC Membranes

Magnet-purified pRBCs or empty "mock" tubes were co-incubated with 0.09% saponin in 1X PBS for 30 s at RT, after which they were washed three times in RPMI containing 2% FCS to remove residual saponin. Saponin lysis of host RBC membrane was confirmed by microscopy. Both saponin-treated and intact parasites were then resuspended in CM and co-incubated with FL-DCs in the presence or absence of 0.5 μM CpG2216. CM or CM and CpG2216 were added to "mock" tubes to control for any potential carry-over of the detergent and added to FL-DCs as separate controls.

FL-DC Culture

Bone marrow cells were stimulated with Flt3-L to induce large quantities of DCs similar in phenotype and function to those found in murine spleen (11, 12, 27) (**Supplementary Figure 1**). Briefly, FL-DCs were obtained as follows: leg bones of C57Bl/6 mice (AMREP Animal Services Precinct Animal Centre, Melbourne, Australia) were dissected out and harvested into RPMI containing 2% v/v FCS. Bones were cut open and bone marrow was flushed with a 22 g needle using 2 mL of RPMI-FCS per bone. After centrifugation at 600 × *g* for 7 min, cells were co-incubated with 1 mL of red cell lysis buffer (Sigma) with constant mixing for 30 s. Cells were washed twice in RPMI1640 containing 2% FCS before resuspending in complete medium and filtering through a 70 μM sieve (Falcon). Cells were resuspended at 1.5×10^6 cells/mL in complete medium containing 100 ng/mL of Flt3-L-Ig (BioXCell) and cultured in vented cap tissue culture flasks (Corning) in a 37°C incubator in 5% CO_2 for 8 days.

Determining the Effect of the Parasite-DC Ratio Upon the DC Response to Purified Blood-Stage *P. falciparum*

After 8 days culture FL-DC were counted and washed in CM. Merozoites and pRBCs were titrated against FL-DCs in round-bottom 96-well-tissue culture plates (Falcon) at a final cell concentration of 0.5×10^6 FL-DC/mL. Additionally, FL-DCs were also cultured with 0.5 μM CpG2216 alone or in addition to parasites, or with media alone or uRBCs as negative controls. All incubations were carried out for 18–20 h at 37°C in 5% CO_2.

Flow Cytometric Analysis

For analysis of surface phenotype, cells were stained in 1X PBS supplemented with 2% v/v FCS and 10% v/v 0.1M EDTA (MACS buffer) with monoclonal antibodies for MHCII, CD11b, CD11c, CD24, CD45R, and CD199. For staining, antibody was diluted in MACS buffer and antibody cocktail was added at $10\mu L/10^6$ cells, with a minimum of 30 μL of cocktail per well or tube, and incubated in the dark at 4°C for 20 min. Cells were washed to remove unbound antibody and analyzed on a BD Fortessa or BD LSRII flow cytometer. DCs were identified as medium-sized cells on forward and side scatter and doublets and PI-positive dead cells excluded. Activation of viable DCs was measured by expression of costimulatory markers MHCII, CD40, CD69, CD80, and CD86 on each DC subset using antibodies outlined in **Supplementary Table 1**.

Cytokine Analysis

Frozen supernatants derived from parasite-FL-DC co-culture experiments were tested for the presence of IFN-γ, IL-1β, IL-2; IL-4, IL-5, IL-9, IL-12p70, IL-13, IL-17a, IL-18, IL-22, IL-23, IL-27, GM-CSF, IP-10, eotaxin, and MIP-1α by ProcartaPlex (eBioscience) multiplex as per manufacturer's instructions. Presence of MIP-2, IL-6, IL-10, GRO-α, MCP-1, MCP-3, MIP-1β, RANTES, and TNF-α were assayed for by both FlowCytomix (eBioScience) and ProcartaPlex. Expression of IFN-α and IFN-β was measured by a separate multiplex (ProcartaPlex).

RESULTS

The Ratio of pRBCs-to-DCs Affects Expression of DC Maturation Markers and This Is Not Rescued in the Presence of TLR9 Ligand

People in endemic malaria regions can have a wide range of parasitemia in peripheral blood. Those with asymptomatic malaria typically have lower levels of parasitemia, ~5,000 *P. falciparum* parasites per mL of peripheral blood on average (28), depending on the setting. This equates to a ratio of ~0.25 parasites to 1 DC in blood. However, significant numbers of asymptomatic people and those with symptomatic malaria have infections over 10^6 parasites per mL, equating to ~50:1 ratio of parasites to blood DC (29, 30).

To model the effect of different parasite concentrations on blood DC we analyzed the response of murine FL-DC to purified pRBCs from a high ratio of 50:1 to a low ratio of 1:1. In replicate, CpG2216 was added to the cultures to ask whether the presence of pRBCs affected the activation of FL-DC by an additional stimuli. The addition of uRBC alone were used to control for responses to RBC alone. To determine cell activation, MHCII and CD40 and CD86 co-stimulation molecule expression was measured upon FL-DCs (**Figure 1**). Analyses of total FL-DC indicated a reduction in CD40 expression at ratios of pRBC:DC of >12.5, and at lower concentrations in the additional presence of TLR9 ligand (CpG2216). Separate analyses of cDC and pDC subsets indicated that high pRBC concentrations led to a significant reduction of co-stimulation marker expression on both $CD24^+$ and $CD11b^+$ cDCs (**Figure 1C**) that was particularly strong for CD40, and also occurred in the additional presence of CpG2216 (**Figure 1A**). While DC viability decreased in response to 50:1 concentrations of pRBC alone, viability was not significantly decreased by pRBC in the presence of CpG yet co-stimulation molecule expression still decreased (**Figure 1B**). In response to low ratios of pRBCs of <12.5 pRBC:DC, cDC expression of co-stimulatory markers was comparable to that induced by CpG2216.

A more complex relationship between MHCII and co-stimulatory marker expression and pRBC ratio was observed in pDCs. Upon stimulation with low ratios of pRBC, pDCs

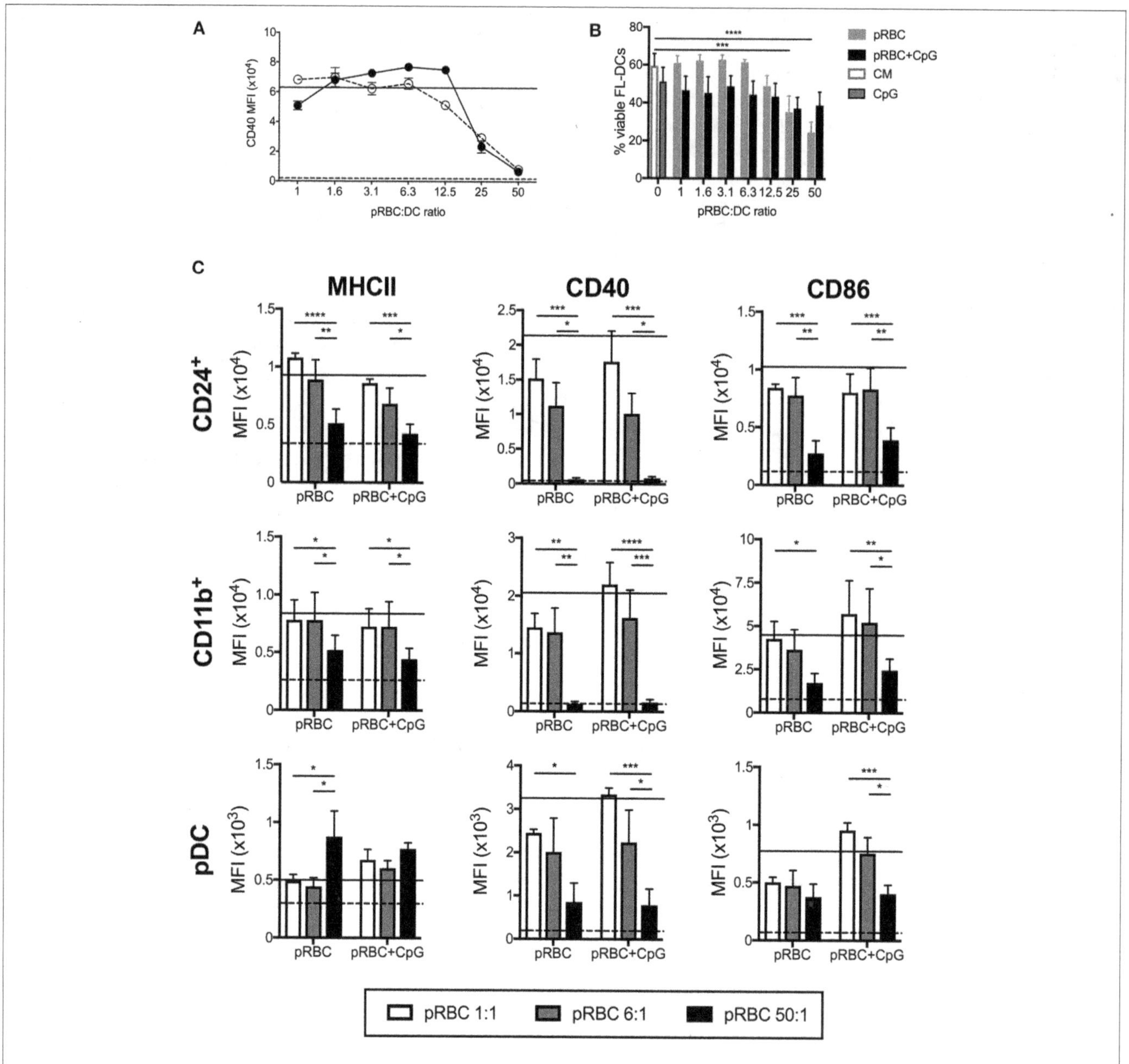

FIGURE 1 | High doses of pRBCs induce poor FL-DC activation and prevent normal TLR9-mediated activation. **(A)** Expression of CD40 on CD24$^+$ cDCs was downregulated in response to high doses of pRBCs alone (solid circles) or pRBCs + CpG2216 (hollow circles). Responses to CpG2216 alone (solid line) and uRBC alone (dashed line) are shown for comparison. **(B)** Viability of total FL-DCs in response to pRBCs alone (gray) or pRBCs + CpG2216 (black). Viability in response to culture medium alone (CM; white with gray border) or CpG2216 alone (CpG; gray with black border) are shown for comparison. **(C)** Expression of MHCII, CD40, and CD86 in response to pRBCs in CD24$^+$ cDC, CD11b$^+$ cDC, and pDCs. Co-stimulatory marker expression is shown in response to pRBC-to-DC ratios of 50:1 (black), 6:1 (gray), and 1:1 (white), as well as in response to CpG2216 (solid line) or uRBCs (dashed line). $^*p < 0.05$, $^{**}p < 0.01$, $^{***}p < 0.001$, $^{****}p < 0.0001$. *P*-values were determined by two-way ANOVA using multiple comparisons. Data shown is from three experiments, each experiment using pooled FL-DC cultures from two mice. Error bars represent SEM of three separate experiments. MFI—geometric mean fluorescence intensity.

expressed MHCII, CD40, and CD86 at elevated levels compared to uRBCs alone, which could be further elevated in the presence of CpG2216. However, upon stimulation of pDC with pRBC ratios >25:1, in the presence or absence of CpG2216, CD40, and CD86 expression was reduced whereas MHCII (**Figure 1C**) and CD80 (data not shown) expression increased to levels above that seen with CpG2216 alone.

The Ratio of pRBCs-to-DCs Alters FL-DC Patterns of Cytokine Production Including in the Presence of TLR9 Ligand

The data of **Figure 1** indicated that at high pRBC:DC ratios, the response of DCs to CpG2216 was inhibited and that overall, DC activation was suppressed. To further investigate the activation of DC across a range of pRBC concentrations we analyzed the production of cytokines in the supernatants of the cultured FL-DC.

Others have previously reported pDC-produced IFN-α in response to *P. falciparum* (19, 31, 32), with conflicting reports on whether the activation of pDCs was inhibited by pRBCs (19, 32). In the FL-DC cultures with pRBCs alone, IFN-α was only detectable in the cultures at ratios of <12.5 parasites per DC (**Figure 2A**). At pRBC:DC ratios of 1:1 and 6:1, we detected high levels of IL-6 and IP-10 (CXCL10) and detectable levels of TNF-α, IL-10, IFN-γ, and MIP-2 (CXCL2, **Figure 2B**). At pRBC-to-DC ratios of 50:1, IL-6, TNF-α and IL-10 production were reduced to the baseline levels induced by uRBCs whilst IP-10, IFN-γ and MIP-2 were produced at levels similar to those observed with ratios of 1:1 pRBC:DC (**Figure 2B**).

We then investigated whether cytokine secretion to pRBCs was boosted in the presence of TLR9 ligand, CpG2216, or if pRBCs were able to suppress CpG2216-induced cytokine secretion. The pDC and pDC-like cells are the only cells capable of producing high levels of IFN-α to CpG oligonucleotides, potent TLR-9 ligands (33). Addition of CpG2216 to pRBC-DC co-incubations increased overall cytokine secretion but a pRBC dose-dependent suppression of TLR9-induced IFN-α, i.e., pDC responses, was observed (**Figure 2A**) from bulk cultures. Reduced production of both TNF-α and IL-10 were also observed with pRBC:DC ratios of 6:1 and above (**Figure 2**). This suppression was marked at pRBC:DC ratios of 50:1 for IL-10, TNF-α, IL-6, and MIP2 production (**Figure 2B**).

Only Freshly Isolated pRBCs Are Suppressors of FL-DC Activation

We compared responses of FL-DCs stimulated with freshly isolated pRBCs and pRBCs previously purified and freeze-thawed. The protocol used for cryopreservation and thawing of pRBCs largely preserves pRBC integrity (34, 35) and is a convenient way of preparing standardized preparations of parasites for research, including experimental human infections (36, 37). However, frozen pRBCs were less efficient at activating the FL-DC (**Figure 3A** and data not shown). Moreover, they were inefficient at suppressing the TLR-9 activation of FL-DC compared to the freshly isolated pRBC (**Figure 3A** and **Supplementary Figure 2**). Therefore, frozen and fresh pRBC preparations were qualitatively different in their fundamental abilities to activate DCs.

Removal of Host RBC Membrane Does Not Prevent Parasite-Induced Suppression of DC Responses

The differences in the ability of fresh vs. frozen and thawed pRBC preparations to affect FL-DC activation suggested that perhaps a reduction in pRBC membrane viability was the cause. To test this, we treated freshly isolated pRBCs with the detergent saponin. Saponin treatment of pRBCs disrupts the RBC membrane and the parasitophorous vacuolar membrane (38). Thus, saponin-treated trophozoites lack expression of malarial proteins normally located on the host red cell membrane, including molecules such as *Pf*EMP1 which have been postulated to inhibit innate immune responses (39–41).

Co-stimulatory marker expression by DCs was similar after stimulation with saponin-treated and untreated pRBCs, with pRBC:DC ratios of 1:1 and 5:1 actually inducing lower levels of activation whilst high doses still led to low CD40 upregulation. In the presence of CpG2216, DCs were similarly activated, regardless of saponin treatment, whilst high doses of saponin-treated pRBC still suppressed the CpG2216-driven CD40 (**Figure 3**) and CD86 upregulation (**Supplementary Figures 3B,C**) on cDC and pDC populations.

Thus, neither the presence of host RBC membrane nor surface-expressed parasite proteins, including *PfEMP1*, appeared to play a major role in suppression of FL-DC activation in the presence of high levels of parasites. Viability was comparable between FL-DCs exposed to saponin-treated and non-treated pRBCs for every ratio of pRBCs to DCs (**Supplementary Figure 3A**). This data also suggested that the differences in DC activation abilities between frozen and freshly isolated pRBC were intrinsic to the trophozoite and not dependent on the host RBC membranes.

Merozoites Are Potent Stimulators of FL-DCs

Merozoites are the extracellular life stage of the malaria parasite. FL-DCs stimulated with ratios of merozoites to DCs from a high ratio of 50:1 to a low ratio of 1:1 were, in the main, highly activated, with dose-dependent increases of all surface activation markers examined (**Figure 4**), although CD11b^{+} FL-DC showed reduced MHCII expression with high concentrations of merozoites (**Figure 4C**). However, in contrast to stimulation with pRBCs, at ratios higher than 12.5 merozoites:DC significant DC death was observed (**Figure 4B**). The rate of cell death at these ratios was high, consistent with excessive activation, and while cell surface activation of the remaining DC by TLR9 ligand was largely not perturbed by high concentrations of merozoites (**Figure 4C**), these results should be viewed in light of the very high rates of DC death at these parasite ratios.

FL-DC Production of Cytokines in Response to Merozoites Generally Increases With Higher Merozoite Dose

In response to increasing doses of merozoites, FL-DCs produced increasing amounts of cytokines (**Figures 5A,B**). This was inverse to the effect observed with pRBCs (**Figure 2**). Merozoites were a potent stimulus for IFN-α production. In the presence of CpG2216, production of TNF-α and IL-6 was reduced with increasing merozoites, potentially due to high merozoites concentrations inducing high DC death (**Figure 4B**). Overall, merozoites appeared to be potent activators of FL-DCs, inducing high levels of cell death at the highest concentrations but apparently not suppressing FL-DC activation by TLR9 ligands.

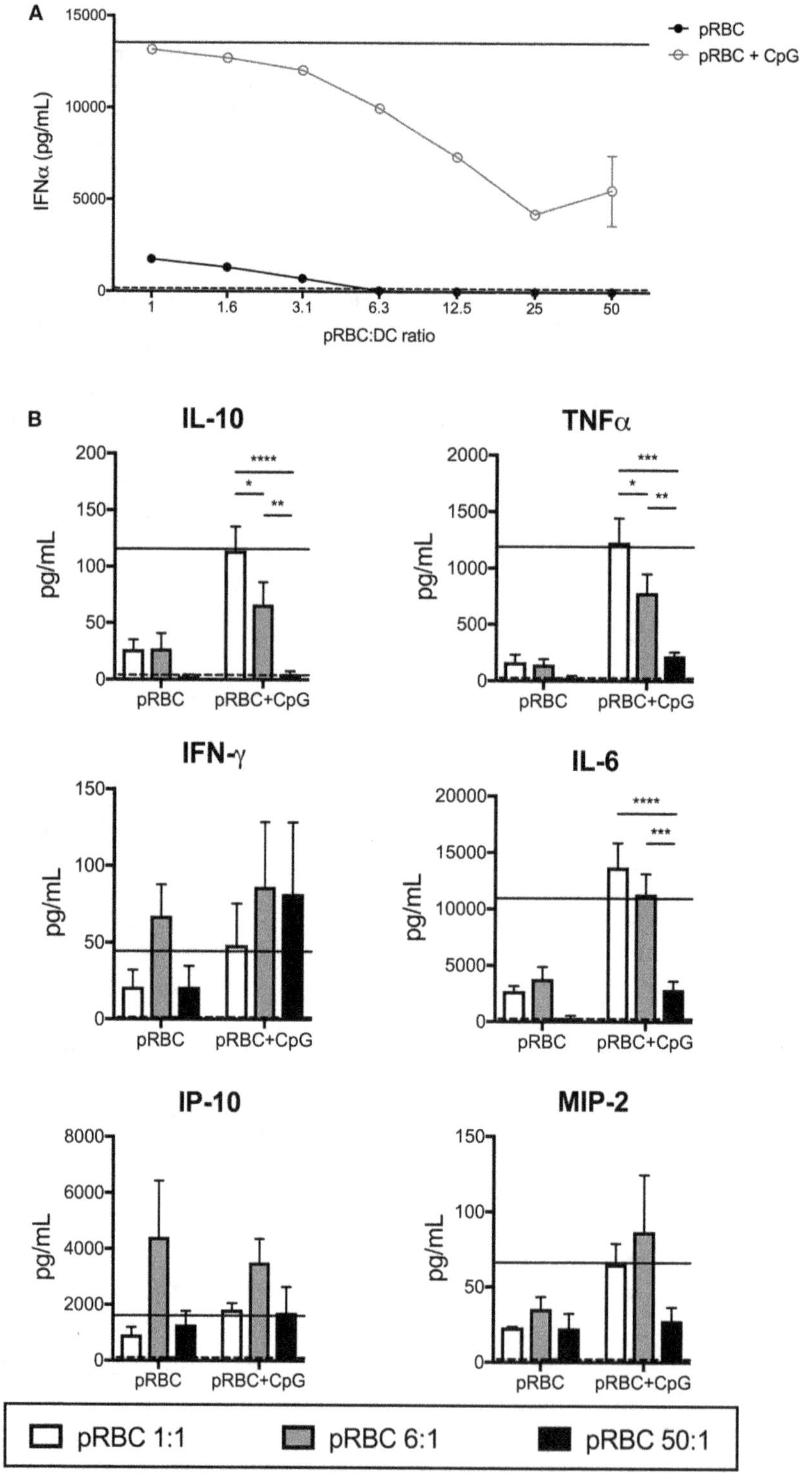

FIGURE 2 | Production of cytokines by FL-DCs is inhibited by high pRBC-to-DC ratios. Supernatants from FL-DC cultures stimulated with pRBCs were assayed for cytokine production using FlowCytomix and ProcartaPlex multiplexes. **(A)** IFN-α expression by FL-DCs was suppressed by the presence of high ratios of pRBCs, even in the presence of TLR9 ligand (pRBC+CpG). **(B)** FL-DC production of cytokines in response to pRBC-to-DC ratios of 1:1 (white), 6:1 (gray), and 50:1 (black) alone, or in the presence of CpG2216. Cytokine expression in response to uRBCs (dashed line) or CpG2216 alone (solid line) are included for comparison. $^{*}p < 0.05$, $^{**}p < 0.01$, $^{***}p < 0.001$, $^{****}p < 0.0001$. *P*-values were determined by two-way ANOVA using multiple comparisons. Data shown is from three experiments with each experiment using pooled FL-DC cultures from two mice. Error bars represent SEM of three separate experiments.

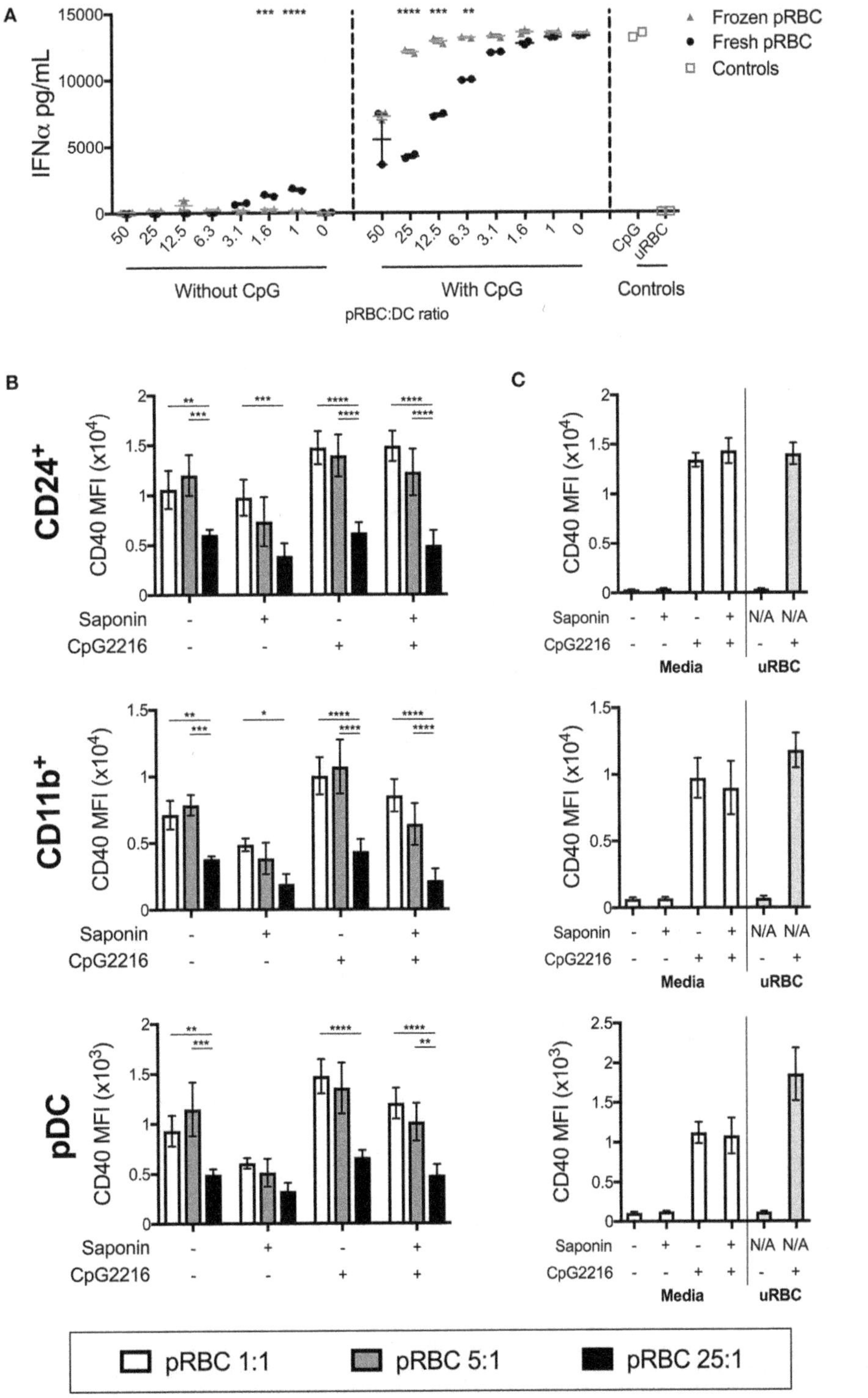

FIGURE 3 | pRBC-induced suppression is dependent on fresh parasites but not on intact host RBC membranes. **(A)** A titration of frozen pRBCs were compared to freshly purified pRBCs for the ability to induce activation and parasite-induced suppression of FL-DC TLR9 responses. Shown are IFN-α responses either to parasites alone or in the additional presence of CpG2216. **(B)** FL-DCs were co-incubated with saponin-treated or untreated *P. falciparum* pRBCs for 18–20 h at three different parasite-to-DC ratios: 1:1 (white), 5:1 (gray), and 25:1 (black), in the presence or absence of CpG2216. DC subpopulations were gated and expression of CD40 is shown. Each bar shows the SEM of three separate experiments, with each experiment using FL-DC cultures derived from pooling two mice. $^{*}p < 0.05$, $^{**}p < 0.01$, $^{***}p < 0.001$, $^{****}p < 0.0001$. *P*-values were determined by two-way ANOVA using multiple comparisons. **(C)** To control for effects of any carry-over saponin, saponin was also added to empty tubes and washed alongside the pRBC samples. Culture medium alone or medium containing CpG2216 were aliquoted into these tubes (designated Saponin +) and used to stimulate FL-DCs. The lack of any suppression of CD40 expression by uRBCs alone (25:1) is shown.

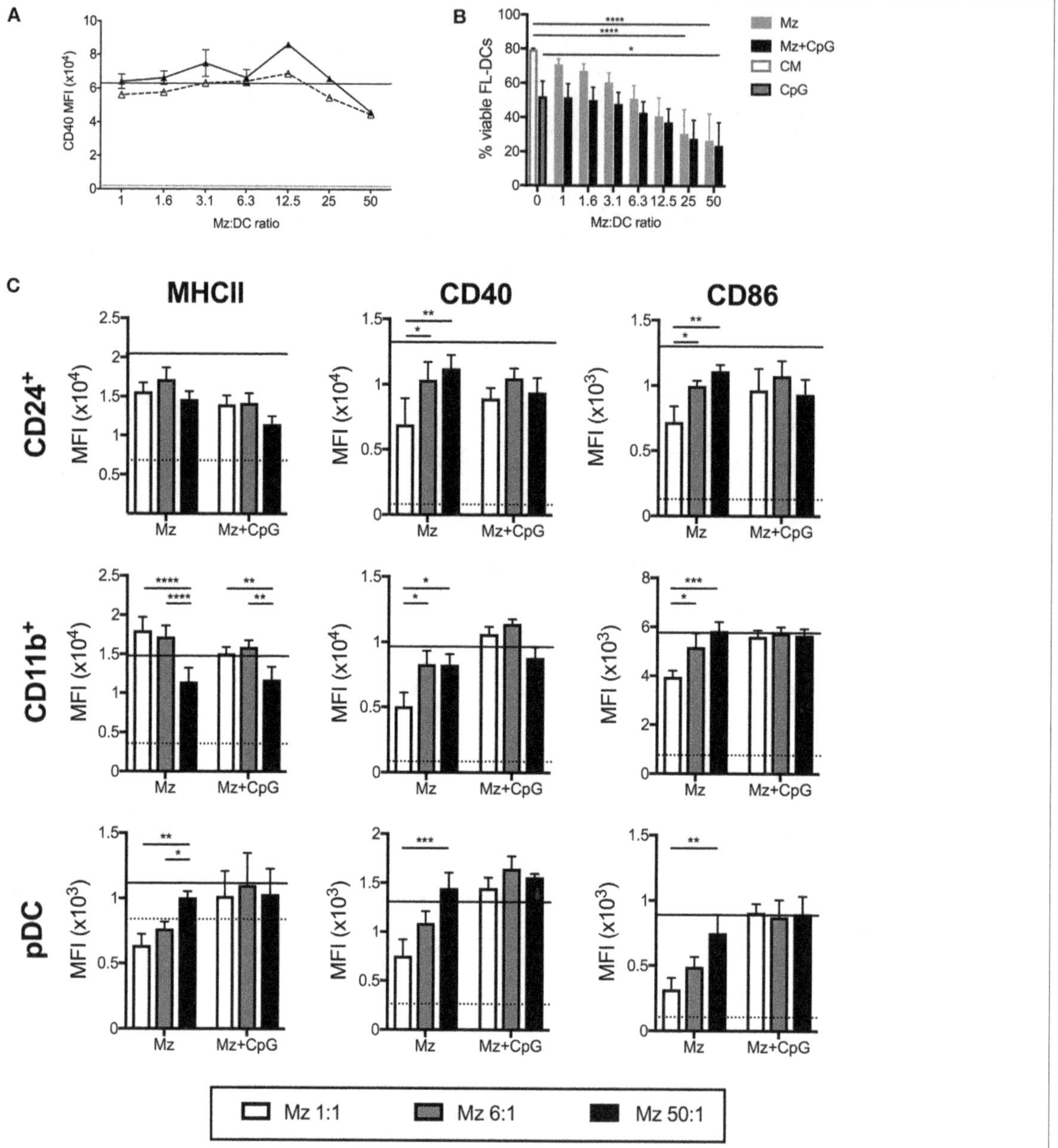

FIGURE 4 | Merozoites induce potent activation but high cell death of FL-DC. **(A)** Surface expression of CD40 on $CD24^+$ cDCs in response to 1–50 merozoites per DC (solid triangles) or in the additional presence of CpG2216 (hollow triangles). Level of CD40 in response to CpG2216 alone (solid line) and media alone (dotted line) are shown for comparison. **(B)** Exposure to high doses of merozoites results in death of up to 90% of FL-DCs after 18 h culture. Viability in response to culture medium alone (CM; white with gray border) or CpG2216 alone (CpG; gray with black border) are shown for comparison. **(C)** MHCII, CD40 and CD86 surface expression on FL-DCs gated for $CD24^+$, $CD11b^+$ or pDC in response to 1:1 (white bars), 6:1 (gray bars), or 50:1 (black bars) merozoites:DC, alone or in the addition presence of CpG2216.). $^*p < 0.05$, $^{**}p < 0.01$, $^{***}p < 0.001$, $^{****}p < 0.0001$. *P*-values were determined by two-way ANOVA using multiple comparisons. Data shown is from three experiments, each experiment using pooled FL-DC cultures from two mice. Error bars represent SEM of three separate experiments.

Merozoites Cannot Rescue FL-DC Suppression Induced by pRBCs

During malaria infection DCs would encounter both trophozoite and merozoite life-stages of the malaria parasite. Since merozoites did not suppress DC activation we tested whether merozoites would rescue the upregulation of CD40 in the presence of pRBCs, with or without TLR9 ligand. A ratio of 25 pRBCs:DCs was used with the addition of equal numbers of merozoites. Ratios of 25 parasites per DC for each life stage were chosen as concentrations that were still inhibitory for pRBCs (**Figure 1A**) but maintained high CD40 levels in response to merozoites alone (**Figure 4A**). Whilst merozoites are potent stimulators of MHC and co-stimulatory molecule expression on FL-DCs (**Figure 4**), they were unable to efficiently activate

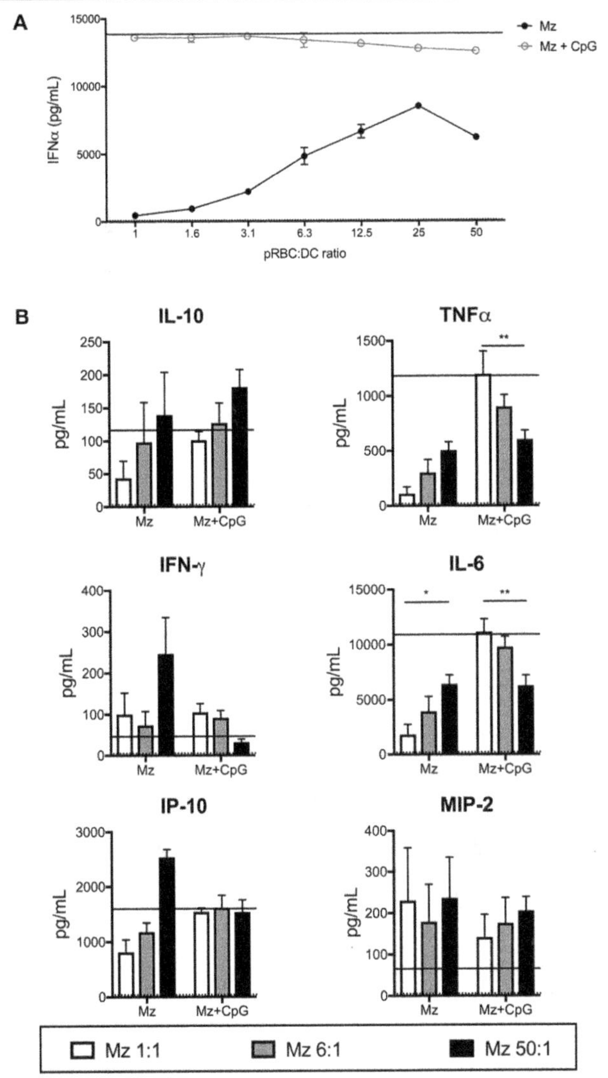

FIGURE 5 | Merozoites induce expression of a range of cytokines from FL-DCs. FL-DCs were incubated for 18 h with merozoites (Mz) and cytokines were measured in the supernatant using FlowCytomix and ProcartaPlex multiplexes. **(A)** High ratios of Mz:DCs induce high expression of IFN-α. **(B)** Mz:DC ratios of 1:1 (white bars), 6:1 (gray bars), or 50:1 (black bars). The expression in response to media alone (dotted line) and CpG2216 alone (solid line) were included for comparison. $^{*}p < 0.05$, $^{**}p < 0.01$. *P*-values were determined by two-way ANOVA using multiple comparisons. Figure shows pooled data from three experiments of FL-DC cultures derived from two mice each.

FL-DCs in the presence of pRBCs, particularly the upregulation of CD40 (**Figure 6**), either when mixed with pRBCs alone or in the additional presence of CpG2216 (**Figure 6**).

DISCUSSION

We have shown that at doses of >6 parasites to 1 DC, *P. falciparum* pigmented trophozoites possess a stage-specific capacity to suppress specific DC functions. This suppressive capacity particularly affects the upregulation of CD40 on all DC subsets and the ability of DCs to produce key cytokines; IFN-α, TNF-α, IL-6, and IL-10. This suppressive capacity of pRBCs is not dependent upon *Pf*EMP1 or other parasite molecules expressed on, or other properties of, the infected host RBC membrane (**Figure 3**).

The pRBCs not only suppressed DC responses to themselves at ratios of >6 per DC but also suppressed the ability of DCs to respond to the potent TLR9 ligand, CpG2216 (**Figure 1**). This included inhibiting the ability of pDCs to produce IFN-α to CpG2216 (**Figure 2A**). Although suppressing TLR9-mediated DC activation, increasing doses of pRBCs did not enhance DC death. Others have previously shown that monocyte-derived DCs, DCs fundamentally different to those investigated herein, also do not require *Pf*EMP1 to be suppressed, though suppression of DC activation at doses of 100:1 were at least in part due to DC apoptosis (42). The data shown herein of suppression of TLR9-mediated FL-DC activation by pRBCs is independent of cell death (**Figure 1**). In the aforementioned study, it was also shown via transwell experiments that cell-cell contact was not required for 100:1 doses of pRBCs to inhibit TLR-mediated upregulation of HLA-DR, CD83, and CD86 (42). Similarly, lysates from pRBCs induced chemokine production from human DCs, similarly to intact pRBCs (32). Both suppression and activation of DCs by pRBCs are therefore mediated by soluble factors, which could potentially be addressed by co-incubating TLR-stimulated DCs with conditioned parasite medium and measuring suppression.

In stark contrast, purified merozoites induced dose-responsive activation of the FL-DCs and high (likely activation-induced) DC death at high doses (**Figures 4, 5**). The merozoites were not able to rescue the activation of FL-DCs in the presence of pRBCs; in fact, pRBCs inhibited the strong merozoite-driven DC activation (**Figure 6**). DC death in malaria is via the apoptotic pathway (4, 42, 43), and it is unclear whether the DC death observed in response to high ratios of parasites in this study is due to parasites directly activating pro-apoptotic signals or whether it is apoptosis as a natural endpoint of DC activation. The increased DC apoptosis may inhibit activation of surrounding DCs by impairing the maturation of immature DCs (44) and polarizing DCs toward a tolerising phenotype (45). Regardless, DC apoptosis is likely a major contributor to the short duration of immune memory to malaria. Determining whether apoptosis is driven by maturation or parasites will help to identify methods of reducing apoptosis and improve downstream DC responses.

In contrast, ratios of 1:1 pRBC potently activated DCs to upregulate co-stimulatory markers (**Figure 1**) and cytokines, including IFN-α (**Figure 3**). Merozoites on the other hand, really showed a dose response effect in their ability to activate DC (**Figures 4, 5**), although ratios of 1 merozoite per DC still activated DC, highest levels of cytokines and cell surface markers were reached with more than 6 merozoites per DC. As merozoites and trophozoites have divergent transcriptomes (46, 47), this may help to identify potential activatory proteins. Furthermore, DC activation by these very low ratios of parasites suggests that even very low parasitaemia may induce potent DC activation, at least initially. Asymptomatic parasitaemia, often

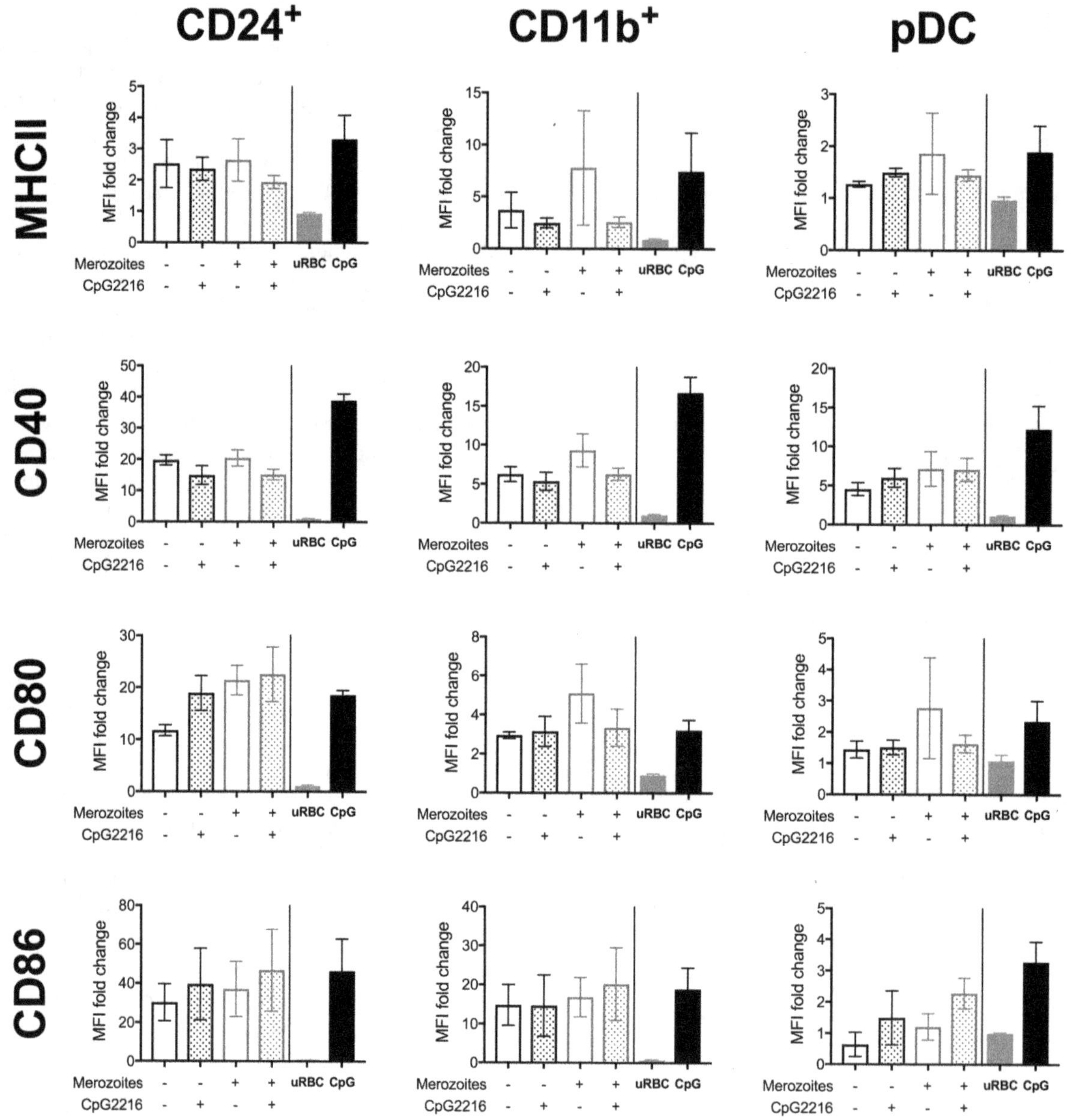

FIGURE 6 | Stimulation with mixed high-dose pRBCs and merozoites in the presence or absence of CpG2216 does not result in recovery of CD40 expression. FL-DCs were stimulated with either pRBCs alone, or pRBCs in the presence of an equivalent ratio of merozoites (Mz), in the presence or absence of CpG2216. All pRBCs and merozoites were added at a ratio of 25 per DC. Neither the addition of merozoites nor the addition of CpG2216 resulted in rescue of CD40 expression, but other markers demonstrated a heterogenous response. Co-stimulatory marker expression is represented as fold increase over media control and each bar represents mean and SEM of two experiments based on pooled FL-DC cultures of two mice.

seen in areas of high transmission, may reflect a pattern where initial potent DC-driven responses are suppressed by subsequent high-parasitaemia infections, leading to immunosuppression and tolerance. In contrast, low-parasitaemia infections may actually induce potent DC responses that lead to the generation of memory.

As regards physiological relevance of the parasite-to-DC ratios examined in this study, there is relatively little information on bioavailability of blood-stage malaria parasites to splenocytes *in vivo*. However, *in vitro* studies suggest that in high-parasitaemia settings a large proportion of merozoites fail to invade (26). This would result in high volumes of merozoites circulating to or being trafficked to the primary lymphoid tissues by migratory DCs, potentially even to the 50:1 ratios reported in this study. It is also observed *in vivo* that the spleen can remove parasites from RBCs without inducing RBC lysis (48–50), and while there is no information at what rate this occurs, splenocytes may encounter membrane-free pRBC at a rate dependent on overall parasite burden. Potentially, splenic DCs may encounter very high ratios of membrane-free pRBC in high parasitaemia settings, and as DC responses are not significantly affected by pRBC membrane, it is possible that the patterns reported in our study reflect physiological phenomena occurring in lymphoid organs.

An important point revealed in this work was that the DC response to frozen and thawed pRBCs is distinct from the response to fresh pRBCs (**Figure 3**). Methods to standardize frozen pRBC preparations have been used to prepare parasite vaccinations for standardization of controlled human malaria infection trials in naïve individuals (36). While this method induces viable parasites, it is likely that a proportion of ring-stage trophozoites would not survive the freezing process and may lead to induction of sub-optimal DC responses or tolerance. Furthermore, it serves as a caution for *in vitro* experiments that may use cryopreserved pRBCs as an immune stimulus. The data shown would argue that a comparison with freshly isolated pRBCs is needed to determine whether responses of human DCs and other innate responses *in vivo* and *in vitro* are qualitatively different when comparing inoculation with freeze-thawed vs. fresh pRBC preparations.

The surface activation marker most consistently suppressed by the presence of pRBCs, in both cDCs and pDCs, was CD40. Ligation of CD40 is crucial as it improves DC survival and enhances antigen presentation, therefore acting as a direct marker for DC activation (3). The interaction of CD40:CD40L between DCs and T cells activates both cell types and provides a vital positive feedback loop for cytokine secretion and co-stimulatory marker upregulation by DCs (3). Loss of CD40 on the surface of pRBC-exposed DCs could result in failure to induce downstream co-stimulatory pathways, resulting in overall failure of DC function. Work by Mukherjee and Chauhan highlights the importance of CD40 signaling for upregulation of other co-stimulatory markers in the moDC:*P. falciparum* context. When CD40L was added to moDCs co-incubated with "suppressive" doses of pRBCs, expression of CD83 was unaltered and expression of CD80 enhanced, rather than suppressed (51). A similar mechanism may be present in *bona fide* DCs. If CD40 expression is restored in DCs exposed to high doses of *P. falciparum*, it may restore their ability to stimulate T and B lymphocytes, which has implications for the design of next generation vaccine adjuvants that either target pRBC mechanisms of CD40 down-regulation or independently lead to enhanced expression of CD40 on DCs.

Murine FL-DC were used as a model for human blood DCs as they could be easily generated in large numbers and consistently produce similar levels of pDCs and cDCs (**Supplementary Figure 4**). FL-DCs also show greater transcriptomic similarities to their human counterparts than moDCs, another model commonly used to study malaria-DC interactions (9). The major difference between murine FL-DCs and human blood DCs is that only pDCs in humans express TLR9 (52). However, findings in human moDCs, which also do not express TLR9, are also suppressed by high doses of pRBCS (42, 53), suggesting high pRBC doses can suppress DC activation by multiple alternate pathways.

The mechanism by which pRBCs inhibit DC activation remains unclear. The effects of hemozoin upon DCs have been debated in the literature (18, 19) but it is unlikely to be the suppressive factor in this model as merozoite preparations were not hemozoin-depleted prior to DC co-incubation, yet still induced potent DC activation. A possible explanation may be found in the proteomic and transcriptomic differences between pRBCs and merozoites. The merozoite transcriptome is 45% smaller than that of the trophozoite. Merozoites lack the expression of many proteins required for hemoglobin digestion, protein export, and parasite metabolism (46, 47). One of these trophozoite-restricted protein families may contain the factor responsible for suppression; alternately, it may be a lipid, RNA byproduct or metabolite of the pigmented trophozoite, which is a very metabolically active life stage.

In conclusion, we demonstrate that pRBCs can suppress specific key DC functions and activation, in contrast to the activatory effect of merozoites. While DCs would interact with both merozoites and pRBCs in the blood, the specific suppressive effect of pRBCs appeared dominant and occurred even in the presence of merozoites. These findings may help partly explain why malaria immunity is typically slow to be acquired through natural exposure, why vaccine efficacy and vaccine-induced immune responses are lower in malaria endemic settings than among malaria-naïve subjects (54), and why immunity to malaria is generally not well-maintained (55). Further research to understand the mechanistic basis for these effects and identifying strategies to overcome them may be crucial for the development of highly efficacious and long-lasting vaccines.

ETHICS STATEMENT

This study was carried out in accordance with NHMRC guidelines and approved by the Animal Ethics Committee at AMREP Animal Services Precinct Animal Centre, Melbourne, Australia and Monash University, Clayton, Australia.

AUTHOR CONTRIBUTIONS

XZY and RJL carried out the research and analyzed the data. GF carried out essential experiments. JP contributed essential technical expertise. MOK and JGB designed and supervised the research and analyzed the data. XZY wrote the first draft. All authors contributed to writing of the manuscript.

FUNDING

Funding was provided by NHMRC (Senior Research Fellowships to JGB and MOK; Early Career Fellowship to RJL; Project grant to MOK). Burnet Institute was supported by the NHMRC Independent Research Institutes Support Scheme and a Victorian State Government Operational Infrastructure Grant. JB and GF are members of the Australian Centre for Research Excellence in Malaria Elimination (ACREME), funded by the NHMRC.

ACKNOWLEDGMENTS

With thanks to staff of the AMREP Flow facility and Monash Flow Cytometry Platform, the technicians and staff of the animal facilities at AMREP and Monash.

REFERENCES

1. Castiglioni P, Lu C, Lo D, Croft M, Langlade-Demoyen P, Zanetti M, et al. CD4 T cell priming in dendritic cell-deficient mice. *Immunology* (2003) 15:127–36. doi: 10.1093/intimm/dxg015
2. Draper SJ, Sack BK, King CR, Nielsen CM, Rayner JC, Higgins MK, et al. Malaria vaccines: recent advances and new horizons. *Cell Host Microbe* (2018) 24:43–56. doi: 10.1016/j.chom.2018.06.008
3. Caux C, Massacrier C, Vanbervliet B, Dubois B, Van Kooten C, Durand I, et al. Activation of human dendritic cells through CD40 cross-linking. *J Exp Med.* (1994) 180:1263–72. doi: 10.1084/jem.180.4.1263
4. Woodberry, Minigo G, Piera KA, Amante FH, Pinzon-Charry A, Good MF, et al. Low-level *Plasmodium falciparum* blood-stage infection causes dendritic cell apoptosis and dysfunction in healthy volunteers. *J Infect Dis.* (2012) 206:333–40. doi: 10.1093/infdis/jis366
5. Kho S, Marfurt J, Handayuni I, Pava Z, Noviyanti R, Kusuma A, et al. Characterization of blood dendritic and regulatory T cells in asymptomatic adults with sub-microscopic *Plasmodium falciparum* or *Plasmodium vivax* infection. *Malar J.* (2016) 15:328. doi: 10.1186/s12936-016-1382-7
6. Breitling LP, Fendel R, Mordmueller B, Adegnika AA, Kremsner PG, Luty AJ. Cord blood dendritic cell subsets in African newborns exposed to *Plasmodium falciparum* in utero. *Infect Immun.* (2006) 74:5725–9. doi: 10.1128/IAI.00682-06
7. Urban BC, Cordery D, Shafi MJ, Bull PC, Newbold CI, Williams TN, et al. The frequency of BDCA3-positive dendritic cells is increased in the peripheral circulation of Kenyan children with severe malaria. *Infect Immun.* (2006) 74:6700–6. doi: 10.1128/IAI.00861-06
8. Sallusto F, Lanzavecchia A. Efficient presentation of soluble antigen by cultured human dendritic cells is maintained by granulocyte/macrophage colony-stimulating factor plus interleukin 4 and downregulated by tumor necrosis factor alpha. *J Exp Med.* (1994) 179:1109–18. doi: 10.1084/jem.179.4.1109
9. Robbins SH, Walzer T, Dembélé D, Thibault C, Defays A, Bessou G, et al. Novel insights into the relationships between dendritic cell subsets in human and mouse revealed by genome-wide expression profiling. *Genome Biol.* (2008) 9:R17 doi: 10.1186/gb-2008-9-1-r17
10. Brawand P, Fitzpatrick DR, Greenfield BW, Brasel K, Maliszewski CR, De Smedt T. Murine plasmacytoid pre-dendritic cells generated from Flt3 ligand-supplemented bone marrow cultures are immature APCs. *J Immunol.* (2002) 169:6711–19. doi: 10.4049/jimmunol.169.12.6711
11. Naik SH, Proietto AI, Wilson NS, Dakic A, Schnorrer P, Fuchsberger M, et al. Cutting edge: generation of splenic CD8+ and CD8- dendritic cell equivalents in Fms-like tyrosine kinase 3 ligand bone marrow cultures. *J Immunol.* (2005) 174:6592–7. doi: 10.4049/jimmunol.174.11.6592
12. Brasel K, De Smedt T, Smith JL, Maliszewski CR. Generation of murine dendritic cells from flt3-ligand-supplemented bonel marrow cultures. *Blood* (2000) 96:3029–39. Available online at: http://www.bloodjournal.org/content/96/9/3029.long?sso-checked=true
13. Kirkling ME, Cytlak U, Lau CM, Lewis KL, Resteu A, Khodadadi-Jamayran A, et al. Notch signaling facilitates *in vitro* generation of cross-presenting classical dendritic cells. *Cell Rep.* (2018) 23:3658–72.e6. doi: 10.1016/j.celrep.2018.05.068
14. Macri C, Pang ES, Patton T, O'Keeffe M. Dendritic cell subsets. *Semin Cell Dev Biol.* (2018) 84:11–21. doi: 10.1016/j.semcdb.2017.12.009
15. O'Keeffe M, Hochrein H, Vremec D, Scott B, Hertzog P, Tatarczuch L, et al. Dendritic cell precursor populations of mouse blood: Identification of the murine homologues of human blood plasmacytoid pre-DC2 and CD11c+ DC1 precursors. *Blood* (2003) 101:1453–9. doi: 10.1182/blood-2002-03-0974
16. O'Keeffe M, Hochrein H, Vremec D, Caminschi I, Miller JL, Anders EM, et al. Mouse plasmacytoid cells: long-lived cells, heterogeneous in surface phenotype and function, that differentiate into CD8(+) dendritic cells only after microbial stimulus. *J Exp Med.* (2002) 196:1307–19. doi: 10.1084/jem.20021031
17. Ank N, Iversen MB, Bartholdy C, Staeheli P, Hartmann R, Jensen UB, et al. An important role for type III interferon (IFN-lambda/IL-28) in TLR-induced antiviral activity. *J Immunol.* (2008) 180:2474–85. doi: 10.4049/jimmunol.180.4.2474
18. Parroche P, Lauw FN, Goutagny N, Latz E, Monks BG, Visintin A, et al. Malaria hemozoin is immunologically inert but radically enhances innate responses by presenting malaria DNA to Toll-like receptor 9. *Proc Natl Acad Sci USA.* (2007) 104:1919–24. doi: 10.1073/pnas.0608745104
19. Wu X, Gowda NM, Kumar S, Gowda DC. Protein-DNA complex is the exclusive malaria parasite component that activates dendritic cells and triggers innate immune responses. *J Immunol.* (2010) 184:4338–48. doi: 10.4049/jimmunol.0903824
20. Pichyangkul S, Gettayacamin M, Miller RS, Lyon JA, Angov E, Tongtawe P, et al. Pre-clinical evaluation of the malaria vaccine candidate P. falciparum MSP1 42 formulated with novel adjuvants or with alum. *Vaccine* (2004) 22:3831–40. doi: 10.1016/j.vaccine.2004.07.023
21. Loughland JR, Minigo G, Sarovich DS, Field M, Tipping PE, Montes de Oca M, et al. Plasmacytoid dendritic cells appear inactive during sub-microscopic *Plasmodium falciparum* blood-stage infection, yet retain their ability to respond to TLR stimulation. *Sci Rep.* (2017) 7:2596. doi: 10.1038/s41598-017-02096-2
22. Wykes MN, Kay JG, Manderson A, Liu XQ, Brown DL, Richard DJ, et al. Rodent blood-stage Plasmodium survive in dendritic cells that infect naive mice. *Proc Natl Acad Sci USA.* (2011) 108:11205–10. doi: 10.1073/pnas.1108579108
23. Moll K, Kaneko A, Scherf A, Wahlgren M. *Methods in Malaria Research.* 5th ed. BioMalPar (2008).
24. Lambros C, Vanderberg JP. Synchronization of *Plasmodium falciparum* erythrocytic stages in culture. *J Parasitol.* (1979) 65:418–20. doi: 10.2307/3280287
25. Goodyer ID, Johnson J, Eisenthal R, Hayes DJ. Purification of mature-stage *Plasmodium falciparum* by gelatine flotation. *Ann Trop Med Parasitol.* (1994) 88:209–11. doi: 10.1080/00034983.1994.11812859
26. Boyle MJ, Wilson DW, Richards JS, Riglar DT, Tetteh KK, Conway DJ, et al. Isolation of viable *Plasmodium falciparum* merozoites to define erythrocyte invasion events and advance vaccine and drug development. *Proc Natl Acad Sci USA.* (2010) 107:14378–83. doi: 10.1073/pnas.1009198107
27. Ding Y, Wilkinson A, Idris A, Fancke B, O'Keeffe M, Khalil D, et al. FLT3-ligand treatment of humanized mice results in the generation of large numbers of CD141+ and CD1c+ dendritic cells *in vivo*. *J Immunol.* (2014) 192:1982–9. doi: 10.4049/jimmunol.1302391
28. Imwong M, Stepniewska K, Tripura R, Peto TJ, Lwin KM, Vihokhern B, et al. Numerical distributions of parasite densities during asymptomatic malaria. *J Infect Dis.* (2016) 213:1322–9. doi: 10.1093/infdis/jiv596
29. Rolling T, Schmiedel S, Wichmann D, Wittkopf D, Burchard GD, Cramer JP. Post-treatment haemolysis in severe imported malaria after intravenous artesunate: case report of three patients with hyperparasitaemia. *Malar J.* (2012) 11:169. doi: 10.1186/1475-2875-11-169
30. Mordmüller B, Kremsner PG. Hyperparasitemia and blood exchange transfusion for treatment of children with falciparum malaria. *Clin Infect Dis.* (1998) 26:850–2. doi: 10.1086/513926
31. Pichyangkul S, Yongvanitchit K, Kum-arb U, Hemmi H, Akira S, Krieg AM, et al. Malaria blood stage parasites activate human plasmacytoid dendritic cells and murine dendritic cells through a Toll-like receptor 9-dependent

pathway. *J Immunol.* (2004) 172:4926–33. doi: 10.4049/jimmunol.172.8.4926
32. Götz A, Tang MS, Ty MC, Arama C, Ongoiba A, Doumtabe D, et al. Atypical activation of dendritic cells by *Plasmodium falciparum. Proc Natl Acad Sci USA.* (2017) 114:E10568–7. doi: 10.1073/pnas.1708383114
33. O'Keeffe M, Fancke B, Suter M, Ramm G, Clark J, Wu L, et al. Nonplasmacytoid, high IFN-a-producing, bone marrow dendritic cells. *J Immunol.* (2012) 188:3774–83. doi: 10.4049/jimmunol.1101365
34. Kinyanjui SM, Howard T, Williams TN, Bull PC, Newbold CI, Marsh K. The use of cryopreserved mature trophozoites in assessing antibody recognition of variant surface antigens of *Plasmodium falciparum*-infected erythrocytes. *J Immunol Methods* (2004) 288:9–18. doi: 10.1016/j.jim.2004.01.022
35. Chan JA, Howell KB, Reiling L, Ataide R, Mackintosh CL, Fowkes FJ, et al. Targets of antibodies against Plasmodium falciparum-infected erythrocytes in malaria immunity. *J Clin Invest.* (2012) 122:3227–38. doi: 10.1172/JCI62182
36. Stanisic DI, Liu XQ, De SL, Batzloff MR, Forbes T, Davis CB, et al. Development of cultured *Plasmodium falciparum* blood-stage malaria cell banks for early phase *in vivo* clinical trial assessment of anti-malaria drugs and vaccines. *Malar J.* (2015) 14:1–10. doi: 10.1186/s12936-015-0663-x
37. Stanisic DI, Gerrard J, Fink J, Griffin PM, Liu XQ, Sundac L, et al. Infectivity of *plasmodium falciparum* in malaria-naive individuals is related to knob expression and cytoadherence of the parasite. *Infect Immun.* (2016) 84:2689–96. doi: 10.1128/IAI.00414-16
38. Elandalloussi LM, Smith PJ. Preparation of pure and intact *Plasmodium falciparum* plasma membrane vesicles and partial characterisation of the plasma membrane ATPase. *Malar J.* (2002) 1:6. doi: 10.1186/1475-2875-1-6
39. Barfod L, Dalgaard MB, Pleman ST, Ofori MF, Pleass RJ, Hviid L. Evasion of immunity to *Plasmodium falciparum* malaria by IgM masking of protective IgG epitopes in infected erythrocyte surface-exposed PfEMP1. *Proc Natl Acad Sci USA.* (2011) 108:12485–90. doi: 10.1073/pnas.1103708108
40. Hsieh FL, Turner L, Bolla JR, Robinson CV, Lavstsen T, Higgins MK. The structural basis for CD36 binding by the malaria parasite. *Nat Commun.* (2016) 7:12837. doi: 10.1038/ncomms12837
41. Sampaio NG, Eriksson EM, Schofield L. *Plasmodium falciparum* PfEMP1 modulates monocyte/macrophage transcription factor activation and cytokine and chemokine responses. *Infect Immun.* (2017) 86:e00447–17. doi: 10.1128/IAI.00447-17
42. Elliott SR, Spurck TP, Dodin JM, Maier AG, Voss TS, Yosaatmadja F, et al. Inhibition of dendritic cell maturation by malaria is dose dependent and does not require *Plasmodium falciparum* erythrocyte membrane protein 1. *Infect Immun.* (2007) 75:3621–32. doi: 10.1128/IAI.00095-07
43. Pinzon-Charry A, Woodberry T, Kienzle V, McPhun V, Minigo G, Lampah DA, et al. Apoptosis and dysfunction of blood dendritic cells in patients with falciparum and vivax malaria. *J Exp Med.* (2013) 210:1635–46. doi: 10.1084/jem.20121972
44. Kushwah R, Oliver JR, Zhang J, Siminovitch KA, Hu J. Apoptotic dendritic cells induce tolerance in mice through suppression of dendritic cell maturation and induction of antigen-specific regulatory T cells. *J Immunol.* (2009) 183:7104–18. doi: 10.4049/jimmunol.0900824
45. Kushwah R, Wu J, Oliver JR, Jiang G, Zhang J, Siminovitch KA, et al. Uptake of apoptotic DC converts immature DC into tolerogenic DC, which induce differentiation of Foxp3+ regulatory T cells. *Eur J Immunol.* (2010) 40:1022–35. doi: 10.1002/eji.200939782
46. Le Roch KG, Johnson JR, Florens L, Zhou Y, Santrosyan A, Grainger M, et al. Global analysis of transcript and protein levels across the *Plasmodium falciparum* life cycle. *Genome Res.* (2004) 14:2308–18. doi: 10.1101/gr.2523904
47. Florens L, Washburn MP, Raine JD, Anthony RM, Grainger M, Haynes JD, et al. A proteomic view of the *Plasmodium falciparum* life cycle. *Nature* (2002) 419:520–6. doi: 10.1038/nature01107
48. Chotivanich K, Udomsangpetch R, Dondorp A, Williams T, Angus B, Simpson JA, et al. The mechanisms of parasite clearance after antimalarial treatment of *Plasmodium falciparum* malaria. *J Infect Dis.* (2000) 182:629–33. doi: 10.1086/315718
49. Chotivanich K, Udomsangpetch R, McGready R, Proux S, Newton P, Pukrittayakamee S, et al. Central role of the spleen in malaria parasite clearance. *J Infect Dis.* (2002) 185:1538–41. doi: 10.1086/340213
50. Angus BJ, Chotivanich K, Udomsangpetch R, White NJ. *In vivo* removal of malaria parasites from red blood cells without their destruction in acute falciparum malaria. *Blood* (1997) 90:2037–40.
51. Mukherjee P, Chauhan VS. Plasmodium falciparum-free merozoites and infected RBCs distinctly affect soluble CD40 ligand-mediated maturation of immature monocyte-derived dendritic cells. *J Leukoc Biol.* (2008) 84:244–54. doi: 10.1189/jlb.0807565
52. Hémont C, Neel A, Heslan M, Braudeau C, Josien R. Human blood mDC subsets exhibit distinct TLR repertoire and responsiveness. *J Leukoc Biol.* (2013) 93:599–609. doi: 10.1189/jlb.0912452
53. Urban BC, Ferguson DJ, Pain A, Willcox N, Plebanski M, Austyn JM, et al. *Plasmodium falciparum*-infected erythrocytes modulate the maturation of dendritic cells. *Nature* (1999) 400:73–7. doi: 10.1038/21900
54. Beeson JG, Kurtovic L, Dobaño C, Opi DH, Chan J-A, Feng G, et al. Challenges and strategies for developing efficacious and long-lasting malaria vaccines. *Sci Transl Med.* (2019) 11:eaau1458. doi: 10.1126/scitranslmed.aau1458
55. Fowkes FJ, Boeuf P, Beeson JG. Immunity to malaria in an era of declining malaria transmission. *Parasitology* (2016) 143:139–53. doi: 10.1017/S0031182015001249

11

Humanized Mice are Instrumental to the Study of *Plasmodium falciparum* Infection

Rajeev K. Tyagi[1,2,3*†], *Nikunj Tandel*[4†], *Richa Deshpande*[4], *Robert W. Engelman*[5], *Satish D. Patel*[6] *and Priyanka Tyagi*[7]

[1] *Division of Gastroenterology, Hepatology and Nutrition, Department of Medicine, Vanderbilt University Medical Center, Nashville, TN, United States,* [2] *Biomedical parasitology Unit, Institute Pasteur, Paris, France,* [3] *Department of Global Health, College of Public Health, University of South Florida, Tampa, FL, United States,* [4] *Institute of Science, Nirma University, Ahmedabad, India,* [5] *Department of Pediatrics, Pathology and Cell Biology, University of South Florida, Tampa, FL, United States,* [6] *Zydus Research Centre, Ahmedabad, India,* [7] *Department of Basic and Applied Sciences, School of Engineering, GD Goenka University, Gurgaon, India*

Correspondence:
Rajeev K. Tyagi
rajeev.tyagi@vumc.org;
rajeev.gru@gmail.com

[†] *Co-first authors*

Research using humanized mice has advanced our knowledge and understanding of human haematopoiesis, non-adaptive and adaptive immunity, autoimmunity, infectious disease, cancer biology, and regenerative medicine. Challenges posed by the human-malaria parasite *Plasmodium falciparum* include its complex life cycle, the evolution of drug resistance against anti-malarials, poor diagnosis, and a lack of effective vaccines. Advancements in genetically engineered and immunodeficient mouse strains, have allowed for studies of the asexual blood stage, exoerythrocytic stage and the transition from liver-to-blood stage infection, in a single vertebrate host. This review discusses the process of "humanization" of various immunodeficient/transgenic strains and their contribution to translational biomedical research. Our work reviews the strategies employed to overcome the remaining-limitations of the developed human-mouse chimera(s).

Keywords: humanized/chimeric mice, malaria, NSG mice, TK/NOG mice, FRG mice, huRBCs, huHep, clodronate loaded liposomes

---

Abbreviations: ACT, Artemisinin-based combination therapy; AIDS, acquired immune deficiency syndrome; anti-Gr1, Anti-granulocyte receptor 1; APCs, antigen presenting cells; cGy, centigray (equals to 0.01 gray); CIMP, Chemical immunomodulation protocol; Clo-lip, Clodronate-loaded liposomes; CYPs, Cytochrom P450s; DCs, Dendritic cells; FAH, fumarylacetoacetate hydrolase; *FoxN1* - forkhead Box N1; FRG, $FAH^{-/-}Rag2^{-/-}IL2R\gamma^{null}$; GCV, ganciclovir; GM-CSF, Granulocyte-macrophage colony-stimulating factor ; GVHD, graft versus host disease; hBMCs, human bone marrow cells; HepG2, human liver carcinoma cells; hESCs, Human embryonic stem cells; hPBLs, human peripheral blood lymphocytes; HSCs, Human hematopoietic stem cells; HSVtk, herpes simplex virus type 1 thymidine kinase; huBMCs, Human bone marrow cells; huHep, Human hepatocytes; huPBLs, Human peripheral blood lymphocytes; huRBCs, Human-red blood cells; IFA, immunofluorescence assay; IFN-γ, interferon gamma; *IL-2rg*, interleukin-2 Receptor ɤ-chain; IP, Intra-peritoneal; iPSC, Induced pluripotent stem cells; IRS, indoor residual spray; IV, Intravenous; KO, knockout; LS, Liver stage; MCP-1, Monocyte chemoattractant protein-1; M-CSF, Macrophage colony-stimulating factor; MP, Malaria pigments; MST, Median survival time; NICC, Neonatal porcine islet cell clusters; NK-cell, Natural killer cells; NOD, Non-obese diabetic; PBMCs, Peripheral-blood mononuclear cells; PHA, Phyto-haemagglutinin; $Prkdc^{SCID}$, Protein kinase, DNA activated, catalytic polypeptide; Severe Combined Immunodeficiency; qRT-PCR, Qualitative reverse transcriptase polymerase chain reaction; *Rag*1/2, Recombination-activating gene 1/2; RBCs/huRBCs, Red blood cells/human-red blood cells; RH5, Reticulocyte-binding protein homolog 5; rhGH, Recombinant human growth hormone; rhuPRL, Recombinant human prolactin; RI/huHep-RI, Repopulation index/huHep-repopulation index; SCID, Severe combined immunodeficiency; SIRPα, Signal regulatory protein alpha; TB, Tubercuosis; TCR- T-cell receptor; TNF-α, Tumor necrosis factor-alpha; TRAP, Thrombospondin-related anonymous protein; Tregs, Regulatory T cells; uPA, Urokinase plasminogen activator; USGI, ultra-sound guided injection; WHO, World Health Organization.

BACKGROUND: THE BURDEN OF MALARIA

Among the numerous infectious diseases, malaria remains a major health challenge. Malaria is a disease which spreads through the bite of female *anopheles* mosquitoes, who carry the infection moieties (sporozoites) of parasites belonging to the *Plasmodium* genus (1). The greater morbidity and mortality related to human malaria infections reported by World Health Organization (WHO), is due to the wide range of hosts, mainly affecting humans with a high host tropism. 216 million cases of malaria infection was reported across the world in 2016, with a death toll of 445,000. In comparison, 237 million cases were reported in 2010 and 211 million cases were reported in 2015 (2). The death incidence rate in Sub-Saharan Africa is more than 85% in children <5 years of age (3).

The pathophysiology and molecular mechanism of malaria has been revealed, contributing to improving our understanding of malaria biology. The routine culture of an asexual blood stage infection of *P. falciparum* was successfully achieved (4). However, various aspects related to the mechanism of cell motility and invasion, changes in cell signaling pathways and the modulation of host cells, escape from the immune system and establishment of an infection into the liver, or to stay in hypnozoite stages, are not very clear. The technological advances in the field of epidemiology and entomology support the research and reduces the burden of understanding the malaria parasitology by staining the vivid stages of all parasites (5–7).

The tens of millions of non-immune individuals from areas where malaria is not transmitted, visit malaria endemic areas, and face the risk of malaria infection (8, 9). The two major weapons against malaria are vector control and chemoprophylaxis/chemotherapy (10). Various treatments such as indoor residual spray (IRS), use of insecticide-treated bed nets, and medical care through antimalarial drugs (artemisinin-based combination therapy-ACT etc) are available to reduce the burden of malaria (11, 12). Unfortunately, attempts to eradicate the disease based on these methods have had only limited success due to wide spread drug resistance by the parasite (13) as well as insecticide resistance of the mosquito vector (14). This bleak situation drives scientist to develop additional control measures such as a malaria vaccine which is both appealing and urgent. However, an effective malaria vaccine development has not been found, despite enormous and continued efforts made in this direction (15).

Biology of Malaria Parasites

The causative agent of the malaria parasite has a complex multi-stage life cycle which commences with the bite of the female anopheles mosquito, a definitive host that carries sporozoites to infect healthy humans (intermediate host) to complete the life cycle of the parasite (**Figure 1**). The disease in humans is caused by one or a combination of *Plasmodium* spp.: *P. vivax, P. falciparum, P. malariae*, and *P. ovale* (7). Also, in geographically limited zones of South-East Asia, the Malaysian island of Borneo in particular, infections caused by *P. Knowlesi*, a zoonosis without visible transmission to other hosts, can be observed (16).

The systemic *P. falciparum* infection causes greater morbidity and mortality due to its severity and poor diagnosis. On the contrary, *P. vivax* infection is less severe, but formation of hypnozoites and their genesis, need to be studied to understand the mechanism of frequent relapses (17).

Malaria infection in humans begins when the sporozoites from the salivary glands of female *anopheles* mosquito enter the bloodstream via the skin and travel to the liver. The sporozoites traverse through blood vessels and reach the liver, and undergoes the tightly regulated signaling mechanism before rendering the infection to the hepatocytes (1). The invaded hepatocytes allow for the replication of sporozoites and leads to the formation of schizonts. This asexual reproduction stage stays inside the liver of human cells and lasts for 7–10 days, depending on the species and strain of the parasite. Each schizont gives rise to several merozoites which are released into the bloodstream, indicating the end of the exoerythrocytic phase of the malaria infection. The infection by *P. vivax* and *P. ovale* is not characterized with this reproduction step since pathogens might reside as hypnozoites within the hepatocytes for a longer duration, until the infection relapses (18).

The merozoites in the bloodstream invade the erythrocytes and the first stage after invasion is the formation of a ring that later evolves into a trophozoite. The trophozoite cannot metabolize heme so it converts heme into a yellow pigment, hemozoin. The globin part of hemoglobin is utilized as a source of amino acids, needed for reproduction. Trophozoite then develops into erythrocytic schizont and each mature erythrocytic schizont gives rise to new merozoites that eventually rupture the erythrocytes which are released into the bloodstream to invade new RBCs. This is the symptomatic stage in which clinical manifestations of the disease begin to appear. Further, unlike the liver stage, the erythrocytic stage of the malaria parasite repeats multiple times (7, 18).

The differentiation of the parasite into male and female non-pathogenic gametocytes (propagation carriers), also takes place within RBCs. If a female Anopheles mosquito takes a blood meal, the gametocytes are taken up and mature into macrogamete (female) and microgamete (male). The microgamete undergoes three divisions producing eight nuclei in the process in the mosquito's gut, and each nucleus fertilizes with a macrogamete resulting in the formation of an ookinete. The ookinete penetrates the midgut wall and becomes encapsulated, forming an oocyst. The ookinete nucleus divides, producing thousands of sporozoites within the oocyst. Toward the end of sporogony, lasting 8–15 days, the oocyst ruptures and sporozoites travel to the salivary gland of mosquito, ready to be injected into a human host during the next blood meal (7, 19).

HUMAN-CHIMERIC MICE (HUMANIZED MICE)

Mice have been used as *in-vivo* models to study a diverse range of infectious pathogens (20). The murine and human

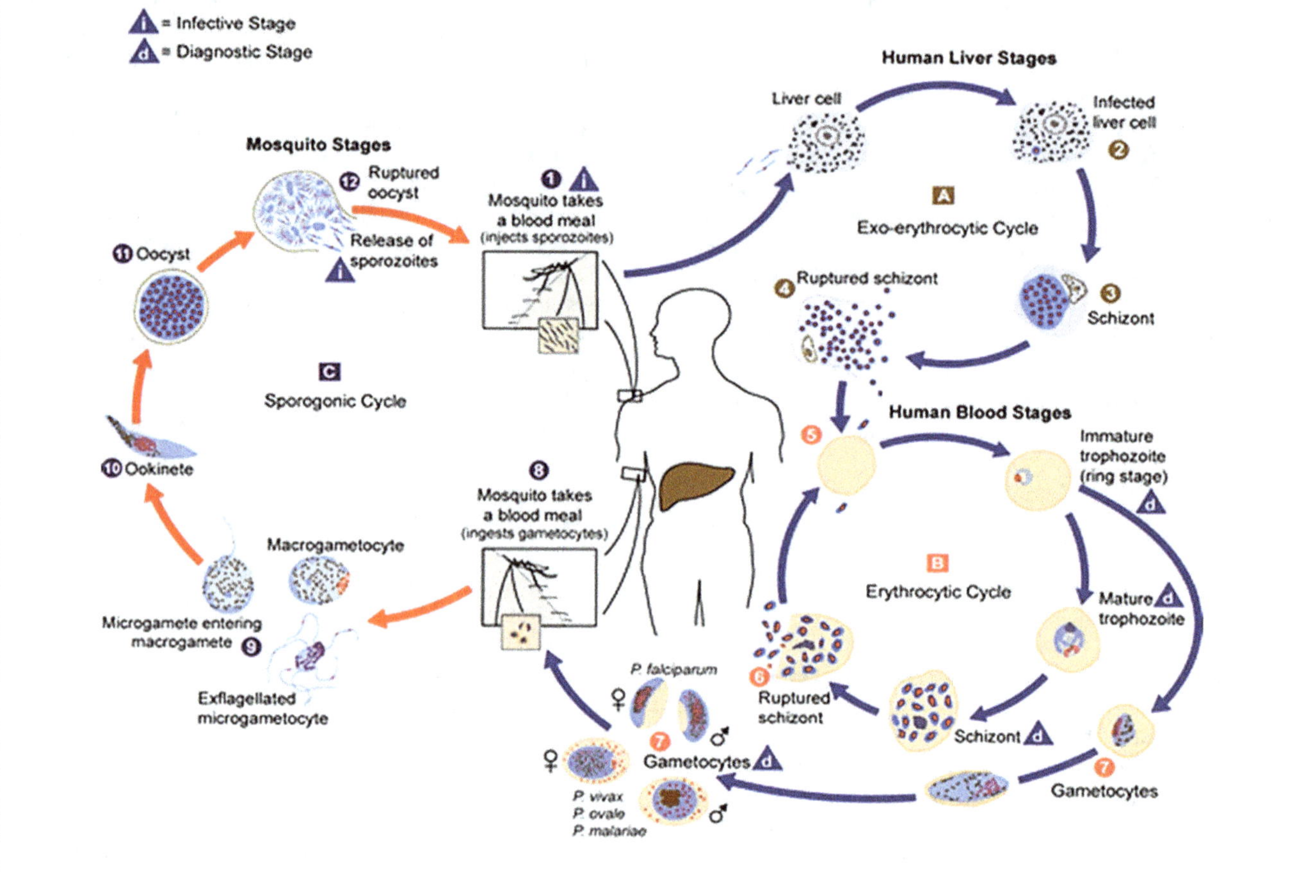

FIGURE 1 | The malaria parasite life cycle (1). Sporozoites infect liver cells (2) and mature into schizonts, which rupture and release merozoites (4). (Of note, in *P. vivax* and *P. ovale* a dormant stage [hypnozoites] can persist in the liver and cause relapses by invading the bloodstream weeks, or even years later.) After this initial replication in the liver (exo-erythrocyticschizogony (A)), the parasites undergo asexual multiplication in the erythrocytes (erythrocyticschizogony (B)). Merozoites infect red blood cells (5)]. The ring stage trophozoites mature into schizonts, which rupture releasing merozoites (5)]. Some parasites differentiate into sexual erythrocytic stages (gametocytes) (7). Blood stage parasites are responsible for the clinical manifestations of the disease. The gametocytes, male (microgametocytes) and female (macrogametocytes), are ingested by an *Anopheles* mosquito during a blood meal (8). The parasites' multiplication in the mosquito is known as the sporogonic cycle (C). While in the mosquito's stomach, the microgametes penetrate the macrogametes generating zygotes (9). The zygotes in turn become motile and elongated (ookinetes) (10) which invade the midgut wall of the mosquito where they develop into oocysts (11). The oocysts grow, rupture, and release sporozoites (12), which make their way to the mosquito's salivary glands. Inoculation of the sporozoites (1) into a new human host perpetuates the malaria life cycle. (Source: https://www.cdc.gov/malaria/about/biology/index.html).

genome shares nearly 85–99% similarity, but due to the complexity of the organization of cells, tissues and organs and specificity of the human immune system (21–23) some mouse strains are less than ideal *in-vivo* models. Recent advances made in translational biomedical research suggest the importance of immunomodulatory agents and target-specificity, and encourage the development of "humanized mouse models" (21, 24).

The theoretical and empirical evidence for the need of "human" mouse models, as well as advancements made in immunological research is the genesis and driving force for the development of chimeric mice. The immunodeficient mice transplanted with human cells or tissues are referred to as "humanized mice," with engraftment and repopulation of a functional human system (25). Since tissue and cell grafts are perceived as foreign and rejected by the host immune system, immunodeficient mice are inevitably required to achieve human cell engraftment followed by their repopulation. Therefore, immunomodulatory agents are administered to modulate the immune response to reduce graft rejection episodes.

Humanized-mice evolved from the origin of athymic (nude) mice with an underdeveloped/impaired thymus. The process of "humanization" of immunodeficient mice has progressed and a variety of immunodeficient mice have been developed by incorporating specific defects in their immune system through genetic engineering approaches. A brief account on immunological and physiological characteristics of some

TABLE 1 | list of various immunodeficient mouse strains.

Mice	Mutation	Mice Information	Character	Application	References
BXN (Beige/Xid/Nude) Developed by the collaborative work of NIH, USA, and referred as "NIH-III"	Beige mutation (*bg*^{J} or *bg*^{2J})	Originally produced at Oak Ridge National Laboratory due to radiation-induced mutation, name represents the color of affected mice Available as a single mutation in C57BL/6J or C3H/HeJ Also available at Jackson Laboratory	Defective and reduced bactericidal activity, absence of NK cells and defects in CTLs and antibody responses to tumor cells Defect in lysosomal enzymes of neutrophils Short life span, low body weight and poor bleeding time	Identical mutant to Chediak-Higashi syndrome in humans which helps in understanding the similar abnormalities To study the role of pigment and their genes in combination with pale ear (*ep* mutation) Study of giant lysosomes an important marker in identification and studying hematopoietic stem cells Most importantly to study the mechanism of metastatic spread of cancer, infectious diseases, hypersensitivity, bone marrow grafts To distinguish between the cytotoxic function of NK cells and NK T cells in normal and beige mice	(32–39)
	Xid mutation	CBA/N mice having X-linked immune deficiency mutation Available at Jackson Laboratory	Depletion in the number of peripheral B-cells and The B cells having less surface IgM to IgD ration which represent the disorder in B-cell maturation Curtail in IgM and IgG3 concentration in the serum, and reduction in capacity (or inactivity) of thymo-independent MHC-II responses	Helpful in understanding the mutation of Bruton's tyrosine kinase gene (*Btk*) which plays an crucial role in B-cell development To study the expression of V_H gene in spleen Reveal the crucial role of IgM in preventing the infection of *Crytococccus neoformans* from lungs to the brain in chronic pulmonary infection model Role of BCR in TACI expression (T cell-independent type 1 Ag such as LPS which stimulate BCR)	(40–44)
	Nude mutation	Mutation in *FOX1* (winged-helix/forkead transcription factor) gene, also called athymic nude Abnormal hair growth First reported at Virus laboratory, Ruchill Hospital, Glasgow by Dr.N.R.Grist Available at Jackson Laboratory	Practical absence of the thymus hairlessness, lack of functional T-cells, and deficiencies in cellular immunity, Partial defect in B cell development However, there is no defect in T-cell precursors and therefore in adult mice some functional T cells can be observed Due to the defect in T helper cell activity, thymus-dependent antigen were detected by IgM only, high NK cell activity	As an experimental model for tumor inoculation to study the metastasis and their growth inhibition by drug treatment Suitable model to study the infectious diseases (*Mycobacterium leprae,* parasite infection of protozoa and worms) Studies of autoimmunity and allergy Model for the liver deficiency study and treatment and xenotransplantation	(40, 45–49)
SCID mice	Mutation in the *Prkdc*^{SCID} gene on chromosome-16	Mutation in an enzyme which has an activity in DNA repair *Prkdc* (protein kinase, DNA activated, catalytic polypeptide) No V(D)J recombination occur *Prkdc*^{SCID}naturally occurred in BALB/c-*Igh*^{b} which are maintained at Institute of Cancer research in Philadelphia Available at Jackson Laboratory	Non-responsiveness of spleen toward T and B cells making them unavailable Ideal host for xenografting cells originating from the myeloid lineage remained unaffected due to their vital role for the survival which enable to generate lymphocytes bearing receptors of restricted diversity called **"leakiness"** Flawed DNA repair mechanismleave them susceptible toward radiation The first mouse strain that reportedly supported the human peripheral blood mononuclear cells (hu-PBMCs) engraftment to study HIV infection	Useful in studies of normal and abnormal lymphocyte development and function, role of nonlymphoid cells in the absence of lymphocytes Humanized SCID used to study the infectious diseases (HIV and EBV) and their therapeutics Suitable for the engraftment of human tissues such as tumor cells and cell lines, skin, pancreatic islets Ideal model for human tumor xenograft growth, pathophysiology and their metastasis Useful in studying the effect of radiation in normal and tumor cells for genetic deficiency and their repair mechanism	(50–54)

(Continued)

TABLE 1 | Continued

Mice	Mutation	Mice Information	Character	Application	References
RAG mice	carrying a deleted recombination activating gene (*rag1* or *rag-2*)	Mutation in *Rag1* and *Rag2* gene which are important for V(D)J gene rearrangement that can produce the antigen receptor in B and T cells Available at Jackson Laboratory	Inhibits B-cell and T-cell differentiation, results into lack of B and T-cells NK-cell activity is prominent, they do not exhibit immunoglobulin leakiness and less sensitivity to radiation Shorter life span, produce higher amount of B cell lymphomas regularly	Commonly used as models to study the role of the immune system in cancer (tumorigenesis and metastases), autoimmunity, and chemotherapy studies as a potential alternative to Nude and *SCID* mice Higher level of engraftment of human HSC and lymphoid cells Study of the gene function in lymphocyte development by blastocyst complementation method	(55–58)
NOD mice	Contain a unique MHC haplotype (H-2^{g7}), and a single nucleotide polymorphism (SNP) in the TNF-α and CTLA-4 genes	Non-obse Diabetic mice (NOD/ShiLtJ strain)	Impaired immune system with hampered maturation of macrophages, wound healing Defects in their natural killer (NK) cells and $CD4^{+}CD25^{+}$ T-cells Deficiencies of NK T-cells and absence of C5a complement	Important model for human type I diabetic study Allow the prolonged engraftment of human cells and tissues used for infectious disease and cancer Useful in the identification of responsible antigen, genes susceptibility for the diseases, effect of environment on the diseases, efficacy of therapeutics, and development of imaging techniques Humanized-NOD mice with higher susceptibility of vivid xenografts make it a suitable model for the translational biomedical research	(59–61)
NOD/SCID mice	Backcross of NOD with SCID mice (such as C3H/HeJ-SCID and C57/BL6-SCID) transferred the *Prkdc*^{SCID} mutation	Developed by the Fox Chase Cancer center via transferring SCID mutation from C.B-17 to non-obese diabetic background Available at Taconic Bioscience/Jackson Laboratory	Unable to develop diabetes with diminished NK-cell activity and suppressed non-adaptive immune responses Capable of accepting a higher level of engraftment of hu-PBMCs, HSCs, liver and lungs No activity of complements and macrophages exhibiting the defects in the expression of cytokine receptors Shows 80-90% engraftment of HSCs in comparison to other strains Short life span of 8-9 months due to the severe thymic lymphomas, required special care and maintenance, paralysis may occur but changes are rare Leakiness is very less compare to other SCID models and chances of increases are less with the age	Usually used for translational biomedical applications and xenograft transplantation Recommended model for the study of the human platelet survival Study of the pathogenesis of drug induced immune thrombocytopenia (DITP) Useful in cancer biology research for the study of tumor formation, metastasis, their therapeutic treatment and regulation, imaging studies of tumor	(62–70)
NOD/SCID/$\beta_2m^{-/-}$ mice	Knockouts for β2-microglobulin gene which drives the expression and function of murine MHC-I molecules	Double homozygous for SCID and beta2m *B2m* mutation was developed by Dr. Beverly Koller and Dr. Oliver Smithies at University of North Carolina followed by *scid* and *B2m* combined mutation at Jackosn laboratory by Dr. Leonard Shultz	Bear the entire set of deficiencies prominent in the NOD/SCID mice along with complete death of NK-cell activity Disrupts the development and function of NK-cells, B and T-cells, this hampers the MHC-I-mediated immunity Several disadvantages for instance, capacity to sustain only limited development of human lymphocytes, restricted number of T-cells constituted and repopulated in the chimeric organs	Most suitable model for the xenograft transplantation (intra-bone marrow) To study the Influenza infection (due to restricted influenza-specific IgG), myelodysplastic syndrome For the vaccine development and the therapeutics for the tumor	(21, 71–74)

(Continued)

TABLE 1 | Continued

Mice	Mutation	Mice Information	Character	Application	References
NOD/SCID/ IL2Rγ mice	Mutations in the *Il-2rg* gene	Referred as NSG mice NOD/schi-SCID Il-2rg$^{-/-}$ (NSG) mice was developed by crossing the NOD/SCID mice with the *Il-2rg*$^{-/-}$ mice: *scid* and *IL2rg*^{null} (SCID mutation in DNA repair complex mechanism and IL2 rg mutation prevent cytokine signaling via different receptors leading to deficiency in NK cell activity) Available at Jackson Laboratory	Impaired development and function of the lymphocytes and abolish NK-cell formation which in turn impedes IFN-γ secretion Absence of mature murine lymphocytes, functional dendritic cells, leakiness, and prolonged lifespan of mice for about 16 months (long-lived) Various immunodeficient mice were crossed with these IL-2rg$^{-/-}$ knockouts to produce strains with further suppression of immunity	They exhibit excellent ability to accept human xenografts, especially PBMCs, stem cells, myeloid cells and progenitors originated from fetal liver, cord blood, bone marrow and PBMCs Exclusively used for the differentiation and development of HSCs, platelets, RBCs, and T-cells used for analyses Optimum mice model to study the mechanism of inflammation, wound healing, allograft transplantation and their rejection for the clinical purpose (specially human skin graft), remodeling of tissues and revascularization	(75–81)

BCR, B-Cell receptor; TACI, transmembrane activator and calciummodulator and cyclophilin ligand interactor; LPS, lipopolysacchride; NK cells, Natural killer cells; CTLs, Cytotoxic T lymphocytes; MHC, Major histocompatibility Complex; hu-PBMC, Human peripheral blood mononuclear cells; HSC, Hematopoietic stem cells; RBCs, Red blood cells; SCID mice, Severe combined immunodeficiency mice; Rag1/2, Recombination activation gene 1/2; NOD, Non-obese diabetic.

immunodeficient mice is given in **Table 1** (26). The creation of human-mouse chimera(s) follows a cascade of different steps and events for the reconstitution of human cells, using various immunomodulatory protocols. All the procedures to prepare the host for human cells/tissue engraftment followed by their repopulation were described in detail (27), and have been reviewed many times (**Figure 2**) (21, 28–30) by multiple experts in the field.

The developed mouse-human chimeras present an efficient pre-clinical *in-vivo* model to study the human immune system and its interaction with infectious pathogens, hematopoiesis, stem cell development and function, tumor formation, cancer biology, and regenerative medicine.

Human-Mouse Chimeras Required to Study Infectious Pathogens

The pathogens relevant to human disease, which do not infect other animal species, required an animal model that could reconstitute or harbor human tissues to replicate the human immune system (82). The study of human infectious diseases is restricted to *in-vitro* models as humanization of immunocompromised mice is difficult, due to the scarce data available on host-pathogen interaction, cell behavioral pattern and the biological complexity of the human body. The *in-vitro* effect of drugs and therapeutic effect in animals differ in their metabolic pathways, and does not give an accurate prediction of drug metabolic pathways for humans (83). Drug metabolism in humans and their physiological differences in animal model(s) also make it arduous to design and formulate the efficient drugs and their targets. The development of disease-specific drugs will be possible only when the pathogenicity as well as molecular and immune mechanisms of infectious pathogen is well understood. The testing of preclinical drugs and candidate vaccines require humanized mice that help predict the drug metabolism and pharmacokinetics.

Humanized mice have been used over a long period of time, which helps understand the mechanism of rejection of human tissues provoked by human immune cells. However, translation of these studies from murine (immunodeficient mice) models to the clinic, has limited success due to numerous reasons which demand precious focus on human immune responses to allogeneic tissues along with their cumbersome usages and required skilled personnel (84). The technology for cell and tissue transplantation has improved the reconstitution of human immune cells/tissue that allows for the successful study of graft vs. host diseases (GVHD), different allograft studies and other human immune system studies which have been established as a robust preclinical model for human-specific therapeutic inventions (30, 81, 84). The human immune system may be engrafted into the immunodeficient mice, where type of human cells [pluripotent stem cells and their derived cell populations, regulatory T cells (Treg)] and tissues (human skin, islet, cardiac tissues, xenografts) are important in engraftment (81). Therefore, a robust small laboratory animal model transplanted with human

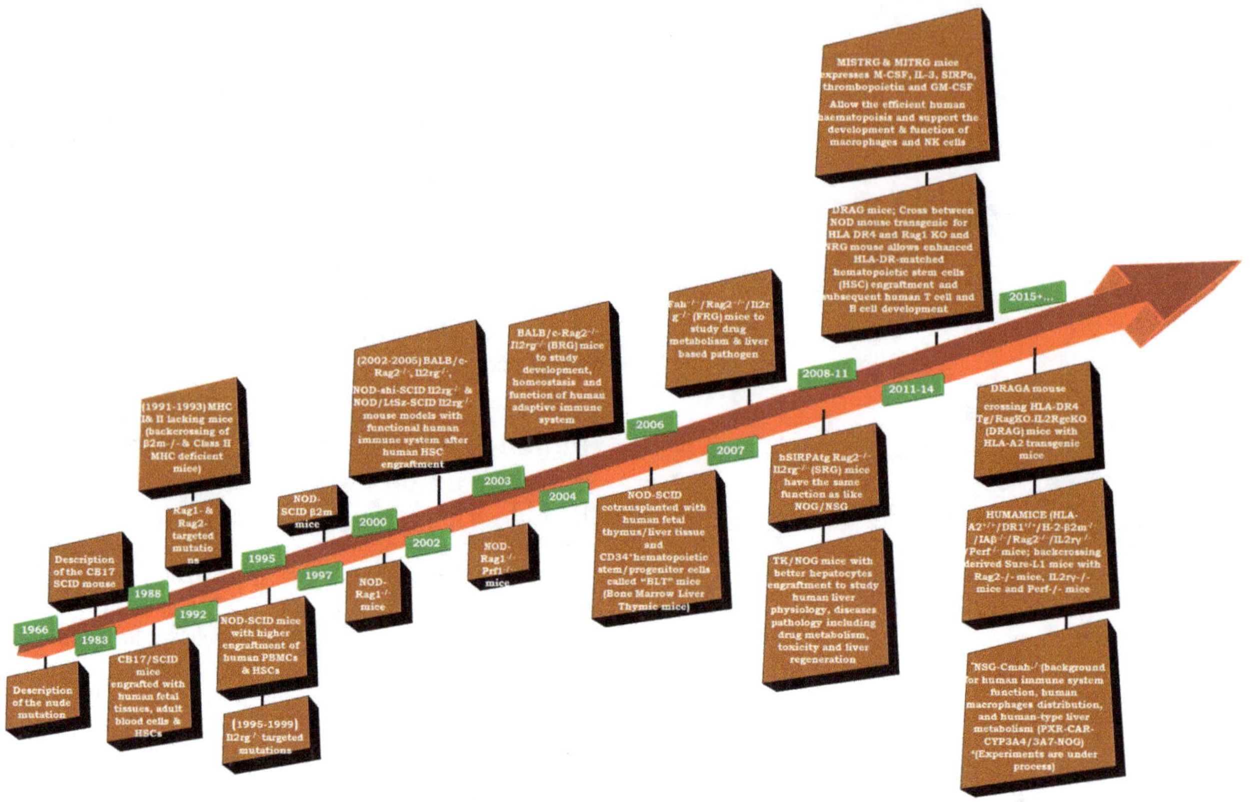

FIGURE 2 | Timeline of important events in the development of humanized mice (adapted and modified from Shultz et al. (31).

hematolymphoid/hematopoietic stem cells is indeed required to advance drug discovery (85).

The liver, an important immunogenic organ, consists of innate immune cells [natural killer (NK) cells, NK-like T cells, Kupffer cells and dendritic cells (DCs)] which play an important role in the local immune surveillance, liver regeneration and pathogenesis of liver diseases (86–88). The enzymes involved in the drug and xenobiotic metabolism and excretion, liver has been the center for the research related to drug mechanism and identifying novel drugs. Hepatotropic viruses and parasitic infections are the cause for a greater rate of mortality in humans, in addition to the toxicity rendered by chemicals. Humanized mice are therefore useful in order to study viral infections with hepatitis B or C and the hepatic stage of the malaria (89) infection. Acute liver failure becomes a predominant issue because of the drug-induced liver injury (90) and uncharacterized behavior of the drug metabolic pathway and clearance from the human body. Therefore, human liver reconstituted immunodeficient mice have been deployed to study the drug metabolic pathways (90, 91). Several approaches have been deployed, including the *in-vitro* culture of human cell lines, transgenic insertions of human genes, cultures of human hepatocytes and chimeric mice with the repopulated humane liver. The *in-vitro* culture has the limitation of continuity which cannot delineate the human liver metabolism. Despite several advantages, expression of transgene, inhibitor and activator proteins of the cells and cofactors required for the reactions derived from the mouse, are some of the limitations (89). To overcome these limitations, investigators have employed human hepatocytes in the culture to investigate the human-relevant drug metabolism processes (89, 92–95). Earlier studies confirmed that hepatocytes are important for the immune tolerogenic properties of the liver (96–98) and their transplantation inhibits allograft rejection (99). Although results obtained by the human hepatocytes with respect to the drug metabolism, studies were limited to the short duration, a maximum of 30–40 days (100, 101). Recently, transgenic mice (TK/NOG) conditioned with ganciclovir (GCV) treatment have shown to deplete a number of mouse hepatocytes to create receptive stroma for the injectable human hepatocytes (huHep). huHep reconstituted humanized mice have been used to test the drugs to predict their pharmacological and toxic nature on human liver (83, 102). It was later observed that human chemokine production by the engrafted huHep is one of the mechanisms that improve the human immune systems reconstitution in the liver of LTH hu-mice (human FTHY and CD34^{+} HSPCs) (103) since they do not, or respond poorly to mouse counterparts (104, 105). These results indicate the improved human immune system reconstitution in the liver of LTH hu-mice (103).

Humanized mice are used to study different diseases, which have been reviewed several times (20, 25, 29–31, 74, 106–109) along with necessary modifications to overcome the limitation of respective models (24, 70, 81).Therefore we did not give a detailed account on mouse models developed to study other diseases, and focused only on the humanized mouse model(s) used to study the biology of *P.falciparum*.

HUMANIZED MICE ARE INSTRUMENTAL TO STUDY THE *P. falciparum*

Advancements made in biomedical research are not sufficient to fight systemic inflammatory diseases such as *P. falciparum* malaria infection in humans. The mouse-human chimeras have been used to study the asexual blood stage, exo-eryhrocytic stages (liver stage), and transition from liver-to-blood stage (17, 110–113) infection of *P. falciparum*. However, specific immune-responses against antigens produced in all stages of the parasite are yet to be explored (114, 115). And, the stage specificity of human parasites does not allow them to grow and develop in murine models (116).

Rodent parasites (*P. berghei* and *P. yoelii*) are used as surrogates to study the pre-erythrocytic infection of human malaria parasites. The species mismatch between the rodent and human parasites makes it difficult to extrapolate (116) their data for human studies. However, there are syntenic proteins such as hepatocytes surface protein CD81 which helps to render the infection in a rodent parasite and *P. falciparum* (117). Similarly, a sporozoites surface protein named thrombospondin-related anonymous protein TRAP is required for liver infection in the human malaria parasite (118) and rodent parasite (*P. berghei*) (119). On the other hand, hepatocytes growth factor receptor (C-Met) plays an important role in the early pre-erythrocytic infection of the liver by *P. berghei* (120). This receptor is not important to study the biology of *P. yoeli* or *P. falciparum* (121). Likewise, a merozoite adhesive erythrocytic protein MAEBL is required for the liver stage infection in *P. falciparum* by sporozoites (122) whereas it is not required in case of *P. berghei* (123). The human malaria parasites were never seen to infect the murine hepatocytes (112). Therefore, a humanized mouse is required to model *P. falciparum* to understand its basic biology, pathophysiology, immunology and pharmacology.

The pre-erythrocytic stage of the parasite life cycle is asymptomatic, and all clinical pathological symptoms are shown because of the progression of the asexual blood stage infection. The erythrocytic stage is routinely studied *in-vitro* by the development of a continuous culture system that allows the replication and growth of an asexual blood stage parasite within human RBCs (4, 124). Recent advancements in the *in-vitro* culture of *P. falciparum* has expanded the knowledge of its blood stage to show the basic parasitology (5) and the development of target specific drugs effective against asexual blood stage infection (125).

The sporogonic stages are generated by feeding the female *Anopheles* mosquitoes on *in-vitro* gametocyte cultures, and the progression of the parasite life cycle in the mosquito as well as subsequent sporozoite accumulation in the salivary gland of the mosquito is allowed. However, the *P. falciparum* liver stage (LS) has proven much more difficult to study even though complete LS development in primary huHep and subsequent transition to *in-vitro* erythrocytic infection was shown over 30 years ago (126) followed by subsequent studies (118, 127–129). The primary human hepatocytes, or HepG2 cells, have been used to study the development of LS infection of *P. vivax* (130, 131). FRG-KO huHep mice were used to study the LS infection and formation of hypnozoites during the *P.vivax* infection (132).

Currently, drug resistance against the *Plasmodium* strains remains the main hurdle in effective vaccine development. However, there is remarkable improvement in the development of novel drug therapies. On the other hand, development of novel tools are a prerequisite of the rapid transition of preclinical drugs to the clinic, along with the fulfillment of SERCaP (Single Exposure Radical Cure and Prophylaxis) guidelines (133). To address the above-mentioned issues, recently developed humanized mice helped investigating the different stages of malaria parasites in detail (6).

Humanized Mice Support the Development and Replication of Asexual Blood Stage Infection of *P. falciparum* (RBC Reconstituted Humanized Mice)

The human-red blood cells (huRBCs) host the asexual blood stage infection of *P. falciparum*. The huRBCs reconstituted immunodeficient NSG mice present nearly an ideal model to develop an understanding of the asexual blood stage infection. The different strains of immunodeficient mice, which were used for the asexual blood stage infection, are listed in **Table 2**. Different strategies provided a humanized environment for the circulation of human immune effecters and huRBCs, maintaining the stable long-term blood chimerism (17). The sizeable and long-term huRBCs grafting (human blood chimerization) and control of inflammatory responses provoked by the parasites are crucial factors contributing to the success of humanized mouse (134). The same humanized mouse (PfhuRBC-NSG-IV) was used to experimentally induce the artesunate resistance and to validate the resistance phenotype (135).

Other Blood Stage Humanized Mouse Models

Tsuji et al. first reported the transplantation of huRBCs into immunodeficient SCID mice (140). To overcome the rapid elimination of huRBCs from the mouse's periphery, they discovered that the intraperitoneal (IP) injection of human serum significantly extended the survival of huRBCs injected intravenously (IV). After the successful and stable engraftment of huRBCs into SCID mice, some of the animals were irradiated (dose of 300 cGray) 2 days prior to *P. falciparum* infection (FUV strain) and a blood smear was drawn for the Giemsa staining. They observed the rapid elimination of infected and non-infected huRBCs from the non-irradiated SCID mice, compared to the irradiated mice with a decrease in the parasitemia during the initial 5 days of infection. The trend of parasitemia remained constant even upon dilution, by administering huRBCs up to 20

TABLE 2 | The developed "humanized mouse model(s)" for asexual blood stage infection of *P. falciparum*.

P. falciparum strain(s)	Humanized mice	Applications	References
NF54 or multiresistant T24	BXN (Beige/Xid/Nude)	First rodent model for *P.falciparum* study, to test the novel compounds for the drug development and evaluation of drug responses, vaccine development	(136–138)
FUP, NF54, 3D7, Dd2 and clinical isolates	SCID (Severe Combined Immunodeficiency) and NOD/SCID	Helpful in *in-vivo* studies of human malaria parasites and vaccine development	(139–141)
Mouse-adapted 3D7	NOD/SCID/$\beta_2$microglobulin $(\beta_2 m)^{-/-}$	*in-vivo* experimental drug/exposure-response assay	(142)
Mouse-adapted 3D7	NOD/SCID/IL-2 receptor γ chain $(IL2R\gamma)^{null}$or NSG mice	To check the response against various antimalarial therapeutics	(143, 144)
Different parasite strains (3D7,UPA and K1) without any prior adaptation	NOD/SCID/IL-2 receptor γ chain $(IL2R\gamma)^{null}$ or NSG mice with an additional treatment of clodronate delivered through liposomes	Most comprehensive humanized mouse model allowing to develop the sexual stage parasites besides the asexual-blood stage development	(134, 145)
NF54, 3D7	HLA-transgenic mice	Discovery of novel protective malaria antigen and immune responses	(146)
NF54	TK/NOG	Used to assess the drug toxicology and metabolism, and *P. falciparum* infection in transplanted human hepatocytes	(6)

TK/NOG, thymidine kinase/NOD/Shi-scid/IL-2Rγnull mice; HLA, human leukocytes antigen; 3D7, NF54, PAM, different P .falciparum strain.

days. This report suggested that *P. falciparum* could grow and develop only in huRBCs (140). However, the SCID mice needed further modifications to establish the hosting of huRBCs. This mouse proved to be a valuable tool for the *in-vivo* study as well as the vaccine development of human malaria parasites.

Similarly, Moore *et al* used the NOD/SCID mice infected with NF54 and 3D7 *P. falciparum* strains, with a single dose of uninfected huRBCs, injected intraperitoneally to see their development in the mouse's circulation. Later, infected and uninfected huRBCs were injected intrapertioneally every day. They observed the stable human blood chimerization and parasitemia in the peripheral blood for 16 days post-infection. Also, the sexual form of parasites (gametocytes) were observed and assessed with respect to their infectivity (139). In conclusion, NOD/SCID mice could also serve as a model for humanization without using any immunomodulatory agent. This might help in understanding the role of the immune response against the *P. falciparum* infection, but the adaptation of parasites and ascetic solutions prior to IP injection was required.

Later, Badell *et al* suggested the use of AB^+ huRBCs to achieve a significant blood chimerism in SCID/NIH III mice for extended periods. However, they used different immunomodulatory agents to deplete the host's residual innate immune effecters. The dichloromethyleneblphosphonate-(Cl_2MBP)-encapsulated liposomes were administered weekly intraperitoneally. The parasitemia was estimated up to 3% and maintained over 0.3% for 17 days. All the developmental stages of asexual erythrocytic cycle were observed. Therefore, this mouse model was used to study the drug(s) at pre-clinical levels for the development of a vaccine (136) and to assess the effect of antimalarial drugs reported for human infection (138). These findings overcame the limitations seen with previous models deploying novel immunomodulation protocols.

To develop an ideal mouse model to carry out wider applications of *P. falciparum,* Sabeter *et al* used CIMP (chemical immunomodulation protocol) in NOD/SCID mice to see whether they are susceptible and receptive to infection. They compared their model with the existing huRBCs-NIH III (BXN) mouse. The CIMP was modified and infected huRBCs, with various stages of parasites injected into the NOD/SCID mice intraperitoneally and followed until the end of the study. PCR and Giemsa staining were used to determine the low-grade parasitaemia together with a histopathological analysis. The infected percentage of NOD/SCID and BXN was estimated at 75 and 8%, respectively for 35 days post-infection. The higher-grade parasitemia in BXN and initial lower parasitemia was the hall mark in NOD/SCID for 7 days. The greater rise in the parasitaemia was seen during the second infectious challenge on day 17. PCR was performed on the DNA extracted from the animals, which showed 100% sensitivity and 67.3% specificity. The histology on different organs such as the bone marrow, spleen, liver, lungs and kidney was carried out. The malaria pigments (MP) inside the phagocytic cells were responsible for the elimination of infected-huRBCs, from the peripheral blood used as an indicator. These results suggested the distribution of MP laden macrophages were dependent on the parasitaemia and mouse strain (149). In brief, treatment of CIMP showed the better engraftment of huRBCs in NOD/SCID mice and supported the development and progression of *P. falciparum* infection. NOD/SCID mice were used to test the anti-malarial activity of novel compounds. The susceptibility of NOD/SCID mice with two different *P. falciparum* strains (3D7 and Dd2) and clinical isolates were assessed using slightly modified immunomodulation protocols. Results showed the parasitaemia of 0.05–8% sustained for 19 days with the development of asexual and sexual stage of parasites. These findings suggest that prior adaptation of parasite to its host is not necessarily required for the growth and development of the parasite (141).

Recent Development and Currently Available Humanized Mice for Asexual Blood Stage

The usage of chemical agents may influence the parasites development as well as the unexplored interaction with antimalarial drugs. Thus, without the use of any additional immunosuppressive agents, the successfully developed NOD/SCID/$\beta_2$microglobulin $(\beta_2 m)^{-/-}$ mice paved the way for the asexual stage of *P. falciparum* to examine the antimalarial compounds and the human response (142).

The mouse-adapted *P. falciparum* strain was used to study the infectious challenge in a novel mouse model "NSG mice" (NOD/SCID/IL-2 receptor γ chain $(IL2R\gamma)^{null}$). These mice supported the ten-fold higher burden of parasitized and non-parasitized huRBCs, compared to the NOD/SCID/$\beta_2$microglobulin $(\beta_2 m)^{-/-}$mice (144). Although administration of huRBCs intraperitoneally presents better engraftment (142, 143), the transperitoneal passage of blood from the peritoneum to the blood stream was one of the major issues observed with the IP model (134). The value of this mouse model was validated by the assessment of the therapeutic potential of antimalarial drugs (147).

The optimal blood stage mouse model was developed by employing different malaria parasite strains, without requiring prior adaptation to the host. The huRBCs injection and infectious challenge were administered through intraperitoneally and intravenously (134, 145), respectively. The high rising and long-standing parasitaemia was achieved in the mouse by controlling the number of monocytes/macrophages through the treatment of clo-lip (**Supplementary Figure 1**). This pharmacological agent was shown (145) to deplete 70–80% murine monocytes/macrophages. The model also demonstrated a higher level of parasite synchronization and partial sequestration of tainted huRBCs in the vasculature, a hallmark marvel observed in malaria patients. The huRBCs reconstituted mouse showing sustained and stable development of asexual blood stage parasites, also supports the development of sexual stages (gametocytes) (**Supplementary Figure 2**) (145). The developed humanized mice was used to induce the experimental induction of high level artesunate resistance in *P. falciparum* and to validate the resistance phenotype (135).

The huRBCs reconstituted NSG mice were challenged with *P. falciparum,* showing the development of gametocytes. Further, the developed mouse model allowed the *in-vivo* experimental drug/exposure-response assay (147). Developed humanized mice, harboring asexual blood stages of *P. falciparum,* more closely resembled the process in humans. Later, huRBCs-NSG mice were used to understand the interaction of gametocytes with the bone marrow and spleen and the efficacy of anti-gametocytidal activity of drug(s). The value of this mouse model was validated by assessing the efficacy of primaquine, which kills the sexual stages of *P. falciparum.* The clearance of gametocytes, compared to that seen in the control, suggests that the immunomodulation protocol does not hinder the assessment activity of drug effectiveness against the transmission stage of the *P. falciparum* infection. This helps better understand the role of drugs on the gametocytes present in the sequestration sites (150).

The supply of human serum and hypoxanthine resulted in the augmentation of a greater huRBCs chimeric index and parasitic growth. The continuous supply of huRBCs with an effective immunomodulatory protocol is inevitable for the effective and successful growth and development of the *P.falciparum* infection in available humanized mice. The issue of poor huRBCs grafting was overcome by the administration of human cytokines (151). The gamma irradiated NSG mice were injected with CD34$^+$ HSC intracardially and showed more than 40% human leukocytes reconstitution administered with the plasmid containing erythropoietin and human IL-3 intravenously (152). Mice showing at least 1.5% huRBCs reconstitutions were used for the subsequent experiments. Purified mature schizonts (3D7 strain) of the *P. falciparum* (*ex-vivo* infection) were added to the blood, maintained in RPMI 1640, supplemented with serum and incubated at 37°C for up-to 64 hrs, followed by the Giemsa staining. Within 16 hrs of infection, ring stages were observed with the parasitaemia of 0.02 to 1.6%. The infected-RBCs harvested from the humanized mice were analyzed by fluorescent activated cell sorting. The infectious challenge in *de-novo* synthesized and reconstituted humanized mice were detected by microscopy, PCR and flow cytometry. This shows the variation in the infection ability of various strains tested. The *P. falciparum* infection in the *de -novo* generated huRBCs as well as re-invasion was observed (151).

Sexual Stages and Blood-to-Mosquito Transmission

To determine the infectivity of the developed sexual parasites in huRBC-reconstituted NOD/SCID mice, *Anopheles stephensi* and *A. freeborni* mosquitoes directly fed on mice showing sexual stages. The oocyst formation in the mid-gut of the mosquitoes 7–10 days post-feeding, indicates the infectivity of sexual parasites and their successful transmission from humanized mice to mosquitoes (139). Similarly, the FRG-NOD huHep mice successfully produced the asexual blood stage parasites when they were challenged with NF54 *P. falciparum* infection. Subsequently, parasites were maintained in a continuous culture and produced gametocytes. The mosquitoes fed on these sexual stages, and upon dissection, the number of oocyst and sporozoites were estimated as the same in the salivary glands of infected mosquitoes (111). Later, the sexual parasites developed in other humanized DRAG mice were investigated for the transmission to mosquitoes via direct infection or through an *in-vitro* culture method. The development of oocyst and sporozoites in *A. stephensi* mosquitoes in both conditions was observed (146). Further, TK/NOG mice showed the development of all stages of gametocytes and maintained it for a longer duration. However, their transmission to mosquitoes required further experimental validation (6).

Liver-Humanized Mice to Study Exoerythrocytic (EE)/Liver Stage Infection of *P. falciparum*

From the multistage life cycle of the human malaria parasite in their primary (mosquitoes) and secondary host (human), the least known stage is the exoerythrocytic (EE)/liver stage. Notably, the exploration of the LS infection of *P. falciparum* in a human host is hampered by the low success rate of a hepatic stage culture, which is limited to a few days and which can be extended up to a month (128). This is possible with *P. falciparum,* by *in-vitro* human hepatocytes alone or through the co-culture (129, 153) in HC-04 cells, but with very low sporozoites infectivity estimated at 0.066% with *P. falciparum,* posing a challenge to study LS infection (127). The infectivity of sporozoites were later seen to increase up-to 0.8% (122, 154) and 1.3–1.4% in the same hepatocytes cells (HC-04) during the study of protein O-fucosylation activity (118), which is still relatively low compared to what could be achieved with primary hepatocytes or with *P. berghei/yoelii* infection in *in-vitro*. Therefore, the development of the more convenient *in-vivo* model will help better understand the liver pathophysiology within a human host. A transgenic and immunodeficient mouse strain showing better control over its non-adaptive immune response is therefore needed. The chimeric mouse model(s), as reported elsewhere (109), facilitates the understanding of LS and mimics humans to develop a further understanding of the various biological phenomena of LS parasites.

Liver Stage Mouse Models: Developments and Recent Advances

Following this direction, the first attempt was made to transplant the huHep in SCID mice (110). huHep were transplanted through open mouse survival surgery, followed by an infectious challenge of infected sporozoites isolated from the *A. stephensi* mosquitoes. The histopathological studies were carried out on sections of various tissues removed on day 3, 7, and 9 post-infectious challenge. Immunofluorescence assays were carried out with circumsporozoite protein (CSP), merozoite surface antigen 1 (MSA-1) and liver stage antigen-1 (LSA-1) to detect the *P. falciparum* infection in transplanted hepatocytes. The success rate of transplanted huHep-SCID mice were estimated at around 95% and infection was detected even 4 months after human hepatocyte transplantation. The results obtained were similar to that of non-human primates such as chimpanzees. However, the rate of sporozoites infection and their correlation with other existing animal models need to be evaluated (110).

Liver with severe chronic disease conditions, can enhance the engraftment of huHep (155). The expression of uPA was back-crossed with SCID or SCID/Beige background which resulted in the better engraftment and repopulation of huHep, measured up to 14 weeks at regular interval post-transplantation. The proteomic analysis was performed to evaluate whether the huHep were functioning properly through COFRADIC^{TM}. uPA/SCID-huHep mice were given the infectious challenge with the *P. falciparum* sporozoites, and the liver of infected animals was extracted for immunofluorescence assay to carry out a gene expression study. Several specific antibodies, reported for parasites, were used to detect the *P. falciparum* infection. Furthermore, RNA was extracted from the liver tissues to see the expression of specific genes such as PfCSP, PfLSA-1, and PfMSP-1, present during the early and late liver stage infection (156). The longer period of survival of parasites within the transplanted huHep were questioned. Therefore, residual innate immune effecters were controlled by the IP injection of clodronate-liposome. Immunohistochemical studies have shown higher engraftment of human hepatocytes within the clusters of hepatocytes. The intravenously injected sporozoites were seen to infect huHep as well as the development of schizonts on day 5 in the sections made from liver tissue and stained with the Hematoxylin-Eosin stain. The use of different antibodies and gene expression studies confirmed the development of liver stage infection (157). The role of sporozoites-expressed genes P52 and P36 (important for the hepatocyte infection) in genetically attenuated parasites (GAPs) showed the development (158) and expression of liver stage antigen-1 (LSA-1) during the *P. falciparum* infection (159) in uPA/SCID humanized mice. Also, uPA/SCID humanized mice were used to better understand the migration of sporozoites inside the human host and to study the escape mechanism of SPECT (sporozoites microneme protein essential for cell traversal) and PLP1 (perforin-like protein 1) employed by *P. falciparum* sporozoites (154). However, the poor breeding efficiency, a limited time-window for transplantation, renal diseases in reconstituted mice (160) and liver injury caused by the plasminogen treatment which leads to the other complications, were major concerns (148). Additionally, mice were not used to study the transition of parasite from liver-to-blood stage infection in one host (147).

Grompe et al developed a model with a mutation in the fumarylacetoacetate hydrolase (FAH) enzyme. These mice however, died within 12 hrs of birth, due to liver complications (161). Therefore, these FAH-KO needed continuous drug (NTBC) pressure to avoid liver damage and associated health complications (162). Thereafter, several mouse models were developed by back-crossing FAH knockout mice with NOD/SCID or RAG1. None were able to repopulate the human hepatocytes. Besides, FAH/nude, and FAH/RAG1 were also unable to engraft the human cells due to the immune rejection (160). Nevertheless, FAH/NOD/SCID mice were grafted with a smaller number of human cells. However, liver failure resulted in the death of animals when NTBC pressure was withdrawn (160).

Liver Stage Mouse Model and Transition From Liver-to-Blood Stage Infection

As $Rag2^{-/-}/Il2rg^{-/-}$ mice have shown the highest engraftment, $FAH^{-/-}$ were backcrossed with Rag 2 and IL2Rγ and resulted in the triple knock-out (KO) of FRG mice ($FAH^{-/-}Rag2^{-/-}IL2R\gamma^{null}$). This mouse model achieved more than 90% engraftment of huHep and several mice survived up to 4 months, even after the withdrawal of the NTBC drug, which was confirmed by histological, immunocytochmeical and RT-PCR analysis specific to human hepatocytes (160). The FRG-huHep chimeric mice were injected with *P. falciparum* sporozoites intravenously. Mice were euthanized on day 3, 5, 6, and 7 post-infection for histopathology, indirect immunofluorescence assays (IFAs) and gene expression studies. Results of all the studies confirmed the successful infection in transplanted huHep, transcripts of *P. falciparum,* which amplified specific genes, and the development of LS infection (111). The formation of mature merozoites followed by the transition to the blood-stage is a very important step, as it allows for the study of a complete life cycle in one host. C57BL/6 background of the FRG mice hindered the engraftment of huRBCs because of incompatibility with SIRPα (163). Therefore, FRG, and NOD/SCID mice were back-crossed to create "FRG-NOD" which was reconstituted with huHep and challenged with *P. falciparum* sporozoites followed by intravenous injection of huRBCs on the 6th and 7th day post LS infectious challenge. The huHep reconstituted mice showed the development of LS infection (111). Subsequently, blood was processed with an *in-vitro P. falciparum* culture medium to cultivate the parasites. The blood smears were drawn from the culture and stained with Giemsa solution every 24 h. The gametocytes along with different asexual stages of parasites were observed. This indicates the successful transition from liver-to-blood-stage infection (111).

FRG-huHep mice were used to assess the humoral immune response against the LS infection of *P. falciparum* (164). The natural infection route (mosquito's bites) was chosen, rather than adopting the conventional route of administration of sporozoites. FRG-huHep mice have revealed the role of inhibitory antibodies against the *P. falciparum* infection. This humanized mouse model could be used to optimize and assess the efficacy of candidate vaccines (164) prior to the clinical trials. Recently, FRG-huHep mice were used to determine the anti-liver stage potential of Atovaquone-Proguanil and Primaquine (165). A novel antimalarial molecule (DSM265), which reportedly selectively targets *Plasmodial* dihydroorotate dehydrogenease (DHODH) *in-vitro* and *in-vivo* blood stage and improve liver stage activity in *in-vitro,* was tested in these mice (166). The oral dose of the drug quantified the log reduction to 2.5 in the liver parasites by *in-vivo* bioluminescent imaging through an IVIS spectrum. The obtained results helped to understand the mechanism of action, the pharmacokinetic or pharmacodynamic study of drugs, before deploying to clinical trials (165).

Likewise, FRG-huHep mice with slight modifications in the administration of huRBCs were used, with the additional treatment of the cytotoxic chemotherapy agent cyclophosphamide with clo-lip, to prevent the phagocytosis of huRBCs (167). This revealed the effective long terms survival of transplanted mice, allowed the infection in huHep, as well as the higher number of infected huRBCs on day 7 post-sporozoite infection challenge, a successful liver to blood stage transition and a sustained asexual blood stage infection of *P. falciparum* with increasing parasitemia. The *P. falciparum* reticulocyte-binding protein homolog 5 (RH5) is an important merozoite invasion ligand which interacts with huRBCs and is essential for the infection of all the parasite strains (168). Therefore, the anti-RH5 antibody in FRG-huHep/huRBC mice were used to determine its efficacy and utility. qRT-PCR, IVIS and parasite multiplication rates (PMRs) were observed to determine the potential of blocking the blood stage infection *in-vivo* while transitioning from the liver stage (167). The FRG mice, despite allowing the successful development of liver and blood stages, and despite being helpful in the assessment of the efficacy of various novel candidate vaccines and drugs, need skilled personnel to maintain the higher level of huRBCs on day 6 post-LS challenge (167).

Next Generation Mouse Models for Exoerythrocytic Stage and Completion of Life Cycle in One Host

To overcome the limitations of uPA/SCID and FRG mice, a transgene called herpes simplex virus type 1 thymidine kinase (HSVtk) was expressed in the hepatocytes of NOG mice (TK/NOG). The host was prepared by GCV conditioning which induces the apoptosis of liver cells to deplete the number of murine hepatocytes. The reconstitution of GCV conditioned TK/NOG mice show the sizeable huHep-repopulation index (huHep-RI) confirmed by the immunohistochemical staining of different antibodies. The value of developing human liver chimeric (huHep-TK/NOG) mice was assessed by determining the efficacy of human specific drug metabolism in these mice. The long-term survival (more than 6 months) without any exogenous drug treatment justifies the value of huHep-TK/NOG to study the LS infection of *P. falciparum.* TK/NOG mice allow the additional dose of GCV even after the human cell repopulates, which helps achieving higher re-population index of human xenografts (148). Additionally, TK/NOG mice hardly require additional drug supplements to suppress the host immune system, except the residual cells of the monocyte-macrophage lineage (169). huHep reconstituted TK/NOG mice favor and support the development of LS and transition to blood stage infection.

Studies were carried out with the huHep-TK/NOG mice to gauge the metabolism of anti-inflammatory drug (diclofenac) in humans (170). These mice revealed the potential for reliable 2-fold engraftment, for all phases of the *P. falciparum* life cycle within one host. huHep-TK/NOG mice supported the huRBCs reconstitution at days 5–6 post sporozoite challenge in the same host, which allowed for the transition from LS–to blood-stage infection of *P. falciparum* (**Figure 3**) to be studied. The added advantage with this mouse model, unlike others (111), is that it does not need two mouse strains to get the complete life cycle in one host.

Soulard V *et al.* and his group used the TK/NOG mice to study the LS infection of *P. falciparum* (6). huHep-TK/NOG mice were injected with sporozoites intravenously and liver sections extracted from the infected mice were analyzed on the 5th and 7th day post-infection. The parasite development was confirmed specifically in the huHep region. huHep reconstituted mice receiving LS infection when administered with huRBCs intraperitoneally daily, reached 50–60% blood chimerism within the 6th day and 80–90% on day 12. On the 6th day post-LS infection, the transition from the liver to blood stage in the same host was observed. The blood sample was collected and maintained in *in-vitro* culture for 8–10 days to reveal the *P. falciparum* blood stage parasites. The aggregate gametocyte numbers could constitute up to 8.5% of total parasites, and 2.5% mature gametocytes (6). It was revealed that the TK/NOG model, most closely resembles human processes and is therefore the most suitable for preclinical drug studies and *in-vivo* LS infection.

Various humanized mouse models used to study liver-stage infection is summarized in **Table 3** (147).

Human-Immune System Repopulated Mouse Models to Study the Liver Stage Infection

Humanized mice with a human immune system (HIS) will help to develop pre-clinical models for the study of infectious diseases. Mice with the HIS expression called DRAG (HLA-DR4.RagKO.IL2RγcKO.NOD) were employed to study the complete life cycle of *P. falciparum* when transplanted with CD34^{+} HSCs (146). After 4 months post-transplantation with human HSC, DRAG mice were challenged with *P. falciparum* sporozoites. The parasitaemia was measured by PCR as well as counted on the Giemsa stained blood smears. The liver sections were observed 5 days later by using immunohistochemistry for HSP70. The blood stage parasites were observed between 10 and 28 days post infectious challenge, followed by the blood stage *in-vitro* culture wherein rings, trophozoites and schizonts were observed (146). The complete life cycle of *P. falciparum* in one host was achieved, but low parasitaemia levels, the development of a functional human immune system and host monocytes (in DRAG mice) and adaptation of the parasite strain(s), are concerns which need to be addressed (6). The recently developed humanized DRAGA mice were injected with the liver *P. falciparum* sporozoites (Pfspz) along with Chloroquine diphosphate pressure (171) to elicit the pre-erythrocytic immunity. These animals were protected against the challenge with infectious Pfspz, but had no protection against the asexual blood stage infection (171). We believe this humice could serve as a pre-clinical tool to study the immunogenic potential of newly discovered malaria candidate vaccines and drugs.

Very recently, NSG mice were transplanted with primed human spleen cells (hu-Spl-NSG) to assess the immune response and to understand the biology of the pathogen, to develop an effective vaccine (172). The two different constructions of the liver stage antigen-3 (LSA-3) (shorter and longer) which express during the liver stage and on the surface of sporozoites used as anti-LSA-3, may prevent the invasion of hepatocytes by sporozoites and protect them. Both constrains of protein have shown the different results, as the shorter form of LSA-3 shows the production of IFN-γ (humoral immune response) which was null in the full length protein, whereas the full length of LSA-3 protein showed the production of T regulatory (Treg) cells, but not a shorter constrain. The similarity of Treg sequences found in the human samples was confirmed. hu-Spl-NSG mice might be used to estimate the immune response, and overcome the limitations of graft vs. host reactions seen in hu-PBMCs reconstituted mice (172).

The complete cycle of (LS to blood stage transition) *P. falciparum* in developed humanized mice, will help performing numerous applications for vaccine development and formal genetic studies. In conclusion, developed human liver chimeric mice will revolutionize translational biomedical research and open doors for the vaccine development and drug therapeutics for other inflammatory diseases such as hepatitis, dengue, cancer, AIDS, and TB.

CONCLUSION AND FUTURE PERSPECTIVES

Considering the importance of humanized mice in biomedical research, coordinated efforts are being made to engineer the advanced immunocompromised mice, to support human cell (HSCs and hepatocytes) grafting. The introduction of genetic immunodeficiency in mice plays a central role during "humanization" to reduce graft rejection episodes. Therefore, various mouse strains have been engineered to deplete the host's immunity, which aims to achieve sizeable grafting of

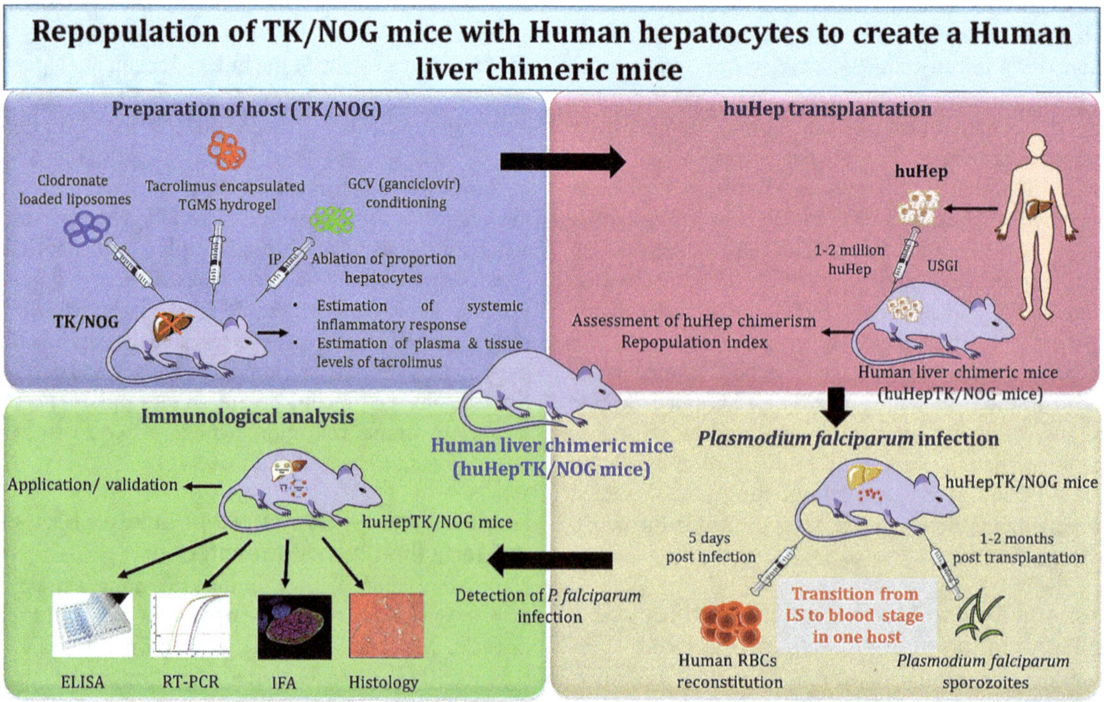

FIGURE 3 | Schema of "creation" for human liver chimeric mice to study LS infection of *P. falciparum* and subsequent transition to blood-stage infection.

TABLE 3 | The comparative analysis of different LS humanized mice to study inflammatory diseases, (Adapted and modified from Vaughan et al. (147).

		Alb-uPA SCID (Beige)	$FAH^{-/-}Rag2^{-/-}IL2R\gamma^{null}$ (FRG)	TK/NOG	HLA-DR4.RagKO.IL2Rγ cKO.NOD (DRAG)
Liver Injury	Mutation	uPA (urokinase-type plasminogen activator) overexpression	Fumarylacetoacetate hydrolase deficiency	Herpes simplex virus type 1 thymidine kinase (HSVtk) transgene expression	NRG mice chimeric with human-mouse class II transgenes encoding the HLA-DR4 genotype fused to the *I-E*^{d} MHC class II molecule
	Occurrence	At birth	At birth and increased by the NTBC treatment	On day 7 and 5 prio to transplantation, liver cells treated with GCV and maintain without any exogenous drug pressure	At birth
Transplantation age		Within 3 weeks of post-birth	Any (adult)	Adult 8-week-old	Four months of post infusion of human HSC
Human Chimerism		up to 100%	up to 90%	more than 90%	High (human cells and HSCs) but human RBCs were less (0.2–1%)
Throughput		Low	Medium	High	Medium
Additional challenges		Continuing and progressive damage to liver parenchymal stage, poor breeding efficiency, renal disease	Development liver carcinomas, under drug exposure for longer duration	No systemic morbidity	Less number of human hepatocytes developments, develop a functional human immune system, development of mouse monocytes
Plasmodium falciparum	Sporozoite infection	Yes	Yes	Yes	Yes
	Liver stage development				
	Early	✓	✓	✓	✓
	Mid	✓	✓	✓	✓
	Late (merozoite release)	✓	✓	✓	✓
	Liver-to-blood stage transition	No	Yes	Yes	Yes
Erythrocyte co-engraftment possible		No	No	Yes	Yes (low)
Unique advantage		No	No	Additional GCV treatment is used twice only prior to huHep transplantation	Fusion with HSC develop human hepatocytes, kupffer cells, liver endothelial cells and erythrocytes, Sustain complete life cycle of *P. falciparum* without exogenous addition of human hepatocytes/RBCs
Stability and reproducibility of humanized liver		human chimerism can only be achieved in homozygous SCID/ Alb-uPA immunodeficient recipients	Long life span through NTBC drug treatment, but other associated complications are seen	Over the 8 months of pro-long period without any drug pressure	Human RBCs can detect for up to 4 months
References		(147)	(147)	(6, 148)	(146)

NTBC, 2-(2-nitro-4-(trifluoromethyl)benzoyl)cyclohexane-1,3-dione; GCV, ganciclovir.

human cells/tissues. A major contribution of these mouse model(s) is to study the erythrocytic stage and liver stage infection of *P. falciparum*. We believe an ideal humanized mouse model will be instrumental to study novel drugs and their targets, assessing the immunogenicity of novel candidate vaccines. Higher immunosuppression and novel transplantation strategies are indeed needed to create a small laboratory, straightforward and reproducible humanized mouse model. This review will help the development of new methods to create a humanized mouse with stable human cell transplantation and repopulation, to study systemic inflammatory diseases.

AUTHOR CONTRIBUTIONS

RT conceived the idea of the study, carried out all experiments related to mouse humanization and modeling *P. falciparum* in humanized mice and wrote the manuscript. NT and RD helped format and write the manuscript. RE reviewed the manuscript. SP provided logistics. PT helped in the preparations of figures and tables and writing of the manuscript.

ACKNOWLEDGMENTS

RT would like to express his gratitude toward Dr. Pierre Druilhe, of Institute Pasteur, Paris, France, for helping with the development of the human-mouse chimera to study asexual blood stage infection of *P. falciparum* during his doctoral thesis program. RT expresses his sincere thanks to Dr. John Adams, of University of South Florida and Dr. Christopher Cutler, of August University, USA for their help during his Postdoctoral training. RT thanks the Department of Science and Technology (DST), Govt. of India for funding part of this study (grant number: ECR/2015/000264).

REFERENCES

1. Cowman AF, Healer J, Marapana D, Marsh K. Malaria: biology and disease. *Cell* (2016) 167:610–24. doi: 10.1016/j.cell.2016.07.055
2. WHO. *World Malaria Report 2017*. Geneva: World Health Organization (2017).
3. UNICEF. *Malaria Mortality Among Children Under Five Is Concentrated in Sub-Saharan Africa*. UNICEF Data: Monitoring the situation of Women and Children (2015). Available online at: https://data.unicef.org/topic/child-health/malaria/
4. Trager W, Jensen JB. Human malaria parasites in continuous culture. *Science* (1976) 193:673–5. doi: 10.1126/science.781840
5. Grüring C, Heiber A, Kruse F, Ungefehr J, Gilberger T-W, Spielmann T. Development and host cell modifications of *Plasmodium falciparum* blood stages in four dimensions. *Nat Commun.* (2011) 2:165. doi: 10.1038/ncomms1169
6. Soulard V, Bosson-Vanga H, Lorthiois A, Roucher C, Franetich J-F, Zanghi G, et al. *Plasmodium falciparum* full life cycle and *Plasmodium* ovale liver stages in humanized mice. *Nat Commun.* (2015) 6:7690. doi: 10.1038/ncomms8690
7. Phillips MA, Burrows JN, Manyando C, Van Huijsduijnen RH, Van Voorhis WC, Wells TNC. Malaria. *Nat Rev Dis Primers* (2017) 3:17050. doi: 10.1038/nrdp.2017.50
8. Huang Z, Tatem AJ. Global malaria connectivity through air travel. *Malar J.* (2013) 12:269. doi: 10.1186/1475-2875-12-269
9. Angelo KM, Libman M, Caumes E, Hamer DH, Kain KC, Leder K, et al. Malaria after international travel: a GeoSentinel analysis, 2003–2016. *Malar J.* (2017) 16:293. doi: 10.1186/s12936-017-1936-3
10. Zofou D, Nyasa RB, Nsagha DS, Ntie-Kang F, Meriki HD, Assob JCN, et al. Control of malaria and other vector-borne protozoan diseases in the tropics: enduring challenges despite considerable progress and achievements. *Infect Dis Poverty* (2014) 3:1. doi: 10.1186/2049-9957-3-1
11. Santos-Magalhães NS, Mosqueira VCF. Nanotechnology applied to the treatment of malaria. *Adv Drug Deliv Rev.* (2010) 62:560–75. doi: 10.1016/j.addr.2009.11.024
12. Tizifa TA, Kabaghe AN, Mccann RS, Van Den Berg H, Van Vugt M, Phiri KS. Prevention efforts for malaria. *Curr Trop Med Rep.* (2018) 5:41–50. doi: 10.1007/s40475-018-0133-y
13. WHO. *Status Report on Artemisinin and ACT Resistance (April 2017)*. Geneva: World Health Organization 11 (2017).
14. WHO. *Global Report on Insecticide Resistance in Malaria Vectors: 2010–2016*. Geneva: World Health Organization (2018).
15. Coelho CH, Doritchamou JYA, Zaidi I, Duffy PE. Advances in malaria vaccine development: report from the 2017 malaria vaccine symposium. *NPJ Vaccines* (2017) 2:34. doi: 10.1038/s41541-017-0035-3
16. Su X-Z. Human malaria parasites: are we ready for a new species? *J Infect Dis.* (2010) 201:1453–4. doi: 10.1086/652238
17. Siu E, Ploss A. Modeling malaria in humanized mice: opportunities and challenges. *Ann N Y Acad Sci.* (2015) 1342:29–36. doi: 10.1111/nyas.12618
18. Alaganan A, Singh P, Chitnis CE. Molecular mechanisms that mediate invasion and egress of malaria parasites from red blood cells. *Curr Opin Hematol.* (2017) 24:208–14. doi: 10.1097/MOH.0000000000000334
19. Ménard R, Tavares J, Cockburn I, Markus M, Zavala F, Amino R. Looking under the skin: the first steps in malarial infection and immunity. *Nat Rev Microbiol.* (2013) 11:701–12. doi: 10.1038/nrmicro3111
20. Walsh NC, Kenney LL, Jangalwe S, Aryee K-E, Greiner DL, Brehm MA, et al. Humanized mouse models of clinical disease. *Ann Rev Pathol.* (2017) 12:187–215. doi: 10.1146/annurev-pathol-052016-100332
21. Shultz LD, Brehm MA, Garcia-Martinez JV, Greiner DL. Humanized mice for immune system investigation: progress, promise and challenges. *Nat Rev Immunol.* (2012) 12:786–98. doi: 10.1038/nri3311
22. Zschaler J, Schlorke D, Arnhold J. Differences in innate immune response between man and mouse. *Crit Rev Immunol.* (2014) 34:433–54. doi: 10.1615/CritRevImmunol.2014011600
23. Perlman RL. Mouse models of human disease An evolutionary perspective. *Evol Med Public Health* (2016) 2016:170–6. doi: 10.1093/emph/eow014
24. Brehm MA, Shultz LD, Luban J, Greiner DL. Overcoming current limitations in humanized mouse research. *J Infect Dis.* (2013) 208:S125–30. doi: 10.1093/infdis/jit319
25. Fujiwara S. Humanized mice: a brief overview on their diverse applications in biomedical research. *J Cell Physiol.* (2017) 233:2889–901. doi: 10.1002/jcp.26022
26. Mcgonigle P, Ruggeri B. Animal models of human disease: challenges in enabling translation. *Biochem Pharmacol.* (2014) 87:162–71. doi: 10.1016/j.bcp.2013.08.006
27. Zhang B, Duan Z, Zhao Y. Mouse models with human immunity and their application in biomedical research. *J Cell Mol Med.* (2009) 13:1043–58. doi: 10.1111/j.1582-4934.2008.00347.x
28. Halban PA, German MS, Kahn SE, Weir GC. Current status of islet cell replacement and regeneration therapy. *J Clin Endocrinol Metab.* (2010) 95:1034–43. doi: 10.1210/jc.2009-1819
29. Denayer T, Stöhr T, Van Roy M. Animal models in translational medicine: Validation and prediction. *New Horiz Transl Med.* (2014) 2:5–11. doi: 10.1016/j.nhtm.2014.08.001
30. Hogenes M, Huibers M, Kroone C, De Weger R. Humanized mouse models in transplantation research. *Transplant. Rev.* (2014) 28:103–10. doi: 10.1016/j.trre.2014.02.002
31. Shultz LD, Ishikawa F, Greiner DL. Humanized mice in translational biomedical research. *Nat Rev Immunol.* (2007) 7:118–30. doi: 10.1038/nri2017
32. Novak EK, Swank RT, Meisler MH. Pigmentation and lysosome function in mice homozygous for both pale ear and beige-J pigment genes. *Genet Res.* (1980) 35:195–204. doi: 10.1017/S001667230001404X

33. Roder JC, Haliotis T, Klein M, Korec S, Jett JR, Ortaldo J, et al. A new immunodeficiency disorder in humans involving NK cells. *Nature* (1980) 284:553. doi: 10.1038/284553a0
34. Ash P, Loutit J, Townsend K. Osteoclasts derive from hematopoietic stem cells according to marker, giant lysosomes of beige mice. *Clin Orthop Relat Res.* (1981) 249–58. doi: 10.1097/00003086-198103000-00039
35. Harrison D, Carlson G. Effects of the beige mutation and irradiation on natural resistance to marrow grafts. *J Immunol.* (1983) 130:484–9.
36. Fodstad Ø, Hansen CT, Cannon GB, Statham CN, Lichtenstein GR, Boyd MR. Lack of correlation between natural killer activity and tumor growth control in nude mice with different immune defects. *Cancer Res.* (1984) 44:4403–8.
37. Galli SJ, Hammel I. Unequivocal delayed hypersensitivity in mast cell-deficient and beige mice. *Science* (1984) 226:710–3. doi: 10.1126/science.6494907
38. Haliotis T, Ball JK, Dexter D, Roder JC. Spontaneous and induced primary oncogenesis in natural killer (NK)-cell-deficient beige mutant mice. *Int J Cancer* (1985) 35:505–13. doi: 10.1002/ijc.2910350414
39. Bannai M, Oya H, Kawamura T, Naito T, Shimizu T, Kawamura H, et al. Disparate effect of beige mutation on cytotoxic function between natural killer and natural killer T cells. *Immunology* (2000) 100:165–9. doi: 10.1046/j.1365-2567.2000.00040.x
40. Azar HA, Hansen CT, Costa J. N: NIH (S) II-nu/nu mice with combined immunodeficiency: a new model for human tumor heterotransplantation 2. *J Natl Cancer Inst.* (1980) 65:421–30.
41. Dighiero G, Lim A, Lembezat MP, Kaushik A, Andrade L, Freitas A. Comparative study of VH gene family usage by newborn xid and non-xid mice, newborn NZB and adult NZB mice, and by splenic and peritoneal cavity B cell compartments. *Eur J Immunol.* (1988) 18:1979–83. doi: 10.1002/eji.1830181217
42. Cancro MP, Sah AP, Levy SL, Allman DM, Schmidt MR, Woodland RT. xid mice reveal the interplay of homeostasis and Bruton's tyrosine kinase-mediated selection at multiple stages of B cell development. *Int Immunol.* (2001) 13:1501–14. doi: 10.1093/intimm/13.12.1501
43. Szymczak WA, Davis MJ, Lundy SK, Dufaud C, Olszewski M, Pirofski L-A. X-linked immunodeficient mice exhibit enhanced susceptibility to Cryptococcus neoformans Infection. *MBio* (2013) 4:e00265–e00213. doi: 10.1128/mBio.00265-13
44. Uslu K, Coleman AS, Allman WR, Katsenelson N, Bram RJ, Alugupalli KR, et al. Impaired B cell receptor signaling is responsible for reduced TACI expression and function in X-linked immunodeficient mice. *J Immunol.* (2014) 1203468. doi: 10.4049/jimmunol.1203468
45. Flanagan S. 'Nude', a new hairless gene with pleiotropic effects in the mouse. *Genet Res.* (1966) 8:295–309.
46. Giovanella BC, Hunter JT. [34] Use of the nude mouse in immunological research. In: Di Sabato G, Langone JJ, Van Vunakis H, editors. *Methods in Enzymology*. Elsevier (1984). p. 348–57.
47. Nehls M, Pfeifer D, Schorpp M, Hedrich H, Boehm T. New member of the winged-helix protein family disrupted in mouse and rat nude mutations. *Nature* (1994) 372:103. doi: 10.1038/372103a0
48. Vidal I, Richert L. The nude mouse as model for liver deficiency study and treatment and xenotransplantation. *Int J Hepatol.* (2012) 2012:140147. doi: 10.1155/2012/140147
49. Szadvari I, Krizanova O, Babula P. Athymic nude mice as an experimental model for cancer treatment. *Physiol Res.* (2016) 65:S441–53.
50. Bosma GC, Custer RP, Bosma MJ. A severe combined immunodeficiency mutation in the mouse. *Nature* (1983) 301:527–30. doi: 10.1038/301527a0
51. Mccune J, Namikawa R, Shih C-C, Rabin L, Kaneshima H. The SCID-hu mouse: a small animal model for HIV infection and antiviral testing. In: Melchers F, Albert ED, von Boehmer H, Dierich MP, Du Pasquier L, Eichmann K, et al., editors. *Progress in Immunology*. Berlin; Heidelberg: Springer (1989). p. 1046–9. doi: 10.1007/978-3-642-83755-5
52. Bosma MJ, Carroll AM. The SCID mouse mutant: definition, characterization, and potential uses. *Annu Rev Immunol.* (1991) 9:323–50. doi: 10.1146/annurev.iy.09.040191.001543
53. Koo GC, Hasan A, O'reilly RJ. Use of humanized severe combined immunodeficient mice for human vaccine development. *Exp Rev. Vaccines* (2009) 8:113–20. doi: 10.1586/14760584.8.1.113
54. Huang P, Westmoreland SV, Jain RK, Fukumura D. Spontaneous nonthymic tumors in SCID mice. *Comp Med.* (2011) 61:227–34.
55. Mombaerts P, Iacomini J, Johnson RS, Herrup K, Tonegawa S, Papaioannou VE. RAG-1-deficient mice have no mature B and T lymphocytes. *Cell* (1992) 68:869–77. doi: 10.1016/0092-8674(92)90030-G
56. Shinkai Y, Lam K-P, Oltz EM, Stewart V, Mendelsohn M, Charron J, et al. RAG-2-deficient mice lack mature lymphocytes owing to inability to initiate V (D) J rearrangement. *Cell* (1992) 68:855–67. doi: 10.1016/0092-8674(92)90029-C
57. Chen J, Lansford R, Stewart V, Young F, Alt FW. RAG-2-deficient blastocyst complementation: an assay of gene function in lymphocyte development. *Proc Natl Acad Sci USA.* (1993) 90:4528–32. doi: 10.1073/pnas.90.10.4528
58. Notarangelo LD, Kim M-S, Walter JE, Lee YN. Human RAG mutations: biochemistry and clinical implications. *Nat Rev Immunol.* (2016) 16:234–46. doi: 10.1038/nri.2016.28
59. Kikutani H, Makino S. The murine autoimmune diabetes model: NOD and related strains. *Adv Immunol.* (1992) 51:285–322. doi: 10.1016/S0065-2776(08)60490-3
60. Chaparro RJ, Dilorenzo TP. An update on the use of NOD mice to study autoimmune (Type 1) diabetes. *Expert Rev Clin Immunol.* (2010) 6:939–55. doi: 10.1586/eci.10.68
61. Pearson JA, Wong FS, Wen L. The importance of the Non Obese Diabetic (NOD) mouse model in autoimmune diabetes. *J Autoimmun.* (2016) 66:76–88. doi: 10.1016/j.jaut.2015.08.019
62. Shultz LD, Schweitzer PA, Christianson SW, Gott B, Schweitzer IB, Tennent B, et al. Multiple defects in innate and adaptive immunologic function in NOD/LtSz-scid mice. *J Immunol.* (1995) 154:180–91.
63. Aharinejad S, Abraham D, Paulus P, Abri H, Hofmann M, Grossschmidt K, et al. Colony-stimulating factor-1 antisense treatment suppresses growth of human tumor xenografts in mice. *Cancer Res.* (2002) 62:5317–24. doi: 10.1158/0008-5472.can-04-0961
64. Bastide C, Bagnis C, Mannoni P, Hassoun J, Bladou F. A Nod Scid mouse model to study human prostate cancer. *Prostate Cancer Prostatic Dis.* (2002) 5:311. doi: 10.1038/sj.pcan.4500606
65. Chen X, Sievers E, Hou Y, Park R, Tohme M, Bart R, et al. Integrin $\alpha\beta3$-targeted imaging of lung cancer. *Neoplasia* (2005) 7:271–9. doi: 10.1593/neo.04538
66. Lam P, Yang W, Amemiya Y, Kahn H, Yee A, Seth A. Genetic analysis of breast cancer metastasis in a human bone NOD/SCID mouse model. In: AACR *Annual Meeting* Los Angeles, CA (2007).
67. Williams SV, Wildt SJ, Brooks AI, Cooper DM. The SHrN^{TM} scid hairless NOD mouse model: Development and characterization. In. *Proceedings: AACR 101st Annual Meeting 2010.* Washington, DC (2010).
68. Van Pham P, Vu NB, Duong TT, Nguyen TT, Truong NH, Phan NLC, et al. Suppression of human breast tumors in NOD/SCID mice by CD44 shRNA gene therapy combined with doxorubicin treatment. *Onco Targets Ther.* (2012) 5:77. doi: 10.2147/OTT.S30609
69. Bakchoul T, Fuhrmann J, Chong BH, Bougie D, Aster R. Recommendations for the use of NOD/SCID mouse model in autoimmune-and drug-induced thrombocytopenia: communication from the SSC of the ISTH. *J Thromb Haemost.* (2015) 13:872. doi: 10.1111/jth.12879
70. Holzapfel BM, Wagner F, Thibaudeau L, Levesque J-P, Hutmacher DW. Concise review: humanized models of tumor immunology in the 21st century: convergence of cancer research and tissue engineering. *Stem Cells* (2015) 33:1696–704. doi: 10.1002/stem.1978
71. Christianson SW, Greiner DL, Hesselton RA, Leif JH, Wagar EJ, Schweitzer IB, et al. Enhanced human CD^{4+} T cell engraftment in beta2-microglobulin-deficient NOD-scid mice. *J Immunol.* (1997) 158:3578–86.
72. Thanopoulou E, Cashman J, Kakagianne T, Eaves A, Zoumbos N, Eaves C. Engraftment of NOD/SCID-β2 microglobulin null mice with multilineage neoplastic cells from patients with myelodysplastic syndrome. *Blood* (2004) 103:4285–93. doi: 10.1182/blood-2003-09-3192
73. Macchiarini F, Manz MG, Palucka AK, Shultz LD. Humanized Mice: Are We There Yet? *J Exp Med.* (2005) 202:1307–11. doi: 10.1084/jem.20051547
74. Belizário JE. Immunodeficient mouse models: an overview. *Open Immunol J* (2009) 2:79–85. doi: 10.2174/1874226200902010079
75. Matthews D, Clark P, Herbert J, Morgan G, Armitage R, Kinnon C, et al. Function of the interleukin-2 (IL-2) receptor gamma-chain in biologic

responses of X-linked severe combined immunodeficient B cells to IL-2, IL-4, IL-13, and IL-15. *Blood* (1995) 85:38–42.
76. Ito M, Hiramatsu H, Kobayashi K, Suzue K, Kawahata M, Hioki K, et al. NOD/SCID/γ mouse: an excellent recipient mouse model for engraftment of human cells. *Blood* (2002) 100:3175–82. doi: 10.1182/blood-2001-1 2-0207
77. Ishikawa F, Yasukawa M, Lyons B, Yoshida S, Miyamoto T, Yoshimoto G, et al. Development of functional human blood and immune systems in NOD/SCID/IL2 receptor γ chain null mice. *Blood* (2005) 106:1565–73. doi: 10.1182/blood-2005-02-0516
78. Ito M, Kobayashi K, Nakahata T. NOD/Shi-scid IL2rgnull (NOG) mice more appropriate for humanized mouse models. *Curr Top Microbial Immunol.* (2008) 324:53–76.
79. Racki WJ, Covassin L, Brehm M, Pino S, Ignotz R, Dunn R, et al. NOD-scid IL2rγnull (NSG) mouse model of human skin transplantation and allograft rejection. *Transplantation* (2010) 89:527–36. doi: 10.1097/TP.0b013e3181c90242
80. Coughlan AM, Harmon C, Whelan S, O'brien EC, O'reilly VP, Crotty P, et al. Myeloid engraftment in humanized mice: impact of granulocyte-colony stimulating factor treatment and transgenic mouse strain. *Stem Cells Dev.* (2016) 25:530–41. doi: 10.1089/scd.2015.0289
81. Kenney L, Shultz LD, Greiner D, Brehm M. Humanized mouse models for transplant immunology. *Am J Transplant.* (2016) 16:389–97. doi: 10.1111/ajt.13520
82. Rämer PC, Chijioke O, Meixlsperger S, Leung CS, Münz C. Mice with human immune system components as *in vivo* models for infections with human pathogens. *Immunol Cell Biol.* (2011) 89:408–16. doi: 10.1038/icb.2010.151
83. Xu D, Peltz G. Can humanized mice predict drug "behavior" in humans? *Annu Rev Pharmacol Toxicol.* (2016) 56:323–38. doi: 10.1146/annurev-pharmtox-010715-103644
84. Brehm MA, Shultz LD. Human allograft rejection in humanized mice: a historical perspective. *Cell Mol Immunol.* (2012) 9:225. doi: 10.1038/cmi.2011.64
85. Theocharides AP, Rongvaux A, Fritsch K, Flavell RA, Manz MG. Humanized hemato-lymphoid system mice. *Haematologica* (2016) 101:5–19. doi: 10.3324/haematol.2014.115212
86. Racanelli V, Rehermann B. The liver as an immunological organ. *Haematology* (2006) 43:S54–62. doi: 10.1002/hep.21060
87. Gao B, Jeong Wi Fau-Tian Z, Tian Z. Liver: an organ with predominant innate immunity. *Hepatology* (2008) 47:729–36. doi: 10.1002/hep.22034
88. Jenne CN, Kubes P. Immune surveillance by the liver. *Nat Immunol.* (2013) 14:996–1006. doi: 10.1038/ni.2691
89. Strom SC, Davila J, Grompe M. Chimeric mice with humanized liver: tools for the study of drug metabolism, excretion, and toxicity. *Methods Mol Biol)* (2010) 640:491–509. doi: 10.1007/978-1-60761-688-7_27
90. Maes M, Vinken M, Jaeschke H. Experimental models of hepatotoxicity related to acute liver failure. *Toxicol Appl Pharmacol.* (2016) 290:86–97. doi: 10.1016/j.taap.2015.11.016
91. Ballet F. Preventing drug-induced liver injury: how useful are animal models? *Dig Dis.* (2015) 33:477–85. doi: 10.1159/000374093
92. Strom SC, Pisarov La Fau-Dorko K, Dorko K Fau-Thompson MT, Thompson Mt Fau-Schuetz JD, Schuetz Jd Fau-Schuetz EG, Schuetz EG. Use of human hepatocytes to study P450 gene induction. *Meth Enzymol.* (1996) 272:388–401. doi: 10.1016/S0076-6879(96)72044-X
93. Pichard-Garcia L, Gerbal-Chaloin S Fau-Ferrini J-B, Ferrini Jb Fau-Fabre J-M, Fabre Jm Fau-Maurel P, Maurel P. Use of long-term cultures of human hepatocytes to study cytochrome P450 gene expression. *Meth Enzymol.* (2002) 357:311–21. doi: 10.1016/S0076-6879(02)57 689-8
94. Pascussi JM, Gerbal-Chaloin S Fau-Drocourt L, Drocourt L Fau-Assenat E, Assenat E Fau-Larrey D, Larrey D Fau-Pichard-Garcia L, Pichard-Garcia L Fau-Vilarem MJ, et al. Cross-talk between xenobiotic detoxication and other signalling pathways: clinical and toxicological consequences. *Xenobiotica* (2004) 34:633–64. doi: 10.1080/00498250412331285454
95. Hewitt NJ, Lechon Mj Fau-Houston JB, Houston Jb Fau-Hallifax D, Hallifax D Fau-Brown HS, Brown Hs Fau-Maurel P, Maurel P Fau-Kenna JG, et al. Primary hepatocytes: current understanding of the regulation of metabolic enzymes and transporter proteins, and pharmaceutical practice for the use of hepatocytes in metabolism, enzyme induction, transporter, clearance, and hepatotoxicity studies. *Drug Metab Rev.* (2007) 39:159–234. doi: 10.1080/03602530601093489
96. Arnold B. Parenchymal cells in immune and tolerance induction. *Immunol Lett.* (2003) 89:225–8. doi: 10.1016/S0165-2478(03)00150-0
97. Okunishi K, Dohi M Fau-Nakagome K, Nakagome K Fau-Tanaka R, Tanaka R Fau-Mizuno S, Mizuno S Fau-Matsumoto K, Matsumoto K Fau-Miyazaki J-I, et al. A novel role of hepatocyte growth factor as an immune regulator through suppressing dendritic cell function. *J Immunol.* (2005) 175:4745–53. doi: 10.4049/jimmunol.175.7.4745
98. Rutella S, Bonanno G Fau-Procoli A, Procoli a Fau-Mariotti A, Mariotti a Fau-De Ritis DG, De Ritis Dg Fau-Curti A, Curti a Fau-Danese S, et al. Hepatocyte growth factor favors monocyte differentiation into regulatory interleukin (IL)-10++IL-12low/neg accessory cells with dendritic-cell features. *Blood* (2006) 108:218–27. doi: 10.1182/blood-2005-0 8-3141
99. Zhang M, Wang H, Tan S, Navarro-Alvarez N, Zheng Y, Yang YG. Donor CD47 controls T cell alloresponses and is required for tolerance induction following hepatocyte allotransplantation. *Sci Rep.* (2016) 6:26839. doi: 10.1038/srep26839
100. Ferrini JB, Pichard L Fau-Domergue J, Domergue J Fau-Maurel P, Maurel P. Long-term primary cultures of adult human hepatocytes. *Chemicobiol Intereact.* (1997) 107:31–45. doi: 10.1016/S0009-2797(97)00072-0
101. Runge D, Kohler C Fau-Kostrubsky VE, Kostrubsky Ve Fau-Jager D, Jager D Fau-Lehmann T, Lehmann T Fau-Runge DM, Runge Dm Fau-May U, et al. Induction of cytochrome P450 (CYP)1A1, CYP1A2, and CYP3A4 but not of CYP2C9, CYP2C19, multidrug resistance (MDR-1) and multidrug resistance associated protein (MRP-1) by prototypical inducers in human hepatocytes. *Biochem Biophys Res Commun.* (2000) 273:333–41. doi: 10.1006/bbrc.2000.2902
102. Kitamura S, Sugihara K. Current status of prediction of drug disposition and toxicity in humans using chimeric mice with humanized liver. *Xenobiotica* (2014) 44:123–34. doi: 10.3109/00498254.2013.868062
103. Guo J, Li Y, Shan Y, Shu C, Wang F, Wang X, et al. Humanized mice reveal an essential role for human hepatocytes in the development of the liver immune system. *Cell Death Dis.* (2018) 9:667. doi: 10.1038/s41419-018-0720-9
104. Rongvaux A, Takizawa H, Strowig T, Willinger T, Eynon EE, Flavell RA, et al. Human hemato-lymphoid system mice: current use and future potential for medicine. *Annu Rev Immunol.* (2013) 31:635–74. doi: 10.1146/annurev-immunol-032712-095921
105. Herndler-Brandstetter D, Shan L, Yao Y, Stecher C, Plajer V, Lietzenmayer M, et al. Humanized mouse model supports development, function, and tissue residency of human natural killer cells. *Proc Natl Acad Sci USA.* (2017) 114:E9626–E9634. doi: 10.1073/pnas.1705301114
106. Brehm MA, Shultz LD, Greiner DL. Humanized mouse models to study human diseases. *Curr Opin Endocrinol Diabetes Obes.* (2010) 17:120. doi: 10.1097/MED.0b013e328337282f
107. Ito R, Takahashi T, Katano I, Ito M. Current advances in humanized mouse models. *Cell Mol Immunol.* (2012) 9:208–14. doi: 10.1038/cmi.2012.2
108. Day C-P, Merlino G, Van Dyke T. Preclinical mouse cancer models: a maze of opportunities and challenges. *Cell* (2015) 163:39–53. doi: 10.1016/j.cell.2015.08.068
109. Ernst W. Humanized mice in infectious diseases. *Comp Immunol Microbiol Infect Dis.* (2016) 49:29–38. doi: 10.1016/j.cimid.2016.08.006
110. Sacci JB, Schriefer ME, Resau JH, Wirtz RA, Detolla LJ, Markham RB, et al. Mouse model for exoerythrocytic stages of *Plasmodium falciparum* malaria parasite. *Proc Natl Acad Sci USA.* (1992) 89:3701–5. doi: 10.1073/pnas.89.9.3701
111. Vaughan AM, Mikolajczak SA, Wilson EM, Grompe M, Kaushansky A, Camargo N, et al. Complete *Plasmodium falciparum* liver-stage development in liver-chimeric mice. *J Clin Invest.* (2012) 122:3618. doi: 10.1172/JCI 62684
112. Kaushansky A, Mikolajczak SA, Vignali M, Kappe SH. Of men in mice: the success and promise of humanized mouse models for human malaria parasite infections. *Cell Microbiol.* (2014) 16:602–11. doi: 10.1111/cmi.12277
113. Minkah NK, Schafer C, Kappe SH. Humanized mouse models for the study of human malaria parasite biology, pathogenesis and immunity. *Front Immunol.* (2018) 9:807. doi: 10.3389/fimmu.2018.00807

114. Arama C, Troye-Blomberg M. The path of malaria vaccine development: challenges and perspectives. *J Intern Med.* (2014) 275:456–66. doi: 10.1111/joim.12223
115. Subudhi AK, Boopathi P, Pandey I, Kohli R, Karwa R, Middha S, et al. *Plasmodium falciparum* complicated malaria: modulation and connectivity between exportome and variant surface antigen gene families. *Mol Biochem Parasitol.* (2015) 201:31–46. doi: 10.1016/j.molbiopara.2015.05.005
116. Orfano AS, Nacif-Pimenta R, Duarte AP, Villegas LM, Rodrigues NB, Pinto LC, et al. Species-specific escape of *Plasmodium* sporozoites from oocysts of avian, rodent, and human malarial parasites. *Malar J.* (2016) 15:394. doi: 10.1186/s12936-016-1451-y
117. Silvie O, Rubinstein E, Franetich J-F, Prenant M, Belnoue E, Rénia L, et al. Hepatocyte CD81 is required for *Plasmodium falciparum* and *Plasmodium yoelii* sporozoite infectivity. *Nat Med.* (2003) 9:93–6. doi: 10.1038/nm808
118. Lopaticki S, Yang AS, John A, Scott NE, Lingford JP, O'neill MT, et al. Protein O-fucosylation in *Plasmodium falciparum* ensures efficient infection of mosquito and vertebrate hosts. *Nat Commun.* (2017) 8:561. doi: 10.1038/s41467-017-00571-y
119. Sultan AA, Thathy V, Frevert U, Robson KJ, Crisanti A, Nussenzweig V, et al. TRAP is necessary for gliding motility and infectivity of *Plasmodium sporozoites. Cell* (1997) 90:511–22. doi: 10.1016/S0092-8674(00)80511-5
120. Carrolo M, Giordano S, Cabrita-Santos L, Corso S, Vigário AM, Silva S, et al. Hepatocyte growth factor and its receptor are required for malaria infection. *Nat Med.* (2003) 9:1363–9. doi: 10.1038/nm947
121. Kaushansky A, Kappe SH. The crucial role of hepatocyte growth factor receptor during liver-stage infection is not conserved among *Plasmodium* species. *Nat Med.* (2011) 17:1180–1. doi: 10.1038/nm.2456
122. Yang AS, Lopaticki S, O'neill MT, Erickson SM, Douglas DN, Kneteman, NM, et al. AMA1 and MAEBL are important for *Plasmodium falciparum* sporozoite infection of the liver. *Cell Microbiol.* (2017) 19:e12745. doi: 10.1111/cmi.12745
123. Kariu T, Yuda M, Yano K, Chinzei Y. MAEBL is essential for malarial sporozoite infection of the mosquito salivary gland. *J Exp Med.* (2002) 195:1317–23. doi: 10.1084/jem.20011876
124. Maitland K, Makanga M, Williams TN. Falciparum malaria: current therapeutic challenges. *Curr Opin Infect Dis.* (2004) 17:405–12. doi: 10.1097/00001432-200410000-00004
125. Miura K. Progress and prospects for blood-stage malaria vaccines. *Expert Rev Vaccines* (2016) 15:765–81. doi: 10.1586/14760584.2016.11 41680
126. Mazier D, Beaudoin RL, Mellouk S, Druilhe P, Texier B, Trosper J, et al. Complete development of hepatic stages of *Plasmodium falciparum in vitro*. *Science* (1985) 227:440–2. doi: 10.1126/science.3880923
127. Sattabongkot J, Yimamnuaychoke N, Leelaudomlipi S, Rasameesoraj M, Jenwithisuk R, Coleman RE, et al. Establishment of a human hepatocyte line that supports *in vitro* development of the exo-erythrocytic stages of the malaria parasites *Plasmodium falciparum* and *P. vivax. Am J Trop Med Hyg.* (2006) 74:708–15. doi: 10.4269/ajtmh.2006.74.708
128. March S, Ng S, Velmurugan S, Galstian A, Shan J, Logan DJ, et al. A microscale human liver platform that supports the hepatic stages of *Plasmodium falciparum* and vivax. *Cell Host Microbe* (2013) 14:104–15. doi: 10.1016/j.chom.2013.06.005
129. Roth A, Maher SP, Conway AJ, Ubalee R, Chaumeau V, Andolina C, et al. A comprehensive model for assessment of liver stage therapies targeting *Plasmodium vivax* and *Plasmodium falciparum*. *Nat Commun.* (2018) 9:1837. doi: 10.1038/s41467-018-04221-9
130. Mazier D, Landau I, Druilhe P, Miltgen F, Guguen-Guillouzo C, Baccam D, et al. Cultivation of the liver forms of *Plasmodium vivax* in human hepatocytes. *Nature* (1984) 307:367–9. doi: 10.1038/307367a0
131. Hollingdale MR, Collins WE, Campbell CC, Schwartz AL. *In vitro* culture of two populations (dividing and nondividing) of exoerythrocytic parasites of *Plasmodium vivax. Am J Trop Med Hyg.* (1985) 34:216–22. doi: 10.4269/ajtmh.1985.34.216
132. Mikolajczak SA, Vaughan AM, Kangwanrangsan N, Roobsoong W, Fishbaugher M, Yimamnuaychok N, et al. *Plasmodium vivax* liver stage development and hypnozoite persistence in human liver-chimeric mice. *Cell Host Microbe* (2015) 17:526–35. doi: 10.1016/j.chom.2015.02.011
133. Raphemot R, Posfai D, Derbyshire ER. Current therapies and future possibilities for drug development against liver-stage malaria. *J Clin Invest.* (2016) 126:2013–20. doi: 10.1172/JCI82981
134. Tyagi RK, Arnold L, Mejia P, Van Rooijen N, Pérignon J-L, Druilhe P. Analysis of innate defences against *Plasmodium falciparum* in immunodeficient mice. *Malar J.* (2010) 9:197. doi: 10.1186/1475-2875-9-197
135. Tyagi RK, Gleeson PJ, Arnold L, Tahar R, Prieur E, Decosterd L, et al. High-level artemisinin-resistance with quinine co-resistance emerges in *P. falciparum* malaria under *in vivo* artesunate pressure. *BMC Med.* (2018) 16:181. doi: 10.1186/s12916-018-1156-x
136. Badell E, Pasquetto V, Druilhe P, Van Rooijen N. A mouse model for human malaria erythrocytic stages. *Parasitol Today* (1995) 11:235–7. doi: 10.1016/0169-4758(95)80088-3
137. Badell E, Oeuvray C, Moreno A, Soe S, Van Rooijen N, Bouzidi A, et al. Human malaria in immunocompromised mice: an *in vivo* model to study defense mechanisms against *Plasmodium falciparum*. *J Exp Med.* (2000) 192:1653–60. doi: 10.1084/jem.192.11.1653
138. Moreno A, Badell E, Van Rooijen N, Druilhe P. Human malaria in immunocompromised mice: new *in vivo* model for chemotherapy studies. *Antimicrob Agents Chemother.* (2001) 45:1847–53. doi: 10.1128/AAC.45.6.1847-1853.2001
139. Moore JM, Kumar N, Shultz LD, Rajan TV. Maintenance of the human malarial parasite, *Plasmodium falciparum*, in scid mice and transmission of gametocytes to mosquitoes. *J Exp Med.* (1995) 181:2265–70. doi: 10.1084/jem.181.6.2265
140. Tsuji M, Ishihara C, Arai S, Hiratai R, Azuma I. Establishment of a SCID mouse model having circulating human red blood cells and a possible growth of *Plasmodium falciparum* in the mouse. *Vaccine* (1995) 13:1389–92. doi: 10.1016/0264-410X(95)00081-B
141. Moreno A, Ferrer E, Arahuetes S, Eguiluz C, Van Rooijen N, Benito A. The course of infections and pathology in immunomodulated NOD/LtSz-SCID mice inoculated with *Plasmodium falciparum* laboratory lines and clinical isolates. *Int J Parasitol.* (2006) 36:361–9. doi: 10.1016/j.ijpara.2005.10.012
142. Angulo-Barturen I, Jiménez-Díaz MB, Mulet T, Rullas J, Herreros E, Ferrer S, et al. A murine model of falciparum-malaria by *in vivo* selection of competent strains in non-myelodepleted mice engrafted with human erythrocytes. *PLoS ONE*(2008) 3:e2252. doi: 10.1371/journal.pone.0002252
143. Jiménez-Díaz MB, Mulet T, Viera S, Gómez V, Garuti H, Ibáñez J, et al. Improved murine model of malaria using *Plasmodium falciparum* competent strains and non-myelodepleted NOD-scid IL2Rγnull mice engrafted with human erythrocytes. *Antimicrob Agents Chemother.* (2009) 53:4533–6. doi: 10.1128/AAC.00519-09
144. Jiménez-Díaz MB, Mulet T, Gómez V, Viera S, Alvarez A, Garuti H, et al. Quantitative measurement of Plasmodium-infected erythrocytes in murine models of malaria by flow cytometry using bidimensional assessment of SYTO-16 fluorescence. *Cytometry A* (2009) 75:225–35. doi: 10.1002/cyto.a.20647
145. Tyagi RK, Arnold L, Meija P, Swetman C, Gleeson J, Pérignon J-L, et al. Further improvements of the *P. falciparum* humanized mouse model. *PLoS ONE* (2011) 6:e18045. doi: 10.1371/journal.pone.0018045
146. Wijayalath W, Majji S, Villasante EF, Brumeanu TD, Richie TL, Casares S. Humanized HLA-DR4. RagKO. IL2RγcKO. NOD (DRAG) mice sustain the complex vertebrate life cycle of *Plasmodium falciparum* malaria. *Malaria J.* (2014) 13:386. doi: 10.1186/1475-2875-13-386
147. Vaughan AM, Kappe SH, Ploss A, Mikolajczak SA. Development of humanized mouse models to study human malaria parasite infection. *Future Microbiol.* (2012) 7:657–65. doi: 10.2217/fmb.12.27
148. Hasegawa M, Kawai K, Mitsui T, Taniguchi K, Monnai M, Wakui M, et al. The reconstituted 'humanized liver'in TK-NOG mice is mature and functional. *Biochem Biophys Res Commun.* (2011) 405:405–10. doi: 10.1016/j.bbrc.2011.01.042
149. Sabater AM, Moreno M, Moreno FJ, Eguiluz C, Van Rooijen N, Benito A. Experimental infection of immunomodulated NOD/LtSz-SCID mice as a new model for *Plasmodium falciparum* erythrocytic stages. *Parasitol Res.* (2005) 95:97–105. doi: 10.1007/s00436-004-1249-7
150. Duffier Y, Lorthiois A, Cisteró P, Dupuy F, Jouvion G, Fiette L, et al. A humanized mouse model for sequestration of *Plasmodium falciparum* sexual

stages and *in vivo* evaluation of gametocytidal drugs. *Sci Rep.* (2016) 6:35025. doi: 10.1038/srep35025

151. Amaladoss A, Chen Q, Liu M, Dummler SK, Dao M, Suresh S, et al. De novo generated human red blood cells in humanized mice support *Plasmodium falciparum* infection. *PLoS ONE* (2015) 10:e0129825. doi: 10.1371/journal.pone.0129825
152. Chen Q, Khoury M, Chen J. Expression of human cytokines dramatically improves reconstitution of specific human-blood lineage cells in humanized mice. *Proc Natl Acad Sci USA.* (2009) 106:21783–8. doi: 10.1073/pnas.0912274106
153. Dembélé L, Franetich J-F, Lorthiois A, Gego A, Zeeman A-M, Kocken CH, et al. Persistence and activation of malaria hypnozoites in long-term primary hepatocyte cultures. *Nat Med.* (2014) 20:307. doi: 10.1038/nm.3461
154. Yang AS, O'neill MT, Jennison C, Lopaticki S, Allison CC, Armistead J S, et al. Cell traversal activity is important for *Plasmodium falciparum* liver infection in humanized mice. *Cell Rep.* (2017) 18:3105–16. doi: 10.1016/j.celrep.2017.03.017
155. Meuleman P, Libbrecht L, De Vos R, De Hemptinne B, Gevaert K, Vandekerckhove J, et al. Morphological and biochemical characterization of a human liver in a uPA-SCID mouse chimera. *Hepatology* (2005) 41:847–56. doi: 10.1002/hep.20657
156. Sacci JB, Alam U, Douglas D, Lewis J, Tyrrell DLJ, Azad AF, et al. *Plasmodium falciparum* infection and exoerythrocytic development in mice with chimeric human livers. *Int J Parasitol.* (2006) 36:353–60. doi: 10.1016/j.ijpara.2005.10.014
157. Morosan S, Hez-Deroubaix S, Lunel F, Renia L, Giannini C, Rooijen NV, et al. Liver-stage development of *Plasmodium falciparum* in a humanized mouse model. *J Infect Dis.* (2006) 193:996–1004. doi: 10.1086/500840
158. Vanbuskirk KM, O'neill MT, De La Vega P, Maier AG, Krzych U, Williams J, et al.. Preerythrocytic, live-attenuated *Plasmodium falciparum* vaccine candidates by design. *Proc Natl Acad Sci USA.* (2009) 106:13004–9. doi: 10.1073/pnas.0906387106
159. Mikolajczak SA, Sacci JBJr, De La Vega P, Camargo N, Vanbuskirk K, Krzych U, et al. Disruption of the *Plasmodium falciparum* liver-stage antigen-1 locus causes a differentiation defect in late liver-stage parasites. *Cell Microbiol.* (2011) 13:1250–60. doi: 10.1111/j.1462-5822.2011.01617.x
160. Azuma H, Paulk N, Ranade A, Dorrell C, Al-Dhalimy M, Ellis E, et al. Robust expansion of human hepatocytes in Fah$^{-/-}$/Rag2$^{-/-}$/Il2rg$^{-/-}$ mice. *Nat Biotechnol.* (2007) 25:903–10. doi: 10.1038/nbt1326
161. Grompe M, Al-Dhalimy M, Finegold M, Ou C-N, Burlingame T, Kennaway NG, et al. Loss of fumarylacetoacetate hydrolase is responsible for the neonatal hepatic dysfunction phenotype of lethal albino mice. *Genes Dev.* (1993) 7:2298–307. doi: 10.1101/gad.7.12a.2298
162. Grompe M, Lindstedt S, Al-Dhalimy M, Kennaway NG, Papaconstantinou J, Torres-Ramos CA, et al. Pharmacological correction of neonatal lethal hepatic dysfunction in a murine model of hereditary tyrosinaemia type I. *Nat Genet.* (1995) 10:453. doi: 10.1038/ng0895-453
163. Hu Z, Van Rooijen N, Yang Y-G. Macrophages prevent human red blood cell reconstitution in immunodeficient mice. *Blood* (2011) 118:5938–46. doi: 10.1182/blood-2010-11-321414
164. Sack BK, Mikolajczak SA, Fishbaugher M, Vaughan AM, Flannery EL, Nguyen T, et al. Humoral protection against mosquito bite-transmitted *Plasmodium falciparum* infection in humanized mice. *NPJ Vaccines* (2017) 2:27. doi: 10.1038/s41541-017-0028-2
165. Flannery EL, Foquet L, Chuenchob V, Fishbaugher M, Billman Z, Navarro MJ, et al. Assessing drug efficacy against *Plasmodium falciparum* liver stages *in vivo*. *JCI Insight* (2018) 3:92587. doi: 10.1172/jci.insight.92587
166. Phillips MA, Lotharius J, Marsh K, White J, Dayan A, White KL, et al. A long-duration dihydroorotate dehydrogenase inhibitor (DSM265) for prevention and treatment of malaria. *Sci Transl Med.* (2015) 7:296ra11. doi: 10.1126/scitranslmed.aaa6645
167. Foquet L, Schafer C, Minkah NK, Alanine DG, Flannery EL, Steel RW, et al. *Plasmodium falciparum* liver stage infection and transition to stable blood stage infection in liver-humanized and blood-humanized FRGN KO mice enables testing of blood stage inhibitory antibodies (reticulocyte-binding protein homolog 5) *in vivo*. *Front Immunol.* (2018) 9:524. doi: 10.3389/fimmu.2018.00524
168. Payne RO, Milne KH, Elias SC, Edwards NJ, Douglas AD, Brown RE, et al. Demonstration of the blood-stage *Plasmodium falciparum* controlled human malaria infection model to assess efficacy of the *P. falciparum* apical membrane antigen 1 vaccine, FMP2. 1/AS01. *J Infect Dis.* (2016) 213:1743–51. doi: 10.1093/infdis/jiw039
169. Peltz G. Can 'humanized'mice improve drug development in the 21st century? *Trends Pharmacol. Sci.* (2013) 34:255–60. doi: 10.1016/j.tips.2013.03.005
170. Kamimura H, Ito S, Nozawa K, Nakamura S, Chijiwa H, Nagatsuka S-I, et al. Formation of the accumulative human metabolite and human-specific glutathione conjugate of diclofenac in TK-NOG chimeric mice with humanized livers. *Drug Metab Dispos.* (2015) 43:309–16. doi: 10.1124/dmd.114.061689
171. Majji S, Wijayalath W, Shashikumar S, Brumeanu TD, Casares S. Humanized DRAGA mice immunized with *Plasmodium falciparum* sporozoites and chloroquine elicit protective pre-erythrocytic immunity. *Malar J.* (2018) 17:114. doi: 10.1186/s12936-018-2264-y
172. Ghosn S, Chamat S, Prieur E, Stephan A, Druilhe P, Bouharoun-Tayoun H. Evaluating human immune responses for vaccine development in a novel human spleen cell-engrafted NOD-SCID-IL2rγNull Mouse Model. *Front Immunol.* (2018) 9:601. doi: 10.3389/fimmu.2018.00601

12

*Pfs*230 and *Pfs*48/45 Fusion Proteins Elicit Strong Transmission-Blocking Antibody Responses Against *Plasmodium falciparum*

Susheel K. Singh[1,2†]*, Susan Thrane*[2†]*, Bishwanath K. Chourasia*[2]*, Karina Teelen*[3]*, Wouter Graumans*[3]*, Rianne Stoter*[3]*, Geert-Jan van Gemert*[3]*, Marga G. van de Vegte-Bolmer*[3]*, Morten A. Nielsen*[2]*, Ali Salanti*[2]*, Adam F. Sander*[2]*, Robert W. Sauerwein*[3]*, Matthijs M. Jore*[3*] *and Michael Theisen*[1,2*]

[1] Department for Congenital Disorders, Statens Serum Institut, Copenhagen, Denmark, [2] Centre for Medical Parasitology at Department of International Health, Immunology and Microbiology, University of Copenhagen and Department of Infectious Diseases, Copenhagen University Hospital, Rigshospitalet, Copenhagen, Denmark, [3] Department of Medical Microbiology, Radboud University Medical Center, Nijmegen, Netherlands

***Correspondence:**
Matthijs M. Jore
Matthijs.Jore@radboudumc.nl
Michael Theisen
mth@ssi.dk

† These authors have contributed equally to this work

The *Plasmodium falciparum Pf*s230 and *Pf*s48/45 proteins are expressed during transmission from man to mosquito and are leading candidates for a malaria transmission blocking vaccine. Individually they generate transmission blocking (TB) antibodies in rodent models. Whether the single protein vaccines are suitable to use in field settings will primarily depend on their potency to elicit functional antibodies. We hypothesized that a combination of both proteins will be more potent than each protein individually. Therefore we designed chimeric proteins composed of fragments of both *Pf*s230 and *Pf*s48/45 as well as single protein fragments, and expressed these in *Lactoccus lactis*. Both the individual *Pf*s230 and *Pf*s48/45 fragments and chimeras elicited high levels of functional antibodies in mice. Importantly, one of the chimeric proteins elicited over threefold higher transmission blocking antibody responses than the single antigens alone. Furthermore the immunogenicity of one of the chimeras could be enhanced through coupling to a virus-like particle (VLP). Altogether these data support further clinical development of these novel constructs.

Keywords: malaria, vaccines, multivalent, transmission blocking, *Lactococcus lactis*

INTRODUCTION

The transmission of *Plasmodium falciparum* from one person to another relies on the generation of male and female gametocytes in the human host that can be picked up and spread by a mosquito. The aim of a malaria transmission blocking vaccine (MTBV) is to effectively block malaria transmission at the population level thereby contributing to malaria elimination.

Several MTBV candidates have been identified by screening monoclonal antibodies generated against *P. falciparum* mosquito stages for TB activity (1–4). Three proteins, *Pf*s48/45, *Pf*s230, and *Pf*s25 are currently targeted as lead candidates for an MTBV. Of these, *Pf*s48/45 and *Pf*s230 are expressed in the gametocyte as it develops from stage III through V in the human host. Shortly, after being taken up by a blood-feeding mosquito, the parasite emerges from the RBC as a gamete and after a few rounds of replication motile males fertilize female gametes to form zygotes. *Pf*s48/45 is expressed on the surface of both male and female gametes where it is bound to the plasma membrane through a GPI-anchor (5) and forms a stable complex with *Pf*s230 (6). Both *Pf*s48/45 and *Pf*s230 are important for male fertility (7).

Humans develop naturally acquired immunity against *P. falciparum* gametocytes (8–10) and antibodies against *Pf*s230 and *Pf*s48/45 have been associated with TB activity in some but not all immune epidemiological studies (11, 12). Recently, we demonstrated that *Pf*s48/45- and *Pf*s230-specific antibodies exhibit strong TB activity in the standard membrane feeding assay (SMFA) (13), the gold standard for assessing transmission blockade *ex vivo* (2, 14–16). Whether such antibodies act synergistically, as observed for combinations of mAbs targeting different epitopes on *Pf*s48/45 (2), is not yet known.

*Pf*s48/45 and *Pf*s230 are members of the six-cysteine (6-Cys) s48/45 protein family and contain three and fourteen 6-Cys domains respectively (17). Each 6-Cys domain contains up to six cysteine residues that are involved in intra-domain disulfide bond formation which results in conformational antibody epitopes. The C-terminal 6-Cys domain of *Pfs*48/45 contains the conformational epitope I, which is targeted by the most potent TB monoclonal antibody described to date, mAb45.1 (18). We have recently used the *Lactococcus lactis* expression system for the production of the C-terminal 6-Cys domain of *Pf*s48/45 (6C) as a fusion protein (R0.6C) with the N-terminal GLURP-R0 region (19, 20). The resulting fusion protein can be produced in high yields of properly folded monomeric protein which elicited high levels of TB antibodies in small rodents (19, 20). In the case of *Pf*s230, the C fragment spanning the N-terminal pro-domain and first three 6-Cys domains has been shown to elicit the most potent TB antibodies (21). The presence of three 6-Cys domains suggests that disulfide bonds may be critical for proper folding of each of these domains. Accordingly, a series of *Pf*s230-specific transmission-blocking monoclonal antibodies did not recognize reduced *Pf*s230 (22). In an attempt to identify the minimal *Pf*s230-domain involved in the generation of TB antibodies, *Pf*s230 constructs containing the Pro, Pro+I, Pro+I,II, and Pro+I,II,III domains were produced individually in the wheat germ cell-free system (23). Interestingly, the N-terminal Pro domain, which lacks cysteines, was sufficient to elicit complement-dependent TB activity in the SMFA, suggesting that TB antibodies may also be directed against non-conformational epitopes (23). With respect to *Pf*s230, the C-fragment was the first construct to elicit TB antibodies; however, oocyst reduction was incomplete suggesting that folding was compromised by an incorrect cysteine connectivity (21). Another construct, *Pf*s230D1, corresponding to amino acid residues 444 to 736 was produced in *Pichia pastoris* as a properly folded protein and elicited TB antibodies in rodents (24).

While clinical trials with *Pf*s230D1 are ongoing (ClinicalTrials.gov Identifier: NCT02334462) and R0.6C is in early clinical development phase, we sought to identify more potent *Pf*s48/45- and *Pf*s230-based immunogens. We hypothesized that a combination of antibodies against both proteins would be more potent than against each antigen individually. Therefore we constructed chimeric proteins composed of fragments of both *Pf*s230 and *Pf*s48/45, expressed these in *L. lactis* and evaluated antibody responses in rodents. A multicomponent hybrid protein containing both *Pf*s48/45 and *Pf*s230 holds the potential to lower the required threshold of functional antibodies and to reduce the risk of escape mutations.

METHODS

Preparation of Constructs

Three different truncated forms of *Pf*s230 from N-terminus, i.e. Pro (pro domain AA 443 to 590), Pro+I (pro domain and domain I, AA 443 to 736) and Pro+I,II,III (pro domain through domain III, AA 443 to 1132) were amplified by PCR from *P. falciparum* 3D7 DNA (GenBank accession number L08135) and cloned into the *Bgl*II restriction site of pSS5 plasmid containing N-terminus Spycatcher (25). *Pf*s48/45$_{291-428}$ (6C) was amplified from an expression vector encoding R0.6C (19, 20) using the forward primer 5′-CCAT<u>GGATCC</u>GAAAAAAAAGTCATACACGGATGTAACTTC-3′ and the reverse primer 5′-CCAT<u>AGATCT</u>TGCTGAATCTATAGTAACTGTCATATAAGC-3′. The amplified PCR product was digested with *Bam*HI and *Bgl*II (underlined) and cloned in frame into plasmids containing the Pro or Pro+I inserts to generate Pro-6C and Pro+I-6C fusion constructs, respectively. All the constructs were verified by DNA sequencing and transformed into *L. lactis* MG1363 by electroporation for expression of recombinant proteins with 6xHis tags.

Fermentation and Protein Purification

Fermentation of *L. lactis* MG1363, containing *Pf*s230 or *Pf*s230-*Pf*s48/45 fusion constructs were carried out as described previously (19, 26). Briefly, cell-free culture-filtrates were concentrated five-fold and buffer exchanged into Tris buffer (50 mM Tris, 50mM NaCl pH 8.0 supplemented with 10mM Imidazole) using a Quix Stand Benchtop system (Hollow fiber cartridge with cutoff at 10,000 or 30,000 Da, surface area 650cm^2, GE Healthcare, Sweden) followed by filtration through a Durapore filter (PVDF, 0.22 μm, Millipore) and applied to a 5 ml HisTrap HP column (GE Healthcare, Sweden). Bound protein was eluted with 500mM Imidazole in Tris buffer pH 8.0 (50 mM Tris, 50mM NaCl) at a flow rate of 4 ml/min. Fractions containing the desired protein were further applied to a 5 ml HiTrap Q HP column (GE Healthcare, Sweden) for purification of monomeric proteins. Bound protein was eluted through step gradient elution in Tris buffer pH 8.0 (50 mM Tris, 1mM EDTA, 1 M NaCl) and fractions containing monomers were concentrated by a VIVA spin column with a 10 or 30 kDa cutoff (Vivascience, Germany), and kept in 50 mM Tris, 250 mM NaCl and 1 mM EDTA, pH 8.0 at −80°C until use. Immune purification for Pro-6C and Pro+I-6C was done as previously described (26). Fractions containing the desired protein were pooled and then concentrated and buffer exchanged against 50 mM Tris, 100 mM NaCl, and 1 mM EDTA, pH 8.0 and kept at −80°C until use. Fractions were analyzed by SDS-PAGE and immune blotting with mAb45.1 against *Pf*s48/45 conformational epitope I. Protein concentrations were measured using a BCA kit (Thermo Fisher Scientific, USA).

Protein Characterization

Analytical size exclusion high-performance liquid chromatography (SE-HPLC) of purified fusion proteins was performed as described previously (19, 20). Briefly, 5 μl of protein was loaded on an Agilent advance Bio SEC 300 Å, 2.7 μm, 4.6 × 300 mm SEC column (Agilent Technologies, GB) and eluted with a 0.1 ml/min flow of elution buffer (phosphate buffer) at room temperature. Protein standards (Sigma Aldrich) were also run using the same conditions mentioned above for sizing of the purified recombinant proteins. The amount of free cysteine residues was measured using Ellman's Reagent (Thermo Fisher Scientific, USA) following the manufacturer's instructions. A standard curve was constructed using known concentrations of free cysteine (Sigma-Aldrich, USA). Folding was determined in the mAb45.1 sandwich ELISA as described (19, 26).

Production of VLPs

SpyTag was genetically fused to the N-terminus of AP205, as previously described (27). In brief, the SpyTag peptide sequence (AHIVMVDAYKPTK) was fused to the gene sequence encoding the major AP205 coat protein (Gene ID: 956335) using a flexible linker (GSGTAGGGSGS) between the two sequences. The SpyTag-AP205 VLPs were expressed in *Escherichia coli* One Shot® BL21 Star™ (DE3) cells (Thermo Fisher Scientific, USA) and purified by ultracentrifugation using an Optiprep™ (Sigma-Aldrich, USA) gradient. For conjugation to VLPs, purified soluble Pro-6C or Pro+I-6C proteins were incubated at a molar ratio of 1:1 (VLP/antigen) in a 1xPBS buffer for 2 h at room temperature. Unbound protein was removed by dialysis against PBS using 1,000 MWCO dialysis tubing (Spectrum Labs, USA). Densitometric analysis of SDS-PAGE gels was used to estimate protein concentrations.

Dynamic Light Scattering

Uncoupled VLP, soluble proteins and proteins conjugated to VLP were adjusted to 0.5–1 mg/ml in PBS and spun at 15,000 g for 10 min. Seventy Microliter sample was loaded into a disposable Eppendorf Uvette cuvette (Sigma-Aldrich, USA) and measured at 25°C on a DynoPro NanoStar (WYATT Technology, USA) equipped with a 658 nm laser. Each sample was measured 20 times and intensity-average size and percentage polydispersity (PD) was estimated using Dynamic software (Version 7.5.0).

Electron Microscopy

Pro-6C or Pro+I-6C coupled to VLP (with concentrations between 0.4 and 0.5 mg/ml based on antigen content) were incubated on carbon-coated and glow-discharged grids and negatively stained with 2% phosphotungstic acid (pH 7.4). The particles were analyzed on a CM 100 BioTWIN electron microscope with an accelerating voltage of 80 kV. Images were acquired using an Olympus Veleta camera and particle size was estimated using iTEM software.

Animals and Immunogenicity Studies

In the first experiment, groups ($n = 5$) of CD-1 mice 5–7 weeks of age (Janvier Labs, Denmark) were immunized 3 times at 3-week interval by the intramuscular injection of equimolar amounts of immune-purified Pro-6C and the individual *Pf*s230 and *Pf*s48/45 recombinant protein constructs formulated with Alhydrogel® (Brenntag, Denmark) to a final concentration of 2 mg/ml Aluminum. Please note that six mice received R0.6C. Each dose contained 128 pmoles of soluble protein (equivalent to 2 μg 6C). Serum was collected on days 14, 35, and 56. In the second experiment, groups ($n = 8$) of CD-1 mice were immunized with 64 pmoles (equivalent to 1 μg 6C) Pro-6C or Pro+I-6C (soluble or conjugated to VLP) as described above for the first experiment. One mouse receiving Pro+I-6C was terminated due to behavioral abnormalities not related to vaccination. All animals were treated in accordance with the regulations and guidelines of the European and National authorities.

Enzyme-Linked Immunosorbent Assay (ELISA) for Antibody Response Measurement

Gametocyte extract ELISA was performed with cultured sexual stage of *Pf* NF54 parasites as previously described (26). Serum immunoglobulin (IgG) subclass levels were measured using ELISA as previously described (28). For antigen-specific ELISA, 96-well plates (Nunc MaxiSorp) were coated with 0.5 μg/well of *Pf*s48/45-6C (25), Pro+I, or Pro+I,II,II as appropriate. Antigen-specific antibodies were detected using HRP-conjugated polyclonal goat anti-mouse IgG (Novex A16072, diluted 1:3000). Antibody midpoint titer (EC50) was calculated using sigmoidal curve fitting. One-sided analysis of variance on the log-transformed values was used to confirm that ELISA data contain essential differences. Mann-Whitney test was then used to investigate whether the chimera elicited higher levels of specific antibodies compared to individual components. *p*-Values are two-sided and quoted without adjustment for multiple testing since the significance of the chimera was the primary problem under investigation. p-values ≤ 0.05 were considered significant. Statistical analysis was conducted using GraphPad Prism 7 (GraphPad Software, USA).

Standard Membrane Feeding Assay (SMFA)

The biological activity of specific antisera was assessed in the SMFA as previously described (26, 29). Depending on availability, wild type *P. falciparum* NF54 gametocytes or transgenic *P. falciparum* NF54 (NF54-HGL) gametocytes expressing luciferase (29) were fed to *Anopheles stephensi* mosquitoes that were reared and maintained at Radboudumc, The Netherlands. Non-heat inactivated mice sera, and active or heat-inactivated human complement was added to the cultured material prior to feeding to mosquitoes. After 6–8 days, oocysts in 20 fed mosquitoes were counted by microscopy, or quantified in four pools of five mosquitoes (NF54-HGL) by measuring luciferase levels (29). Samples were tested in two independent SMFA experiments. Luminescence-based TRA estimates from two independent feeds with each of four pools of five mosquitoes were made using generalized linear mixed models (GLMMs) without zero-inflated negative binomial error structure (30, 31). Microscopy-based estimates from two feeds with 20 mosquitoes each were made using GLMMs with zero-inflated negative binomial error structure (30, 31). Statistical differences between test samples were determined using General Linear Mixed Regression analysis. Statistical analyses were performed using R studio (v. 3.2.4, The R Foundation, Boston, USA). Pre-immune pooled mice serum samples were also tested in a single independent SMFA experiment (**Figure S2**).

Depletion of Antigen-Specific IgGs

*Pf*s230- and *Pf*s48/45-specific antibodies were depleted from serum using *Pf*s230-CMB (32) and R0.10C-containing columns respectively, as previously described (13). The *Pf*s230-CMB fragment contains AA 444-730 and thus covers the Pro+I fragment expressed in *L. lactis*. To test if all antigen-specific IgGs were depleted, the flow through serum (depleted serum) was tested in ELISA using plates coated with *Pf*s230-CMB or SpyC-6C as appropriate (25, 26).

RESULTS

Expression of a Multivalent *Pf*s230-*Pf*s48/45 Chimera in *L. Lactis*

To test whether a multivalent vaccine targeting *Pf*s48/45 and *Pf*s230 is immunogenic, we generated a chimeric construct containing the Pro domain of *Pf*s230 fused to the 6C fragment of *Pf*s48/45 (**Figure 1A**). We anticipated that this Pro-6C fusion protein would express well in *L. lactis* since the *Pf*s230-Pro domain is glutamate-rich, does not contain cysteines, and is similar to the R0 domain which previously enhanced expression of properly-folded 6C in *L. lactis* (25, 26). In addition to Pro-6C, we made constructs that either contained *Pf*s48/45 or *Pf*s230 fragments (**Figure 1A**). *L. lactis* MG1363 harboring these constructs were grown in a 1L bioreactor and the respective recombinant proteins were purified from the clarified supernatant through the C-terminal His-tag by immobilized metal affinity chromatography and ion exchange chromatography (**Figure 1B**). As expected, protein yields decreased with increasing number of *Pf*s230 domains

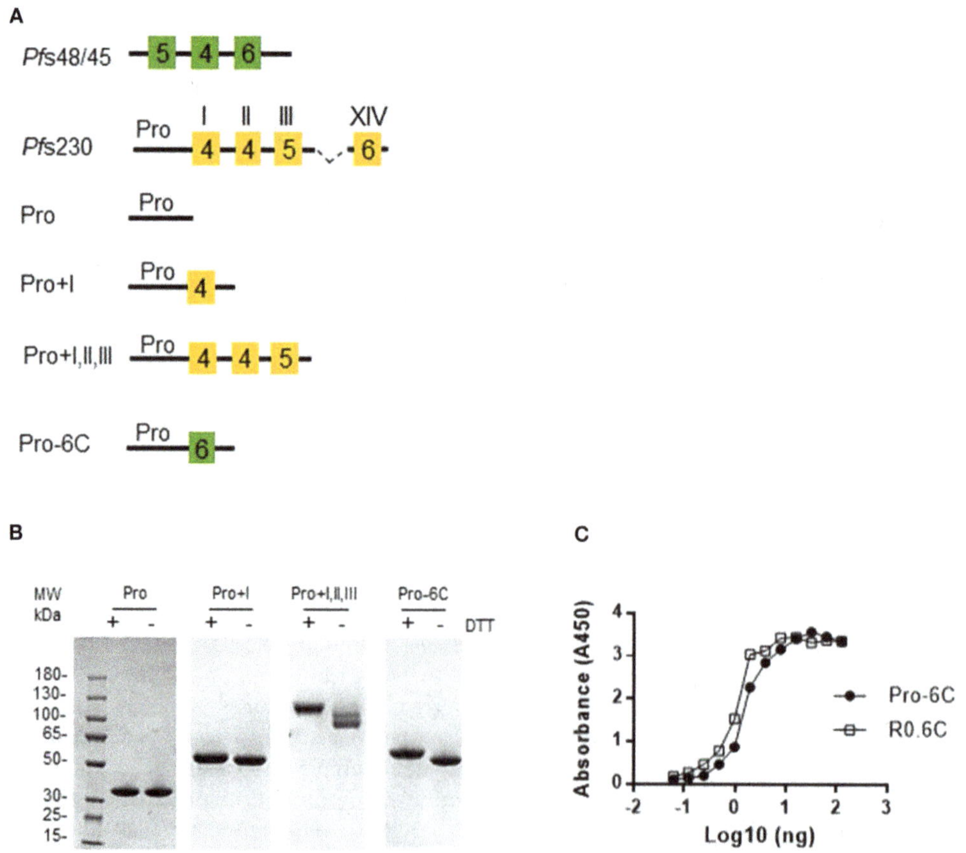

FIGURE 1 | Production of recombinant *Pf*s230 and *Pf*s48/45. **(A)** Schematic representation of *Pf*s230 constructs and *Pf*s230-*Pf*s48/45 chimera. Each construct contains the SpyCatcher sequence at the N-terminus and a His-tag at the C-terminus. 6-Cys domains are shown as boxes and numbers indicate the number of cysteines. The Pro-domain does not contain cysteines. **(B)** Coomassie blue stained 4–12.5% polyacrylamide gel of conventionally purified *Pf*s230 constructs and immune-purified Pro-6C chimera. Protein was loaded in each lane with (+) or without (–) DTT (10 mM). The sizes (kDa) of the molecular mass markers are indicated. **(C)** Sandwich ELISA of purified Pro-6C chimera. The antigens were captured with mAb45.1 and detected with anti-His-HRP. Immune purified R0.6C were used as a reference. X-axis is shown on a logarithmic scale.

(**Table S1**). Pro-6C was further immune-purified on a mAb 45.1-column to enrich for properly folded protein species (**Figure 1B**). The yield of immune-purified Pro-6C was 15 mg/L, similar to that of R0.6C. Conformational mAb 45.1 against the *Pf*s48/45 epitope I reacted with Pro-6C and this binding was equivalent to that of immune-purified R0.6C, suggesting that they exhibit similar cysteine-connectivity (**Figure 1C**).

Immunogenicity of Soluble *Pf*s48/45 and *Pf*s230 Protein Constructs

Groups of mice were immunized 3 times at 3-week interval with equimolar amounts of Pro-6C and individual *Pf*s230 and *Pf*s48/45 recombinant protein constructs formulated on Alhydrogel®. We used a suboptimal antigen dose to detect differences in immunogenic properties between protein constructs. Chimeric Pro-6C elicited significantly higher levels of gametocyte-specific antibodies than those obtained with the individual Pro domain (Mann-Whitney test, $p = 0.0079$) and levels comparable to those obtained with Pro+I, and R0.6C (**Figure 2A**). We found that levels of specific antibodies against the Pro and 6C domains were similar in mice immunized with Pro-6C compared to mice immunized with the individual Pro and 6C (R0.6C) antigens, suggesting that these domains do not exhibit antigenic competition (**Figures 2B,C**). As expected, levels of *Pf*s230-specific antibodies increased with *Pf*s230 fragment length (**Figure 2C**). The functional activity of vaccine-induced antibodies was determined by testing pooled antisera from each group in serial dilutions in the SMFA. All proteins except the Pro domain, elicited a TB response of >80% at a 1/9 dilution. Interestingly, Pro-6C induced higher levels of functional

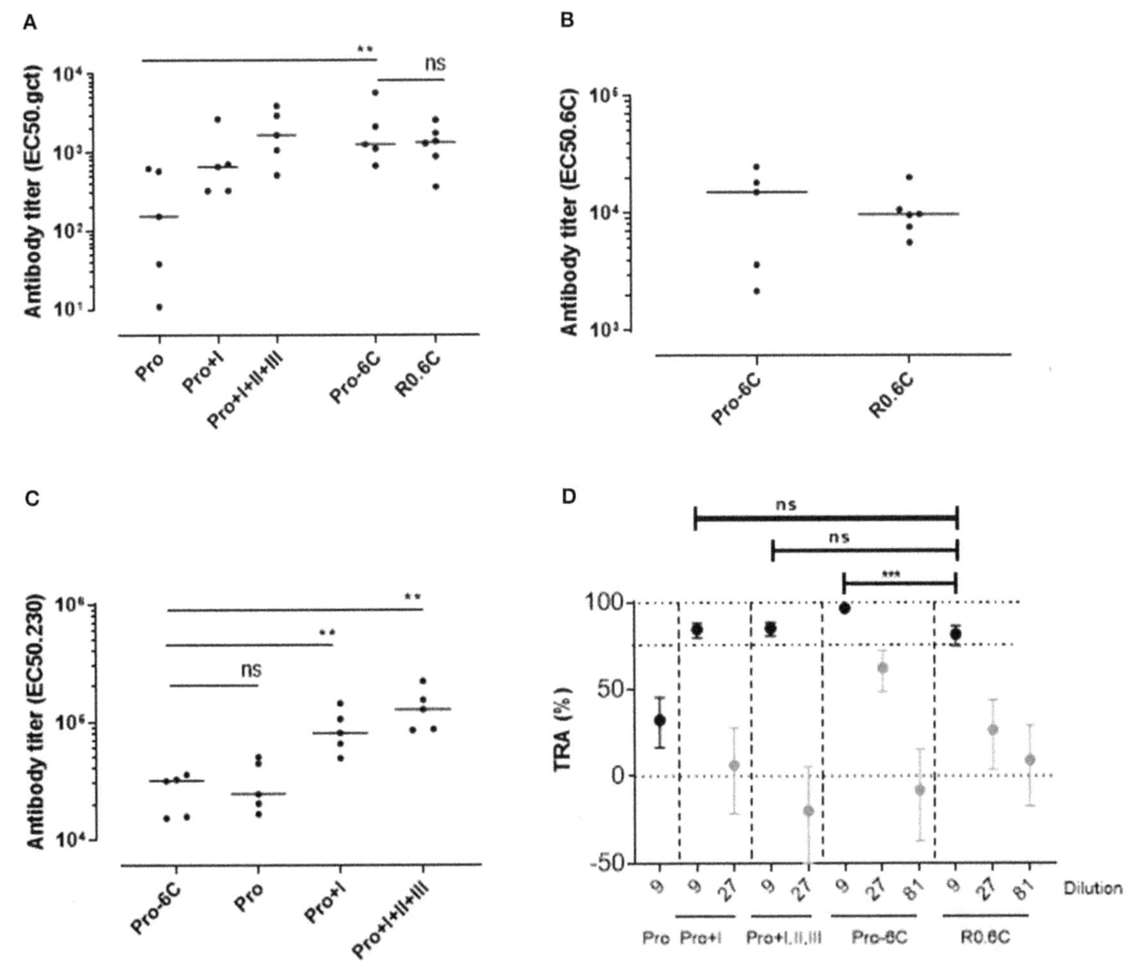

FIGURE 2 | Immunogenicity of Pro-6C and individual fragments. Groups of mice ($n = 5$) were immunized with immune purified Pro-6C in a comparative study with individual Pro, Pro+I, Pro+I,II,III and R0.6C constructs. Day 56 serum was tested for antibody reactivity on ELISA plates coated with **(A)** gametocyte extract, **(B)** *Pf*s48/45-6C or **(C)** *Pf*s230 Pro+I,II,III. Antibody titers (dots represent individual mice) are expressed as EC50 values. Horizontal lines represent median values. The asterisks represent statistical significance determined by Mann-Whitney test (**$p < 0.01$, ns not significant). **(D)** Functional activity of serial dilutions of pooled sera in the SMFA. Transmission reducing activity (TRA) is the reduction of oocyst numbers compared to a serum control. All samples were tested in the presence of active complement. Data points are best estimates of two independent SMFA experiments and error bars represent 95% confidence intervals. Comparison between test samples was done using General Linear Mixed Regression analysis (***$p < 0.005$, ns, not significant).

antibodies than the other recombinant proteins including R0.6C ($p < 0.001$) (**Figure 2D**), supporting further investigation of multi-component *Pf*s230-*Pf*s48/45 vaccines.

Generation of Soluble and VLP-Based Chimeric Constructs

Next, we tested whether the potency of Pro-6C could be further increased by including the first 6-Cys domain of *Pf*s230 (Pro+I-6C) (**Figure 3A**). The Pro+I-6C chimera was purified following the same workflow developed for Pro-6C. The yield of immune-purified Pro+I-6C was 5 mg/L, which was 3-fold lower than that of Pro-6C most likely due to the additional cysteine residues (**Table S1**). The folding of both chimera was similar as determined in the mAb45.1 sandwich ELISA (**Figure 3B**). Disulfide-bonding was confirmed by demonstrating very low levels of free thiol groups (<1%) under native conditions (data not shown). Immune purified Pro-6C and Pro+I-6C eluted as single peaks by analytical size exclusion chromatography demonstrating that they form homogeneous solutions of monomeric protein species (**Figures 3C,D**). Before starting *in vivo* immunogenicity studies with both soluble constructs, we also coupled Pro-6C and Pro+I-6C to virus-like particles (VLPs) to see if this would further increase the immunogenicity of the chimeras. Both Pro-6C and Pro+I-6C contained a SpyCatcher domain allowing covalent coupling to SpyTag-decorated AP205 VLPs (25, 33). Spy-Catcher Pro-6C and Pro+I-6C coupled to SpyTag VLPs efficiently (**Figure 4A**) and properly folded *Pf*s48/45 epitope I was retained during conjugation, as shown by western blot and mAb45.1 sandwich ELISA (**Figures 4A,B**). Both VLPs formed homogenous populations of non-aggregated antigen-VLP complexes as demonstrated by transmission electron microscopy (**Figure 4C**). Furthermore, the VLP-particles displaying Pro-6C and Pro+I-6C demonstrated a low percentage of polydispersity (<16%) measured by dynamic light scattering (DLS) experiments and an average size of 71.8 and 73.7 nm, respectively (**Figure 4D**).

Immunogenicity of Soluble and VLP-Based Chimeric Constructs

The immunogenicity of soluble Pro-6C and Pro+I-6C, and of Pro-6C and Pro+I-6C coupled to VLPs was assessed *in vivo*.

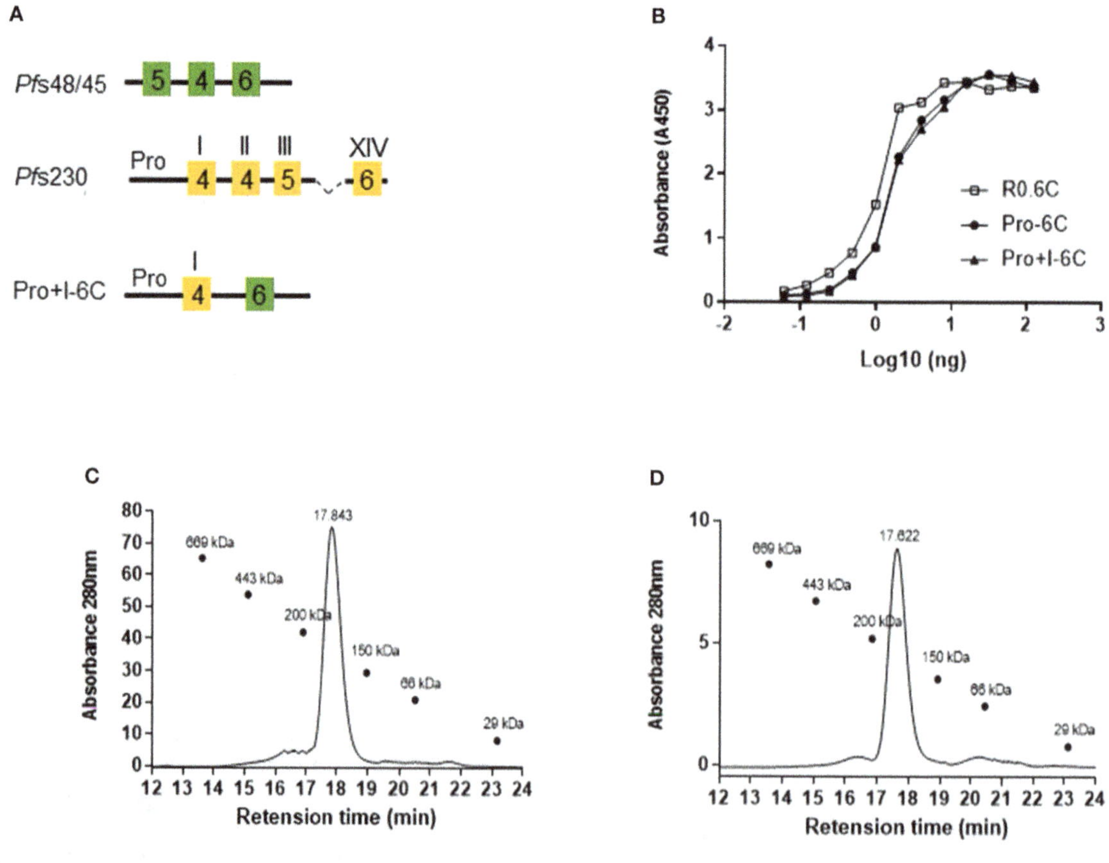

FIGURE 3 | Design and characterization of a multi-domain *Pfs*230-*Pfs*48/45 chimera. **(A)** Schematic representation of the Pro+I-6C chimera. This protein contains the SpyCatcher sequence at the N-terminus and a His-tag at the C-terminus. 6-Cys domains are shown as boxes and numbers indicate the number of cysteines. The Pro-domain does not contain cysteines. **(B)** Sandwich ELISA of purified chimera. Immune purified R0.6C was used as a reference. Size exclusion chromatography analysis of **(C)** Pro-6C and **(D)** Pro+I-6C. SE-HPLC was performed under native conditions in a phosphate buffer of pH 7.2 to determine the amount of monomer in the sample. The sizes (kDa) of the molecular mass markers are indicated.

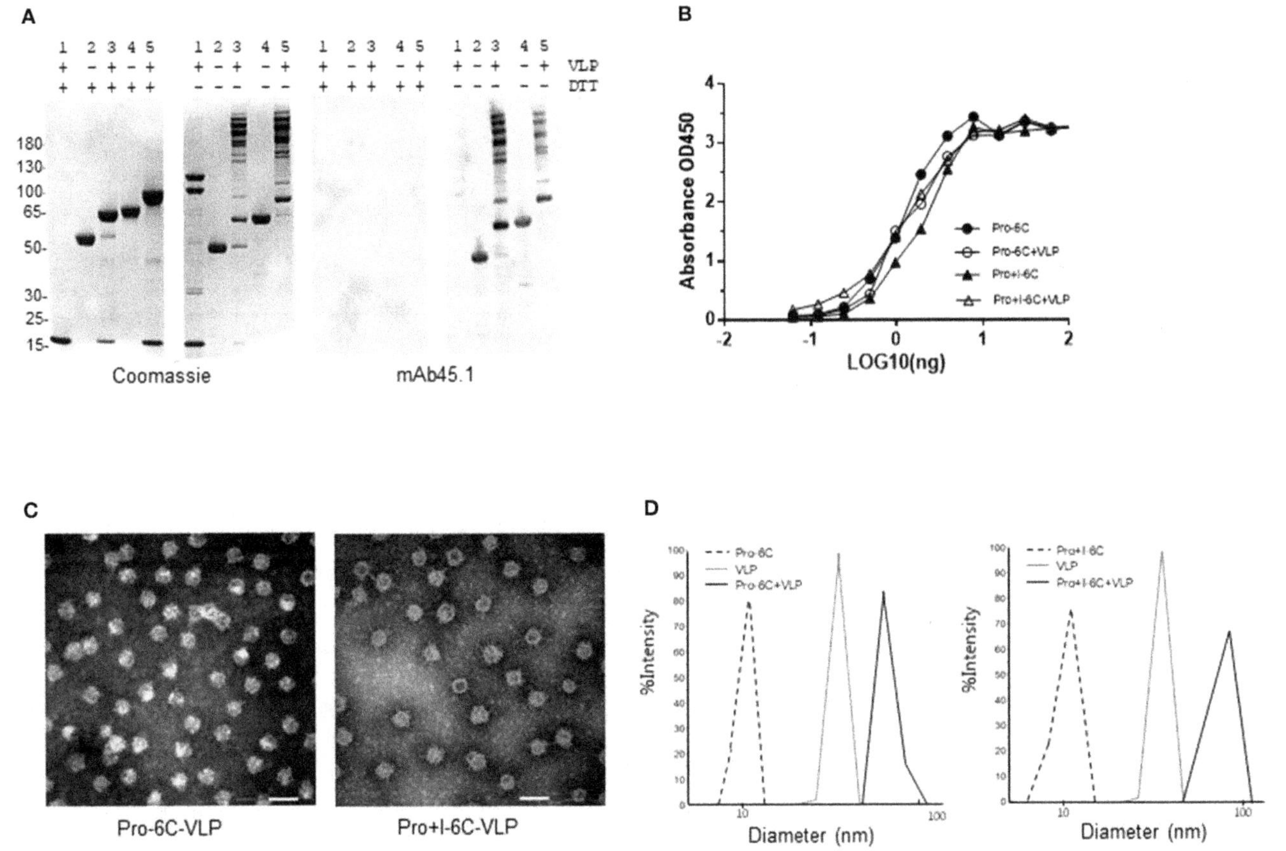

FIGURE 4 | Characterization of virus-like particle-based vaccines. SpyCatcher tagged Pro-6C and Pro+I-6C were mixed with SpyTag-AP205 resulting in a unidirectional display of the chimeras on the VLP surface. **(A)** Reduced and non-reduced SDS-PAGE gel and western blot. The gels (left) are stained with coomassie blue, while the western blots (right) are developed with mAb45.1 as primary antibody. The following was loaded corresponding to the numbers; Lane 1: AP205 (VLP); lane 2: Pro-6C; lane 3: Pro-6C-VLP; lane 4: Pro+I-6C; Lane 5: Pro+I-6C-VLP. **(B)** Sandwich ELISA, using mAb 45.1 as the solid phase capture antibody. **(C)** Transmission electron microscopy images (negative stain) of the VLP-based vaccines after assembly. Both Pro-6C-VLPs and Pro+I-6C-VLPs appear non-aggregated, uniformly dispersed and have an estimated size of 30 nm. Scale bar 100 nm. **(D)** Dynamic light scattering (DLS) profile of the vaccine components Pro-6C [10.5 nm, polydispersity (PD) 10.7%], Pro+I-6C (10.8 nm, PD 20.7%), VLP (25.6 nm, PD 16.8%) and the purified vaccine products; Pro-6C-VLP (71.8 nm, PD 11.5%), and Pro+I-6C-VLP (73.7 nm, PD 15.8%).

Groups of CD-1 mice ($n = 8$) were immunized 3 times at 3-week intervals with equimolar amounts of antigen adjuvanted on Alhydrogel®. Soluble Pro+I-6C elicited significantly (Mann-Whitney test, $p = 0.0079$) higher levels of *Pf*s230-specific responses than soluble Pro-6C (**Figure 5A**). However, this increase was not associated with higher levels of gametocyte-specific antibodies (**Figure 5C**), possibly due to the difference in Pfs230-specific antibody levels being masked by higher 6C-specific signals in the gametocyte ELISA, as observed for single antigen constructs (**Figure 2A**). The functional activity of pooled anti-sera from each group was then tested at serial dilutions in the SMFA. Antibodies against soluble Pro+I-6C promoted higher SMFA activity than antibodies against Pro-6C at a 1/27 dilution ($p < 0.001$) (**Figure 5D**), in line with the SMFA results obtained with the single domain constructs (**Figure 2D**). VLP display did not provide an increase in gametocyte-, *Pf*s48/45-, or *Pf*s230-specific antibodies for both Pro-6C and Pro+I-6C (**Figures 5A–C**). VLP-display of Pro-6C enhanced (Mann-Whitney test, $p < 0.001$) the production of functional antibodies as demonstrated in the SMFA while there was no such effect for Pro+I-6C (**Figure 5D**).

Functional Activity of Domain Specific Antibodies in the SMFA

To investigate the functional activity of domain-specific antibodies, pooled sera from mice immunized with soluble Pro+I-6C (no VLP) were depleted for *Pf*s230- and *Pf*s48/45-specific antibodies using affinity columns with immobilized *Pf*s230 and *Pf*s48/45 respectively, as previously described for human antibodies (13). Antibody depletion was confirmed by ELISA (data not shown). The functional activity of antibody-depleted sera was then tested in the SMFA in 2-fold serial dilutions in the presence of complement. Sera depleted of *Pf*s230-specific or *Pf*s48/45-specific antibodies retained transmission blocking activity at 9- and 18-fold dilutions, respectively, demonstrating that functional antibodies against both proteins are induced by the Pro+I-6C construct

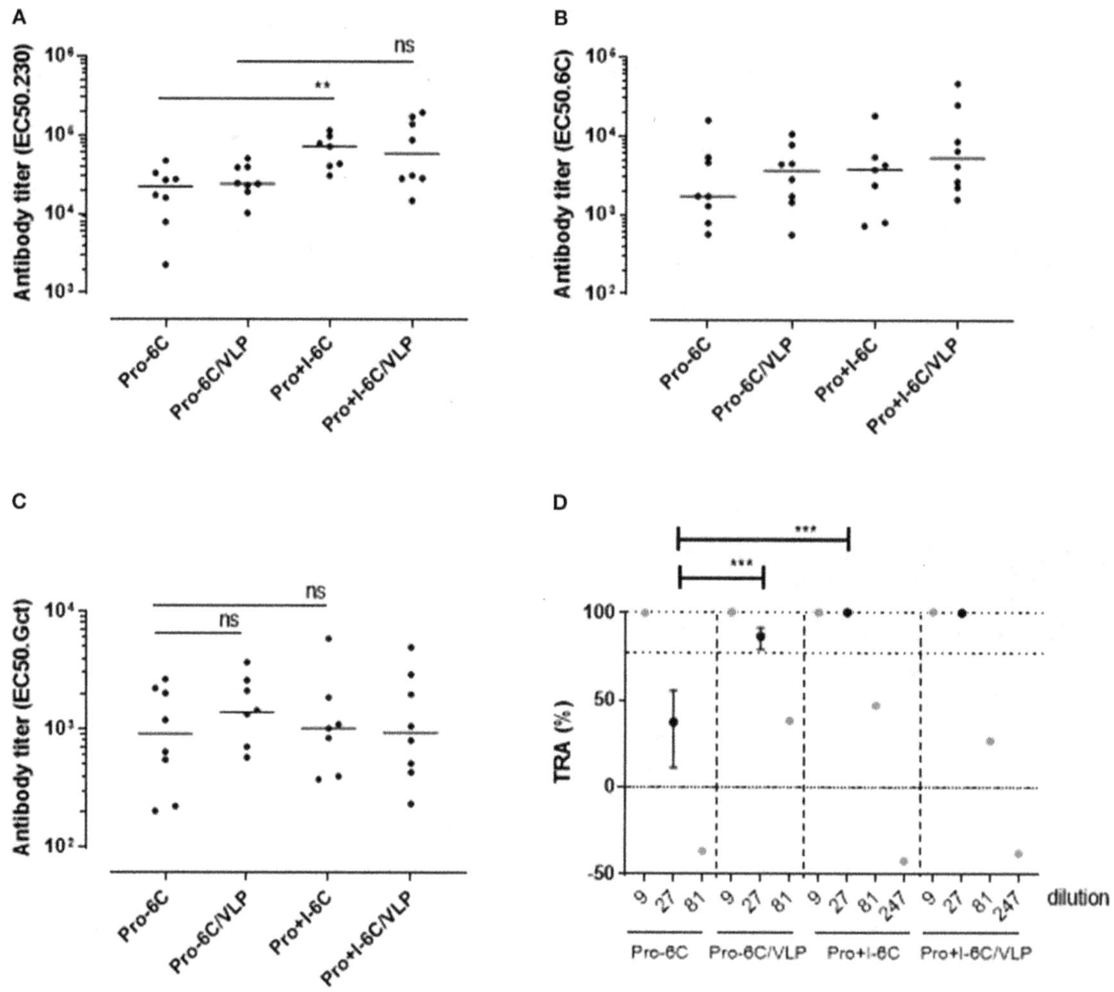

FIGURE 5 | VLP-delivery of Pro-6C and Pro+I-6C. Groups of mice ($n = 8$) were immunized with soluble Pro-6C and Pro+I-6C or bound to AP205. Day 56 serum was tested for antibody reactivity on ELISA plates coated with **(A)** *Pf*s230 Pro+I,II,III **(B)**, *Pf*s48/45-6C or **(C)** gametocyte extract. Antibody titers (dots represents individual mice) are expressed as EC_{50} values. Horizontal lines represent median values. The asterisks represent statistical significance determined by Mann-Whitney test (**$p < 0.01$, ns not significant). **(D)** Functional activities of serial diluted sera were assessed in the SMFA. Transmission reducing activity (TRA) is the reduction of oocyst load compared to a serum control. All samples are tested in the presence of active complement. Data points are best estimates of two independent SMFA experiments and error bars represent 95% confidence intervals. Note that 1/81 and 1/247 samples were tested in SMFA only once and therefore no confidence intervals are given. Comparison between samples was done using General Linear Mixed Regression analysis (***$p < 0.005$, ns, not significant).

(**Figure 6A**). Since the TB activity of *Pf*s230-specific antibodies depends on complement (22), depleted anti-sera were re-tested in SMFA with and without active complement. As expected, *Pf*s230-specific antibodies (Δ6C) lost their functional activity in the absence of active complement (**Figure 6B**). Since complement fixation is dependent on specific antibody subclasses (34), we determined the IgG subclass profile elicited by the Pro+I-6C formulation. The chimera elicited predominantly IgG1 antibodies, and to a lower extent IgG2a and IgG2b antibodies (**Figure S1**). Altogether, these data show that functional antibodies are generated against both domains of the chimeric construct and that *Pf*s230-specific antibodies are complement dependent.

DISCUSSION

*Pf*s230 and *Pf*s48/45 are expressed during the *P. falciparum* sexual stages in humans and elicit antibodies which effectively prevent parasite multiplication in the infected mosquito (13). Promising *Pf*s230- and *Pf*s48/45-based MTBV candidates are currently entering clinical development individually. Here we set out to produce constructs with higher potency and to this end produced and tested chimeric proteins based on both vaccine candidates. To the best of our knowledge, this is the first study that explores a multivalent MTBV based on *Pf*s230 and *Pf*s48/45. Our chimeric proteins induce antibodies that have >80% transmission reducing activity in the SMFA, which is high

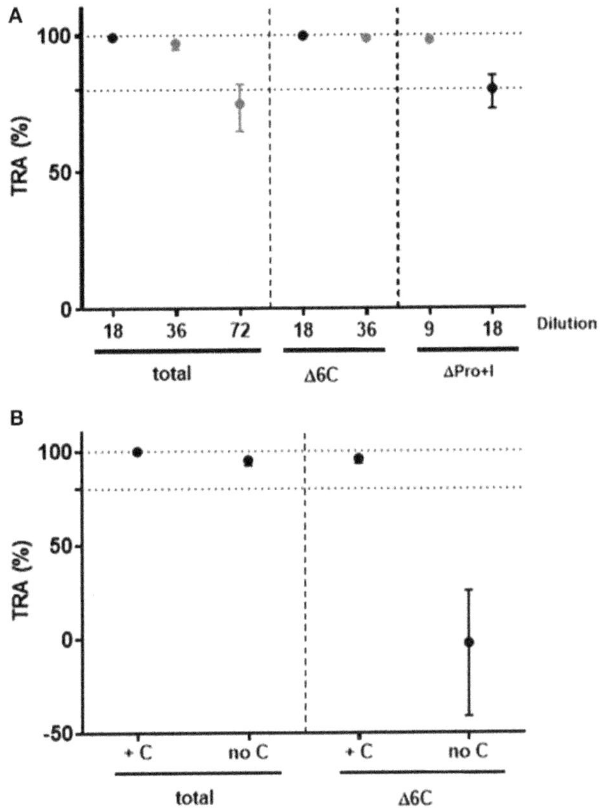

FIGURE 6 | Functional activity of domain-specific antibodies generated by Pro+I-6C. Domain-specific antibodies were depleted from pooled sera of mice immunized with Pro+I-6C, using columns containing *Pf*s230-Pro+I and *Pf*s48/45-10C (13), to generate sera that recognize either 6C or Pro+I respectively. **(A)** Serial dilutions of sera containing Pro+I antibodies only (Δ6C) and sera containing 6C antibodies only (ΔPro+I) were tested in the SMFA, in the presence of active complement. **(B)** Total sera and sera containing Pro+I antibodies only were re-tested with (+C) and without (no C) active complement at a dilution of 1/9. Transmission reducing activity (TRA) is the reduction of oocyst numbers compared to a serum control. Data points are best estimates of two independent SMFA experiments and error bars represent 95% confidence intervals.

enough to meet the no/go decision criterion for selection and further vaccine development (35). Overall, our data show that these chimeric proteins elicited antibodies with higher TB activity in the SMFA than the single proteins alone (**Figures 2D, 5D**) and are therefore attractive next generation vaccine candidates.

One concern when generating multivalent vaccines is that one of the components is immunodominant and that responses against the other component are therefore compromised (36, 37). To investigate this we tested specific antibody responses against the individual domains by ELISA and demonstrated that these are not affected when the domains are presented as part of chimeric proteins. Moreover, the depletion experiments showed that antibodies against the Pro+I- and 6C-domains are functional in the SMFA. Interestingly, the Pro+I-6C chimera elicited higher levels of functional *Pf*s230-specific antibodies than the Pro+I domain alone; sera from Pro+I immunized mice showed no TRA in the SMFA at 1/27 dilution, whereas sera depleted of 6C-specific antibodies from mice immunized with Pro+I-6C still retained 99% TRA at 1/36 dilution. This apparent difference was not reflected in levels of specific antibodies detected in the *Pf*s230-ELISA indicating that functional activity in the SMFA is not only dependent on quantity but also the quality of antibodies. Importantly, there was no difference in levels of functional antibodies against the *Pf*s48/45-6C-domain when comparing Pro+I-6C and R0.6C immunized mice suggesting that the increase in functional activity of *Pf*s230-specific antibodies is, at least in part, related to a better presentation of antibody epitopes in the *Pf*s230 domain I of the Pro+I-6C chimera.

Adjuvants with the ability to enhance antigen immunogenicity are critical components of an efficacious subunit vaccine. In the case of chimeras that include *Pf*s230, it is particularly important that vaccination elicit antibodies with complement-fixing activity. Here we show that Pro+I-6C formulated on Alhydrogel® elicited high levels of IgG1 antibodies, but also Pro+I specific IgG2a and IgG2b antibodies in mice. Murine IgG2a and IgG2b are subclasses of IgG that bind with high affinity to human complement (34). The activation of complement may subsequently trigger lysis of gametes in the infected mosquito (22). It remains to be determined whether the Pro+I-6C chimera may also elicit complement-fixing antibodies in humans.

Both *Pf*s230- and *Pf*s48/45-based vaccine constructs are rich in cysteine and proper disulfide bond formation is critical for functional antibody responses (22, 38). Therefore, successful construction and production of chimeric proteins depend on the maintenance of conformational integrity of immunologically relevant regions of the individual domains. The mAb45.1 is a conformational mAb (2) that reacts with properly folded *Pf*s48/45 but not disulphide reduced *Pf*s48/45 (38). Its reactivity with the fusion proteins indicate proper cysteine connectivity of the *Pf*s48/45 domain. Accordingly, our results from ELISA and immunoblotting analysis showed that the purified chimeras expressed in *L. lactis* were strongly recognized by mAb45.1 and had thus retained conformational epitope I in the *Pf*s48/45-6C domain. It was particularly encouraging that recombinant Pro+I-6C reacted with mAb45.1 since *Pf*s230 domain I contains four cysteine residues which may potentially interfere with disulfide bonding of the *Pf*s48/45-6C domain. While disulphide bond studies have not been completed on the two chimera, the positive reactivity with mAb45.1, indicate that the *Pf*s230 sequence does not disrupt the proper disulphide formation of the *Pf*s48/45 6C domain contained within. Correct folding was further supported by antibody depletion experiments showing that both domains of the chimeras elicited functional antibodies. The data thus demonstrate that *L. lactis* is not only suitable for expression of *Pf*s48/45 fragments (19), but also for *Pf*s230 fragments and fusions thereof. The immune purification of the two chimeras used here is not compliant with cGMP manufacturing since a monoclonal antibody of rat origin was used. However, a purification process based on conventional chromatographic procedures is currently being developed. Although yields and purity remain to be determined, it is likely that high product yields can be obtained through upscaling the fermentation process which is straightforward since there is no requirement for oxygen and vigorous stirring during fermentation (39). Additionally, yields of properly folded protein species may also be increased through protein refolding processes as those developed for R0.6C (20).

In conclusion, we have produced two chimeras composed of leading vaccine candidates against the transmission stages of *P. falciparum*. Both chimera elicited high levels of functional antibodies in rodents and outperformed the corresponding individual protein fragments. Previously, rodents have been immunized with *Pf*s25 administered together with either *Pf*s28 or *Pf*s230C (40). In contrast to our findings for Pfs48/45-Pfs230 chimeras, the *Pf*s25-based dual-antigen vaccines did not elicit higher levels of functional antibodies than the corresponding single antigen vaccines (40). Together these data demonstrate that additive effects can only be achieved for certain antigen combinations. Our results do not only support the use of chimeric proteins for MTBV development but also for malaria vaccine development in general (26, 28, 41, 42). Another advantage of multi-component vaccines is that the production of antibodies against multiple antigens might help reduce the spread of potential escape mutants in the population. Such escape mutants may compromise overall vaccine efficacy as exemplified with the RTS,S malaria vaccine (43). This multivalent strategy is thus conceptually attractive and will constitute a novel means toward control and eventually eradication of malaria once clinical efficacy has been demonstrated.

ETHICS STATEMENT

The animal studies were approved by the Danish Animal Experiments Inspectorate. Approval number: 2013-15-2934-00902/BES.

AUTHOR CONTRIBUTIONS

SS, ST, BC, KT, RS, WG, G-JvG, MvdV-B, and MJ: performed the experiments. ST, MN, AS, and AFS: designed the VLP constructs. SS, MT, and MJ: designed the experiments. MT, MJ, and RWS: wrote the manuscript. All authors reviewed the manuscript.

FUNDING

This work was supported by the Danish Ministry of Foreign Affairs (DFC file no.14-P01-GHA), the Danish Council for Strategic research (grant 13127) and by the European Union's Horizon 2020 research and innovation program under grant agreement No. 733273. The funders had no role in the study design, data collection and analysis, decision to publish, or preparation of the manuscript.

ACKNOWLEDGMENTS

The authors would like to thank Tenna Jensen and Magnus Friis Søndergaard for technical assistance with protein purification and characterization and Laura Pelser, Jolanda Klaassen, Astrid Pouwelsen, and Jacqueline Kuhnen for mosquito infection and dissection work.

SUPPLEMENTARY MATERIAL

Figure S1 | Subclass-specific antibody responses in mice immunized with Pro+I-6C. Day 56 sera were tested for antibody reactivity on ELISA plates coated **(A)** Pro+I or **(B)** 6C. Results for individual mice are shown, and a horizontal bar represents each median value.

Figure S2 | Pre-immune mouse serum contains low intrinsic TRA. Pooled mouse serum from each group was tested at 1/9 dilution in a single SMFA experiment. TRA is the reduction of oocyst numbers compared to a serum control. Error bars represent 95% confidence intervals. TRA values below 50% have large confidence intervals and this can explain the observed variation between different groups. The mean TRA of all groups is 21% (CIs: 5.7–34.1%) demonstrating that mouse serum has low intrinsic TRA.

Table S1 | Production and quantification of *Pf*s230 and *Pf*s230/*Pf*s48/45 chimeric protein in *L. lactis*.

REFERENCES

1. Carter R, Transmission blocking malaria vaccines. *Vaccine.* (2001) 19:2309–14. doi: 10.1016/S0264-410X(00)00521-1
2. Vermeulen AN, Ponnudurai T, Beckers PJ, Verhave JP, Smits MA, Meuwissen JH. Sequential expression of antigens on sexual stages of *Plasmodium falciparum* accessible to transmission-blocking antibodies in the mosquito. *J Exp Med.* (1985) 162:1460–76. doi: 10.1084/jem.162.5.1460
3. Vermeulen AN, Roeffen WF, Henderik JB, Ponnudurai T, Beckers PJ, Meuwissen JH. *Plasmodium falciparum* transmission blocking monoclonal antibodies recognize monovalently expressed epitopes. *Dev Biol Stand.* (1985) 62:91–7.
4. Nikolaeva D, Draper SJ, Biswas S. Toward the development of effective transmission-blocking vaccines for malaria. *Expert Rev Vaccines.* (2015) 14:653–80. doi: 10.1586/14760584.2015.993383
5. Kocken CH, Jansen J, Kaan AM, Beckers PJ, Ponnudurai T, Kaslow DC, et al. Cloning and expression of the gene coding for the transmission blocking target antigen *Pf*s48/45 of *Plasmodium falciparum*. *Mol Biochem Parasitol.* (1993) 61:59–68. doi: 10.1016/0166-6851(93)90158-T
6. Kumar N. Target antigens of malaria transmission blocking immunity exist as a stable membrane bound complex. *Parasite Immunol.* (1987) 9:321–35. doi: 10.1111/j.1365-3024.1987.tb00511.x
7. van Dijk MR, Janse CJ, Thompson J, Waters AP, Braks JA, Dodemont HJ, et al. A central role for P48/45 in malaria parasite male gamete fertility. *Cell.* (2001) 104:153–64. doi: 10.1016/S0092-8674(01)00199-4
8. Drakeley CJ, Bousema JT, Akim NI, Teelen K, Roeffen W, Lensen AH, et al. Transmission-reducing immunity is inversely related to age in *Plasmodium falciparum* gametocyte carriers. *Parasite Immunol.* (2006) 28:185–90. doi: 10.1111/j.1365-3024.2005.00818.x

9. Bousema JT, Drakeley CJ, Sauerwein RW. Sexual-stage antibody responses to *P. falciparum* in endemic populations. *Curr Mol Med.* (2006) 6:223–9. doi: 10.2174/156652406776055140
10. Crompton PD, Kayala MA, Traore B, Kayentao K, Ongoiba A, Weiss GE, et al. A prospective analysis of the Ab response to *Plasmodium falciparum* before and after a malaria season by protein microarray. *Proc Natl Acad Sci USA.* (2010) 107:6958–63. doi: 10.1073/pnas.1001323107
11. Theisen M, Jore MM, Sauerwein R. Towards clinical development of a *Pf*s48/45-based transmission blocking malaria vaccine. *Expert Rev Vaccines.* (2017) 16:329–36. doi: 10.1080/14760584.2017.1276833
12. Stone WJ, Dantzler KW, Nilsson SK, Drakeley CJ, Marti M, Bousema T, et al. Naturally acquired immunity to sexual stage *P. falciparum* parasites. *Parasitology.* (2016) 143:187–98. doi: 10.1017/S0031182015001341
13. Stone WJR, Campo JJ, Ouedraogo AL, Meerstein-Kessel L, Morlais I, Da D, et al. Unravelling the immune signature of *Plasmodium falciparum* transmission-reducing immunity. *Nat Commun.* (2018) 9:558. doi: 10.1038/s41467-018-03769-w
14. Carter R, Graves PM, Keister DB, Quakyi IA. Properties of epitopes of *Pf*s 48/45, a target of transmission blocking monoclonal antibodies, on gametes of different isolates of *Plasmodium falciparum. Parasite Immunol.* (1990) 12:587–603. doi: 10.1111/j.1365-3024.1990.tb00990.x
15. Rener J, Graves PM, Carter R, Williams JL, Burkot TR. Target antigens of transmission-blocking immunity on gametes of *Plasmodium falciparum. J Exp Med.* (1983) 158:976–81. doi: 10.1084/jem.158.3.976
16. Ponnudurai T, Lensen AH, Van Gemert GJ, Bensink MP, Bolmer M, Meuwissen JH. Infectivity of cultured *Plasmodium falciparum* gametocytes to mosquitoes. *Parasitology.* (1989) 98(Pt 2):165–73. doi: 10.1017/S0031182000062065
17. Gerloff DL, Creasey A, Maslau S, Carter R. Structural models for the protein family characterized by gamete surface protein Pfs230 of *Plasmodium falciparum. Proc Natl Acad Sci USA.* (2005) 102:13598–603. doi: 10.1073/pnas.0502378102
18. Roeffen W, Teelen K, van As J, vd Vegte-Bolmer M, Eling W, Sauerwein R. *Plasmodium falciparum*: production and characterization of rat monoclonal antibodies specific for the sexual-stage *Pf*s48/45 antigen. *Exp Parasitol.* (2001) 97:45–9. doi: 10.1006/expr.2000.4586
19. Singh SK, Roeffen W, Andersen G, Bousema T, Christiansen M, Sauerwein R, et al. A *Plasmodium falciparum* 48/45 single epitope R0.6C subunit protein elicits high levels of transmission blocking antibodies. *Vaccine.* (2015) 33:1981–6. doi: 10.1016/j.vaccine.2015.02.040
20. Singh SK, Roeffen W, Mistarz UH, Chourasia BK, Yang F, Rand KD, et al. Construct design, production, and characterization of *Plasmodium falciparum* 48/45 R0.6C subunit protein produced in *Lactococcus lactis* as candidate vaccine. *Microbial Cell Factories.* (2017) 16:97. doi: 10.1186/s12934-017-0710-0
21. Williamson KC, Keister DB, Muratova O, Kaslow DC. Recombinant Pfs230, a *Plasmodium falciparum* gametocyte protein, induces antisera that reduce the infectivity of *Plasmodium falciparum* to mosquitoes. *Mol Biochem Parasitol.* (1995) 75:33–42. doi: 10.1016/0166-6851(95)02507-3
22. Read D, Lensen AH, Begarnie S, Haley S, Raza A, Carter R. Transmission-blocking antibodies against multiple, non-variant target epitopes of the *Plasmodium falciparum* gamete surface antigen Pfs230 are all complement-fixing. *Parasite Immunol.* (1994) 16:511–9. doi: 10.1111/j.1365-3024.1994.tb00305.x
23. Tachibana M, Wu Y, Iriko H, Muratova O, MacDonald NJ, Sattabongkot J, et al. N-terminal prodomain of Pfs230 synthesized using a cell-free system is sufficient to induce complement-dependent malaria transmission-blocking activity. *Clin Vaccine Immunol.* (2011) 18:1343–50. doi: 10.1128/CVI.05104-11
24. MacDonald NJ, Nguyen V, Shimp R, Reiter K, Herrera R, Burkhardt M, et al. Structural and immunological characterization of recombinant 6-cysteine domains of the *Plasmodium falciparum* sexual stage protein Pfs230. *J Biol Chem.* (2016) 291:19913–22. doi: 10.1074/jbc.M116.732305
25. Singh SK, Thrane S, Janitzek CM, Nielsen MA, Theander TG, Theisen M, et al. Improving the malaria transmission-blocking activity of a *Plasmodium falciparum* 48/45 based vaccine antigen by SpyTag/SpyCatcher mediated virus-like display. *Vaccine.* (2017) 35:3726–32. doi: 10.1016/j.vaccine.2017.05.054
26. Theisen M, Roeffen W, Singh SK, Andersen G, Amoah L, van de Vegte-Bolmer M, et al. A multi-stage malaria vaccine candidate targeting both transmission and asexual parasite life-cycle stages. *Vaccine.* (2014) 32:2623–30. doi: 10.1016/j.vaccine.2014.03.020
27. Thrane S, Janitzek CM, Matondo S, Resende M, Gustavsson T, de Jongh WA, et al. Bacterial superglue enables easy development of efficient virus-like particle based vaccines. *J Nanobiotechnol.* (2016) 14:30. doi: 10.1186/s12951-016-0181-1
28. Lousada-Dietrich S, Jogdand PS, Jepsen S, Pinto VV, Ditlev SB, Christiansen M, et al. A synthetic TLR4 agonist formulated in an emulsion enhances humoral and Type 1 cellular immune responses against GMZ2–a GLURP-MSP3 fusion protein malaria vaccine candidate. *Vaccine.* (2011) 29:3284–92. doi: 10.1016/j.vaccine.2011.02.022
29. Vos MW, Stone WJ, Koolen KM, van Gemert GJ, van Schaijk B, Leroy D, et al. A semi-automated luminescence based standard membrane feeding assay identifies novel small molecules that inhibit transmission of malaria parasites by mosquitoes. *Sci Rep.* (2015) 5:18704. doi: 10.1038/srep18704
30. Churcher TS, Blagborough AM, Delves M, Ramakrishnan C, Kapulu MC, Williams AR, et al. Measuring the blockade of malaria transmission–an analysis of the standard membrane feeding assay. *Int J Parasitol.* (2012) 42:1037–44. doi: 10.1016/j.ijpara.2012.09.002
31. Bolker BM, Brooks ME, Clark CJ, Geange SW, Poulsen JR, Stevens MH, et al. Generalized linear mixed models: a practical guide for ecology and evolution. *Trends Ecol Evol.* (2009) 24:127–35. doi: 10.1016/j.tree.2008.10.008
32. Farrance CE, Rhee A, Jones RM, Musiychuk K, Shamloul M, Sharma S, et al. A plant-produced Pfs230 vaccine candidate blocks transmission of *Plasmodium falciparum. Clin Vaccine Immunol.* (2011) 18:1351–7. doi: 10.1128/CVI.05105-11
33. Veggiani G, Zakeri B, Howarth M. Superglue from bacteria: unbreakable bridges for protein nanotechnology. *Trends Biotechnol.* (2014) 32:506–12. doi: 10.1016/j.tibtech.2014.08.001
34. Stewart WW, Johnson A, Steward MW, Whaley K, Kerr MA. The activation of C3 and C4 in human serum by immune complexes containing mouse monoclonal antibodies of different isotype and affinity: effects on solubilisation. *Mol Immunol.* (1988) 25:1355–61.
35. Sauerwein RW, Bousema T. Transmission blocking malaria vaccines: assays and candidates in clinical development. *Vaccine.* (2015) 33:7476–82. doi: 10.1016/j.vaccine.2015.08.073
36. Theisen M, Cox G, Hogh B, Jepsen S, Vuust J. Immunogenicity of the *Plasmodium falciparum* glutamate-rich protein expressed by vaccinia virus. *Infect Immun.* (1994) 62:3270–5.
37. Johansson BE, Kilbourne ED. Dissociation of influenza virus hemagglutinin and neuraminidase eliminates their intravirionic antigenic competition. *J Virol.* (1993) 67:5721–3.
38. Outchkourov N, Vermunt A, Jansen J, Kaan A, Roeffen W, Teelen K, et al. Epitope analysis of the malaria surface antigen *pf*s48/45 identifies a subdomain that elicits transmission blocking antibodies. *J Biol Chem.* (2007) 282:17148–56. doi: 10.1074/jbc.M700948200
39. Singh SK, Tiendrebeogo RW, Chourasia BK, Kana IH, Singh S, Theisen M. *Lactococcus lactis* provides an efficient platform for production of disulfide-rich recombinant proteins from *Plasmodium falciparum. Microbial Cell Factories.* (2018) 17:55. doi: 10.1186/s12934-018-0902-2
40. Menon V, Kapulu MC, Taylor I, Jewell K, Li Y, Hill F, et al. Assessment of antibodies induced by multivalent transmission-blocking malaria

vaccines. *Front Immunol.* (2017) 8:1998. doi: 10.3389/fimmu.2017.01998

41. Pan W, Huang D, Zhang Q, Qu L, Zhang D, Zhang X, et al. Fusion of two malaria vaccine candidate antigens enhances product yield, immunogenicity, and antibody-mediated inhibition of parasite growth *in vitro*. *J Immunol.* (2004) 172:6167–74. doi: 10.4049/jimmunol.172.10.6167
42. Kalra A, Edula JR, Gupta PK, Pandey AK, Chauhan VS. Antigenicity of a bacterially expressed triple chimeric antigen of *Plasmodium falciparum* AARP, MSP-311 and MSP-119: PfAMSP-Fu35. *PLoS ONE.* (2016) 11:e0165720. doi: 10.1371/journal.pone.0165720
43. Neafsey DE, Juraska M, Bedford T, Benkeser D, Valim C, Griggs A, et al. Genetic diversity and protective efficacy of the RTS,S/AS01 malaria vaccine. *N Engl J Med.* (2015) 373:2025–37. doi: 10.1056/NEJMoa1505819

13

Dendritic Cell Responses and Function in Malaria

Xi Zen Yap [1,2†‡], Rachel J. Lundie [1,3*†‡], James G. Beeson [1,2,4] and Meredith O'Keeffe [1,3]*

[1] Burnet Institute, Melbourne, VIC, Australia, [2] Department of Medicine, Dentistry, and Health Sciences, The University of Melbourne, Parkville, VIC, Australia, [3] Department of Biochemistry and Molecular Biology, Biomedicine Discovery Institute, Monash University, Clayton, VIC, Australia, [4] Department of Microbiology and Central Clinical School, Monash University, Clayton, VIC, Australia

***Correspondence:**
Xi Zen Yap
zen.yap@radboudumc.nl
Rachel J. Lundie
lundie.r@wehi.edu.au

†These authors have contributed equally to this work

‡Present Address:
Xi Zen Yap,
Radboud University Medical Centre, Nijmegen, Netherlands
Rachel J. Lundie,
The Walter and Eliza Hall Institute of Medical Research, Parkville, VIC, Australia

Malaria remains a serious threat to global health. Sustained malaria control and, eventually, eradication will only be achieved with a broadly effective malaria vaccine. Yet a fundamental lack of knowledge about how antimalarial immunity is acquired has hindered vaccine development efforts to date. Understanding how malaria-causing parasites modulate the host immune system, specifically dendritic cells (DCs), key initiators of adaptive and vaccine antigen-based immune responses, is vital for effective vaccine design. This review comprehensively summarizes how exposure to *Plasmodium* spp. impacts human DC function *in vivo* and *in vitro*. We have highlighted the heterogeneity of the data observed in these studies, compared and critiqued the models used to generate our current understanding of DC function in malaria, and examined the mechanisms by which *Plasmodium* spp. mediate these effects. This review highlights potential research directions which could lead to improved efficacy of existing vaccines, and outlines novel targets for next-generation vaccine strategies to target malaria.

Keywords: dendritic cells, malaria, *Plasmodium falciparum*, *Plasmodium vivax*, vaccines

INTRODUCTION: MALARIA

Malaria remains one of the greatest challenges to public health in the developing world. It is caused by infection with the *Plasmodium* species of Apicomplexans, which have a complex life cycle spanning multiple organ sites (**Figure 1**), facilitated by multiple morphologically and antigenically distinct life stages, and expression of multiple antigens (1–5).

The *Plasmodium* life cycle bridges two hosts: mosquitoes, where sexual replication occurs, and humans, where the parasite undergoes asexual replication. The latter begins when an infected mosquito injects sporozoite-stage parasites from mosquito salivary glands into the skin (**Figure 1**). A small fraction of sporozoites will travel to the liver, where the sporozoite will traverse hepatic tissue until it locates a suitable hepatocyte. The subsequent exoerythrocytic form will release merozoites into the bloodstream upon rupture (6). *Plasmodium vivax* can also enter a dormant liver stage known as the hypnozoite, which can mature and produce merozoites weeks to years after the initial infection (7, 8). Despite being only 1 μm in size, the merozoite expresses a range of parasite proteins that ligate host red blood cell (RBC) ligands to drive invasion. After invasion the merozoite forms a parasitophorous vacuole in host cells, where it begins to mature into a trophozoite (9).

From 18 to 32 h post-invasion, the trophozoite increases DNA replication and metabolic activity. The mid-trophozoite stage exports various parasite proteins, including those crucial to host pathology, such as the *P. falciparum* erythrocyte membrane protein 1 (*Pf*EMP1) (10). At 34 h post-invasion, the parasite becomes a

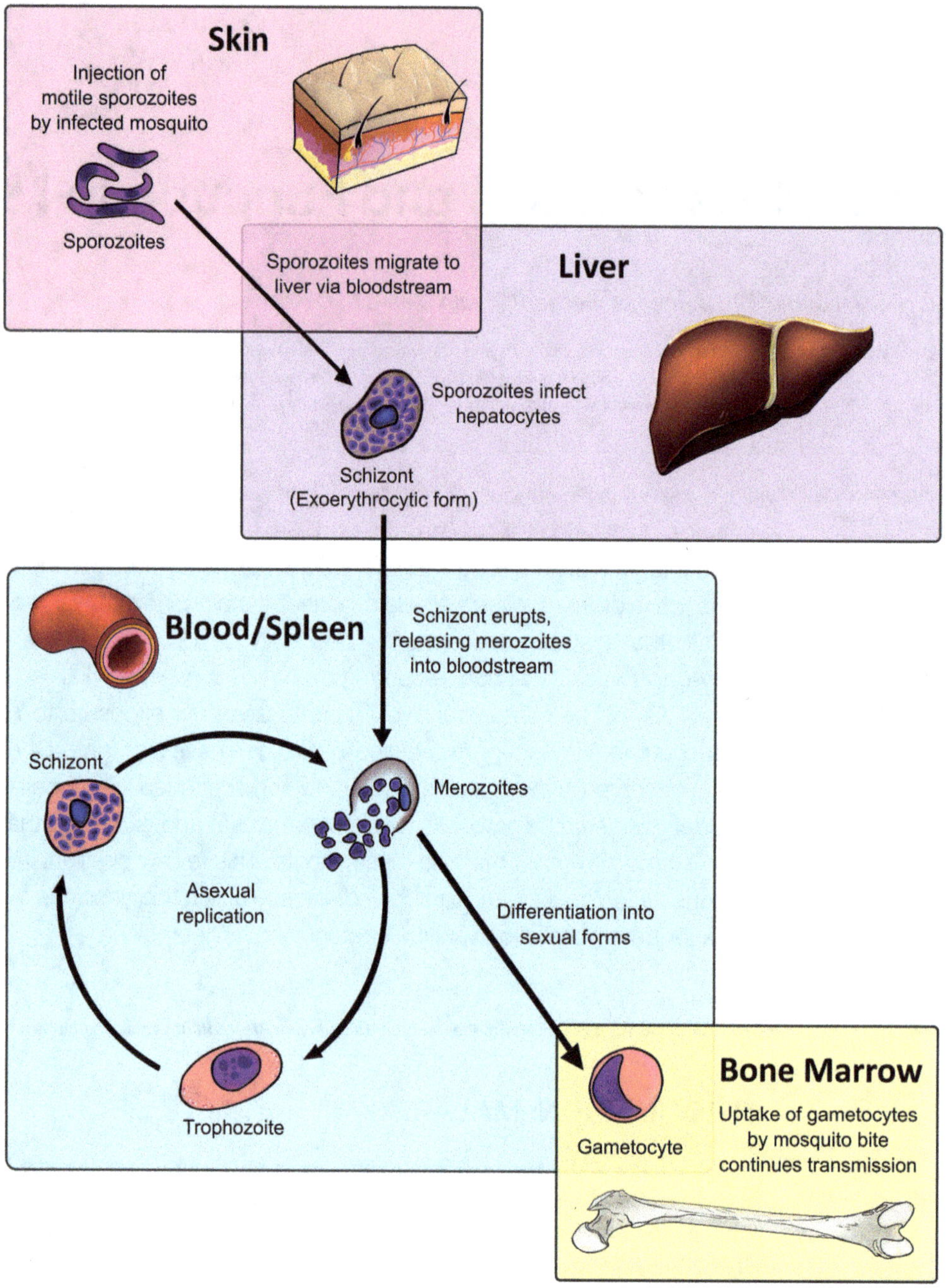

FIGURE 1 | Dendritic cells, located throughout the body at various stages of maturity, interact with all stages of the malaria parasite life cycle within the human host. The *Plasmodium* life cycle encompasses multiple life stages across a range of tissues. The asexual life cycle in the human host begins when mosquitoes inject sporozoites, the highly motile infectious life stage, into the host's skin. The sporozoite migrates to the liver, where it traverses multiple host cells before entering into an exoerythrocytic form. The exoerythrocytic form matures into a multinucleate schizont, which releases merozoites into the bloodstream upon lysis. Merozoites infect host red blood cells and mature into intraerythrocytic life stages known as trophozoites, which are highly metabolically active. After DNA replication the trophozoite will become a blood-stage schizont, which will lyse and release daughter merozoites into the bloodstream, resuming the process. Instead of becoming trophozoites, a fraction of merozoites will instead differentiate into sexual stages known as gametocytes, which sequester in the bone marrow. Only at the end of their maturation process do gametocytes re-enter the bloodstream, where they are taken up by mosquito bite to commence sexual replication in the mosquito host and continue the cycle.

multinucleate, segmented stage known as the schizont. After 48 h of intracellular maturation and replication, the schizont ruptures, destroying the erythrocyte and releasing parasite metabolites, waste products, and between 16 to 32 daughter merozoites are released into the bloodstream (9), where the cycle will begin afresh.

After 7–15 days in circulation, a small proportion of *P. falciparum* trophozoites will commit to sexual replication, where the process of schizogony is replaced by the formation of sexual stages known as gametocytes (11, 12). Generation of *P. vivax* gametocytes is much faster, with gametocytes being detectable in circulation from 3 days post-infection (13, 14). Gametocytes undergo five maturation stages: stages I-IV preferentially sequester in the bone marrow (BM) and spleen (15–17) while stage V gametocytes re-enter the circulation, where they can be taken up by the bite of infected mosquitoes (18).

The effect of each malaria life stage on host immune function is not well understood, nor are the broader underlying mechanisms of antimalarial immunity. It is frequently observed that individuals living in highly endemic regions develop clinical immunity against symptomatic disease, but generally do not develop sterilizing immunity that completely protects against infection. Antibodies are a crucial component of naturally acquired clinical immunity, as passive transfer of immunoglobulins from malaria immune to non-immune individuals is sufficient to reduce parasitaemia and resolve symptoms (19). Furthermore, clinical immunity appears in most cases to be relatively short-lived and broadly declines in the absence of boosting [reviewed in (20)]. An improved understanding of antimalarial immunity will enable development of future vaccines which can accelerate acquisition of clinical immunity, or better yet, induce sterile immunity.

Malaria Vaccines

The most advanced malaria vaccine candidate to date is RTS,S, which targets the circumsporozoite protein (CSP) of *P. falciparum*. RTS,S has shown modest efficacy in Phase III clinical trials, with 29 and 36% efficacy in young infants and young children, respectively over 3–4 years, with a booster dose given at 20 months (21). The sub-optimal efficacy of RTS,S and its failure to elicit protective immunity in many recipients is poorly understood (21–23). To elucidate the immunological responses that future malaria vaccines should aim to induce or improve upon, it is vital to understand how different parasite life stages modulate the host immune system. This review focuses specifically on the interactions between malaria parasites and dendritic cells (DCs), sentinel antigen presenting cells of the immune system that are crucial for generating effective immune responses and immunological memory.

Dendritic Cells

DCs function as a crucial bridge between innate and adaptive immunity. In a healthy individual, DCs constitute only 1% of all peripheral blood mononuclear cells (PBMC) (24–26), yet they exert potent regulatory effects on both the innate and adaptive immune system (**Figure 2**). Upon encountering foreign antigens in the presence of pathogen associated molecular patterns (PAMPs), DCs undergo a process of maturation and migrate to the spleen and draining lymph nodes where they interact with pathogen-specific T cells. In addition to presenting antigen via major histocompatibility complex (MHC) surface molecules, DCs express co-stimulatory molecules required for naïve T cell proliferation and differentiation into effector cells, including CD40, CD80 (B7-1), and CD86 (B7-2). Through secretion of cytokines and chemokines, DCs recruit other immune cells and influence the nature of the adaptive T and B cell response, ultimately leading to clearance of infected cells and extracellular pathogens (**Figure 2**). Crucially, DCs are present at all clinically relevant sites for the development of *Plasmodium* life stages, namely the skin, blood, bone marrow, spleen, and liver (**Figure 1**).

Based on the expression of CD11c and CD123, human DCs can be broadly classified into plasmacytoid DCs (pDC; $Lin^{-}HLA\text{-}DR^{+}CD11c^{-}CD123^{+}$) and conventional DCs (cDC; $Lin^{-}HLA\text{-}DR^{+}CD11c^{+}CD123^{-}$) populations. The pDCs are the body's major producers of the anti-viral interferon (IFN)-α, though they constitute only 0.35% of PBMCs (25, 26). These cells are crucial in antiviral responses. The cDCs specialize in priming and presenting antigen to T cells (27), and constitute 0.6% of PBMCs (25, 26). Using the blood dendritic cell antigen (BDCA) markers, it is possible to further differentiate cDC populations into cDC1 ($BDCA\text{-}3^{+}/CD141^{+}$) and cDC2 ($BDCA\text{-}1^{+}/CD1c^{+}$) subsets, while pDCs express BDCA-2 (CD303) and BDCA-4 (CD304) (28–30).

Given the central role of DCs in sensing infection and orchestrating immune responses, it is not surprising that many pathogens have evolved immune evasion strategies which specifically target DCs in order to interfere with innate and adaptive immune responses (31–34). Thus, understanding how DCs initiate and maintain effective immune responses against malaria parasites, whilst minimizing detrimental and life-threatening immunopathology, is imperative for vaccine development.

AT THE MEETING POINTS: SITES OF DC AND *PLASMODIUM* SPP. INTERACTION

Interactions between DCs and *Plasmodium* parasites occur at every stage of the parasite life cycle within the human host: skin (35), liver (36), and most importantly within the blood and spleen (37), where the majority of host pathology occurs. Recent studies have also revealed that the bone marrow (BM) compartment is a major tissue reservoir for gametocyte development and proliferation of malaria parasites (38–41). Tissue-resident DCs in each of these sites have the potential to endocytose parasite components and initiate the development of specific adaptive immune responses to *Plasmodium* infection. Importantly, DCs in these tissues exist in different maturation states and thus vary in their ability to influence adaptive and innate immune responses and induce inflammatory responses. Within the liver, DCs are thought to induce tolerogenic responses to prevent induction of harmful immunopathology (42, 43), whilst in spleen, DCs propagate strong immune responses, and blood DCs have an intermediate phenotype with a lower capacity for inducing inflammation compared to their splenic counterparts (44).

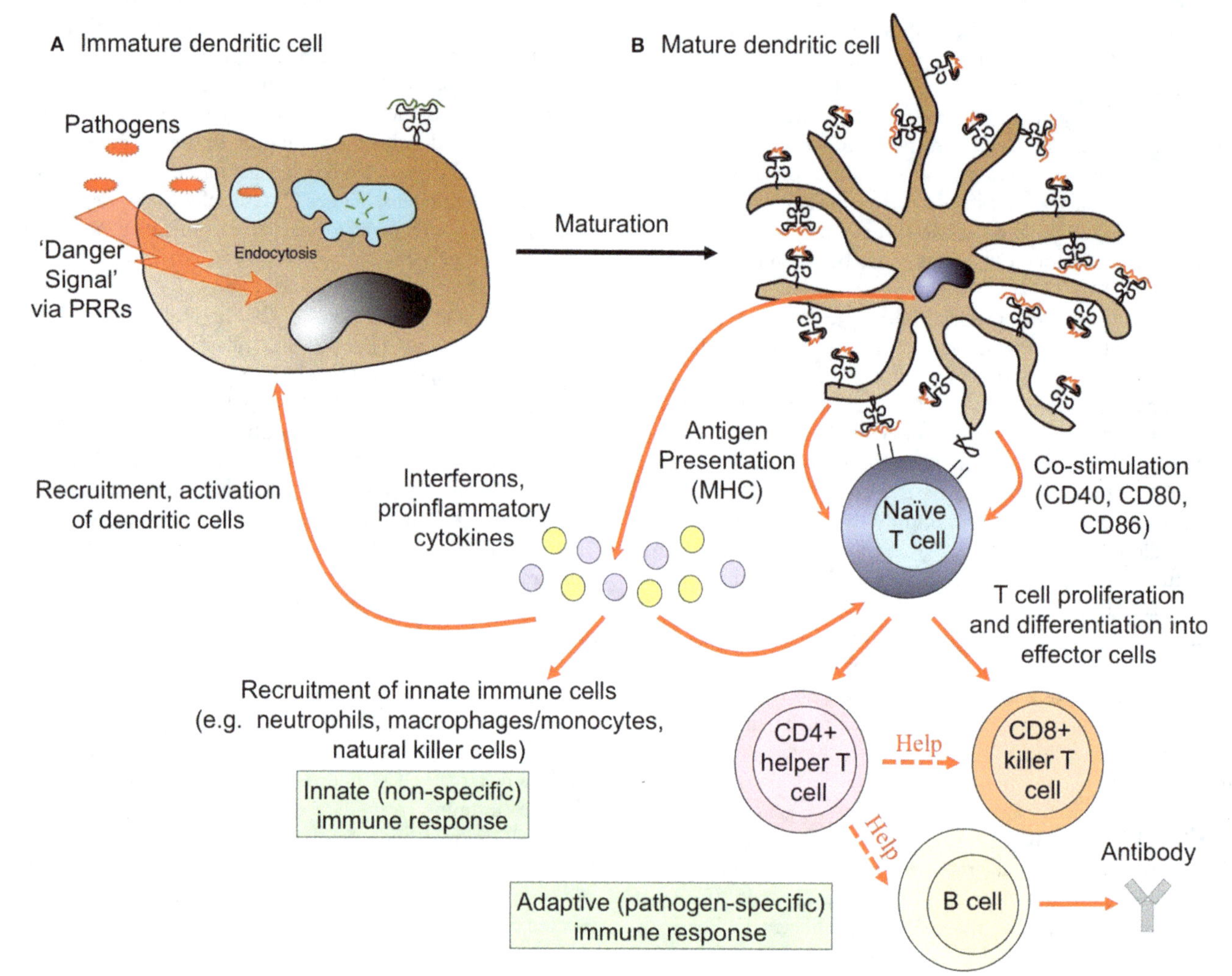

FIGURE 2 | Dendritic cells link innate and adaptive arms of the immune system. **(A)** Uptake of pathogens and recognition of pathogen-associated "danger signals" by pattern recognition receptors (PRRs) triggers dramatic morphological and functional changes in DCs, termed maturation. These changes involve the formation of dendrites, down-regulation of antigen uptake, and redistribution of major histocompatibility complex (MHC) molecules from intracellular endocytic compartments to the cell surface. **(B)** Mature DCs migrate to draining lymph nodes and present information about the invading pathogen in the form of processed peptides loaded onto MHC molecules to naïve T cells. Upregulation of MHC and co-stimulation molecules enables activated DCs to initiate adaptive T and B cell immune responses, the nature of which are determined by the cytokine milieu. This initiates the cascade to an adaptive immune response, leading to clearance of infected cells, and extracellular pathogens. Activated mature DCs also secrete interferons and proinflammatory cytokines that recruit circulating innate immune cells to provide rapid defense against infection.

Skin and Liver DC Interactions With Sporozoites: Lessons From Murine Models

The skin is the site of first contact between DCs and *Plasmodium* spp. Studies in mice have demonstrated that sporozoites remain in the skin for up to 60 min prior to entering the circulation, after which they lose motility (45). Remarkably, up to 50% of sporozoites become trapped in the dermis, while 30% of those that succeed in entering the circulation enter lymphatic rather than blood vessels (45). Thus, the majority of sporozoites fail to reach the bloodstream and are instead phagocytosed by DCs in the skin-draining lymph nodes, which prime protective $CD4^+$ (46–48) and $CD8^+$ T cell responses (49, 50). It is likely that a substantial proportion of immunity to sporozoite stages arises predominantly in response to these "failed" sporozoites.

Interestingly, there is some evidence that sporozoites which arrest within the liver may promote induction of limited liver-stage immunity. A murine study demonstrated that apoptosing hepatocytes infected by irradiated sporozoites triggered recruitment of circulating blood DCs to the liver (51). These DCs phagocytosed apoptotic hepatocytes and migrated to lymph nodes, where they induced protective IFN-γ-producing $CD8^+$ T cell responses (50).

Importantly, in the above study, infiltrating DCs from the cutaneous lymph nodes initiated immune responses, not liver-resident DCs (50). In humans (52) and mice (53), tissue-resident liver DCs are reportedly less mature than blood DCs, as they are poor at antigen processing and express only low levels of costimulatory markers. While liver DCs in humans are capable of inducing allogeneic T cell responses, they are less effective at this than their blood counterparts, and therefore promote a T cell phenotype that is less responsive to subsequent stimulation (52, 54). When considered in conjunction with their high capacity for IL-10 secretion (52), the liver DC phenotype may be one that promotes a more tolerogenic environment, favorable to sporozoite survival. This could partly explain why sterile immunity rarely occurs in response to natural infection, with tolerogenic liver-resident DCs acting to suppress inflammatory responses which would induce protection. Studies using mouse models with humanized livers have shown promise for investigating *Plasmodium* spp. skin-to-liver transfer (55, 56). In combination with FMS-like tyrosine kinase 3 ligand (Flt3-L)-treated cord blood engrafted humanized mice, which produce large quantities of human DCs similar to those seen in blood (57), combined liver-immune system humanized mice could be a useful avenue to investigate DC involvement in liver-stage immunity.

The Bone Marrow As a Reservoir for Gametocytes

A similar phenomenon of immune tolerance may occur in the BM, which emerging evidence suggests is a privileged developmental niche for the transmission stages of *Plasmodium*. Autopsy studies have indicated that both *P. vivax* and *P. falciparum* (15, 58–61) gametocytes sequester in the BM, the latter of which is supported by the presence of a *Pf*EMP1 type capable of binding BM endothelium (62). Poor immune responses to parasites in this milieu may be due to tolerogenic potential of the BM microenvironment. There is very little data on BM DCs. One non-human primate study indicated that BM-derived $CD123^{+}HLA\text{-}DR^{+}$ pDCs had a decreased capacity to express co-stimulatory molecules in response to pathogens relative to blood DCs (63), while $CD11c^{+}$ BM cells in a murine study had a similar capacity for T cell stimulation relative to their blood and spleen counterparts (64). However, it is not clear whether the $CD11c^{+}$ population in the latter study was comprised solely of DCs.

No studies to date have examined how DCs in the BM respond to sequestered parasites, although one murine study has reported that pDCs, present in the BM at frequencies 20 times higher than in the blood or spleen, are the major producers of IFN-α during *P. yoelii 17X YM* infection (65). If the BM is indeed a reservoir for infection, as is suggested by recent primate studies (41), studying whether BM DCs are capable of initiating antimalarial immune responses will be important for achieving elimination.

Blood and Spleen DC Interactions With Malaria Blood-Stages

Blood-stage parasitaemia provides multiple opportunities for blood and splenic DCs to interact with parasites. The parasite spends the majority of the asexual blood-stage cycle within the host RBC. While *P. vivax* exclusively infects reticulocytes, which express surface MHC and can therefore be cleared by $CD8^{+}$ T cells (66), *P. falciparum* also infects mature RBCs, which do not express surface MHC molecules, thus enabling host immune evasion. Despite this, the blood-stage is an antigenically rich phase of the *Plasmodium* life cycle [reviewed in (67, 68)], affecting a large proportion of host cells and triggering potent inflammatory immune responses that cause most of the symptoms of malaria. Maturation of parasitized RBCs (pRBCs) culminates in lysis of the host RBC, releasing merozoites into the circulation. Merozoites that fail to invade a new RBC will remain in the circulation where they are directly phagocytosed (69) or circulate to the spleen for clearance. The *Pf*EMP1 molecule, which is expressed on the pRBC surface, may play a dual role in this life stage. While it is a prime target for antibodies in naturally acquired immunity (70), one report suggests it may also modulate immune function via binding to CD36 on APCs, including DCs (71). Furthermore, *Pf*EMP1-mediated sequestration in the periphery is long held to be a parasite adaptation aimed at avoiding splenic clearance (72).

DCs play a vital role in initiating and regulating adaptive immunity to blood-stage malaria (73–75). However, there is strong evidence that *Plasmodium* parasites modulate DC maturation and function to interfere with the development of protective immune responses. Data from mouse models indicate that blood-stage infection suppresses both existing and developing liver-stage immunity by inhibiting DC activation (76), and inhibits DCs from responding to subsequently encountered pathogens (77–79). Importantly, murine studies suggest that DCs also play a role in the induction of immune-mediated pathology, including the life-threatening syndrome of cerebral malaria (80, 81). Thus, it is of vital importance that we understand the factors governing the ability of DCs to alter the balance between protection and pathology.

DCs, Malaria, and Unanswered Questions

The majority of DC-*Plasmodium* interactions in humans have been studied in two ways: (1) studying peripheral blood DCs from currently or previously infected individuals, or (2) measuring DC responses to parasite stimuli *in vitro*. In the first method, DCs were isolated from the blood of individuals who were naturally or experimentally infected with malaria. The surface phenotype and function of these DCs was compared to uninfected controls, either the same individuals prior to or post-infection, or a matched control group (82–102). In the second method, DCs from malaria-naïve individuals were stimulated with *Plasmodium* products to assess the resulting phenotype. The majority of reports which used the latter generated DCs from monocytes *in vitro* using GM-CSF and IL-4 (71, 103–106), while a minority reported responses from *bona fide* DCs from blood (83, 85, 107, 108).

As such, there is limited knowledge about how naïve DC subsets resident in different human tissues and blood respond to *Plasmodium*, and what factors influence this response. This knowledge is vitally important for designing vaccine strategies which specifically enhance the ability of DCs to induce protective responses while limiting induction of immunopathology. Understanding how naïve DC function is altered by *Plasmodium* exposure will provide insight into how DCs are affected in infected individuals, and therefore what vaccine strategies will be required to overcome this altered phenotype.

PERIPHERAL BLOOD DC RESPONSES TO NATURAL OR EXPERIMENTAL *PLASMODIUM* INFECTION

A total of 24 *ex vivo* studies to date have examined how natural or experimental exposure to *Plasmodium* spp. affects the activation phenotype and function of human peripheral blood DCs, in both acute infection and after prior exposure (summarized in **Table 1**). The following sections analyse these studies in detail, according to species infection.

DC Phenotypes and Responses During *P. falciparum* Infection

Plasmodium falciparum is responsible for a high burden of morbidity and mortality in pregnant women and children, and can cause severe and fatal disease outcomes including cerebral malaria, miscarriage, and multiple organ failure (110). Infected persons typically present to hospital when blood-stage infection becomes symptomatic, which can occur nine to 30 days after the initial infection (111). Classifying malaria cases as mild/uncomplicated vs. severe is based on specific clinical features, including but not limited to coma, haemoglobinuria, vital organ dysfunction, or respiratory distress (110). The majority of *ex vivo* studies have been carried out in settings of high *P. falciparum* transmission, focusing on the phenotype and function of DCs in high-risk groups including children and pregnant women (**Table 1**).

DCs and *P. Falciparum* in Children in High-Transmission Settings

In a DC study comparing infected children to non-infected controls in a holoendemic setting, Kenyan children hospitalized with mild vs. severe malaria exhibited decreased HLA-DR expression on DCs and reduced DC numbers in circulating blood, regardless of disease severity (82). A subsequent study which followed children during malaria and after treatment showed that malaria specifically decreased HLA-DR expression on cDC but not pDC subsets, and reduced the ability of DCs to induce allogeneic T cell proliferation in mixed leucocyte reactions (MLR) (96). Furthermore, infection correlated to an increase in absolute numbers of circulating BDCA-3^+ cDC1s. Importantly, these effects of *P. falciparum* on DC phenotype and function were still observed 14 days after hospital discharge and curative treatment (96), suggesting that malaria-induced immunosuppression can persist for some time after parasite clearance.

A subsequent study was conducted in Mali, another holoendemic setting, where DC function was compared between infected and non-infected children from the Fulani and Dogon ethnic groups. DCs from children aged 2–10 years displayed reduced HLA-DR expression after malaria exposure (100). Infection was also associated with increased proportions of circulating BDCA-2^+ pDC and BDCA-3^+ cDC1 populations, with reduced CD86 expression in the former (100). In this study genetic differences were proposed to play a role in clinical outcomes of *P. falciparum* infection due to differences in cytokine production between the 2 ethnic groups, with PBMCs from Dogon children displaying significantly impaired cytokine production, correlating with more severe fever and higher parasitaemia (100). These responses could be attributed in part to reduced DC function, including a reduction of pDC-derived IFN-α production in response to TLR9 ligands.

More recently, Guermonprez et al. reported that children with malaria, regardless of disease severity, had an increased frequency of the BDCA-3^+ cDC1 population (102). This correlated with increased serum concentrations of the DC growth factor Flt3-L that preferentially increases pDC and cDC1 *in vivo* (112, 113). During malaria, Flt3-L is produced by mast cells in response to uric acid metabolism by *Plasmodium* parasites (102).

Together, these studies suggest that malaria in children in high-transmission settings negatively impacts DC activation marker expression and modulates DC function. The low activation status of peripheral DCs may be due to sequestration of activated DCs in affected tissues. Moreover, an increased number of circulating BDCA-3^+ cDC1s appears to be a common feature of malaria in this setting. Urban et al. also showed that DC dysfunction persisted after the resolution of malaria (96), leaving these individuals vulnerable to co-infections. The apparent contradiction between reduced DC numbers in the first study (82) and elevated numbers of BDCA-3^+ cDC1s in the second study (96) is likely due to more sophisticated gating strategies in the latter, enabling discrimination of individual DC subsets (96), rather than classifying all HLA-DR^+ cells as DCs (82). Rigorous and well-defined flow cytometry gating strategies that use an appropriate combination of antibodies to DC subset-specific surface markers are imperative for DC research and may help to resolve some of the apparent discrepancies in the literature.

DCs and *P. Falciparum* in Pregnancy in High-Transmission Settings

Four studies evaluating changes in DC populations in infection during pregnancy have yielded conflicting results. Two studies, one from Gabon (94) and one from Benin and Tanzania (101), observed that overall DC numbers were decreased in pregnant women infected with *P. falciparum* compared to uninfected matched pregnant controls, while a study from Senegal (97) reported a decrease in the pDC population only relative to non-pregnant uninfected controls. Another study from Benin (109) did not observe any difference in DC numbers between infected and non-infected pregnant women. Changes in surface activation marker expression varied across studies (**Table 1**).

Again, different gating strategies may underlie some of the differences observed between these studies. Simply gating on $CD123^+$ or $CD11c^+$ populations may run a risk of false positives if isolation and lineage staining is not extensive enough. Use of cord blood (94, 97) or placenta-derived (97) DCs may also

TABLE 1 | *In vivo* exposure to *Plasmodium* species modulates human DC responses.

References	Cohort demographic	Transmission intensity (country)	DC subset gating strategy (phenotype)	Changes in surface molecule expression	Serum /plasma cytokines	Other effects
P. falciparum						
Urban et al. (82)	Children	Holoendemic (Kenya)	HLA-DR$^+$, CD83$^+$	Decreased: HLA-DR No change: CD83	Increased: TNF-α IL-10	Decreased DC numbers
Pichyangkul et al. (83)	Hospitalized adults	Mesoendemic (Thailand)	cDC (HLA-DR$^+$CD11c$^+$) pDC (HLA-DR$^+$CD123$^+$)		Increased: IFN-α	Reduced numbers of circulating pDC
Breitling et al. (94)	Pregnant women	Holoendemic (Gabon)	cDC (BDCA1$^+$) pDC (BDCA2$^+$)	No change: HLA-DR*		Decrease in overall DC numbers
Urban et al. (96)	Children	Holoendemic (Kenya)	cDC (CD11c$^+$BDCA1$^+$, CD11c$^+$BDCA3$^+$) pDC (CD123$^+$BDCA2$^+$)	Decreased: HLA-DR (cDC)	Increased: TNF-α IL-10 IL-12	Elevated number of BDCA-3$^+$ cDC1 in circulating blood during and after malaria infection Decreased cDC ability to induce allogeneic T cell proliferation
Diallo et al. (97)	Pregnant women	Hypoendemic (Senegal)	cDC (CD11c$^+$CD123^{lo}) pDC (CD11c$^-$CD123^{hi}) Less differentiated DC (CD11c$^-$CD123^{lo})	No change: CD83* Decreased: HLA-DR*	Increased: TNF-α IFN-γ IL-10	Women who have had malaria have higher percentages of less differentiated DC Decreased circulating pDC in infected pregnant women
Loharungsikul et al. (98)	Hospitalized adults	Mesoendemic (Thailand)	cDC (BDCA1$^+$, BDCA3$^+$) pDC (BDCA2$^+$)	Increased: TLR2 (cDC) Decreased: TLR9 (pDC) No change: TLR4 (cDC)		Decreased fraction of TLR2$^+$ cDC in peripheral blood during infection
Fievet et al. (109)	Pregnant women	Mesoendemic (Benin)	cDC (BDCA1$^+$, BDCA3$^+$) pDC (BDCA2$^+$)	Increased: HLA-DR (BDCA1, BDCA2) No change: CD86* HLA-DR (BDCA3)	No change: TNF-α IFN-γ IL-10 IL-12 IL-6 MIP-1α	Increased percentage of HLA-DR positive BDCA2$^+$ cells during infection Decreased absolute number of all DCs from women with ≥3 pregnancies Increased pDC number in women with ≥3 pregnancies
Gonçalves et al. (99)	Clinic admission	Hypo- to mesoendemic (Brazil)	cDC (HLA-DR$^+$CD11c$^+$) pDC (HLA-DR$^+$CD123$^+$)	No change: CD86*	Increased: IFN-γ TNF-α IL-10	Decreased cDC number Decreased total DC number

(Continued)

TABLE 1 | Continued

References	Cohort demographic	Transmission intensity (country)	DC subset gating strategy (phenotype)	Changes in surface molecule expression	Serum /plasma cytokines	Other effects
Arama et al. (100)	Children	Mesoendemic (Mali)	cDC (HLA-DR$^+$BDCA1$^+$, HLA-DR$^+$BDCA3$^+$, HLA-DR$^+$CD16$^+$) pDC (HLA-DR$^+$BDCA2$^+$)	Decreased: HLA-DR* CD86 (pDC)	Decreased: IFN-γ	Increased BDCA-2$^+$ pDC and BDCA-3$^+$ cDC1 populations in peripheral blood Impairment of TLR signaling in DC during malaria results in more severe clinical symptoms
Ibitokou et al. (101)	Pregnant women	Mesoendemic (Benin) Holoendemic (Tanzania)	cDC (HLA-DR$^+$BDCA1$^+$) pDC (HLA-DR$^+$BDCA2$^+$)	Decreased: HLA-DR (cDC) Increased: CD86 (pDC)		Decreased pDC and cDC fraction in peripheral blood
Guermonprez et al. (102)	Children	Holoendemic (Kenya)	cDC (CD11c$^+$BDCA1$^+$, CD11c$^+$BDCA3$^+$) pDC (CD123$^+$BDCA2$^+$)		Increased: Flt3L	Increased BDCA-3$^+$ cDC1 fraction in peripheral blood Increased CD8$^+$ T cell activation in peripheral blood
Pinzon-Charry et al. (84)	Infected adults	Holoendemic (Papua)	cDC (HLA-DR$^+$CD11c$^+$) pDC (HLA-DR$^+$CD123$^+$) iDC (HLA-DR$^+$CD123$^-$CD11c$^-$)	Decreased: HLA-DR CD83 CD86	Increased: TNF-α IFN-γ IL-2 IL-4 IL-6 IL-10	Decreased pDC and cDC fractions Increased fraction of immature DC Increased DC apoptosis Decreased ability to induce T cell proliferation Decreased antigen uptake
Restimulation of DCs from naturally *P. falciparum*-infected individuals[†]						
Fievet et al. (109)	Pregnant women	Mesoendemic (Benin)	cDC (BDCA1$^+$, BDCA3$^+$) pDC (BDCA2$^+$)	No change: HLA-DR (cDC)	Increased: IFN-γ TNF-α IL-10 No change: IFN-α IL-6 IL-12 MIP-1α	Increased production of proinflammatory cytokines by women ≤25 years independent of gravidity
Götz et al. (85)	Adults	Holoendemic (Mali)	cDC (HLA-DR$^+$BDCA1$^+$, HLA-DR$^+$BDCA3$^+$, HLA-DR$^+$CD16$^+$)	Increased: HLA-DR CD86 No change: CD40 CD80	Increased: CCL2 CXCL9 CXCL10 No change: IL-1β IL-6 IL-10 TNF-α CCL5	

(Continued)

TABLE 1 | Continued

References	Cohort demographic	Transmission intensity (country)	DC subset gating strategy (phenotype)	Changes in surface molecule expression	Serum /plasma cytokines	Other effects
P. vivax						
Jangpatarapongsa et al. (86)	Hospitalized adults	Mesoendemic (Thailand)	cDC (HLA-DR^+CD11c^+) pDC (HLA-DR^+CD123^+)		Increased: IL-10	Decreased fraction of cDC and pDC during infection Increased numbers of $FOXP3^+$ T_{REG} during infection
Gonçalves et al. (99)	Clinic admission	Hypo- to mesoendemic (Brazil)	cDC (HLA-DR^+CD11c^+) pDC (HLA-DR^+CD123^+)	*Decreased*: CD86*	Increased: TNF-α IL-10	Increased pDC fraction Decreased cDC number Decreased total DC number
Pinzon-Charry et al. (84)	Infected adults	Holoendemic (Papua)	cDC (HLA-DR^+CD11c^+) pDC (HLA-DR^+CD123^+) iDC (HLA-$DR^+CD123^-CD11c^-$)	Decreased: HLA-DR CD83 CD86	Increased: TNF-α IFN-γ IL-2 IL-4 IL-6 IL-10	Decreased pDC and cDC fractions Increased fraction of immature DC Increased DC apoptosis Decreased T cell proliferation Decreased antigen uptake
***P. falciparum* and *P. vivax* coinfection**						
Gonçalves et al. (99)	Clinic admission	Hypo- to mesoendemic (Brazil)	cDC (HLA-DR^+CD11c^+) pDC (HLA-DR^+CD123^+)	No change: CD86*	Increased: TNF-α IL-10	Decreased cDC fraction Increased pDC fraction
Kho et al. (87)	Children, adults, hospitalized children, and adults	Holoendemic (Papua)	cDC (HLA-DR^+BDCA1^+, HLA-DR^+BDCA3^+) pDC (HLA-DR^+BDCA2^+)	Increased: HLA-DR* Decreased: HLA-DR (cDC)		Increased pDC fraction during asymptomatic *P. vivax* but not *P. falciparum* infection Decrease in BDCA-1^+ cDC2 fraction during asymptomatic infection with either species or during uncomplicated malaria
Kho et al. (88)	Adults	Holoendemic (Papua)	cDC (HLA-DR^+BDCA1^+, HLA-DR^+BDCA3^+) pDC (HLA-DR^+BDCA2^+)	Decreased: HLA-DR		Decreased numbers of circulating pDC and BDCA-1^+ cDC2 during symptomatic infections but not during subpatent infections Reduced $CD4^+$ T cell proportion Decreased proportion of activated and resting T_{REG}
Controlled human malaria infection with *P. falciparum*						
Woodberry et al. (89)	Healthy adult males	N/A (CHMI)	cDC (HLA-DR^+CD11c^+) pDC (HLA-DR^+CD123^+)	Decreased: HLA-DR (pDC)	No change: TNF-α IL-6 IL-10 IL-12	Increased DC apoptosis Decreased overall DC numbers Decreased phagocytic activity

(Continued)

TABLE 1 | Continued

References	Cohort demographic	Transmission intensity (country)	DC subset gating strategy (phenotype)	Changes in surface molecule expression	Serum /plasma cytokines	Other effects
Teirlinck et al. (90)	Healthy adults	N/A (CHMI)	cDC (HLA-DR$^+$BDCA1$^+$, HLA-DR$^+$BDCA3$^+$) pDC (HLA-DR+BDCA2$^+$) CD16$^+$ DC (HLA-DR$^+$CD16$^+$ CD14$^-$)	Increased: HLA-DR (CD16$^+$, pDC) CD86 (CD16$^+$) CD16 (CD16$^+$, BDCA-1$^+$, pDC) CD1c (CD16$^+$, BDCA-1$^+$, pDC) No change: HLA-DR (cDC) CD86 (cDC, pDC)		Increased expression of BDCA-1 and CD16 on all subsets except BDCA-3$^+$ cDC1 Increased CD1c/BDCA-1 and CD16 expression on monocytes after treatment
Loughland et al. (91)	Healthy adults	N/A (CHMI)	cDC (HLA-DR$^+$CD11c$^+$ BDCA-1$^+$)	Decreased: HLA-DR CD86	Increased: TNF-α No change: IL-12	Increased DC apoptosis Decreased antigen uptake Decreased overall DC numbers
Loughland et al. (92)	Healthy adults	N/A (CHMI)	pDC (HLA-DR$^+$CD11c$^-$CD123$^+$)	Decreased: HLA-DR No change: HLA Class I	No change: TNF-α Increased: IFN-α	Reduced circulating pDC at and 24 h after peak parasitaemia Increased caspase-3 expression in pDCs Increased expression of *NLRC5*, *C14orf119* and *TSG101* Decreased expression of *DMBT1*, *AREGB*, *RNF139*, *CRYM*, and *BAG3*
Loughland et al. (93)	Healthy adults	N/A (CHMI)	CD16$^+$ DC (HLA-DR$^+$CD14$^-$CD11c$^+$BDCA-1$^-$CD16$^+$CD86$^+$)	Decreased: CD16 Increased: HLA-DR CD86	Increased: TNF-α IL-10	Increased proportion of CD16$^+$ DCs among all CD11c$^+$ DCs Non-parasite-specific loss of CD16 when DCs are in culture
Controlled human malaria infection with *P. vivax*						
Woodberry et al. (95)	Healthy adults	N/A (CHMI)	cDC (HLA-DR$^+$CD11c$^+$ BDCA1$^+$, HLA-DR$^+$CD11c$^+$ BDCA3$^+$) pDC (HLA-DR$^+$CD123$^+$) CD16$^+$ DC (HLA-DR$^+$CD11c$^+$ CD16$^+$)	Decreased: HLA-DR (cDC) CD123* No change: HLA-DR (pDC)	Increased: IFN-γ	Reduced circulating pDC, BDCA-1$^+$ and BDCA-3$^+$ DC Increased caspase-3 expression in pDC, CD16$^+$, and BDCA-1$^+$ cDC Increased numbers of activated T_{REG} during infection Increased indoleamine 2,3-dioxygenase metabolism drives T_{REG} differentiation

Transmission intensity, reported intensity of transmission in the catchment area at the time of sample collection; DC subset gating strategy, subsets and markers used to define the subsets which were examined in the study; changes in surface molecule expression, change in activation marker expression after exposure to Plasmodium, relative to healthy controls; serum/plasma cytokines, cytokines assayed for in serum or plasma, change measured relative to healthy controls (no stimulation/no exposure); other effects, other observed changes in cell populations, numbers, or function. *All DC subsets affected. †Surface molecule expression and cytokine secretion for DCs in these studies were measured in supernatants of purified DC cultures after restimulation with pRBCs (85) or TLR ligands (109), as opposed to direct measurement of DC phenotypes from whole blood.*

contribute to phenotypic differences between these DCs and peripheral blood DCs, due to the unique microenvironments of these pregnancy-associated tissues. Gravidity can also be an important contributing factor. Since primigravid women are at the highest risk of severe inflammatory disease [reviewed in (114)], the proportion of women in their first pregnancy should always be accounted for in immunological studies. Inclusion of pregnant non-infected controls is also imperative to determine whether pregnancy itself is a confounding factor affecting DC function during malaria.

Function of DCs From Naturally Exposed Individuals

Three studies of adults with symptomatic malaria carried out in Thailand (98), Brazil (99), and Papua (84) provide insights into how *P. falciparum* immunity develops in lower-transmission settings. Within the Thailand cohort, activation marker expression was not assessed, but circulating numbers of pDCs were significantly reduced in both mild and severe malaria compared to healthy controls. IFN-α levels in the serum increased (83), but it was not established whether this directly correlated with pDC function. The percentage of immature HLA-DR^{+}CD11c^{-}CD123^{-} cells in circulation increased, while the fractions of circulating CD11c^{+} cDCs and CD123^{+} pDCs were decreased. DCs from infected participants were apoptotic (upregulated the apoptotic marker Annexin-V) and were defective at antigen uptake and induction of naïve T cell proliferation in allogeneic T cell activation assays (84). All three cohorts were recruited via clinical admissions, which self-selects for individuals with lower pre-existing immunity and perhaps a more naïve phenotype.

In short, it appears that while impairment is more pronounced in high-transmission settings due to frequent re-infection and higher overall parasite burden, downregulation of DC function is a common feature of malaria. Considering that malaria induces potent inflammation, this DC phenotype may therefore be comparable to what is seen in other inflammatory diseases such as bacterial sepsis (115), HIV (116), or HCV (117). In these patients it is also common to observe reductions in circulating DC numbers (115, 116) and reduced HLA-DR (117) or CD86 (115, 117) expression. Persistent systemic inflammation may therefore explain this reduction in DC function in naturally malaria-infected persons. Again, more rigorous classification of cDC1, cDC2, and pDCs may clarify some of the discrepancies amongst different reports.

Stimulation of DCs From Naturally Exposed Individuals

In a study examining DC responses to TLR stimulation after natural *P. falciparum* infection, DCs from naturally exposed pregnant women in Benin were collected from cord blood (109). Whole PBMC cultures were stimulated with TLR4 ligand LPS, TLR3 ligand polyinosinic:polycytidylic acid (polyI:C), or TLR9 ligand CpG-A ODN to stimulate BDCA-1^{+} cDC2, BDCA-3^{+} cDC1, or pDCs, respectively, due to the high expression of each TLR on these specific DC subsets (118). Synthetic hemozoin prepared from haemin chloride was also used for DC stimulation. There was no difference in HLA-DR expression between infected and non-infected women upon stimulation with either TLR ligands or hemozoin. PBMCs from infected women produced more TNF-α and IL-10 in response to CpG-A stimulation, more IFN-γ in response to polyI:C, and more TNF-α in response to hemozoin relative to non-infected women (109).

Only one study to date has stimulated DCs from naturally exposed individuals using pRBCs (85). DCs were purified from the blood of adults from a highly endemic region in Mali at the end of the transmission season and DC activation was compared to that in naïve controls. All exposed individuals were PCR-negative for infection at the time of enrolment (85). When stimulated with pRBCs at a ratio of 3 pRBCs per DC, DCs from these individuals upregulated expression of HLA-DR and CD86 and expressed CCL2, CXCL9, and CXCL10, but did not produce any IL-1β, IL-6, IL-10, or TNF-α (85). In Section 4, this review outlines how a lack of cytokine secretion is commonly observed in *in vitro* studies of *bona fide* DC, and therefore should not necessarily be considered a sign of DC suppression. However, it is interesting that when DCs isolated from malaria-exposed individuals were stimulated with pRBCs following cessation of high malaria transmission (85), DCs could express an activatory surface phenotype in response to stimulation. Thus, it may be that sustained reductions in transmission allow restoration of DC function.

TLR Modulation in DCs by *P. falciparum*

Only one study to date has investigated the ability of *P. falciparum* to modulate TLR expression on DCs as a potential mechanism of immune suppression (98). In this study, individuals with severe or mild *P. falciparum* infection exhibited increased TLR2 expression on cDCs but decreased TLR9 expression on pDCs, with no observable change in TLR4 expression (98) compared to healthy controls. The severity of infection did not impact these changes in TLR expression. Moreover, the fraction of TLR2^{+} DCs in the periphery decreased during infection (98). TLR2, TLR4, and TLR9 have all been implicated in sensing of *Plasmodium*-derived "danger signals." Namely, TLR2 and TLR4 recognize glycophospholipid (GPI) anchors for merozoite surface proteins (119), and TLR9 detects *Plasmodium* DNA (120). As this is the only study to assess TLR expression profiles during *Plasmodium* infection, it is unclear whether this effect is a common feature of malaria. Nevertheless, it suggests that even low-level *Plasmodium* infections can modulate host responses by downregulating the signals required for APC activation.

The Effects of Natural *P. vivax* Infection on DC Phenotype and Function

Plasmodium vivax is the second major malaria pathogen. It inhabits a broader geographical range than *P. falciparum*, posing a risk to more than 3.2 billion individuals worldwide (121). Its pathogenic potential is enhanced by its ability to become a latent hypnozoite in the liver (7), but as it exclusively infects reticulocytes (122), it is difficult to maintain in culture and remains relatively understudied. Immunity to *P. vivax* has primarily been studied in symptomatic persons who present to healthcare. As the geographical ranges of *P. vivax* and *P. falciparum* transmission overlap, it is often difficult to exclude the immunological impact of prior *P. falciparum* exposure. Nonetheless, it is possible to describe the acute effects of *P. vivax* single-species infection, even though an individual's infection history may be unclear, if diagnosis is sufficiently rigorous. The gold standard for species-specific diagnosis is PCR. However, in resource-poor settings rapid diagnostic tests are typically used.

Due to the paucity of studies from *P. vivax*-exposed individuals it is difficult to conclude the effects of *P. vivax* malaria on DC function. DC numbers decreased during infection, both as a fraction (84, 86) and as total numbers (99). In the latter study, the pDC fraction was increased while cDC numbers decreased (99). Another study observed a decrease in both pDC and cDC fractions, as well as increased DC apoptosis (84). *Plasmodium vivax* malaria has also been reported to down-regulate CD86 expression on DCs (84, 99).

The Effect of Mixed *Plasmodium* Infections on DC Function

Phenotypic analyses of peripheral blood DC from individuals co-infected with two *Plasmodium* spp. support similar reductions in overall DC numbers as seen in individuals experiencing single infections (87, 88, 99). However, it is not yet known whether this correlates to impairments in DC function. A study from Gonçalves et al. in a mesoendemic area of Brazil found that asymptomatic individuals infected with both *P. falciparum* and *P. vivax* had decreased circulating cDCs but increased circulating pDCs (99). Studies in a holoendemic region of Papua found that pDC fractions increased during asymptomatic *P. vivax* but not *P. falciparum* infection, with pDC and BDCA-1$^+$ cDC2 fractions decreasing during acute infection with either species (87, 88). No changes were observed in the BDCA-3$^+$ cDC1 fraction in children or adults during acute or asymptomatic infection with either species (87, 88), in contrast to the findings in African cohorts (96, 100, 102). HLA-DR expression on DCs was increased during asymptomatic *P. vivax* infection (87), but decreased during acute mixed or single-species infections (87, 88).

It is interesting that HLA-DR expression on DCs was positively correlated with parasitaemia in children with asymptomatic *P. vivax* infection, but negatively correlated with parasitaemia in adults with asymptomatic *P. falciparum* infection (87). Thus, it may be that the two major pathogenic *Plasmodium* species polarize the immune system in different ways. This data also suggests fundamental differences in how childrens' and adults' DCs respond to *Plasmodium* exposure—an important factor to keep in mind considering the at-risk populations for either species.

Insights From Controlled Malaria Infection Models

Controlled Human Malaria Infection With *P. falciparum*

The development of a controlled human malaria infection model (CHMI) has produced valuable insights into antimalarial immunity. In one CHMI model which has been used to study DC in malaria, healthy volunteers who are typically malaria-naïve were inoculated with an ultra-low (<180) or low (1,800) dose of *P. falciparum* pRBCs thawed from a pre-prepared biobank. Atovaquone/proguanil or artemether/lumefantrine treatment was administered 6 days post-infection (ultra-low-dose group) or when parasitaemia reached 1,000 parasites per mL (low-dose group). Despite the low parasite biomass of the inoculum in the low-dose group, an estimated 20 times lower than the number of merozoites released from an infected hepatocyte after sporozoite replication (123), DC numbers were significantly decreased in the low-dose group due to increased DC apoptosis (89). Intriguingly, infection-induced apoptosis appeared to be exclusive to HLA-DR$^+$ cells, including DCs. Furthermore, the decrease in DC numbers coincided with the peak of symptomatic malaria, and while cDC numbers recovered to pre-infection levels after drug treatment, pDC numbers remained at 47% of baseline 60 h post-cure (89). HLA-DR expression on pDCs was also impaired. Importantly, DCs from the low-dose group displayed impaired phagocytosis, which persisted for 36 h after drug cure. In contrast, the ultra-low-dose group experienced no symptoms and no DC impairment (89). This study suggests that a certain parasite biomass is required for functional impairment of DCs. However, since the ultra-low-dose group were treated prior to development of symptoms, it is unclear whether an ultra-low dose is sufficient to induce immunity that can control sub-symptomatic parasitaemia, or whether immune impairment would have eventuated if parasitaemia had been allowed to develop.

Function of pDCs and BDCA-1$^+$ cDC2s during CHMI

A second controlled infection study from Loughland et al. utilized a similar low- (1800 pRBCs) and ultra-low (150 pRBCs) dose to more closely study BDCA-1$^+$ cDC2 activation (91) and pDC function (92) after controlled infection. Unlike the prior study, patients were treated upon reaching a parasitaemia of 1000 pRBCs per mL, regardless of initial parasite inoculum. Importantly, both groups experienced a decrease in HLA-DR expression on BDCA-1$^+$ cDC2s that coincided with peak parasitaemia but also persisted 24 h after drug treatment (91). However, only the high-dose group exhibited decreased DC numbers, increased DC apoptosis, and reduced phagocytic capacity relative to baseline (91, 92). A positive association was also observed between phagocytic activity and HLA-DR expression at peak parasitaemia (91).

The ability of DCs to respond to TLR stimulation after exposure to malaria was also evaluated in these studies (91) by restimulating DCs taken from participants during peak parasitaemia. Interestingly, the BDCA-1$^+$ cDC2 from individuals in the high-dose group were impaired in their capacity to upregulate HLA-DR and CD86 in response to stimulation with TLR1/2, TLR4, and TLR7 ligands or whole pRBCs. This impairment was DC-specific, as monocytes' capacity for activation marker expression was unaltered by malaria exposure (91). In contrast, pDCs restimulated with TLR7 and TLR9 ligands upregulated expression of HLA-DR, CD123, and IFN-α, and upregulated CD86 in response to TLR7 stimulation (92). The cDC1 subset was not examined in these studies. These results were similar to TLR stimulations of cord blood

DCs from pregnant women, where CpG-A stimulation of pDCs showed enhancement of cytokine production in infected individuals (109), though caution must be taken when comparing naïve CHMI participants to naturally-exposed pregnant women in Benin.

Together, these studies suggest that a single infection is sufficient to impair cDC function, while pDC function is more resilient. As discussed further on, this highlights a need to further study pDC function during malaria and the potential role of this subset in immunopathology.

CD16$^+$ DC function in CHMI

The CD16$^+$ DC subset's status as a steady-state DC rather than a monocyte subset that acquires DC-like characteristics during inflammation remains unclear (27, 124, 125). Improved strategies for distinguishing "true" CD16$^+$ DCs from CD16$^+$CD14$^-$ monocytes have not yet been established, although a recent single-cell RNAseq study highlighted a population of BDCA-1$^-$BDCA-3$^-$CD16$^+$ cDCs that is transcriptomically distinct from monocytes (126). However, two studies have examined the role of CD16$^+$ "DCs" in malaria, both in CHMI. Both studies observed that relative to pre-CHMI levels HLA-DR and CD86 expression in these DCs increased after curative treatment (90, 93) and 24 h prior to peak parasitaemia (93). At peak parasitaemia CD16$^+$ DCs had an increased ability to spontaneously produce TNF-α, IL-10, and IL-12. CD16$^+$ DCs collected at peak parasitaemia and restimulated with pRBCs expressed higher levels of IL-10 relative to baseline (93). When restimulated with TLR1/2 or TLR4 ligands, these CD16$^+$ DCs produced high levels of TNF-α and moderate amounts of IL-10 and IL-12. When restimulated with TLR7 ligands, the CD16$^+$ DCs produced TNF-α only (93). While caution must be taken in ascribing *bona fide* DC status to the CD16$^+$ DCs, these studies indicate that these cells are activated during infection and in the highly inflammatory environment post-treatment. Their high production of both TNF-α and IL-10, which may aid in killing or suppression of DCs, respectively, suggest that they could be major contributors to DC modulation, including that seen many days post-treatment and clearance of infection (96).

CHMI With *P. vivax*

Due to the technical difficulty of maintaining *P. vivax* in continuous culture, to date only one CHMI has been published using *P. vivax* (95). In this study, peripheral DC numbers were significantly reduced during acute infection relative to baseline, though this was concurrent with an overall reduction in circulating PBMC (95). All subsets (BDCA-3$^+$ cDC1s, BDCA-1$^+$ cDC2s, pDCs, and CD16$^+$ cDCs) upregulated caspase-3 during acute infection and after treatment, suggesting that the reductions in DC numbers in the periphery could also be due to increased apoptosis. Overall, DC impairment by *P. vivax* CHMI was largely similar to what was observed with *P. falciparum* (89, 91); HLA-DR expression on BDCA-1$^+$ cDC was reduced during acute infection and 24 h after treatment (95).

Ex vivo DCs in *Plasmodium* Infection: What Do We Know?

In summary, *Plasmodium* infection can result in reduced DC numbers in the periphery, both as an absolute number (89, 91, 94, 99) and as a proportion of total leucocytes (82, 97, 101), reportedly due to increased DC apoptosis (84, 89, 91). DC capacity for phagocytosing antigen is also decreased (89, 91), which correlates with DC activation (127), yet their ability to induce T cell proliferation in allogeneic T cell stimulation assays is impaired (84, 89, 96). HLA-DR expression is generally decreased (87–89, 91, 92, 95–97, 100, 101), with some variability between DC subsets (**Table 1**). It is not clear whether the reduction in HLA-DR is due to an increase in new immature DCs in the circulation, or direct downregulation by parasites. There is little consensus regarding other markers: reports on CD83 (84, 97) and CD86 expression are contradictory, though CD86 tends to be elevated on pDCs and decreased on DCs as a total population (83, 84, 91, 100, 101).

It is also unclear whether the decrease in the number of circulating DCs is due to cell death, as suggested by the upregulation of caspase-3 (89, 91, 95) or annexin V (84), or due to increased migration to lymphoid tissues. Decreased DC numbers in both natural and experimental infection, however, coincided with increased serum levels of IL-10 (82, 84, 86, 96, 97, 99) and TNF-α (82, 84, 91, 96, 97, 99), indicating a potential cytokine-mediated mechanism of DC loss. One subset in particular defied this trend: proportions of BDCA-3$^+$ cDC1s were increased during *P. falciparum* infection (96, 100, 102), and remained elevated for some time after acute infection (96). The BDCA-3$^+$ cDC1 subset is associated with the initiation of CD8$^+$ killer T cell responses and the secretion of IL-12 (128). It is likely that increases in serum Flt3-L lead to increased numbers of these DC in the periphery during infection, but these circulating DC do not appear to be capable of inducing functional responses. Further complicating the matter, the BDCA-3$^+$ cDC1 subset is not elevated in single or mixed infections from Papua, where transmission intensity is comparable (87, 88).

Overall, the different methods and markers that have been used to study DCs in this variety of settings makes it difficult to clearly define universal parameters of DC loss of function. It is possible that the DC downregulation described in these studies is a feedback loop promoting regulatory mechanisms in the face of severe malaria-induced inflammation, and that DC downregulation in malaria is not necessarily detrimental to host survival. However, the presence of functional DCs is required for effective vaccine responses, and it is still not clear how malaria-induced DC downregulation affects survival to other pathogens. There is an overall need to understand how these DC phenotypes correlate to clinical outcomes, or at minimum, how malaria directly affects DC function. It will be important to clarify whether DC downregulation during natural infection translates to suppression, namely loss of generalized immune function against non-malaria pathogens or inflammatory stimuli.

In light of this, *in vitro* studies of DC function are vital for three purposes: (1) clarifying the phenotype of DC suppression, (2) determining precisely how malaria modulates DC function, and (3) identifying whether this is through direct interaction with DCs or indirectly through soluble mediators, including cytokines such as TNF-α.

DEFINING THE INTERACTIONS BETWEEN DCS AND *PLASMODIUM* SPP. *IN VITRO*

To date, relatively few studies have investigated direct interactions between *Plasmodium* spp. and human DCs *in vitro*. The majority of these studies have examined the responses of human monocyte-derived DCs (moDCs), since they can be easily generated in large numbers from $CD14^+$ PBMCs or BM monocytes by co-culture with GM-CSF ± IL-4 (129, 130). MoDC are themselves heterogeneous and contain cells with a cDC-like phenotype with high expression of MHC class I and II, BDCA-1, CD40, CD80, and CD11c (129), and macrophage-like cells (131). Transcriptomic analysis indicates that moDC are highly distinct from blood $CD16^+$, cDC2 (BDCA-1^+), and cDC1 (BDCA-3^+) cDC subsets and therefore do not accurately represent the diversity of DC populations or their functions *in vivo* (124). Other recent findings indicate that monocyte-derived inflammatory DCs in humans are more similar to macrophages than to *bona fide* DCs [reviewed in (27, 125)]. Thus, moDCs may not be a representative model for investigating *bona fide* human DC responses. These caveats must be considered when interpreting the data from *in vitro* studies (summarized in **Table 2**).

MoDCs and Intracellular *P. falciparum* Blood-Stage Parasites

Initially, *P. falciparum* pRBCs were thought to suppress moDC function *in vitro* (103) as, when co-cultured with moDCs at a concentration of 100 parasites per DC, they impaired moDC activation via contact-dependent CD36-mediated mechanisms (103). In this study, DCs co-incubated with CD36-binding parasite lines displayed decreased expression of co-stimulatory markers CD40, CD54/ICAM-1, CD80, CD83, and CD86 in response to LPS stimulation, and had a low capacity for inducing allogeneic T cell proliferation (103). Co-incubation with non-CD36 binding parasite lines did not induce the same inhibition. However, a subsequent study found that a high ratio of pRBCs to DCs (100:1) inhibited LPS-induced DC maturation, cytokine production, and allogeneic T cell stimulation regardless of whether the parasite strain had a CD36-binding phenotype, and low doses of parasite (10:1) induced modest DC maturation and autologous T cell proliferation (104). This inhibition of LPS-induced DC maturation with high doses of pRBCs was co-incident with high levels of DC death *in vitro* (104).

Another study reported that a ratio of 10 pRBCs per moDC did not trigger upregulation of HLA-DR, CD83, or CCR7 on moDCs (132), contradicting the findings of Elliott et al. (104). However, the 100:1 ratio induced secretion of IL-1β, IL-6, IL-10, TNF-α, and upregulation of the pro-migratory chemokine receptor CXCR4 (132). Another report indicated that even at a ratio of 25 pRBCs per moDC, moDCs upregulated HLA-DR, CD40, CD80, and CD83 and secreted significantly higher levels of TNF-α, IL-6, and IL-10 (105). At higher pRBC-to-DC ratios, there was a corresponding increase in DC death (105).

Addition of CD40L to pRBC-stimulated moDCs enhanced HLA-DR and CD80 expression while CD86 expression was greatly reduced relative to CD40L alone (105). Secretion of TNF-α, IL-12, and IL-6 was also enhanced, while IL-10 secretion was unchanged relative to CD40L alone (105). In another study, exposure to schizont lysate triggered moDCs to upregulate CD86 but not CD80 or HLA-DR (106). These lysate-stimulated moDCs were capable of inducing allogeneic T cell differentiation into T_H1 and regulatory T cells (T_{REG}), both of which secreted high levels of IFN-γ. T_{REG} induced in this fashion also secreted high levels of IL-10 and TGFβ. Pre-incubating moDCs with parasite lysate did not affect their ability to undergo LPS-driven maturation (106). Lastly, moDCs stimulated with whole schizonts did not upregulate HLA-DR, CD80, or CD86, nor did they express cytokines or chemokines (**Table 2**) (85).

One explanation proposed by Elliott et al. (104) for the conflicting literature on the effect of pRBCs on moDC activation is that high ratios of pRBCs suppress DC function, while low ratios activate DCs (104), though in a recent study moDCs were not activated by stimulation with 3 pRBCs per DC (85). Alternately, variations in methodology are likely to contribute to some of the differences observed: different parasite strains and co-culture periods were used across all studies (**Table 2**). Moreover, the heterogeneity of moDC preparations can vary widely amongst different laboratories. Schizont lysate is also not a proxy for pRBCs as the lytic process produces a mixture of parasite membrane proteins, metabolites, and merozoites (107). The matter is further complicated by the multiple ways of defining "inhibition": whether pRBCs truly block DC activation in response to an external stimulus, and which stimuli in particular are susceptible to this manner of inhibition. Alternatively, it must be clarified whether pRBCs induce higher levels of DC death.

In summary, while a dose-dependent relationship between pRBC dose and moDC inhibition is suggested, this relationship must be substantiated by further studies examining the individual roles that different parasite stimuli, strains, and methodological factors have on the final DC phenotype, preferably focusing on *bona fide* DCs in future studies. A more rigorous definition of moDCs and how "activation" and "inhibition" are defined in these cells, particularly given how different groups have used different activatory cytokine stimulation methods to drive DC-like cells to begin with, will be imperative to resolve existing conflicts.

Monocyte-Derived DCs and Other *Plasmodium* Life Stages

Human DC responses to other *Plasmodium* life stages have been poorly investigated. Only one study has investigated moDC responses to *P. falciparum* merozoites (105). In this study, co-incubation with merozoites resulted in moDC secretion of TNF-α, IL-16, and large amounts of IL-10, despite no changes in costimulatory marker expression (105). Co-incubating merozoites with moDCs in the presence of

TABLE 2 | DC responses after *in vitro* exposure to *P. falciparum*.

References	DC type	Parasite strains	Stimulus type	Post-stimulation phenotype	Cytokines detected	Other effects	Proposed mechanism of action
Monocyte-derived DCs*							
Urban et al. (103)	Monocyte-derived	ITO/A4 ITO/C24 MC T9/96	Whole trophozoite	Decreased: CD40 ICAM-1 CD80 CD83 CD86		Suppressed DC ability to induce T cell activation DC suppression mediated by CD36 binding	CD36 ligation by *PfEMP1*
Urban et al, (71)	Monocyte-derived	ITO/C24 MC	Whole trophozoite	Decreased: HLA-DR CD83	Increased: IL-10 TNF-α Decreased: IFN-γ IL-4 IL-12 No change: TGF-β	Suppressed DC ability to induce T cell activation Co-incubation with CD40L does not restore DC function Apoptotic, but not necrotic cells have similar suppressive function	CD36 ligation by *PfEMP1*
Elliott et al, (104)	Monocyte-derived	ItG E8B CS2 3D7/upsCSBP1-KO	Whole trophozoite	Decreased: HLA-DR CD40 CD80 CD83 CD86	Decreased: IL-10 IL-12	pRBC lysate does not suppress LPS-mediated DC activation and can activate DCs High-dose pRBCs induce DC apoptosis Both CSA- and CD36-binding pRBCs inhibit LPS-mediated T cell proliferation	Parasite-to-DC ratio; *PfEMP1*-independent
Mukherjee and Chauhan, (105)	Monocyte-derived	3D7	Whole trophozoite	Increased: HLA-DR CD80 Decreased: CD86	Increased: TNF-α IL-6 IL-12 No change: IL-10	Stimulate CD4$^+$ T cells to produce IFN-γ, IL-5, and IL-10	Phosphorylation of p38MAPK
			Free merozoite	Decreased: HLA-DR CD80 CD83 No change: CD86	Increased: IL-10 Decreased: IL-12 No change: TNF-α IL-6	Decreased phosphorylation of p38MAPK Stimulate CD4$^+$ T cells to produce IL-10, low amounts of IFN-γ	Modulation of IL-10/IL-12 secretion via altering ERK1/2 signaling
Clemente et al. (106)	Monocyte-derived	3D7	Schizont lysate	Increased: CD86 No change: HLA-DR CD80	No change: IL-10 IL-12	Malaria-exposed DCs induce naive T cell differentiation into T_H1 and T_{REG} subsets	

(Continued)

TABLE 2 | Continued

References	DC type	Parasite strains	Stimulus type	Post-stimulation phenotype	Cytokines detected	Other effects	Proposed mechanism of action
Götz et al. (85)	Monocyte-derived	3D7	Intact schizont	No change: HLA-DR CD80 CD86	No change: CCL2 CCL5 CXCL9 CXCL10 IL-1β IL-6 IL-10 TNFα		
***Bona fide* DCs**[†]							
Pichyangkul et al. (83)	Blood pDC (HLA-DR$^+$CD123$^+$)	TM267R GR MRU LA PH	Intact schizont Schizont lysate	Increased: CD86 CCR7 No change: CD40	Increased: IFN-α No change: TNF-α	Schizont-stimulated pDCs can induce γδ T-cell proliferation and IFN-γ production	
Wu et al. (107)	Blood cDC (HLA-DR$^+$BDCA1$^+$) Blood pDC (HLA-DR$^+$BDCA2$^+$)	3D7	Merozoite lysate		Increased: TNF-α IL-12p40 IFN-α	pDC-cDC cross-signaling is required for cytokine secretion by DCs	Cell-to-cell contact between DC subsets and other immune cells
Gowda et al. (108)	Blood cDC (HLA-DR$^+$BDCA1$^+$) Blood pDC (HLA-DR$^+$BDCA4$^+$)	3D7	Intact trophozoite	Increased: CD36	Increased: TNF-α No change: IL-12p40	DCs internalize CD36-binding pRBCs more efficiently	CD36 ligation by *PfEMP1*
Götz et al. (85)	Blood cDC (HLA-DR$^+$BDCA1$^+$) Blood pDC (HLA-DR$^+$BDCA4$^+$)	3D7	Intact schizont Schizont lysate	Increased: HLA-DR CD40 CD80 CD86	Increased: CCL2 CXCL9 CXCL10 IFN-α No change: CCL5 IL-1β IL-6 IL-10 TNF-α	Low ratios of pRBCs do not suppress DC activation by LPS pRBC-primed DCs induce T_H1-like responses pDC-cDC cross-signaling is required for production of IFN-α, CXCL9 and CXCL10	NFκB- and PPARγ-independent

DC type, how DCs used in this study were derived; Parasite strain(s), P. falciparum laboratory strains used for stimulation; Stimulus type, parasite life stage used in this study and whether parasites were purified or processed.
[*]Monocyte-derived DCs, induced by co-incubating adherent precursors from whole blood with IL-4 and GM-CSF for 24 h (129). [†]Bona fide DCs, DCs which have full DC function after purification from donor tissues, without requiring any cytokine maturation.

CD40L induced high CD86 expression but no increase in other costimulatory surface markers (105). CD40L also induced merozoite-stimulated moDCs to produce high levels of IL-10 (105).

Likewise, only a single study to date has assessed moDC responses to *P. vivax* sporozoites (36). Prior to co-culture, moDCs were matured with TNF-α and LPS and primed, or not, with sporozoite extract. Primed moDC were more efficient than their unprimed counterparts at eliciting IFN-γ secretion and autologous T cell proliferation in DC-T cell co-cultures, and $CD8^{+}$ T cells stimulated by primed moDCs had greater cytotoxic effector activity against infected HC04 hepatocyte lines (36). It is not yet known how DCs respond to other liver-stage parasites such as hypnozoites, exo-erythrocytic forms, or sexual-stage gametocytes.

Interactions Between *Bona fide* Human DCs and *P. falciparum*

Due to the technical challenges in obtaining large numbers of viable *bona fide* human DCs from peripheral blood, relatively few studies have investigated direct interactions between *ex vivo* blood DCs from healthy donors and *P. falciparum* merozoites or pRBCs (**Table 2**). To date, studies have focused on $BDCA\text{-}1^{+}$ cDC2 and pDC populations. None have examined the $BDCA\text{-}3^{+}$ cDC1 subset, likely owing to the rarity of this population. Both merozoites and pRBCs have been shown to induce blood DCs to upregulate CD40, CD80, and CD86 (83, 85), and to secrete IFN-α (83, 85, 107), indicating that *P. falciparum* is capable of activating naïve DCs. Merozoites also triggered production of IL-12p40 and TNF-α (107). Additionally, a ratio of 3 pRBCs per DC resulted in upregulation of HLA-DR and increased expression of the chemokines CCL2, CXCL9, and CXCL10 (IP-10) (85), but did not trigger production of IL-1β, IL-6, IL-10, or TNF-α. Contrary to findings in moDCs, pRBCs did not suppress cytokine responses to LPS in *bona fide* DC, although this may be attributable to the lower pRBC-to-DC ratio used in this study (85). While the authors did not assess whether high doses of pRBCs modulated the ability of *bona fide* DCs to prime naïve T cells, as was shown for moDCs, *bona fide* DCs exposed to low doses of pRBCs were fully functional in their antigen presenting ability, inducing naive T cell proliferation and polarization toward an IFN-γ-producing T_H1 phenotype (85). This does suggest, congruent with moDC studies (104, 106) and some CHMI studies (89, 91), that single, low-parasitaemia blood-stage infections of 10 pRBCs per DC or fewer, equivalent to 200 pRBCs/μL, may induce beneficial DC activation.

It is likely that cross-talk between different DC subsets plays an important role in immune responses to *P. falciparum*. Two studies that have examined this process indicate that DC cross-talk is required for production of TNF-α, IL-12p40 (107), IFN-α, CXCL9, and CXCL10 (also known as IP-10) (85) in response to pRBCs. In the context of antimalarial responses, DC activation appears to be contact-mediated and independent of IFN-α, although partially mediated by the TLR9 pathway (85, 107), expressed by just the pDC subset of human DCs. While cDCs alone are sufficient for inducing T cell activation to pRBCs, the presence of pDCs affects the ability of activated T cells to proliferate and produce cytokines (85). When a mixed culture of pDC and cDC was used in pRBC-primed autologous T cell stimulations, T cells trended toward reduced proliferation and production of IL-10, TNF-α, IFN-γ, and IL-5, but increased IL-2 secretion (85). It is possible that since the overall number of DCs for T cell stimulations was kept constant, reduced T cell activation was a consequence of the reduced proportion of cDCs.

These data highlight a need for future studies to investigate not only the individual roles of *bona fide* DC subsets in immunity to malaria, but also to consider the complexity of the immune response and the influence of cell-to-cell interactions. This should be reflected in the establishment of better *in vitro* models and cell-based systems that more realistically mimic the dynamic interactions and cell behaviors that occur over the course of an immune response *in vivo*.

DC Interactions With Parasite by-Products

The cycle of parasite reproduction is fuelled by a range of host nutrients, not least of which is intraerythrocytic hemoglobin. Hemoglobin breakdown causes accumulation of toxic heme, which the parasite neutralizes by aggregating heme crystals into hemozoin (133). Hemozoin has been proposed to have both suppressive and activatory effects on DCs.

Initial studies reported that purified hemozoin induced CD1a, CD80, and CD83 upregulation and IL-12 secretion from moDCs, whereas monomeric heme and synthetic hemozoin (β-hematin) did not (134). However, these results were contradicted by a subsequent study demonstrating impaired upregulation of HLA-DR, CD40, CD80, CD83, ICAM-1, and CD1a in moDCs pre-incubated with *P. falciparum* hemozoin (135). These conflicting results may be due to the use of different hemozoin sources. Depending on the method of purification, parasite hemozoin can be contaminated with parasite proteins, nucleic acids, and other by-products that can activate alternate pathways. It is possible for even purified hemozoin to adhere to environmental contaminants after purification (133). The altered activity of hemozoin on treatment with phospholipase D (135) and DNAse (136) indicate that contamination with nucleic acids or other parasite metabolites is a likely explanation for the observed variations, particularly since hemozoin has been shown to be a carrier for *Plasmodium* DNA (136).

Murine models have been vital in establishing how hemozoin-malaria DNA complexes activate DCs. Murine Flt3-ligand-induced DCs (137) stimulated with hemozoin chelated to *P. falciparum* DNA secreted high levels of RANTES, IL-12, and TNF-α. In this system, hemozoin assisted in trafficking parasite DNA to intracellular endosomes, and activated DCs via a TLR9- and MyD88-dependent signaling pathway (136). Hemozoin in isolation bound strongly to the murine TLR9 ectodomain while β-hematin, a synthetic form of hemozoin, was unable to activate DCs in this study (136). A subsequent study in humans did observe CD80, CD83, and CXCR4 upregulation on human moDCs after β-hematin stimulation (132), but the β-hematin-induced DCs were unable to induce allogeneic T cell proliferation (132).

Uric acid, another toxic product of *P. falciparum* metabolism, has also been found to upregulate expression of CD80, CD86, and CD11c and to downregulate HLA-DR on purified human blood DCs (138). Uric acid also reportedly stimulated mast cells to produce high levels of the DC growth factor Flt3-L in mice (102). Interestingly, DNAse treatment of uric acid abrogated its activatory effects on DCs (138), similar to what is seen with hemozoin. While uric acid is known to drive inflammation during *Plasmodium* infection through activation of the inflammasome [reviewed in (139)], the role of the inflammasome in anti-malaria DC responses and activation has not been investigated.

Together these studies highlight an important role for *P. falciparum* DNA as an activatory ligand, particularly in activating pDCs and driving production of IFN-α (107). Since only the pDC subset in humans expresses TLR9 [reviewed in (140)], ligation of TLR9 by *P. falciparum* DNA and subsequent cytokine production by pDCs may be one of the primary mechanisms by which human DCs are activated by *Plasmodium* (107, 136). Cytoplasmic pattern recognition receptors for *Plasmodium* DNA, which are expressed in all DC subsets, may also play a prominent role in anti-*Plasmodium* interferon responses (141, 142). Of particular interest are the role of STING-dependent responses in DCs and their role in anti-malaria responses. Considering the wide distribution of *Plasmodium* DNA throughout the host during infection (143), the human DC response to malarial DNA *ex vivo* and *in vitro* is one of the key gaps in knowledge that remains unaddressed.

Murine studies have identified a number of other immunostimulatory *Plasmodium* products, but their role in DC activation has not yet been investigated. Glycosylphosphatidylinositol (GPI) molecules, membrane anchors for *Plasmodium* surface proteins, are known ligands for TLR2 (144), expressed on human cDCs (118). Parasite RNA is known to induce type I IFN via TLR7/MyD88-dependent signaling (145), and TLR7 is highly expressed on human pDCs (118), the major producers of type I IFN. Finally, microvesicles are small organelles of 1 μm of less in size, derived by blebbing of the plasma membrane, which are generated in high volumes during *Plasmodium* infection (146, 147). They can contain a range of parasite material, and are able to induce cytokine secretion from murine (148) and human (149) macrophages. In summary, considering the wide range of immunostimulatory molecules produced by *Plasmodium* spp., it remains interesting that the DC response to malaria is not always activatory. While further studies should continue to identify *Plasmodium* ligands that drive DC activation, this must be studied in combination with the factors that underlie DC suppression in malaria.

DCS AND *PLASMODIUM*: OUTSTANDING QUESTIONS AND FUTURE DIRECTIONS

Immunity to *Plasmodium* is complex, and many aspects of cellular immunity remain poorly understood, particularly the impact of malaria on DC function. A better understanding of DC responses to *Plasmodium* will provide insight into the low efficacy and relative short duration of protection of the current malaria vaccine RTS,S, as well as the slow acquisition of natural immunity in malaria-exposed individuals. One of the most important unresolved questions is one of DC "suppression": namely, whether exposure to *Plasmodium* spp., particularly *P. falciparum*, inhibits the ability of DCs to initiate and orchestrate effective immune responses. Determining precisely how DCs are modulated by *P. falciparum* is crucial for understanding the development of immunity to malaria.

Some of the most interesting insights into the effects of malaria-induced DC impairment come from field studies that stratified patients by severity of infection. Studies that analyzed mild vs. severe malaria cases separately did not observe significant differences in DC phenotype between the groups (82, 102), suggesting that there may be a "tipping point" beyond which DC dysfunction is altered regardless of the severity of clinical presentation. This is underscored by the similarities in DC phenotype between natural exposure and CHMI. The latter are a naïve population, but during acute infection and for at least 24 h after treatment they exhibited similar DC phenotypes to those seen in naturally infected cohorts. Repeated infections could lead to sustained downregulation of DC function. Considering that successful induction of vaccine responses requires DC involvement, the failure of multiple malaria vaccines when transitioning from naïve populations to endemic populations (21, 150) may be due to impaired DC function in these endemic populations prior to vaccination.

Some valuable insights could be obtained by investigating differences in DC impairment between asymptomatic and symptomatic malaria cases. The systemic inflammation characteristic of symptomatic malaria undoubtedly contributes to DC dysfunction. While asymptomatic cases seem to experience similar loss of DC function short-term (87, 88, 99), it may be that they exhibit better recovery of DC function long-term. The phenotypic differences between high- and low-dose inoculation cohorts in CHMI studies (89, 91, 92) suggest that administering curative treatment while parasitaemia is still very low is also effective at limiting DC impairment. The similarities between naturally infected cohorts (**Figure 3**) also suggest that transmission intensity does not have a major impact on DC dysfunction beyond a certain threshold. Studies that follow the long-term effects of malaria exposure on DC function will be essential to clarify whether DC impairment persists after malaria elimination, especially in unstable transmission settings.

Variations in methodology have made it difficult to ascertain the effects *Plasmodium* parasites have on DCs *in vitro*. Particularly, care must be taken when stating that *P. falciparum* "suppresses" DC function *in vitro*: levels of activation lower than that seen in response to positive controls is not necessarily indicative of suppression. True suppression should be defined by an inability of DCs to become activated by known activatory stimuli, particularly pattern recognition receptor ligands. Analyses should also always account for increased cell death, which may result in false reports of suppression. Overall, the data indicates that DC function is not universally suppressed (**Figure 3**). Rather, *Plasmodium* appears to target specific pathways, among them the ones crucial for inducing

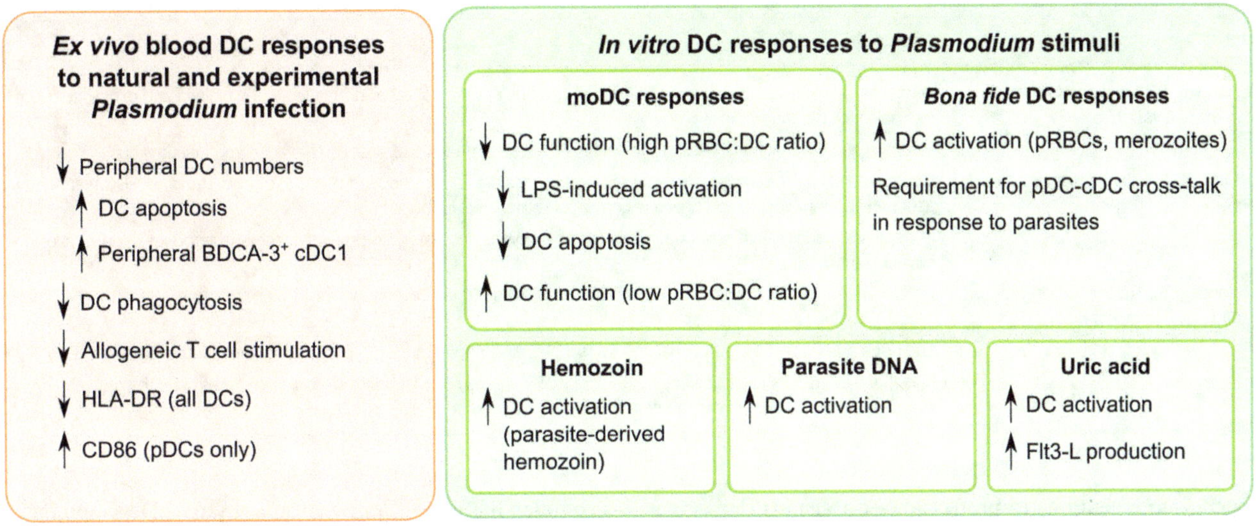

FIGURE 3 | A summary of dendritic cell responses to *Plasmodium*. While the dendritic cell response is heterogeneous, certain trends are evident when examining the entirety of the current literature. Downregulation of dendritic cell function is commonly observed in field studies of infected humans. *In vitro* studies have yielded insight into the complexities of dendritic cell activation by *Plasmodium*, particularly the types of ligands that can trigger an inflammatory response.

naïve T cell proliferation (82, 103, 104), while still allowing DCs to polarize responses toward a T_H1-like phenotype (85, 106). Research into whether the functionality of these T cells is affected relative to other pathogens which induce T_H1 polarization will be important to understand the uniquely *Plasmodium* factors that delay the development of antimalarial immunity.

There also appears to be an important role for DC cross-talk between pDC and cDC subsets (85, 107). This has two crucial implications: first, it warrants further study of how individual DC subsets respond to *Plasmodium* spp. without grouping them into a monolithic conglomeration of HLA-DR^{hi}Lin^{-} cells. In particular, elevation of the circulating BDCA-3^{+} cDC1 subset is a commonly reported phenomenon in field studies but, due to the low frequencies of this rare population, its function in malaria has not been extensively investigated. More rigorous strategies, including cell sorting, should be employed to study how purified subsets respond to malaria. Secondly, pDC cross-talk is essential for production of cytokines such as CXCL10 and IFN-α. CXCL10, also known as IP-10, is majorly implicated in malaria pathogenesis (151–153), and IFN-α has recently been shown to downregulate antimalarial immunity (154, 155). As pDC help is required for production of both of these cytokines, and pDCs are the major producers of IFN-α in malaria (65, 155), strategies to reduce pDC activation in malaria might be beneficial for the longevity of antimalarial immunity. Moreover, malarial DNA has proven to be a potent inflammatory ligand (107, 136), and since only pDCs express TLR9 in humans (118), detection of malarial DNA by pDCs may play a significant role in detrimental cytokine responses, making pDCs an ideal target for strategies to reduce pathogenicity.

Moreover, *ex vivo* and *in vitro* studies depict a complex effect of malaria on the pDC subset. Numbers of circulating pDCs were reduced during natural infection (83, 84, 86, 97, 99) and CHMI (92, 95), though it is unclear whether this is due to pDC death or sequestration. One murine study indicated that pDC could be infected with or endocytose parasites (156). Whether a similar situation exists for human pDC is not known, but it is plausible that large numbers of parasites within pDC could kill these cells, leading to lower circulating numbers. Malaria infection also triggers the upregulation of CCR7 on pDCs (83), suggesting that homing to lymphoid tissues is enhanced during infection. Thus, circulating pDCs may not be the subsets responding to infection, which could explain why pDC activation has not been reported in most field studies. Multiple other factors could also contribute to this perceived lack of pDC activation. Firstly, sustained parasitaemia in malaria-endemic regions may downregulate expression of activatory ligands on circulating pDCs. Secondly, non-conservative gating of pDCs may misrepresent the activation state of this DC population. Thirdly, no field studies to date have measured IFN-α production, which is a direct and functional read-out of pDC activation. *In vitro* studies have observed IFN-α production when pDCs were directly stimulated with parasite products (83, 85, 107). This reinforces the need to study pDC function during malaria to understand whether a loss of pDC numbers in the periphery is associated with a concomitant loss of function.

When interpreting existing literature, it must be kept in mind that the majority of studies have focused on pRBCs and only a minority have examined responses to extracellular forms of the parasite such as merozoites. Considering that DC responses change depending on the parasite life stage (85, 105, 107), even within the relatively limited scope of the blood stages, it will be vital to study the differences between responses to each life stage. Since it is unlikely that a single vaccine will be able to target the entire *Plasmodium* life cycle, understanding the type of responses induced by each life stage is essential for designing new

TABLE 3 | Research priorities in DCs and malaria.

Priority	Approach
Understanding DC functionality to improve malaria vaccines	*In vitro* assays to understand which DC signaling pathways are activated or unaffected by malaria and exploit adjuvant technologies that target these pathways
	Incorporating DC functional assays into vaccine trials as a measure of vaccine relevance and functionality
Correlating DC function in malaria to protection	Controlled human malaria infection studies in naïve and previously exposed cohorts to understand how DC responses are altered by prior exposure and how this correlates with clinical immunity
	In-depth data analyses of how changes in DC phenotypes correlate with protective immune responses and/or overall clinical immunity
Understanding the mechanism of DC modulation by *Plasmodium* spp.	Development of small animal or *in vitro* models to assess human DC responses
	Thorough mapping of the functional and transcriptional changes that DC undergo upon encountering *Plasmodium* spp.
	Measuring DC responses to different *Plasmodium* life stages and determining which life stages have the greatest immunostimulatory potential to facilitate vaccine development

therapeutic interventions to protect the host against damaging immunopathology. A two-pronged "big data" approach could be particularly informative, with the use of RNAseq or proteomics on the DC side to examine immune pathways induced by each parasite life stage, and conversely a proteomics or other—omics-based approach examining the potential immunogens expressed by each parasite life stage. In particular, understanding the pattern recognition receptor signaling pathways which are inhibited or activated by pRBCs would enable more targeted therapies to reverse their suppressive effects. This would inform functional studies, and therefore form a roadmap for vaccine strategies or other therapeutic approaches that could induce potent, long-lasting antimalarial immunity.

A primary caveat of the current literature on human DC responses to malaria, particularly in field studies of infected individuals, is that all studies have looked at circulating blood DCs. It may be that mature DCs migrate into the tissues while immature DCs remain in circulation. Therefore, care should be taken not to generalize the phenotype of these circulating DCs to the responses of liver, spleen or bone marrow tissue-resident DCs, which may have greater functional relevance. Understandably, obtaining tissue-resident cells directly from humans is difficult and ethically challenging. Thus, models such as humanized mice, which produce DCs functionally similar to those found in humans (57, 157), are a promising system to study DCs with a tissue-resident phenotype. While a humanized mouse that is able to support the entire *Plasmodium* life cycle is still out of reach, recent technological improvements have enabled development of models that allow study of immunity to specific life stages [reviewed in (158)]. For example, humanized liver mice could shed light on the elusive phenomenon of liver-stage immunity, while mice with humanized immune systems could provide better insight into cell-mediated mechanisms of protection against the blood stage. Development of a complete humanized mouse model for *Plasmodium* would be invaluable for human immunological research and vaccine development.

Organoids, miniature models of organ function, have proven useful in studying tissues such as the liver (159) and intestine (160). An intestinal organoid model has already been used to study transcriptomic regulation of another Apicomplexan with a complex life cycle, *Cryptosporidium* (161). Development of a splenic organoid could be used for development of functional tissue DCs and enable further study of blood-stage malaria, as well as other blood-borne diseases (162). Liver and skin organoids would also be invaluable for studying the pre-symptomatic phase of the life cycle, and aid development of a vaccine that confers sterile immunity.

Finally, data from *in vitro* studies using moDCs as a model may not be representative of the interactions between *Plasmodium* and steady-state DCs. Both moDCs and *bona fide* DCs show pro- and non-inflammatory responses to *Plasmodium* stimulation, but phenotypic and transcriptomic differences between them highlight that the moDC phenotype is pronouncedly different and may not necessarily be generalizable (125). It was previously thought that moDCs might be analogous to $CD16^+$ DCs. However, recent findings outline that moDCs and $CD16^+$ DCs exist as separate populations in the steady-state (124, 125), and while they may have convergent functions during inflammation, this has not yet been conclusively shown. Therefore, caution should be taken when describing DC-parasite interactions using results generated with moDCs: while it is likely that moDC-like APCs are generated during the course of *Plasmodium* infection, moDCs may not accurately reflect the behavior of steady-state DC populations.

This review has outlined many facets of DC function in malaria that are not well understood (**Table 3**). Firstly, DCs from naïve individuals appear to respond differently to each malaria life stage. These responses should be compared to those seen in exposed individuals for a better understanding of how prolonged malaria exposure affects immune recognition. Secondly, we must further develop an understanding of how the DC phenotypes we observe *ex vivo* and *in vitro* translate into effectiveness, duration, and quality of antimalarial responses. Including DC studies in vaccine trials would help to address which elements best describe a beneficial DC response. This should be supplemented by more studies of DCs in natural infection against comparable non-exposed donors. Thirdly, there is a need for better models to examine DC function in malaria. DC studies of the future should focus as much as possible upon *bona fide* DCs, and seek to develop new models that will permit a more in-depth study of how DC function is altered by the malaria parasite.

To conclude, the complexities of DCs make them a relatively understudied cell type in the context of malaria, where they have a potentially pivotal role in the regulation of antimalarial immunity. Many gaps in knowledge remain to be addressed, and there is a prominent need for novel technologies to bridge the gap. A deeper, more rigorous understanding of how *ex vivo* and *in vitro Plasmodium*-exposed DC phenotypes correlate with effective immunity, and the mechanisms that regulate DC interactions with *Plasmodium* will grant valuable insight into the acquisition of immunity, and form a basis for the development of better vaccines.

AUTHOR CONTRIBUTIONS

XZY wrote the first draft of the manuscript, which was reviewed and edited by RJL, JGB, and MOK. XZY and RJL prepared tables and figures. All authors have read and revised the manuscript.

FUNDING

Funding was provided by NHMRC (Senior Research Fellowships to JGB and MOK; Early Career Fellowship to RJL; Program Grant to JGB; Project grant to MOK). Burnet Institute was supported by the NHMRC Independent Research Institutes Support Scheme and a Victorian State Government Operational Infrastructure Grant. JGB is a member of the Australian Center for Research Excellence in Malaria Elimination (ACREME), funded by the NHMRC.

ACKNOWLEDGMENTS

We would like to thank Ms. G. Stuart for providing graphical elements for **Figure 1**.

REFERENCES

1. Laveran A. *Un Nouveau Parasite Trouvé Dans le Sang de Malades Atteints de Fièvre Palustre: Origine Parasitaire des Accidents de L'impaludisme.* Paris: Bulletins et mémoires de la Société Médicale des Hôpitaux (1881) p. 158–64.
2. Grassi B. *Studi di uno Zoologo Sulla Malaria.* Rome: R. Accademia dei Lincei. (1900). Available online at: https://archive.org/details/studidiunozoolog00gras/page/n8
3. Shortt HE, Garnham PCC. The pre-erythrocytic stage of human malaria, *Plasmodium vivax. Br Med J.* (1948) 1:547.
4. Shortt HE, Fairley NH, Covell G, Shute PG, Garnham PCC. Pre-erythrocytic stage of *Plasmodium falciparum. BMJ.* (1949) 2:1006–1008. doi: 10.1136/bmj.2.4635.1006
5. Florens L, Washburn MP, Raine JD, Anthony RM, Grainger M, Haynes JD, et al. A proteomic view of the *Plasmodium falciparum* life cycle. *Nature.* (2002) 419:520–6. doi: 10.1038/nature01107
6. Bejon P, Andrews L, Andersen RF, Dunachie S, Webster D, Walther M, et al. Calculation of liver-to-blood inocula, parasite growth rates, and preerythrocytic vaccine efficacy, from serial quantitative polymerase chain reaction studies of volunteers challenged with malaria sporozoites. *J Infect Dis.* (2005) 191:619–26. doi: 10.1086/427243
7. Krotoski W. Discovery of the hypnozoite and a new theory of malarial relapse. *Trans R Soc Trop Med Hyg.* (1985) 79:1–11.
8. Mueller I, Galinski MR, Baird JK, Carlton JM, Kochar DK, Alonso PL, et al. Key gaps in the knowledge of *Plasmodium vivax*, a neglected human malaria parasite. *Lancet Infect Dis.* (2009) 9:555–66. doi: 10.1016/S1473-3099(09)70177-X
9. Cowman AF, Crabb BS. Invasion of red blood cells by malaria parasites. *Cell.* (2006) 124:755–66. doi: 10.1016/j.cell.2006.02.006
10. McMillan PJ, Millet C, Batinovic S, Maiorca M, Hanssen E, Kenny S, et al. Spatial and temporal mapping of the PfEMP1 export pathway in *Plasmodium falciparum. Cell Microbiol.* (2013) 15:1401–18. doi: 10.1111/cmi.12125
11. Thomson D. I.-A research into the production, life and death of crescents in malignant tertian malaria, in treated and untreated cases, by an enumerative method. *Ann Trop Med Parasitol.* (1911) 5:57–81. doi: 10.1080/00034983.1911.11686341
12. Day KP, Hayward RE, Dyer M. The biology of *Plasmodium falciparum* transmission stages. *Parasitology.* (1998) 116(Suppl.):S95–109.
13. Boyd M, Kitchen S. On the infectiousness of patients infected with *Plasmodium vivax* and *Plasmodium falciparum. Am J Trop Med Hyg.* (1937) 17:253–62.
14. McKenzie FE, Jeffery GM, Collins WE. Gametocytemia and fever in human malaria infections. *J Parasitol.* (2007) 93:627–33. doi: 10.1645/GE-1052R.1
15. Smalley ME, Abdalla S, Brown J. The distribution of *Plasmodium falciparum* in the peripheral blood and bone marrow of Gambian children. *Trans R Soc Trop Med Hyg.* (1981) 75:103–5.
16. Thomson D. The origin and development of gametes (Crescents) in malignant tertian malaria: some observations on flagellation, etc. *Ann Trop Med Parasitol.* (1914) 8:85–104. doi: 10.1080/00034983.1914.11687643
17. Thomson JG, Robertson A. The structure and development of *plasmodium falciparum* gametocytes in the internal organs and peripheral circulation. *Trans R Soc Trop Med Hyg.* (1935) 29:31–40. doi: 10.1016/S0035-9203(35)90015-3
18. Lensen A, Bril A, van de Vegte M, van Gemert GJ, Eling W, Sauerwein R. *Plasmodium falciparum*: infectivity of cultured, synchronized gametocytes to mosquitoes. *Exp Parasitol.* (1999) 103:101–3. doi: 10.1006/expr.1998.4354
19. Cohen S, McGregor IA, Carrington SP. Gamma-globulin and acquired immunity to human malaria. *Nature.* (1961) 192:733–7. doi: 10.1038/192733a0
20. Fowkes FJI, Boeuf P, Beeson JG. Immunity to malaria in an era of declining malaria transmission. *Parasitology.* (2016) 143:139–53. doi: 10.1017/S0031182015001249
21. Olotu A, Fegan G, Wambua J, Nyangweso G, Leach A, Lievens M, et al. Seven-year efficacy of RTS,S/AS01 malaria vaccine among young African children. *N Engl J Med.* (2016) 374:2519–29. doi: 10.1056/NEJMoa1515257
22. Neafsey DE, Juraska M, Bedford T, Benkeser D, Valim C, Griggs A, et al. Genetic diversity and protective efficacy of the RTS,S/AS01 malaria vaccine. *N Engl J Med.* (2015) 373:2025–37. doi: 10.1056/NEJMoa1505819
23. White MT, Verity R, Griffin JT, Asante KP, Owusu-Agyei S, Greenwood B, et al. Immunogenicity of the RTS,S/AS01 malaria vaccine and implications for duration of vaccine efficacy: Secondary analysis of data from a phase 3 randomised controlled trial. *Lancet Infect Dis.* (2015) 15:1450–8. doi: 10.1016/S1473-3099(15)00239-X
24. Freudenthal PS, Steinman RM. The distinct surface of human blood dendritic cells, as observed after an improved isolation method. *Proc Natl Acad Sci USA.* (1990) 87:7698–702. doi: 10.1073/pnas.87.19.7698
25. Orsini G, Legitimo A, Failli A, Massei F, Biver P, Consolini R. Enumeration of human peripheral blood dendritic cells throughout the life. *Int Immunol.* (2012) 24:347–56. doi: 10.1093/intimm/dxs006
26. Chen XQ, Liu XF, Liu WH, Guo W, Yu Q, Wang CY. Comparative analysis of dendritic cell numbers and subsets between smoking and control subjects in the peripheral blood. *Int J Clin Exp Pathol.* (2013) 6:290–6.
27. Macri C, Pang ES, Patton T, O'Keeffe M. Dendritic cell subsets. *Semin Cell Dev Biol.* (2018) 84:11–21. doi: 10.1016/j.semcdb.2017.12.009

28. Dzionek A, Fuchs A, Schmidt P, Zysk M, Miltenyi S, Buck DW, et al. BDCA-2, BDCA-3, and BDCA-4: three markers for distinct subsets of dendritic cells in human peripheral blood. *J Immunol.* (2000) 165:6037–46. doi: 10.4049/jimmunol.165.11.6037
29. Summers KL, Hock BD, McKenzie JL, Hart DN. Phenotypic characterization of five dendritic cell subsets in human tonsils. *Am J Pathol.* (2001) 159:285–95. doi: 10.1016/S0002-9440(10)61694-X
30. MacDonald KPA, Munster DJ, Clark GJ, Dzionek A, Schmitz J, Hart DNJ, et al. Characterization of human blood dendritic cell subsets. *Blood.* (2002) 100:4512–20. doi: 10.1182/blood-2001-11-0097
31. Hambleton S, Salem S, Bustamante J, Bigley V, Boisson-Dupuis S, Azevedo J, et al. IRF8 mutations and human dendritic-cell immunodeficiency. *N Engl J Med.* (2011) 365:127–38. doi: 10.1056/NEJMoa1100066
32. Meera S, Madhuri T, Manisha G, Ramesh P. Irreversible loss of pDCs by apoptosis during early HIV infection may be a critical determinant of immune dysfunction. *Viral Immunol.* (2010) 23:241–9. doi: 10.1089/vim.2009.0112
33. Ku C-L, von Bernuth H, Picard C, Zhang S-Y, Chang H-H, Yang K, et al. Selective predisposition to bacterial infections in IRAK-4-deficient children: IRAK-4-dependent TLRs are otherwise redundant in protective immunity. *J Exp Med.* (2007) 204:2407–22. doi: 10.1084/jem.20070628
34. Bigley V, Haniffa M, Doulatov S, Wang X-N, Dickinson R, McGovern N, et al. The human syndrome of dendritic cell, monocyte, B and NK lymphoid deficiency. *J Exp Med.* (2011) 208:227–34. doi: 10.1084/jem.20101459
35. da Silva HB, Caetano SS, Monteiro I, Gómez-Conde I, Hanson K, Penha-Gonçalves C, et al. Early skin immunological disturbance after Plasmodium-infected mosquito bites. *Cell Immunol.* (2012) 277:22–32. doi: 10.1016/j.cellimm.2012.06.003
36. Vichchathorn P, Jenwithisuk R, Leelaudomlipi S, Tungpradabkul S, Hongeng S, Cui L, et al. Induction of specific immune responses against the *Plasmodium vivax* liver-stage via *in vitro* activation by dendritic cells. *Parasitol Int.* (2006) 55:187–93. doi: 10.1016/j.parint.2006.04.001
37. Menezes RG, Pant S, Kharoshah MA, Senthilkumaran S, Arun M, Nagesh KR, et al. Autopsy discoveries of death from malaria. *Leg Med.* (2012) 14:111–115. doi: 10.1016/j.legalmed.2012.01.007
38. Farfour E, Charlotte F, Settegrana C, Miyara M, Buffet P. The extravascular compartment of the bone marrow: a niche for *Plasmodium falciparum* gametocyte maturation? *Malar J.* (2012) 11:285. doi: 10.1186/1475-2875-11-285
39. Rogers NJ, Hall BS, Obiero J, Targett G a, Sutherland CJ. A model for sequestration of the transmission stages of *Plasmodium falciparum*: adhesion of gametocyte-infected erythrocytes to human bone marrow cells. *Infect Immun.* (2000) 68:3455–62. doi: 10.1128/IAI.68.6.3455-3462.2000
40. Malleret B, Li A, Zhang R, Tan KSW, Suwanarusk R, Claser C, et al. *Plasmodium vivax*: restricted tropism and rapid remodeling of CD71-positive reticulocytes. *Blood.* (2015) 125:1314–1324. doi: 10.1182/blood-2014-08-596015
41. Obaldia N, Meibalan E, Sa JM, Ma S, Clark MA, Mejia P, et al. Bone marrow is a major parasite reservoir in *Plasmodium vivax* infection. *MBio.* (2018) 9:e00625-18. doi: 10.1128/mBio.00625-18
42. Xia S, Guo Z, Xu X, Yi H, Wang Q, Cao X. Hepatic microenvironment programs hematopoietic progenitor differentiation into regulatory dendritic cells, maintaining liver tolerance. *Blood.* (2008) 112:3175–85. doi: 10.1182/blood-2008-05-159921
43. Goddard S, Youster J, Morgan E, Adams DH. Interleukin-10 secretion differentiates dendritic cells from human liver and skin. *Am J Pathol.* (2004) 164:511–9. doi: 10.1016/S0002-9440(10)63141-0
44. Mittag D, Proietto AI, Loudovaris T, Mannering SI, Vremec D, Shortman K, et al. Human dendritic cell subsets from spleen and blood are similar in phenotype and function but modified by donor health status. *J Immunol.* (2011) 186:6207–17. doi: 10.4049/jimmunol.1002632
45. Hopp CS, Chiou K, Ragheb DRT, Salman AM, Khan SM, Liu AJ, et al. Longitudinal analysis of plasmodium sporozoite motility in the dermis reveals component of blood vessel recognition. *Elife.* (2015) 4:1–21. doi: 10.7554/eLife.07789
46. Roestenberg M, Teirlinck AC, McCall MBB, Teelen K, Makamdop KN, Wiersma J, et al. Long-term protection against malaria after experimental sporozoite inoculation: an open-label follow-up study. *Lancet.* (2011) 377:1770–6. doi: 10.1016/S0140-6736(11)60360-7
47. Roestenberg M, McCall MBB, Hopman J, Wiersma J, Luty AJF, van Gemert GJ, et al. Protection against a malaria challenge by sporozoite inoculation. *N Engl J Med.* (2009) 361:468–77. doi: 10.1056/NEJMoa0805832
48. Bijker EM, Teirlinck AC, Schats R, Van Gemert GJ, Van De Vegte-Bolmer M, Van Lieshout L, et al. Cytotoxic markers associate with protection against malaria in human volunteers immunized with *plasmodium Falciparum* Sporozoites. *J Infect Dis.* (2014) 210:1605–15. doi: 10.1093/infdis/jiu293
49. Amino R, Thiberge S, Martin B, Celli S, Shorte S, Frischknecht F, et al. Quantitative imaging of Plasmodium transmission from mosquito to mammal. *Nat Med.* (2006) 12:220–4. doi: 10.1038/nm1350
50. Chakravarty S, Cockburn IA, Kuk S, Overstreet MG, Sacci JB, Zavala F. CD8+ T lymphocytes protective against malaria liver stages are primed in skin-draining lymph nodes. *Nat Med.* (2007) 13:1035–41. doi: 10.1038/nm1628
51. Leiriao P, Mota MM, Rodriguez A. Apoptotic *Plasmodium*- infected hepatocytes provide antigens to liver dendritic cells. *J Infect Dis.* (2005) 191:1576–81. doi: 10.1086/429635
52. Bamboat ZM, Stableford JA, Plitas G, Burt BM, Nguyen HM, Welles AP, et al. Human liver dendritic cells promote T cell hyporesponsiveness. *J Immunol.* (2009) 182:1901–11. doi: 10.4049/jimmunol.0803404
53. Pillarisetty VG, Shah AB, Miller G, Bleier JI, DeMatteo RP. Liver dendritic cells are less immunogenic than spleen dendritic cells because of differences in subtype composition. *J Immunol.* (2004) 172:1009–17. doi: 10.4049/jimmunol.172.2.1009
54. Bosma BM, Metselaar HJ, Mancham S, Boor PPC, Kusters JG, Kazemier G, et al. Characterization of human liver dendritic cells in liver grafts and perfusates. *Liver Transplant.* (2006) 12:384–93. doi: 10.1002/lt.20659
55. Sack BK, Mikolajczak SA, Fishbaugher M, Vaughan AM, Flannery EL, Nguyen T, et al. Humoral protection against mosquito bite-transmitted *Plasmodium falciparum* infection in humanized mice. *Npj Vaccines.* (2017) 2:27. doi: 10.1038/s41541-017-0028-2
56. Yang ASP, O'Neill MT, Jennison C, Lopaticki S, Allison CC, Armistead JS, et al. Cell traversal activity is important for *Plasmodium falciparum* liver infection in humanized mice. *Cell Rep.* (2017) 18:3105–16. doi: 10.1016/j.celrep.2017.03.017
57. Ding Y, Wilkinson A, Idris A, Fancke B, O'Keeffe M, Khalil D, et al. FLT3-ligand treatment of humanized mice results in the generation of large numbers of CD141+ and CD1c+ dendritic cells *in vivo*. *J Immunol.* (2014) 192:1982–9. doi: 10.4049/jimmunol.1302391
58. Aguilar R, Magallon-Tejada A, Achtman AH, Moraleda C, Joice R, Cisteró P, et al. Molecular evidence for the localization of *Plasmodium falciparum* immature gametocytes in bone marrow. *Blood.* (2014) 123:959–66. doi: 10.1182/blood-2013-08-520767
59. Joice R, Nilsson SK, Montgomery J, Dankwa S, Egan E, Morahan B, et al. *Plasmodium falciparum* transmission stages accumulate in the human bone marrow. *Sci Transl Med.* (2014) 6:244re5. doi: 10.1126/scitranslmed.3008882
60. Wickramasinghe SN, Phillips RE, Looareesuwan S, Warrell DA, Hughes M. The bone marrow in human cerebral malaria: parasite sequestration within sinusoids. *Br J Haematol.* (1987) 66:295–306.
61. Ru Y, Mao B-Y, Zhang F, Pang T, Zhao S, Liu J, et al. Invasion of erythroblasts by *Pasmodium vivax*: a new mechanism contributing to malarial anemia. *Ultrastruct Pathol.* (2009) 33:236–42. doi: 10.3109/01913120903251643
62. Avril M, Brazier AJ, Melcher M, Sampath S, Smith JD. DC8 and DC13 var genes associated with severe malaria bind avidly to diverse endothelial cells. *PLoS Pathog.* (2013) 9:e1003430. doi: 10.1371/journal.ppat.1003430
63. Reeves RK, Fultz PN. Characterization of plasmacytoid dendritic cells in bone marrow of pig-tailed macaques. *Clin Vaccine Immunol.* (2008) 15:35–41. doi: 10.1128/CVI.00309-07
64. Feuerer M, Beckhove P, Garbi N, Mahnke Y, Limmer A, Hommel M, et al. Bone marrow as a priming site for T-cell responses to blood-borne antigen. *Nat Med.* (2003) 9:1151–7. doi: 10.1038/nm914
65. Spaulding E, Fooksman D, Moore JM, Saidi A, Feintuch CM, Reizis B, et al. STING-licensed macrophages prime type I IFN production by plasmacytoid dendritic cells in the bone marrow during severe *Plasmodium yoelii* malaria. *PLoS Pathog.* (2016) 12:e1005975. doi: 10.1371/journal.ppat.1005975

66. Junqueira C, Barbosa CRR, Costa PAC, Teixeira-Carvalho A, Castro G, Sen Santara S, et al. Cytotoxic CD8+T cells recognize and kill *Plasmodium vivax*-infected reticulocytes. *Nat Med.* (2018) 24:1330–6. doi: 10.1038/s41591-018-0117-4
67. M Eriksson E, Sampaio NG, Schofield L. Toll-like receptors and malaria – sensing and susceptibility. *J Trop Dis.* (2013) 2:1–7. doi: 10.4172/2329-891X.1000126
68. Gazzinelli RT, Kalantari P, Fitzgerald KA, Golenbock DT. Innate sensing of malaria parasites. *Nat Rev Immunol.* (2014) 14:744–57. doi: 10.1038/nri3742
69. Trubowitz S, Masek B. *Plasmodium falciparum*: phagocytosis by polymorphonuclear leukocytes. *Science.* (1968) 162:273–4. doi: 10.1126/science.162.3850.273
70. Chan J, Howell KB, Reiling L, Ataide R, Mackintosh CL, Fowkes FJI, et al. Targets of antibodies against *Plasmodium falciparum*-infected erythrocytes in malaria immunity. *J Clin Invest.* (2012) 122:3227–38. doi: 10.1172/JCI62182
71. Urban BC, Willcox N, Roberts DJ. A role for CD36 in the regulation of dendritic cell function. *Proc Natl Acad Sci USA.* (2001) 98:8750–5. doi: 10.1073/pnas.151028698
72. Miller LH, Baruch DI, Marsh K, Doumbo OK. The pathogenic basis of malaria. *Nature.* (2002) 415:673–9. doi: 10.1038/415673a
73. Lundie RJ, de Koning-Ward TF, Davey GM, Nie CQ, Hansen DS, Lau LS, et al. Blood-stage Plasmodium infection induces CD8+ T lymphocytes to parasite-expressed antigens, largely regulated by CD8alpha+ dendritic cells. *Proc Natl Acad Sci USA.* (2008) 105:14509–14. doi: 10.1073/pnas.0806727105
74. Jung S, Unutmaz D, Wong P, Sano G-I, De los Santos K, Sparwasser T, et al. *In vivo* depletion of CD11c+ dendritic cells abrogates priming of CD8+ T cells by exogenous cell-associated antigens. *Immunity.* (2002) 17:211–20. doi: 10.1016/S1074-7613(02)00365-5
75. Voisine C, Mastelic B, Sponaas AM, Langhorne J. Classical CD11c+ dendritic cells, not plasmacytoid dendritic cells, induce T cell responses to *Plasmodium chabaudi* malaria. *Int J Parasitol.* (2010) 40:711–9. doi: 10.1016/j.ijpara.2009.11.005
76. Ocaña-Morgner C, Mota MM, Rodriguez A. Malaria blood stage suppression of liver stage immunity by dendritic cells. *J Exp Med.* (2003) 197:143–51. doi: 10.1084/jem.20021072
77. Wilson NS, Behrens GMN, Lundie RJ, Smith CM, Waithman J, Young L, et al. Systemic activation of dendritic cells by Toll-like receptor ligands or malaria infection impairs cross-presentation and antiviral immunity. *Nat Immunol.* (2006) 7:165–72. doi: 10.1038/ni1300
78. Millington OR, Gibson VB, Rush CM, Zinselmeyer BH, Phillips RS, Garside P, et al. Malaria impairs T cell clustering and immune priming despite normal signal 1 from dendritic cells. *PLoS Pathog.* (2007) 3:1380–7. doi: 10.1371/journal.ppat.0030143
79. Lundie RJ, Young LJ, Davey GM, Villadangos J a, Carbone FR, Heath WR, et al. Blood-stage *Plasmodium berghei* infection leads to short-lived parasite-associated antigen presentation by dendritic cells. *Eur J Immunol.* (2010) 40:1674–81. doi: 10.1002/eji.200939265
80. Piva L, Tetlak P, Claser C, Karjalainen K, Renia L, Ruedl C. Cutting edge: Clec9A+ dendritic cells mediate the development of experimental cerebral malaria. *J Immunol.* (2012) 189:1128–32. doi: 10.4049/jimmunol.1201171
81. deWalick S, Amante FH, McSweeney K a, Randall LM, Stanley AC, Haque A, et al. Cutting edge: conventional dendritic cells are the critical APC required for the induction of experimental cerebral malaria. *J Immunol.* (2007) 178:6033–7. doi: 10.4049/jimmunol.178.10.6033
82. Urban BC, Mwangi T, Ross A, Kinyanjui S, Mosobo M, Kai O, et al. Peripheral blood dendritic cells in children with acute *Plasmodium falciparum* malaria. *Blood.* (2001) 98:2859–61. doi: 10.1182/blood.V98.9.2859
83. Pichyangkul S, Yongvanitchit K, Kum-arb U, Hemmi H, Akira S, Krieg AM, et al. Malaria blood stage parasites activate human plasmacytoid dendritic cells and murine dendritic cells through a Toll-like receptor 9-dependent pathway. *J Immunol.* (2004) 172:4926–33. doi: 10.4049/jimmunol.172.8.4926
84. Pinzon-Charry A, Woodberry T, Kienzle V, McPhun V, Minigo G, Lampah DA, et al. Apoptosis and dysfunction of blood dendritic cells in patients with falciparum and vivax malaria. *J Exp Med.* (2013) 210:1635–46. doi: 10.1084/jem.20121972
85. Götz A, Tang MS, Ty MC, Arama C, Ongoiba A, Doumtabe D, et al. Atypical activation of dendritic cells by *Plasmodium falciparum*. *Proc Natl Acad Sci USA.* (2017) 114:E10568–77. doi: 10.1073/pnas.1708383114
86. Jangpatarapongsa K, Chootong P, Sattabongkot J, Chotivanich K, Sirichaisinthop J, Tungpradabkul S, et al. *Plasmodium vivax* parasites alter the balance of myeloid and plasmacytoid dendritic cells and the induction of regulatory T cells. *Eur J Immunol.* (2008) 38:2697–705. doi: 10.1002/eji.200838186
87. Kho S, Marfurt J, Noviyanti R, Kusuma A, Piera KA, Burdam FH, et al., Preserved dendritic cell HLA-DR expression and reduced regulatory T cell activation in asymptomatic *Plasmodium falciparum* and *P. vivax* infection. *Infect Immun.* (2015) 83:3224–32. doi: 10.1128/IAI.00226-15
88. Kho S, Marfurt J, Handayuni I, Pava Z, Noviyanti R, Kusuma A, et al. Characterization of blood dendritic and regulatory T cells in asymptomatic adults with sub-microscopic *Plasmodium falciparum* or *Plasmodium vivax* infection. *Malar J.* (2016) 15:328. doi: 10.1186/s12936-016-1382-7
89. Woodberry T, Minigo G, Piera K a, Amante FH, Pinzon-Charry A, Good MF, et al. Low-level *Plasmodium falciparum* blood-stage infection causes dendritic cell apoptosis and dysfunction in healthy volunteers. *J Infect Dis.* (2012) 206:333–40. doi: 10.1093/infdis/jis366
90. Teirlinck AC, Roestenberg M, Bijker EM, Hoffman SL, Sauerwein RW, Scholzen A. *Plasmodium falciparum* infection of human volunteers activates monocytes and CD16+ dendritic cells and induces upregulation of CD16 and CD1c expression. *Infect Immun.* (2015) 83:3732–9. doi: 10.1128/IAI.00473-15
91. Loughland JR, Minigo G, Burel J, Tipping PE, Piera KA, Amante FH, et al. Profoundly reduced CD1c + myeloid dendritic cell HLA-DR and CD86 expression and increased tumor necrosis factor production in experimental human blood-stage malaria infection. *Infect Immun.* (2016) 84:1403–12. doi: 10.1128/IAI.01522-15
92. Loughland JR, Minigo G, Sarovich DS, Field M, Tipping PE, Montes de Oca M, et al. Plasmacytoid dendritic cells appear inactive during sub-microscopic *Plasmodium falciparum* blood-stage infection, yet retain their ability to respond to TLR stimulation. *Sci Rep.* (2017) 7:2596. doi: 10.1038/s41598-017-02096-2
93. Loughland JR, Woodberry T, Boyle MJ, Tipping PE, Piera KA, Amante FH, et al. *Plasmodium falciparum* activates CD16+ dendritic cells to produce TNF and IL-10 in subpatent malaria. *J Infect Dis.* (2018) 219:660–71. doi: 10.1093/infdis/jiy555
94. Breitling LP, Fendel R, Mordmueller B, Adegnika AA, Kremsner PG, Luty AJF. Cord blood dendritic cell subsets in African newborns exposed to *Plasmodium falciparum* in utero. *Infect Immun.* (2006) 74:5725–9. doi: 10.1128/IAI.00682-06
95. Woodberry T, Loughland JR, Minigo G, Burel JG, Amante FH, Piera KA, et al. Early immune regulatory changes in a primary controlled human *Plasmodium vivax* infection: CD1c + myeloid dendritic cell maturation arrest, induction of the kynurenine pathway, and regulatory T cell activation. *Infect Immun.* (2017) 85:e00986-16. doi: 10.1128/IAI.00986-16
96. Urban BC, Cordery D, Shafi MJ, Bull PC, Newbold CI, Williams TN, et al. The frequency of BDCA3-positive dendritic cells is increased in the peripheral circulation of Kenyan children with severe malaria. *Infect Immun.* (2006) 74:6700–6. doi: 10.1128/IAI.00861-06
97. Diallo M, Aldebert D, Moreau J-C, Ndiaye M, Jambou R. Decrease of lymphoid dendritic cells in blood from malaria-infected pregnant women. *Int J Parasitol.* (2008) 38:1557–65. doi: 10.1016/j.ijpara.2008.04.013
98. Loharungsikul S, Troye-Blomberg M, Amoudruz P, Pichyangkul S, Yongvanitchit K, Looareesuwan S, et al. Expression of toll-like receptors on antigen-presenting cells in patients with falciparum malaria. *Acta Trop.* (2008) 105:10–5. doi: 10.1016/j.actatropica.2007.08.002
99. Gonçalves RM, Salmazi KC, Santos BAN, Bastos MS, Rocha SC, Boscardin SB, et al. CD4+ CD25+ Foxp3+ regulatory T cells, dendritic cells, and circulating cytokines in uncomplicated malaria: do different parasite species elicit similar host responses? *Infect Immun.* (2010) 78:4763–72. doi: 10.1128/IAI.00578-10
100. Arama C, Giusti P, Boström S, Dara V, Traore B, Dolo A, et al. Interethnic differences in antigen-presenting cell activation and TLR responses in Malian children during *Plasmodium falciparum* malaria. *PLoS ONE.* (2011) 6:e18319. doi: 10.1371/journal.pone.0018319

101. Ibitokou S, Oesterholt M, Brutus L, Borgella S, Agbowaï C, Ezinmègnon S, et al. Peripheral blood cell signatures of *Plasmodium falciparum* infection during pregnancy. *PLoS ONE.* (2012) 7:e49621. doi: 10.1371/journal.pone.0049621
102. Guermonprez P, Helft J, Claser C, Deroubaix S, Karanje H, Gazumyan A, et al. Inflammatory Flt3l is essential to mobilize dendritic cells and for T cell responses during Plasmodium infection. *Nat Med.* (2013) 19:730–8. doi: 10.1038/nm.3197
103. Urban BC, Ferguson DJ, Pain A, Willcox N, Plebanski M, Austyn JM, et al. *Plasmodium falciparum*-infected erythrocytes modulate the maturation of dendritic cells. *Nature.* (1999) 400:73–7. doi: 10.1038/21900
104. Elliott SR, Spurck TP, Dodin JM, Maier AG, Voss TS, Yosaatmadja F, et al. Inhibition of dendritic cell maturation by malaria is dose dependent and does not require *Plasmodium falciparum* erythrocyte membrane protein 1. *Infect Immun.* (2007) 75:3621–32. doi: 10.1128/IAI.00095-07
105. Mukherjee P, Chauhan VS. *Plasmodium falciparum*-free merozoites and infected RBCs distinctly affect soluble CD40 ligand-mediated maturation of immature monocyte-derived dendritic cells. *J Leukoc Biol.* (2008) 84:244–54. doi: 10.1189/jlb.0807565
106. Clemente AM, Fadigati G, Caporale R, Marchese DG, Castronovo G, Sannella AR, et al. Modulation of the immune and inflammatory responses by *Plasmodium falciparum* schizont extracts: role of myeloid dendritic cells in effector and regulatory functions of CD4+ lymphocytes. *Infect Immun.* (2013) 81:1842–51. doi: 10.1128/IAI.01226-12
107. Wu X, Gowda NM, Kumar S, Gowda DC. Protein-DNA complex is the exclusive malaria parasite component that activates dendritic cells and triggers innate immune responses. *J Immunol.* (2010) 184:4338–48. doi: 10.4049/jimmunol.0903824
108. Gowda NM, Wu X, Kumar S, Febbraio M, Gowda DC. CD36 contributes to malaria parasite-induced pro-inflammatory cytokine production and NK and T cell activation by dendritic cells. *PLoS ONE.* (2013) 8:e77604. doi: 10.1371/journal.pone.0077604
109. Fievet N, Varani S, Ibitokou S, Briand V, Louis S, Perrin RX, et al. *Plasmodium falciparum* exposure in utero, maternal age and parity influence the innate activation of foetal antigen presenting cells. *Malar J.* (2009) 8:1–12. doi: 10.1186/1475-2875-8-251
110. World Health Organisation. *Guidelines of the Treatment of Malaria.* Geneva (2010).
111. Bartoloni A, Zammarchi L. Clinical aspects of uncomplicated and severe malaria. *Mediterr J Hematol Infect Dis.* (2012) 4:e2012026. doi: 10.4084/MJHID.2012.026
112. Maraskovsky E, Brasel K, Teepe M, Roux ER, Lyman SD, Shortman K, et al. Dramatic increase in the numbers of functionally mature dendritic cells in Flt3 ligand-treated mice: multiple dendritic cell subpopulations identified. *J Exp Med.* (1996) 184:1953–62. doi: 10.1084/jem.184.5.1953
113. Waskow C, Liu K, Darrasse-Jèze G, Guermonprez P, Ginhoux F, Merad M, et al. The receptor tyrosine kinase Flt3 is required for dendritic cell development in peripheral lymphoid tissues. *Nat Immunol.* (2008) 9:676–83. doi: 10.1038/ni.1615
114. Umbers AJ, Aitken EH, Rogerson SJ. Malaria in pregnancy: small babies, big problem. *Trends Parasitol.* (2011) 27:168–75. doi: 10.1016/j.pt.2011.01.007
115. Elsayh KI, Zahran AM, Lotfy Mohamad I, Aly SS. Dendritic cells in childhood sepsis. *J Crit Care.* (2013) 28:881.e7–13. doi: 10.1016/j.jcrc.2013.05.007
116. Macatonia SE, Lau R, Patterson S, Pinching AJ, Knight SC. Dendritic cell infection, depletion and dysfunction in HIV-infected individuals. *Immunology.* (1990) 71:38–45.
117. Averill L, Lee WM, Karandikar NJ. Differential dysfunction in dendritic cell subsets during chronic HCV infection. *Clin Immunol.* (2007) 123:40–9. doi: 10.1016/j.clim.2006.12.001
118. Hémont C, Neel A, Heslan M, Braudeau C, Josien R. Human blood mDC subsets exhibit distinct TLR repertoire and responsiveness. *J Leukoc Biol.* (2013) 93:599–609. doi: 10.1189/jlb.0912452
119. Nebl T, de Veer M, Schofield L. Stimulation of innate immune responses by malarial glycosylphosphatidylinositol via pattern recognition receptors. *Parasitology.* (2005) 130(Suppl.):S45–62: doi: 10.1017/S0031182005008152
120. Coban C, Ishii KJ, Kawai T, Hemmi H, Sato S, Uematsu S, et al. Toll-like receptor 9 mediates innate immune activation by the malaria pigment hemozoin. *J Exp Med.* (2005) 201:19–25. doi: 10.1084/jem.20041836
121. World Health Organization. *World Malaria Report 2018.* Geneva (2018).
122. Kitchen S. The infection of reticulocytes by *Plasmodium vivax. Am J Trop Med Hyg.* (1938) 1–18:347–59.
123. McCarthy JS, Sekuloski S, Griffin PM, Elliott S, Douglas N, Peatey C, et al. A pilot randomised trial of induced blood-stage *Plasmodium falciparum* infections in healthy volunteers for testing efficacy of new antimalarial drugs. *PLoS ONE.* (2011) 6:e21914. doi: 10.1371/journal.pone.0021914
124. Robbins SH, Walzer T, Dembélé D, Thibault C, Defays A, Bessou G, et al. Novel insights into the relationships between dendritic cell subsets in human and mouse revealed by genome-wide expression profiling. *Genome Biol.* (2008) 9:R17. doi: 10.1186/gb-2008-9-1-r17
125. Collin M, Bigley V. Human dendritic cell subsets: an update. *Immunology.* (2018) 154:3–20. doi: 10.1111/imm.12888
126. Villani A-C, Satija R, Reynolds G, Sarkizova S, Shekhar K, Fletcher J, et al. Single-cell RNA-seq reveals new types of human blood dendritic cells, monocytes, and progenitors. *Science.* (2017) 356:eaah4573. doi: 10.1126/science.aah4573
127. Steinman RM. The Dendritic Cell System and its Role in Immunogenicity. *Annu Rev Immunol.* (1991) 9:271–96. doi: 10.1146/annurev.iy.09.040191.001415
128. Jongbloed SL, Kassianos AJ, McDonald KJ, Clark GJ, Ju X, Angel CE, et al. Human CD141+ (BDCA-3)+ dendritic cells (DCs) represent a unique myeloid DC subset that cross-presents necrotic cell antigens. *J Exp Med.* (2010) 207:1247–60. doi: 10.1084/jem.20092140
129. Sallusto F, Lanzavecchia A. Efficient presentation of soluble antigen by cultured human dendritic cells is maintained by granulocyte/macrophage colony-stimulating factor plus interleukin 4 and downregulated by tumor necrosis factor alpha. *J Exp Med.* (1994) 179:1109–18.
130. Romani N, Gruner S, Brang D, Kämpgen E, Lenz A, Trockenbacher B, et al. Proliferating dendritic cell progenitors in human blood. *J Exp Med.* (1994) 180:83–93.
131. Helft J, Böttcher J, Chakravarty P, Zelenay S, Huotari J, Schraml BU, et al. GM-CSF mouse bone marrow cultures comprise a heterogeneous population of CD11c^{+}MHCII^{+} macrophages and dendritic cells. *Immunity.* (2015) 42:1197–211. doi: 10.1016/j.immuni.2015.05.018
132. Giusti P, Urban BC, Frascaroli G, Albrecht L, Tinti A, Troye-Blomberg M, et al. *Plasmodium falciparum*-infected erythrocytes and beta-hematin induce partial maturation of human dendritic cells and increase their migratory ability in response to lymphoid chemokines. *Infect Immun.* (2011) 79:2727–36. doi: 10.1128/IAI.00649-10
133. Boura M, Frita R, Góis A, Carvalho T, Hänscheid T. The hemozoin conundrum: is malaria pigment immune-activating, inhibiting, or simply a bystander? *Trends Parasitol.* (2013) 29:469–76. doi: 10.1016/j.pt.2013.07.005
134. Coban C, Ishii KJ, Sullivan DJ, Kumar N. Purified malaria pigment (Hemozoin) enhances dendritic cell maturation and modulates the isotype of antibodies induced by a DNA vaccine. *Infect Immun.* (2002) 70:3939–43. doi: 10.1128/IAI.70.7.3939-3943.2002
135. Skorokhod OA, Alessio M, Mordmüller B, Arese P, Schwarzer E. Hemozoin (malarial pigment) inhibits differentiation and maturation of human monocyte-derived dendritic cells: a peroxisome proliferator-activated receptor-gamma-mediated effect. *J Immunol.* (2004) 173:4066–74. doi: 10.4049/jimmunol.173.6.4066
136. Parroche P, Lauw FN, Goutagny N, Latz E, Monks BG, Visintin A, et al. Malaria hemozoin is immunologically inert but radically enhances innate responses by presenting malaria DNA to Toll-like receptor 9. *Proc Natl Acad Sci USA.* (2007) 104:1919–24. doi: 10.1073/pnas.0608745104
137. Brasel K, Smedt T De, Smith JL, Maliszewski CR. Generation of murine dendritic cells from flt3-ligand-supplemented bone marrow cultures. *Blood.* (2000) 96:3029–39. Available online at: http://www.bloodjournal.org/content/96/9/3029
138. van de Hoef DL, Coppens I, Holowka T, Ben Mamoun C, Branch O, Rodriguez A. *Plasmodium falciparum*-derived uric acid precipitates induce maturation of dendritic cells. *PLoS ONE.* (2013) 8:e55584. doi: 10.1371/journal.pone.0055584

139. Gallego-Delgado J, Ty M, Orengo JM, van de Hoef D, Rodriguez A. A Surprising role for uric acid: the inflammatory malaria response. *Curr Rheumatol Rep.* (2014) 16:401. doi: 10.1007/s11926-013-0401-8
140. Hochrein H, O'Keeffe M. Dendritic cell subsets and toll-like receptors. In: Bauer S, Hartmann G, editors. *Handbook of Experimental Pharmacology.* Berlin; Heidelberg: Springer (2008). p. 153–79. doi: 10.1007/978-3-540-72167-3
141. Gallego-Marin C, Schrum JE, Andrade WA, Shaffer SA, Giraldo LF, Lasso AM, et al. Cyclic GMP–AMP synthase is the cytosolic sensor of *Plasmodium falciparum* genomic DNA and activates type I IFN in malaria. *J Immunol.* (2017) 200:768–74. doi: 10.4049/jimmunol.1701048
142. Sisquella X, Ofir-Birin Y, Pimentel MA, Cheng L, Abou Karam P, Sampaio NG, et al. Malaria parasite DNA-harbouring vesicles activate cytosolic immune sensors. *Nat Commun.* (2017) 8:1985. doi: 10.1038/s41467-017-02083-1
143. Nwakanma DC, Gomez-Escobar N, Walther M, Crozier S, Dubovsky F, Malkin E, et al. Quantitative detection of *Plasmodium falciparum* DNA in saliva, blood, and urine. *J Infect Dis.* (2009) 199:1567–74. doi: 10.1086/598856
144. Krishnegowda G, Hajjar AM, Zhu J, Douglass EJ, Uematsu S, Akira S, et al. Induction of proinflammatory responses in macrophages by the glycosylphosphatidylinositols of *Plasmodium falciparum*: cell signaling receptors, glycosylphosphatidylinositol (GPI) structural requirement, and regulation of GPI activity. *J Biol Chem.* (2005) 280:8606–16. doi: 10.1074/jbc.M413541200
145. Baccarella A, Fontana MF, Chen EC, Kim CC. Toll-like receptor 7 mediates early innate immune responses to malaria. *Infect Immun.* (2013) 81:4431–42. doi: 10.1128/IAI.00923-13
146. Campos FM, Franklin BS, Teixeira-Carvalho A, Filho AL, de Paula SC, Fontes CJ, et al. Augmented plasma microparticles during acute *Plasmodium vivax* infection. *Malar J.* (2010) 9:327. doi: 10.1186/1475-2875-9-327
147. Nantakomol D, Dondorp AM, Krudsood S, Udomsangpetch R, Pattanapanyasat K, Combes V, et al. Circulating red cell-derived microparticles in human malaria. *J Infect Dis.* (2011) 203:700–6. doi: 10.1093/infdis/jiq104
148. Couper KN, Barnes T, Hafalla JCR, Combes V, Ryffel B, Secher T, et al. Parasite-derived plasma microparticles contribute significantly to malaria infection-induced inflammation through potent macrophage stimulation. *PLoS Pathog.* (2010) 6:e1000744. doi: 10.1371/journal.ppat.1000744
149. Mantel PY, Hoang AN, Goldowitz I, Potashnikova D, Hamza B, Vorobjev I, et al. Malaria-infected erythrocyte-derived microvesicles mediate cellular communication within the parasite population and with the host immune system. *Cell Host Microbe.* (2013) 13:521–34. doi: 10.1016/j.chom.2013.04.009
150. Laurens MB, Thera MA, Coulibaly D, Ouattara A, Kone AK, Guindo AB, et al. Extended safety, immunogenicity and efficacy of a blood-stage malaria vaccine in Malian children: 24-month follow-up of a randomized, double-blinded phase 2 trial. *PLoS ONE.* (2013) 8:e79323. doi: 10.1371/journal.pone.0079323
151. Wilson NO, Jain V, Roberts CE, Lucchi N, Joel PK, Singh MP, et al. CXCL4 and CXCL10 predict risk of fatal cerebral malaria. *Dis Markers.* (2011) 30:39–49. doi: 10.3233/DMA-2011-0763
152. Jain V, Singh PP, Silawat N, Patel R, Saxena A, Bharti PK, et al. A preliminary study on pro- and anti-inflammatory cytokine profiles in *Plasmodium vivax* malaria patients from central zone of India. *Acta Trop.* (2010) 113:263–8. doi: 10.1016/j.actatropica.2009.11.009
153. Herbert F, Tchitchek N, Bansal D, Jacques J, Pathak S, Bécavin C, et al. Evidence of IL-17, IP-10, and IL-10 involvement in multiple-organ dysfunction and IL-17 pathway in acute renal failure associated to *Plasmodium falciparum* malaria. *J Transl Med.* (2015) 13:369. doi: 10.1186/s12967-015-0731-6
154. Kempaiah P, Anyona SB, Raballah E, Davenport GC, Were T, Hittner JB, et al. Reduced interferon (IFN)-α conditioned by IFNA2 (−173) and IFNA8 (−884) haplotypes is associated with enhanced susceptibility to severe malarial anemia and longitudinal all-cause mortality. *Hum Genet.* (2012) 131:1375–91. doi: 10.1007/s00439-012-1175-1
155. Montes de Oca M, Kumar R, Rivera F de L, Amante FH, Sheel M, Faleiro RJ, et al. Type I interferons regulate immune responses in humans with blood-stage *Plasmodium falciparum* infection. *Cell Rep.* (2016) 17:399–412. doi: 10.1016/j.celrep.2016.09.015
156. Wykes MN, Kay JG, Manderson A, Liu XQ, Brown DL, Richard DJ, et al. Rodent blood-stage Plasmodium survive in dendritic cells that infect naive mice. *Proc Natl Acad Sci USA.* (2011) 108:11205–10. doi: 10.1073/pnas.1108579108
157. Vuckovic S, Abdul Wahid FS, Rice A, Kato M, Khalil D, Rodwell R, et al. Compartmentalization of allogeneic T-cell responses in the bone marrow and spleen of humanized NOD/SCID mice containing activated human resident myeloid dendritic cells. *Exp Hematol.* (2008) 36:1502–12. doi: 10.1016/j.exphem.2008.06.011
158. Minkah NK, Schafer C, Kappe SHI. Humanized mouse models for the study of human malaria parasite biology, pathogenesis, and immunity. *Front Immunol.* (2018) 9:807. doi: 10.3389/fimmu.2018.00807
159. Broutier L, Mastrogiovanni G, Verstegen MM, Francies HE, Gavarró LM, Bradshaw CR, et al. Human primary liver cancer–derived organoid cultures for disease modeling and drug screening. *Nat Med.* (2017) 23:1424–35. doi: 10.1038/nm.4438
160. Spence JR, Mayhew CN, Rankin SA, Kuhar MF, Vallance JE, Tolle K, et al. Directed differentiation of human pluripotent stem cells into intestinal tissue *in vitro. Nature.* (2011) 470:105–9. doi: 10.1038/nature09691
161. Heo I, Dutta D, Schaefer DA, Iakobachvili N, Artegiani B, Sachs N, et al. Modelling Cryptosporidium infection in human small intestinal and lung organoids. *Nat Microbiol.* (2018) 3:814–23. doi: 10.1038/s41564-018-0177-8
162. Klotz C, Aebischer T, Seeber F. Stem cell-derived cell cultures and organoids for protozoan parasite propagation and studying host-parasite interaction. *Int J Med Microbiol.* (2012) 302:203–9. doi: 10.1016/j.ijmm.2012.07.010

14

Immune Responses to the Sexual Stages of *Plasmodium falciparum* Parasites

Jonas A. Kengne-Ouafo[1]*, Colin J. Sutherland*[2]*, Fred N. Binka*[3]*, Gordon A. Awandare*[1]*, Britta C. Urban*[4] *and Bismarck Dinko*[5*]

[1] *West African Centre for Cell Biology of Infectious Pathogens, University of Ghana, Accra, Ghana,* [2] *Department of Immunology and Infection, Faculty of Infectious and Tropical Diseases, London School of Hygiene and Tropical Medicine, London, United Kingdom,* [3] *Department of Epidemiology and Biostatistics, School of Public Health, University of Health and Allied Sciences, Ho, Ghana,* [4] *Faculty of Biological Sciences, Liverpool School of Tropical Medicine, Liverpool, United Kingdom,* [5] *Department of Biomedical Sciences, School of Basic and Biomedical Sciences, University of Health and Allied Sciences, Ho, Ghana*

Correspondence:
Bismarck Dinko
bdinko@uhas.edu.gh

Malaria infections remain a serious global health problem in the world, particularly among children and pregnant women in Sub-Saharan Africa. Moreover, malaria control and elimination is hampered by rapid development of resistance by the parasite and the vector to commonly used antimalarial drugs and insecticides, respectively. Therefore, vaccine-based strategies are sorely needed, including those designed to interrupt disease transmission. However, a prerequisite for such a vaccine strategy is the understanding of both the human and vector immune responses to parasite developmental stages involved in parasite transmission in both man and mosquito. Here, we review the naturally acquired humoral and cellular responses to sexual stages of the parasite while in the human host and the *Anopheles* vector. In addition, updates on current anti-gametocyte, anti-gamete, and anti-mosquito transmission blocking vaccines are given. We conclude with our views on some important future directions of research into *P. falciparum* sexual stage immunity relevant to the search for the most appropriate transmission-blocking vaccine.

Keywords: *Plasmodium falciparum*, gametocytes, humoral immunity, cellular immunity, mosquito immunity

INTRODUCTION

Malaria is one of the most important parasitic infections with the highest burden of mortality and morbidity in sub-Saharan Africa. Despite progress and advances in the strategies to control the disease, malaria claimed the lives of approximately 445,000 people from among 216 million clinical cases globally in 2016; mostly in children under 5 years and pregnant women as reported by WHO (1). The increasing challenges posed by the emergence of resistance to antimalarials by malaria parasites and to insecticides by mosquitoes (2, 3) suggest the need for additional interventions aiming at transmission reduction such as vaccines. Moreover, targeting of multiple stages of the parasites might be the best strategy for any successful malaria vaccine (4), further highlighting the need for continuous identification and validation of alternative and effective targets.

Transmission blocking interventions either targeting gametocytes while in the human host or gametes in the mosquito are considered an essential part of malaria control strategies especially in the quest to eradicate malaria (5, 6). Malaria parasites (sporozoites) are transmitted through the bite of Anopheline mosquitoes. Once in the human system, the sporozoites migrate to the liver where they undergo pre-erythrocytic multiplication (schizogony) leading to the production of merozoites that move into the bloodstream (erythrocytic stage; **Figure 1**). The pathology results from red blood cell (RBCs) invasion and further asexual replication of parasites within RBCs (erythrocytic schizogony) leading to massive RBC lysis, disrupted blood flow due to cytoadherence of parasite-infected RBCs to endothelial surfaces, anemia, and inflammation that may be lethal if untreated. Gametocytes are specialized stages of *Plasmodium* parasites that are essential for transmission from humans to mosquitoes. Initially, a certain proportion of the erythrocytic stage parasites undergoes a permanent differentiation also referred to as sexual commitment into both male (microgametocyte) and female (macrogametocyte) gametocytes (**Figure 1**). This process is known as gametocytogenesis (7, 8).

Sexually committed ring stage trophozoites from erythrocytic stages in peripheral circulation (9, 10) progress into gametocyte developmental stages 1 to IV while sequestered in bone marrow compartments (11–14). This constitutes the main reason why only late gametocyte stages are found in peripheral circulation. Early gametocytes are thought to sequester in tissues such as spleen and bone marrow through parasite-host interactions via parasite molecules less elucidated but probably PfEMP1, STEVORS, or RIFINS (14–16). The human host endothelial receptors mediating sequestration of developing gametocytes in the bone marrow and other organs however remain unidentified (17). Differentiation of male and female gametocytes occur during sexual commitment where the asexual precursor, schizont, give rise to either male or female gametocytes (7, 8).

After about 10–12 days of sequestered development, mature, male, and female gametocytes emerge and circulate in peripheral blood for a variable amount of time until taken up by mosquitoes (18, 19). Gametocytes do not replicate; however, hemoglobin digestion continues until they reach stage IV (20). In addition, gametocyte-specific mRNAs are produced and a subset of these, important for their stage development in the mosquito, are translationally repressed until gametocytes are taken up by the vector when they go back to peripheral circulation (21). The phenomenon governing the return of mature gametocytes in the peripheral blood is not clearly understood. Once ingested, gametocytes rapidly transform into male (microgamete) and female gametes (macrogamete) in response to environmental cues such as a rise in pH, reduction in temperature and exposure to xanthurenic acid (22). Exflagellation (male gamete induction) is followed by the expression of gamete-specific proteins (23). Fertilization of macrogametocytes by microgametes is preceded by 3 rounds of DNA replication by male gametocytes giving rise to 8 motile microgametes resulting in a zygote (**Figure 1**). The zygote elongates to form an ookinete which crosses the midgut wall to develop into an oocyst. Further cell divisions and development of the oocyst give rise to sporozoites. Following oocyst capsule rupture, thousands of sporozoites emerge and invade the mosquito salivary glands which then render the vector infectious to humans during a bloodmeal, thus completing the transmission cycle (24–26) (**Figure 1**).

The infectiousness and transmission potential of gametocytes is influenced by their prevalence and density (27), degree of maturity (28), and both mosquito and human immune responses (29, 30). Furthermore, the efficiency of transmission depends on the generation of sporozoites and therefore level of infectivity or sporozoite dose transmitted (31). Moreover, the sporogonic stages are exposed to the vector's natural immune responses (32–34). It should be pointed out that gametocyte infectiousness refers to the amount of mature gametocytes that can potently infect the mosquito (demonstrated by their ability to undergo further development) after ingestion whereas sporozoite infectivity refers to the dose of potent sporozoites capable of being transmitted to humans during subsequent blood meals.

Here, we review the available evidence for naturally acquired human immune responses against the sexual stages of *Plasmodium* parasites targeting gametocytes and gametes in human and mosquito hosts, respectively. The mosquito immune responses against the development of these sexual stages in the midgut are also discussed, and propositions are made for future research directions toward the design of appropriate transmission blocking vaccines.

NATURALLY ACQUIRED ANTIBODY RESPONSES TO GAMETOCYTE AND GAMETE ANTIGENS

For over three decades now there have been some efforts to illuminate antibody responses to gametocyte and gamete development in mosquitoes and their potential for transmission reducing immunity (TRI). TRI is based on observations of naturally acquired antibodies against gametocytes that are produced in the human host in response to proteins of gametocytes that were not taken up by mosquitoes (35). When these gametocytes die, they release intracellular proteins/antigens into the host circulation. Among these are proteins produced in gametocytes which are crucial for the extracellular parasite development in the mosquito midgut (36, 37). These antigens are then processed and presented by antigen presenting cells eventually eliciting humoral immune responses, which can cause substantial or complete blockade of parasite development (gametogenesis, fertilization) in the mosquito. This is the essence of TRI and forms the basis for the development of transmission-blocking vaccines (TBV). TRI occurs when human antibodies, taken up by a mosquito in a potentially infectious blood-meal containing male and female gametocytes, are able to prevent fertilization and/or development of ookinetes/oocyts/sporozoites in the mosquito and thus infection of the mosquito (38, 39).

Extensively studied antigens to date include gametocyte/gamete proteins such as Pfs230 and Pfs45/48 and the zygote/ookinete proteins Pfs25 and Pfs28 (37) also known as the TBV candidate (30, 37, 40–43). Anti-Pfs230 and Pfs48/45 antibodies target the so-called pre-fertilization phase while anti-Pfs25 and anti-Pfs28 antibodies represent the post-fertilization phases marked by the differences in the parasite stage and target antigens. As such parasite proteins are referred to as Pre- and post-fertilization antigens, respectively. Binding of these antibodies to their antigen either blocks their function

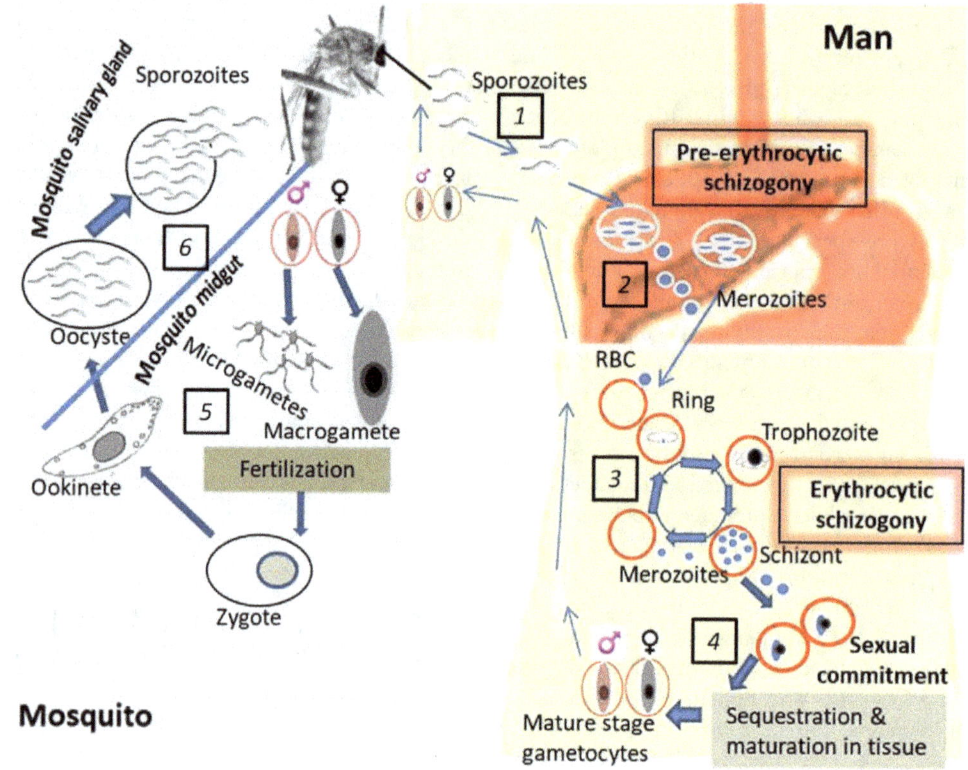

FIGURE 1 | Life cycle of *P. falciparum* development in the human host and mosquito vector. **(1)**. Mosquito's bite and release sporozoites into the human host followed by migration into the liver. **(2)**. Pre-erythrocytic schizogony: infection of hepatocytes and asexual multiplication of the parasites in the liver. **(3)**. Erythrocytic schizogony: translocation of parasites from the liver into the bloodstream accompanied by asexual multiplication and release of merozoites upon RBC rupture. **(4)**. Gametocyte generation: sexual commitment, sequestration of early gametocytes, maturation in tissues and release of mature gametocytes in blood (ready to be picked up by the vector). **(5)**. Parasite development in the mosquito midgut: exflagellation of male gametocytes prior to fertilization which yields the zygote which undergoes further development into a motile ookinete. **(6)**. Parasite development in the mosquito salivary gland: oocyst formation, sporozoite development, and release in the mosquito salivary gland (ready to be transmitted to the human host during subsequent mosquito bites).

essential for parasite development or facilitates complement-mediated gamete killing as shown for antibodies against Pfs230 (44).

Naturally occurring antibodies targeting Pfs230 and Pfs45/48 have been observed in field studies in The Gambia, Kenya, and Cameroon and were associated with reduced malaria transmission (30, 45). However, other studies reported that transmission reduction correlated with antibody responses to Pfs230 only (46) or with anti-Pfs48/45 antibodies only (6, 42, 43). These conflicting results may be due to differences in the history of exposure of study participants or existence of other co-infections.

A recent study by Stone et al. using field-based mosquito-feeding assays found mosquito infection rate to be significantly reduced for people harboring naturally acquired anti-Pfs48/45 and anti-Pfs230 antibodies. In addition, these antibodies were shown to be host gametocyte density-dependent and mechanistically associated with transmission reducing activity (TRA) (47, 48). In the same study, using protein microarray, 43 novel gametocyte proteins whose specific antibodies were associated with TRA were also identified (48). Among these 43 proteins, 16 predicted to be surface-expressed showed responses more similar to those of Pfs48/45 and Pfs230 in terms of TRA and as such warrant further investigations and characterization as TBV candidates (48, 49). However, the increase of natural seroprevalence to Pfs48/45 and Pfs230 with age found by Stone and colleagues did not corroborate a previous study by Ouedraogo et al. (50).

It is worth noting that antibodies against the post-fertilization antigens Pfs25 and Pfs28 have not been observed because these antigens are not exposed to the human immune system. If utilized in a vaccine, post-fertilization antibodies would not be boosted by natural malaria infections in vaccinated individuals. Nevertheless, antibodies against Pfs28 and Pfs25 have shown promise in blocking mosquito stage development and therefore transmission in *in vitro* experiments and are currently being evaluated in clinical trials (51).

The development and evaluation of antibody responses to all gametocyte/gamete-specific antigens and their effect on sexual stages in the mosquito face several challenges (51). First, evaluation of transmission reducing immunity relies heavily on mosquito feeding experiments, otherwise known as standard membrane feeding assays, where gametocyte-infected blood is fed to mosquitoes with or without antibodies to the respective antigens. Dissection of mosquitoes 7 days after blood feeding for oocyt counts is used as an indirect measure of transmission blocking activity. These assays are time-consuming and labor-intensive. Second, it is not known what ingested antibody levels in the mosquito are required that would lead to a subsequent transmission blockade. The identification and validation of gametocyte surface antigens as vaccine candidates with transmission reducing activity (TRA) directly measurable in the human host will overcome these challenges, complement and strengthen current transmission blocking vaccine efforts (6, 52).

NATURALLY ACQUIRED ANTIBODY RESPONSES TO THE SURFACE OF GAMETOCYTE-INFECTED ERYTHROCYTES

It has been difficult to elucidate naturally acquired antibody responses to gametocyte-infected erythrocyte surface antigens (GSAs), distinct from those recognizing internally expressed gametocyte and gamete antigens, in natural human infections. This is largely due to the indirect effect of asexual stage immunity on the prevalence and density of gametocytes.

Naturally acquired sexual stage antibodies are known to be produced against *P. falciparum* gametocyte-infected erythrocyte surface antigens in human peripheral circulation (anti-gametocyte immunity) (4, 53). There are very few studies on human immune responses recognizing gametocyte-infected erythrocyte surface antigens referred to as anti- gametocyte immunity. This is in contrast to anti-gamete immunity which is raised against intracellular proteins of dead gametocytes which have some function at the gamete stages, or more broadly immune responses to gamete surface antigens (4, 6, 31, 52–54).

In the first investigation of its kind, plasma antibodies from gametocytemic Gambian children donated after antimalarial treatment were used to detect antigens on the surface of 3D7 cultured mature stage V gametocytes. Surprisingly, no antibody recognition of the surface of erythrocytes infected with developing gametocytes, stages I-IV, representing the stages known to be sequestered in deep tissues, were found (44, 54). In addition, children harboring these anti-GSA antibody responses were significantly less likely to carry gametocytes after subsequent infections suggesting an ability to control gametocytemia in these patients. It was also shown that malaria patient plasma samples with strong anti-GSA plasma antibody recognition of the mature gametocyte-infected erythrocyte surface were not more likely to recognize the surface of erythrocytes infected with asexual parasites and vice versa (54).

This was a proof of concept for the rationale to develop an anti-GSA transmission blocking vaccine. It derived its basis from epidemiological observations of specific immune suppression of gametocytes in Indonesia (53). *P. falciparum* gametocyte rates were reduced among semi-immune native Papuans, independent of immune control of asexual parasitemia, when compared to a transmigrant Javanese population with a history of lower malaria exposure. These findings suggest specific immune control of gametocytemia as the observations could not be explained by differences in the frequency or grade of parasitemia, illness or by known patterns of antimalarial treatment. Further, immunofluorescence tests with acetone-fixed whole gametocytes showed a correlation between antibody levels and reduced gametocytemia among the native Irianese (53).

The important observations by Saeed et al. (54), the ability of patient plasma to recognize GSA and the significant association with reduced gametocyte carriage, required further investigation. In order to rule out the fact that patient plasma antibody recognition of GSA on mature stage V gametocytes was not a deficiency or artifact of the 3D7 clone, we carried out recognition studies in plasma antibody samples from Ghanaian school children from a high endemicity region, against both a recent isolate and 3D7. In this study, plasma from asymptomatic school children collected over 5 sampling times at weekly intervals were tested against the surface of 3D7 mature gametocyte-infected erythrocytes as well as mature gametocytes derived from a 2012 clinical isolate of Kenyan origin, HL1204. Interestingly, we found plasma antibodies from all children bind to GSA of gametocytes derived from both clones to at least some extent. It was striking to note that plasma from Ghanaian children recognized the GSA on mature gametocytes of Kenyan origin, suggesting that perhaps the antigens detected might be conserved across geographical locations. Immature gametocytes from the clinical isolate were also tested against a selected number of plasma samples from Ghanaian children with strong anti-GSA antibody responses. Similar to the observations of Saeed et al. (54), no detectable recognition of GSA to asynchronous immature gametocytes was observed. These findings were corroborated by some gametocyte adhesion studies (15, 55), which posit that maturing gametocytes do not, as previously thought, sequester from peripheral circulation through adhesion to human bone marrow-derived endothelial surfaces and receptors (56–58). Nevertheless, further studies with tightly synchronized immature gametocyte preparations are required before we can rule out the possibility that developing gametocytes express adhesins involved in parasite ligand-host receptor interactions which mediates sequestration and elicit gametocyte-specific immunity (4).

To further test the prevalence of anti-GSA antibodies in the general endemic population, plasma donated by microscopically-confirmed parasite negative individuals were tested for antibody recognition to GSA. Forty-eight percent (24/50) of parasite-negative children and adults recognized the surface of mature gametocyte-infected erythrocytes (4, 59). Since submicroscopic gametocytemia could not be excluded, anti-GSA antibody carriage in cohort studies utilizing sensitive gametocyte detection methods such as RT-qPCR or QT-NASBA are needed to fully illuminate this relationship. Moreover, testing plasma donated from both gametocyte positive and negative children showed that our findings could possibly represent the general malaria-infected population. In addition, evidence was found that children who harbored anti-GSA antibodies were significantly but weakly associated with lower risk of gametocyte carriage (4). In addition, preliminary indirect evidence suggest that anti-GSA antibodies may be maintained over a period of time (4, 59).

CELLULAR IMMUNE RESPONSES TO GAMETOCYTES WHILE IN THE HUMAN HOST

Studies aiming at evaluating the cellular immune responses to the sexual stages compared to asexual ones of *Plasmodium* species are limited. However, there is evidence that such immunity exists. The transfer of T-cells from gamete-immunized mice was shown in the 1980s to markedly reduce gametocytemia in the recipient mice using the rodent species *P. yoelii nigeriensis* (60). Recipient mice also failed to effectively infect the mosquito vector *A. stephensi* as demonstrated by direct blood feeding (up to 95% transmission reduction) suggesting the direct impact of T-cells on transmission. However, the T-cell transfer had no effects on asexual stages (60). Good et al. (61) further showed that peripheral blood from non-exposed individuals contains T cells (clone) which proliferate and up-regulate interferon-gamma production upon stimulation with mature gametocyte-infected RBCs lysate. Similar results were also obtained in a hyper-endemic region in The Gambia by stimulation of peripheral blood mononuclear cells (PBMCs) of volunteers by gametocyte lysate (62). The detection of gametocyte-specific antibodies in the study participants by ELISA implied previous exposure to sexual stage parasites. Findings from this study suggest a T cell-dependent suppression of gametocytes or T cells helping B cells to fight against the malaria infection. Both asexual and sexual stage-specific antigens have equally been shown to elicit polyclonal T-cell responses in malaria non-exposed individuals (63). However, the reaction is not peculiar to gametocytes since it has been demonstrated that CD4 T Cells from non-exposed individuals react with PfEMP-1 via a Major Histocompatibility Complex (MHC) Class II-T cell receptor-independent Pathway (64). This could be associated to cross-reactivity from other infections. Whether this phenomenon is protective in children is not known.

In other studies, an increase in cytokine production such as TNF-α and IFN-γ was demonstrated in monkeys and humans infected with *P. cynomolgi* and *P. vivax*, respectively (65, 66). The increase in cytokine secretion correlated with the decrease in parasitemia and the inability of gametocytes to infect the mosquito vector and as such, cytokines and other PMBC-derived components (nitric oxide, antibodies) were believed to play a role in the loss of infectivity (66, 67). In their study in 1993, Naotunne et al. showed that the effect of PBMC-derived components on gametocyte infectivity was closely linked to the presence of white blood cells as no effect was seen in their absence (67). This negative effect on the infectivity of gametocytes appeared to be reversed in the presence of high concentration of an L-arginine analog (NGL-monomethyl arginine acetate) (68). This suggests that gametocyte inactivation in the presence of WBCs is achieved through an L-arginine-associated pathway mechanism. In the same line, an *in vitro* study conducted by Smith et al. (69) revealed that *P. falciparum* stage I and IIA gametocytes are to a large extent eliminated from the circulation by non-opsonic phagocytosis mediated by monocytes and macrophages. They showed through antibody inhibition assays and enzyme treatment that the interaction of PfEMP-1 and CD36 plays a major role in this innate defense against early gametocytes stages. This is in line with a previous study reporting the interaction of *P. falciparum* early gametocytes with CD36 receptor (70). A recent study conducted in India demonstrated a significant negative association between gametocytemia and IFN-γ in children (71).

Gametocyte-specific exoantigens (from gametocyte culture supernatants) have been shown to be able to stimulate the proliferation and activation of lymphocytes from *P. falciparum* exposed individual (72). In this study, T cell receptors gamma/delta (TCR $\gamma\delta$+), and CD3$^+$ CD8$^+$ and CD3$^+$ CD4$^-$ CD8$^-$ T cells were found to be up-regulated upon sensitization with these exoantigens. Particularly, the expression of the activation marker CD25$^+$ increased on stimulated CD3$^+$ and $\gamma\delta$ T cells. The frequency of $\gamma\delta$ T cells had previously been found to increase in the course of acute malaria (73). However, it is difficult to ascertain the specificity of the exoantigens because they could as well be coming from ruptured or dead asexual parasite iRBCs. As already indicated, there is a paucity of information on cellular immunity to gametocytes. Therefore, further investigations into the role of cellular immune responses to gametocytes and malaria transmission; and the identification/validation of the antigens involved, in a bid to contribute toward the development of an effective transmission blocking vaccine are required.

CELLULAR IMMUNITY TO SEXUAL STAGES WHILE IN THE MOSQUITO VECTOR

In the mosquito vector, killing of malaria parasites is not only mediated by vertebrate host-derived molecules but also by mosquito components as has previously been demonstrated (32–34). Studies have shown that only a small proportion of gametocytes ingested in the blood meal by the mosquito vector is transformed into oocysts and sporozoites; and only about 38% of mosquitoes that take gametocyte-containing blood become infected (32, 33, 74). This is largely due to the peritrophic membrane or matrix (PM) which constitutes a physical barrier to *Plasmodium species* and other pathogens (33, 75, 76). This membrane is formed after the ingestion of a potentially infectious blood meal by the mosquito and surrounds the ingested blood. It prevents direct contact between the pathogens in the blood and the midgut epithelium and by so doing interferes with midgut invasion (33, 76). However, ookinetes secrete the enzyme chitinase which destroys the chitineous PM and allows it to invade the midgut (33, 77). The midgut epithelial cells are also thought to secrete high amounts of nitric oxide synthase and peroxidases, which in turn leads to nitration of the gut epithelium with subsequent tagging of ookinetes for destruction by the complement system (33, 78, 79).

The innate immune response in the malaria mosquito vector is mediated mainly by hemocytes which eliminate pathogens such as bacteria, fungi, and protozoa by phagocytosis (80–82). The *Anopheles* species and other insects are known to have a complement C3-like protein called thioester-containing proteins (TEP) (80). TEP of *A. gambiae* (AgTEP1) has been shown to be valuable for the initiation of immune defense against *P. berghei*. TEP1 plays the role of opsonins and facilitates the interaction between the parasite and the hemocytes with subsequent encapsulation, and killing of the parasite (80). Double knock-out of the TEP1 gene renders genetically selected refractory *Anopheles* strain susceptible to infection and increases the infectivity rates in susceptible *A. gambiae* (80). This vector defense mechanism has been shown recently to be by-passed by *P. falciparum* through its 6-cysteine protein P47-like (83). This protein is invaluable for *P. berghei* female gamete fertility (84) but in *P. falciparum*, it promotes the gametocyte-to-ookinete development and protects the ookinete from complement-dependent lysis (83).

In addition, infection of *A. gambiae* mosquito by ookinetes of *P. berghei* has been demonstrated to modulate the mosquito's immune system by up-regulating the expression of the antibacterial peptide defensin and a putative gram-negative bacteria-binding protein (85), and a TNF-α factor-like transcription factor (LL3) (86). Silencing of the LL3 gene was found to be associated with an increase in parasite survival, confirming its role in conferring mosquito resistance to the *Plasmodium* parasite. LL3 also affects the expression of another protein, a serine protease inhibitor (SRPN6), which equally confers resistance to invasion by *Plasmodium* (86).

Genomic and transcriptomic analyses of bacterial lipopolysaccharide-stimulated *A. gambiae* mosquitos revealed 23 immune-regulated genes which include putative protease inhibitors, serine proteases, and regulatory molecules (87). Interestingly, the protease inhibitor α-2-macroglobulin was found to be more specific in response to malaria parasite than bacterial infection as observed with mosquitoes fed on a *P. berghei*-infected hamster. This suggests that the immune response mounted by the mosquito vector may be pathogen specific, and other authors have reported similar findings (88). RNA gene interference (RNAi) experiments on *P. falciparum*- and *P. berghei*-infected *An. gambiae* revealed some common genes that confer resistance to both parasite species. However, other genes were found to exhibit species-specificity, conferring resistance only to one parasite species, namely a pattern recognition receptor (MD2-like receptor, AgMDL1) and an immunolectin, FBN39 for *P. falciparum* and the antimicrobial peptide gambicin and a novel putative short secreted peptide, IRSP5 for *P. berghei* (88). Together, these findings show that mosquitoes express molecules with anti-plasmodial properties which act as self-defense mechanism in the vector.

ANTI-GAMETOCYTE AND ANTI-GAMETE TRANSMISSION BLOCKING VACCINES

Up to date, it has been a difficult task developing an effective vaccine against malaria. This is due both to the complexity of the *Plasmodium* parasite life cycle and the polymorphic nature of its antigens (89, 90). However, the hope that an effective malaria vaccine is feasible is based on the observation that in endemic regions, clinically immune adults are protected from severe malaria and death compared to children (89). This could be attributed to the fact that natural immunity in adults is probably complex and dependent on immune responses to many stages. Interestingly, sera from immune individuals have been shown to inhibit gamete fertilization and development in the mosquito vector thereby interfering with disease transmission (91–93). This constitutes the basis of the development of malaria transmission blocking vaccines (TBVs). An emerging concept is to develop vaccines against antigens expressed solely in the mosquito's midgut to which the host immune system is not naturally exposed. Antibodies against those antigens from vaccinated individuals and animals have been shown to interfere with parasite viability and development in the mosquito midgut interaction (94–96).

As a limitation, TBVs are different from the other vaccine types (liver and blood stage vaccines) in the sense that they do not protect against disease in the vaccinees. However, they reduce the risk of transmission to other people by the mosquito vector and by so doing favor herd immunity; as such they have sometimes been referred to as altruistic vaccines (95). Two groups of target antigens (gene superfamilies) exist, namely pre-fertilization and post-fertilization antigens (**Table 1** and **Figure 2**) (48, 97, 107–111, 121). The list (**Table 1**) is not exhaustive both for pre- and post-fertilization antigens as some proteins remain unidentified to date. Some of these target antigens were characterized back in 1983 by Kaushal et al. (98), among them, Pfs48/45, Pfs47, Pfs230, and Pfs25 are immunogenic and less polymorphic, making them good vaccine candidates (122). Their use in combination with strong adjuvants or carrier proteins has been shown to boost their immunogenicity. Some of the adjuvants/carrier proteins used included Maltose Binding Protein (MBP)—Exoprotein A (EPA) from *P. aeruginosa*—Outer Membrane Protein Complex (OMPC)—modified Lickenase carrier (LiKM)—Virus-like particle (VLP)—Alhydrogel. Only two of these vaccine candidates, namely Pfs 230 and Pfs25, have entered clinical trial stage (123) and are reviewed in this paper. The potential of the other antigens (e.g., Pfs48/45) as TBV candidates has been recently reviewed by Chaturvedi et al. (122). Although Pfs 45/48 has not yet attained the clinical trial phase, previous studies demonstrated that antibodies against this antigen elicit up to 99% inhibition of oocyst intensity and 85% inhibition of oocyst prevalence (99). Hence the necessity to pursue studies with the Pfs 48/45 TBV candidate. Moreover, recent studies have identified new sexual stage antigens that require more attention (48, 121)

Pfs230 is a 363 kDa protein and a potent antigen of malaria TBV. It is a main component in the fertilization process as male gametes with impaired Pfs230 gene are incapable of interacting with red blood cells (RBCs) and forming exflagellation centers (100). This results in marked reduction in oocyst production and mosquito infectivity. Similar observations were made with genetically modified *P. falciparum* with a truncated chitinase 1 (PfCHT1) gene which could be due to the inability of affected ookinetes to invade the mosquito midgut (106). Administration of recombinant Pfs230 + Alhydrogel induced high titers of antibodies in rabbits which were found to have significant transmission reducing activity (101). It should be pointed out that only certain fragments of the recombinant Pfs230 antigen induce responses that lead to TRA (99). Significant associations between suppression of mosquito infectivity and anti-Pfs230

TABLE 1 | Sexual stage antigens in the human host and mosquito vector with transmission reducing activity/potentials.

Type	Antigen name	Function/role	References
Parasite pre-fertilization antigens	Pfs48/45	Male gamete attachment to female gamete	(6, 30, 42, 43, 97, 98)
	Pfs47	Fertilization process	(97, 98)
	Pfs230	Main component in the male fertilization process	(30, 41, 98–101)
	STEVORS	Sequestration of early gametocytes and deformability of mature gametocytes	(14–16)
	Plasmodium falciparum surface related antigen (PfSRA)	Erythrocyte invasion, unknown role in gametocytes	(102)
	Plasmodium falciparum LCCL domain-containing protein (CCP)	Parasite development in the mosquito	(103)
	Plasmodium falciparum CX3CL1-binding protein 2	Cytoadherence to host cells	(104)
	Plasmodium falciparum Gametocyte EXported Protein-5 (PfGEXP5)	Gametocyte switching	(105)
Parasite post-fertilization antigens	Pf25	Parasite survival and interactions with mosquito midgut	(37, 51, 98)
	Pfs28	Parasite survival and interactions with mosquito midgut	(37, 51, 98)
	Chitinase 1	Parasite invasion of the midgut	(33, 77, 106)
	Von Willebrand factor-A domain-related protein (WARP)	Ookinete attachment to the mosquito midgut, differentiation of ookinete to oocyst	(107)
	Circumsporozoite and thrombospondin-related anonymous protein (CTRP)	Transition from ookinetes into oocysts in the vector	(108)
	Membrane-attack ookinete protein (MAOP)	Ookinete midgut invasion in vector	(109)
	Secreted ookinete adhesive protein (SOAP)	Ookinete midgut invasion and oocyst development	(110)
	Cell-traversal protein for ookinetes and sporozoites (CelTOS)	Establishment of malaria infections in both vector and vertebrate hosts	(111)
Vector antigens	Midgut-specific alanyl aminopeptidase (AnAPN1)	Ookinete midgut invasion in vector	(75, 112–115)
	Carboxypeptidase B1	Parasite development in the vector	(116, 117)
	Serine protease inhibitors (serpins)	Regulation of the vector innate immune responses	(118)
	Saglin proteins	Vector salivary gland invasion	(119, 120)

antibody levels were also found using membrane feeding assays with sera collected from African populations (43, 45, 46, 124) and in mice (99). This vaccine candidate (125) has entered a phase 1 clinical trial in which the Safety and Immunogenicity of Pfs230D1M-EPA/Alhydrogel is being evaluated in adults in the US and Mali (data unpublished, https://clinicaltrials.gov/ct2/show/NCT02334462).

Pf25 is relevant for parasite survival and interactions with mosquito midgut molecules prior to invasion. Anti-Pf25 antibodies have been shown to halt parasite growth within the mosquito in membrane feeding assays as reviewed by Chaturvedi et al. (122). This vaccine candidate has undergone clinical trial phase 1 in combination with different carriers and adjuvants. Administration of Pf25-Viral-like-particles plus Alhydrogel® to mice resulted in high antibody titers with 100% transmission reducing activity (TRA) throughout the study (126). A clinical trial phase 1a with this combination was recently carried out in the United States (https://clinicaltrials.gov/ct2/show/NCT02013687). It appeared that the combination is safe with no serious adverse reactions observed in healthy volunteers even when higher doses are administered. However, the antibodies generated showed low TRA hence the necessity to prioritize vaccine adjuvant formulations for further investigations (127).

Another combination of Pfs25 and EPA (Pseudomonas aeruginosa ExoProtein A) plus Alhydrogel® was also demonstrated to be well tolerated by naïve individuals after several doses in a phase 1a dose-response clinical trial in the US which correlated with antibody titers (128). A Phase 1b trial of Pfs25-EPA/Alhydrogel® is currently ongoing in Malian adults (122). New promising multimeric Pf25-based Vaccine Candidates ChAd63 Pfs25-IMX313 and MVA Pfs25-IMX313 have recently been developed with promising results (129) and are now undergoing clinical trial phase 1a in the UK. These vaccine candidates consist of attenuated viruses (ChAd63-chimpanzee adenovirus 63 and MVA- modified vaccinia Ankara) encoding the parasite protein Pf25, which are fused to a carrier protein (IMX313-multimerization technology) as adjuvant (NCT02532049). In mouse models, Chad63Pfs25-IMX313 was safe and significantly more immunogenic with higher TRA than monomeric Pfs25 (130). Similar results were obtained with the *P. vivax* antigen (Pvs25H/Alhydrogel), and the *P. falciparum* ortholog Pfs25 in a mouse model. Anti-Pvs25H antibody

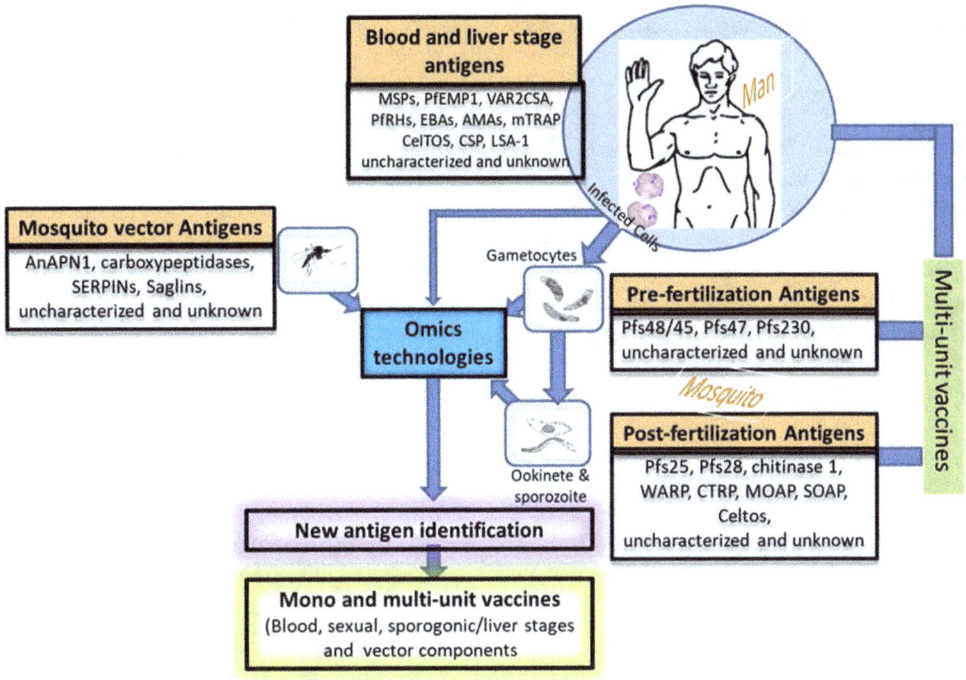

FIGURE 2 | Potential approaches for new vaccine candidate identification and vaccine development. This figure describes in a nutshell the life cycle of the *Plasmodium* species providing different stage-specific antigens and the strategies that could be used to develop more efficacious vaccine by combining potential vaccine candidates from various stages (host's and vector's). Uncharacterized and unknown antigens refer to proteins of unknown functions or proteins that have only been partially characterized such as the multigene families (*var, rif, and stevor*). The function of the proteins encoded by these multigene families have been tremendously studied in the asexual stages of *Plasmodium* but poorly exploited in their sexual counterparts. We propose that more attention should be paid to the sexual stages in terms of vaccine candidate identification and characterization. Nowadays, this could easily be done with the advent of Omics technologies. PfEMP-1, *Plasmodium falciparum* erythrocyte membrane protein-1; RIFINs, repetitive interspersed families of polypeptides; STEVORs, Subtelomeric variable open reading frame polypeptides; MSPs, Merozoite surface proteins; VAR2CSA, A variant of PfEMP-1 with high affinity to placental tissues; PfRHs, *Plasmodium falciparum* reticulocyte binding protein homologs; EBAs, Erythrocyte binding antigens; AMAs, Apical membrane antigens; CSP, Circumsporozoite protein; LSA-1, Liver-Stage Antigen; mTRAP, Merozoite thrombospondin-related anonymous protein; Pfs (230, 48/45, 25,28), *Plasmodium falciparum* gamete surface proteins (molecular weight in dalton); WARP, von Willebrand factor-A domain-related protein; CTRP, Circumsporozoite and TRAP-related protein; MAOP, Membrane-attack ookinete protein; SOAP, Secreted ookinete adhesive protein; CelTos, Cell-traversal protein for ookinetes and sporozoites; AnAPN1, *An. Gambiae* alanyl aminopeptidase; serpins, Serine protease inhibitors; *saglin* proteins.

levels peaked after the third vaccination and vaccine-induced antibodies were functional, giving significant TRA (96). This combination has proven to be safe in humans in a clinical trial phase 1 with similar immunogenicity and TRA as previously shown in mice (131).

The main limitations of these sexual stage vaccine candidates have been the systemic reactogenicity observed in some clinical trials, short-lasting antibody responses owing to the fact that the host has no or limited exposure to the antigens requiring multiple boosting doses and strong adjuvants. In addition the recombinant antigens are difficult to express in their native form (122). To circumvent the issue of limited exposure of pre-fertilization and post-fertilization antigens to the human immune system, it might be good to develop DNA or viral vector-based vaccines containing different antigens (132, 133). This ensures continuous production of the antigens of interest in the host hence permanent stimulation of the immune system, thus bypassing the necessity for multiple immunizations (132, 133). However, the main problem is that the attenuated virus used can revert and cause infections, it can also get integrated in the vaccinee's genome and lead to unforeseen consequences with the associated ethical issues. It would be valuable to make use of high class adjuvants such as the Polymeric nanoparticle- and microparticle-based adjuvant systems that ensure long term delivery of the antigen to the host system when administered (134). It would be good also to include some blood and liver stage antigens to such combinations so that the vaccinee benefits from the process (**Figure 2**).

ANTI-MOSQUITO TRANSMISSION BLOCKING VACCINES

Some mosquito components are invaluable for the sporogonic development of malaria parasites as they are involved in parasite invasion through interaction with parasite receptors. Antibodies raised against these components could be very useful in blocking parasite development in the mosquito vector (95). Thus, these components constitute another class of TBV candidates as their inhibition would likely minimize the risk of new infection in the community (135). An alternative transmission blocking vaccine strategy could be to interfere with the interactions between the parasite and the midgut molecules of the mosquito vector which will lead to the inhibition of ookinete invasion and the development of mosquito stages. Many of such molecules have been identified and characterized (**Table 1** and **Figure 2**). These molecules have been shown to be more conserved than the parasite antigens and are immunogenic in non-human primates (75, 112–115).

Midgut-specific alanyl aminopeptidase (AnAPN1) is a Glycosylphosphatidyl inositol (GPI)-anchored antigen which plays a valuable role in ookinete invasion in *A. gambiae* as previously shown by Dinglasan et al. (113). Administration of a recombinant fragment of rAnAPN160–195 with Alhydrogel has been demonstrated to stimulate a sustained production of antibodies with transmission blocking activities as revealed by membrane feeding assays (112). The TRA was dose dependent with higher antibody levels attaining 100% efficacy, and functional in both the chromosomal M and S forms of *A. gambiae* vectors. Moreover, the *P. falciparum*-infected blood samples used for membrane feeding assays were collected directly from gametocyte positive individuals and the results obtained exceeded those that had been reported previously with laboratory strains (113). More importantly, anti rAnAPN160–195 antibodies had effects on both *P. falciparum* and *P. vivax* and based on that evidence the AnAPN1 TBV has been recommended for phase I clinical trials (112). This antigen is immunogenic in mice and rabbits even in the absence of adjuvants (113, 115). However, it is worth mentioning that another study by Kapulu et al. failed to replicate the finding reported here. In their study, anti-AgAPN1 IgG had no significant impact on oocyst prevalence (99). Antibodies to another GPI-anchored vector midgut protein, α-AgSGU, were also confirmed to have an effect on *P. falciparum* and *P. vivax* development in *An. gambiae* and *An. Dirus* (114). However, high doses of α-AgSGU antibodies were required to achieve 80% TRA rendering *α-AgSGU* less promising as a TBV target.

In the same line, the midgut carboxypeptidase gene of *A. gambiae* (cpbAg) has been shown to be up-regulated following *P. falciparum* gametocyte ingestion by the vector (116). In addition, anti-CPBAG antibodies were shown to inhibit the development of both *P. falciparum and P. berghei* in the vector's midgut. Antibodies directed against CPBA have also been demonstrated to be vector-unspecific in the sense that they also inhibit the development of the *P. falciparum* gametocytes in *A. stephensi* mosquitoes, which is the main malaria vector in Iran and neighboring countries (117). This confirmed the conserved nature of molecules across different vector as predicted using genomic and proteomic approaches (117) and implies that a vaccine designed with CPBA could provide cross-species protection. Thus, CPBA constitutes another promising TBV candidate.

The interaction between the *Plasmodium* sporozoite Thrombospondin Related Anonymous Protein (TRAP) and the mosquito Saglin proteins is a prerequisite for vector salivary gland invasion (119). This has been confirmed by *in vivo* down regulation experiments of *saglin* gene expression which revealed a negative association with salivary gland invasion (119). Moreover, *in silico* analysis of *saglin* revealed the presence of a signal peptide suggesting that it may be a secreted protein. If verified *in vitro* and *in vivo*, Saglin proteins could constitute a new promising candidate for TBV design (120). Similarly, RNA interference silencing and knock-down experiments have demonstrated the essentiality of the serine protease inhibitors (serpins) in the survival of *An. gambiae* and *An. stephensi* as well as in the development of parasites (*P. berghei*) within these vectors (136, 137). Serpins are regulators of the vector innate immune responses and they are involved in the clearance of protozoan parasites (137). Antibodies raised against the *An. gambiae* serpin-2 (AgSRPN2) have been shown to be *P. berghei*-specific in *An. gambiae* and *An. stephensi* as they failed to interfere with *P. falciparum* oocyst formation (118). This study demonstrated that mosquito innate immune response-related molecules could be used as targets for TBV design; however, further investigations are needed to identify and/or validate the right antigens. A limitation here will be that all of these proteins are likely to suffer from the same problems as gamete/ookinete antigens in the sense that several booster doses are required and antibodies may be short-lived.

FUTURE DIRECTIONS IN SEXUAL STAGE IMMUNITY AND VACCINE DEVELOPMENT

Apart from studies reported in these reviews (60–62, 69, 72, 73), studies on host cellular and humoral immunity to gametocytes are scarce if not inexistent. Given promising results in clinical trials of TBV experimental vaccines for malaria eradication, the antigens involved should be characterized further to explore their suitability as vaccine candidates. The generation of long-lived antibodies depends on the generation of long-lived plasma cells and memory B cells (MBCs) within germinal centers (GCs) of secondary lymphoid organs (138). The prerequisite for plasma cells and MBCs is the interaction between follicular T helper cells and B cells. Further investigations of these cell types vis-à-vis the identified antigens in the context of malaria infections are needed. Similarly, further studies aiming at identifying new antigens (mainly vector-, gametocyte-, ookinete-, and/or oocyste-related) using genomics, transcriptomics and proteomics approaches, the Sanger center parasite gene knock-out library and other bioinformatics strategies are warranted (139–141) (**Figure 2**). These approaches take advantage of next generation sequencing (NGS) and the availability of growing numbers of *P. falciparum* whole genome sequences to identify new antigens (142). These methods are relatively fast and high throughput, leading to the identification of a plethora of essential genes or antigens through comparative analyses (139, 141–143). The implications of omics in the fight against infectious disease was recently reviewed by Bah et al. (144). But this would be strengthened by the concomitant ability to cultivate the sequenced lines and generate sexual stages from them for phenotypic studies. Bioinformatic strategies can also overcome some of the difficulties in studying parasites such as *Plasmodium spp.* or *Trypanosoma spp.* which are genetically diverse (140, 145–147). In addition, computer-based algorithms have been developed to delineate T-cell epitopes on essential parasite proteins directly from genome sequence data (148–150). Vaccine developers should consider designing multi-unit or multi-stage TBVs with components from both the parasite (precisely gametocyte antigens) and the vector as this will broaden their spectrum of action.

As far as the search for a vaccine is concerned, much has been done to understand the multigene family PfEMP-1. However, the other multigene family proteins such as RIFIN and STEVOR also constitute an important class of parasite molecules that deserve attention. These form part of the uncharacterized or partially characterized parasite antigen repertoire with respect to the sexual stages (**Figure 2**). The *stevor* multicopy family is made up of a set of 39 genes with 2–3 copies expressed at a time (151) while about 150–200 genes code for RIFINs with many copies expressed at a time as well (152). STEVOR and RIFIN proteins were recently shown to be implicated in rosetting which is a phenomenon associated with sequestration and clinical complications of the malaria (153–157). STEVORs are suspected to be implicated in the sequestration of early gametocytes in tissues such as the bone marrow and spleen as well as the deformability of the mature gametocytes (14–16). There is also evidence that STEVORs alter RBC membrane rigidity since RBC deformability has been shown to be linked to STEVOR dissociation from the mature gametocyte-infected RBC membrane (15). This implies that inhibiting the functions of STEVORS might negatively affect the development of gametocytes and by so-doing will also reduce disease transmission due to a reduced number of sexual stages being ingested by the mosquito vector during its blood meal. Despite their variable nature, the putative role of STEVORs in gametocyte development and sequestration certainly make this family a possible new class of TBV vaccine targets. Humoral responses to these antigens have been demonstrated (158). We therefore recommend further characterization (both humoral and cellular) of anti-STEVOR immune response, in the hope of finding additional clues in the search for efficient TBVs. However, the most pressing task is to develop further STEVOR-specific reagents demonstrating their relevance in anti-gametocyte immune responses and therefore transmission reducing immunity/activities.

In addition to STEVORS, many other Plasmodium antigens such as LCCL domain-containing protein family (103), *Plasmodium falciparum* Surface Related Antigen (PfSRA) (102), CX3CL1-binding protein 2 (104), Gametocyte EXported Protein-5 (PfGEXP5) (105) have been described as potential TBV candidates and as such deserve further characterizations.

AUTHOR CONTRIBUTIONS

JK-O and BD designed and drafted the manuscript. CS, FB, GA, and BU reviewed and edited the manuscript. All authors approved the final version of manuscript for publication.

FUNDING

JK-O is supported by a DELTAS Africa grant (DEL-15-007: Awandare). The DELTAS Africa Initiative is an independent funding scheme of the African Academy of Sciences (AAS)'s Alliance for Accelerating Excellence in Science in Africa (AESA) and supported by the New Partnership for Africa's Development Planning and Coordinating Agency (NEPAD Agency) with funding from the Wellcome Trust (107755/Z/15/Z: Awandare) and the UK government. BD is funded by a Wellcome Trust Training Fellowship in Public Health and Tropical Medicine (110090/Z/15/Z). The views expressed in this publication are those of the authors and not necessarily those of AAS, NEPAD Agency, Wellcome Trust or the UK government.

ACKNOWLEDGMENTS

We are grateful to Prof. Kirk W. Deitsch of Weill Cornell Medical College, New York, for providing critical reviews of the manuscripts which helped improve it.

REFERENCES

1. WHO. *World Malaria Day 2018 "Ready to Beat Malaria": key messages*. No. WHO/CDS/GMP/*2018.06, World Health Organization* (2018).
2. Ashley EA, Dhorda M, Fairhurst RM, Amaratunga C, Lim P, Suon S, et al. Spread of artemisinin resistance in *Plasmodium falciparum* malaria. *N Engl J Med.* (2014) 371:411–23. doi: 10.1056/NEJMoa1314981
3. Dondorp AM, Nosten F, Yi P, Das D, Phyo AP, Tarning J, et al. Artemisinin resistance in *Plasmodium falciparum* malaria. *N Engl J Med.* (2009) 361:455–67. doi: 10.1056/NEJMoa0808859
4. Dinko B, King E, Targett GA, Sutherland CJ. Antibody responses to surface antigens of *Plasmodium falciparum* gametocyte-infected erythrocytes and their relation to gametocytaemia. *Parasite Immunol.* (2016) 38:352–64. doi: 10.1111/pim.12323
5. Alonso PL, Brown G, Arevalo-Herrera M, Binka F, Chitnis C, Collins F, et al. A research agenda to underpin malaria eradication. *PLoS Med.* (2011) 8:e1000406. doi: 10.1371/journal.pmed.1000406
6. Gebru T, Ajua A, Theisen M, Esen M, Ngoa UA, Issifou S, et al. Recognition of *Plasmodium falciparum* mature gametocyte-infected erythrocytes by antibodies of semi-immune adults and malaria-exposed children from Gabon. *Malar J.* (2017) 16:176. doi: 10.1186/s12936-017-1827-7
7. Sinha A, Hughes KR, Modrzynska KK, Otto TD, Pfander C, Dickens NJ, et al. A cascade of DNA-binding proteins for sexual commitment and development in *Plasmodium*. *Nature* (2014) 507:253. doi: 10.1038/nature12970
8. Smith T, Lourenco P, Carter R, Walliker D, Ranford-Cartwright L. Commitment to sexual differentiation in the human malaria parasite, *Plasmodium falciparum*. *Parasitology* (2000) 121:127–33. doi: 10.1017/S0031182099006265
9. Dinko B, Ansah F, Agyare-Kwabi C, Tagboto S, Amoah LE, Urban BC, et al. Gametocyte development and carriage in Ghanaian individuals with uncomplicated *Plasmodium falciparum* malaria. *Am J Trop Med Hyg.* (2018) 99:57–64. doi: 10.4269/ajtmh.18-0077
10. Pelle KG, Oh K, Buchholz K, Narasimhan V, Joice R, Milner DA, et al. Transcriptional profiling defines dynamics of parasite tissue sequestration during malaria infection. *Genome Med.* (2015) 7:19. doi: 10.1186/s13073-015-0133-7
11. Aguilar R, Magallon-Tejada A, Achtman AH, Moraleda C, Joice R, Cisteró P, et al. Molecular evidence for the localization of *Plasmodium*

falciparum immature gametocytes in bone marrow. *Blood* (2014) 123:959–66. doi: 10.1182/blood-2013-08-520767

12. Farfour E, Charlotte F, Settegrana C, Miyara M, Buffet P. The extravascular compartment of the bone marrow: a niche for *Plasmodium falciparum* gametocyte maturation? *Malar J.* (2012) 11:285. doi: 10.1186/1475-2875-11-285
13. Joice R, Nilsson SK, Montgomery J, Dankwa S, Egan E, Morahan B, et al. *Plasmodium falciparum* transmission stages accumulate in the human bone marrow. *Sci Transl Med.* (2014) 6:244re245. doi: 10.1126/scitranslmed.3008882
14. Smalley M, Abdalla S, Brown J. The distribution of *Plasmodium falciparum* in the peripheral blood and bone marrow of Gambian children. *Trans R Soc Trop Med Hyg.* (1981) 75:103–5. doi: 10.1016/0035-9203(81)90019-5
15. Tibúrcio M, Niang M, Deplaine G, Perrot S, Bischoff E, Ndour PA, et al. A switch in infected erythrocyte deformability at the maturation and blood circulation of *Plasmodium falciparum* transmission stages. *Blood* (2012) 119:e172–e180. doi: 10.1182/blood-2012-03-414557
16. Tibúrcio M, Silvestrini F, Bertuccini L, Sander AF, Turner L, Lavstsen T, et al. Early gametocytes of the malaria parasite *Plasmodium falciparum* specifically remodel the adhesive properties of infected erythrocyte surface. *Cell Microbiol.* (2013) 15:647–59. doi: 10.1111/cmi.12062
17. Messina V, Valtieri M, Rubio M, Falchi M, Mancini F, Mayor A, et al. Gametocytes of the malaria parasite *Plasmodium falciparum* interact with and stimulate bone marrow mesenchymal cells to secrete angiogenetic factors. *Front Cell Infect Microbiol.* (2018) 8:50. doi: 10.3389/fcimb.2018.00050
18. Bruce M, Alano P, Duthie S, Carter R. Commitment of the malaria parasite *Plasmodium falciparum* to sexual and asexual development. *Parasitology* (1990) 100:191–200. doi: 10.1017/S0031182000061199
19. Silvestrini F, Alano P, Williams J. Commitment to the production of male and female gametocytes in the human malaria parasite *Plasmodium falciparum*. *Parasitology* (2000) 121:465–71. doi: 10.1017/S0031182099006691
20. Hanssen E, Knoechel C, Dearnley M, Dixon MWA, Le Gros M, Larabell C, et al. Soft X-ray microscopy analysis of cell volume and hemoglobin content in erythrocytes infected with asexual and sexual stages of *Plasmodium falciparum*. *J Struct Biol.* (2012) 177:224–32. doi: 10.1016/j.jsb.2011.09.003
21. Mair GR, Lasonder E, Garver LS, Franke-Fayard BM, Carret CK, Wiegant JC, et al. Universal features of post-transcriptional gene regulation are critical for *Plasmodium* zygote development. *PLoS Pathog.* (2010) 6:e1000767. doi: 10.1371/journal.ppat.1000767
22. Billker O, Shaw M, Margos G, Sinden R. The roles of temperature, pH and mosquito factors as triggers of male and female gametogenesis of *Plasmodium berghei in vitro*. *Parasitology* (1997) 115:1–7. doi: 10.1017/S0031182097008895
23. Billker O, Lindo V, Panico M, Etienne A, Paxton T, Dell A, et al. Identification of xanthurenic acid as the putative inducer of malaria development in the mosquito. *Nature* (1998) 392:289. doi: 10.1038/32667
24. Sinden R. The cell biology of sexual development in *Plasmodium*. *Parasitology* (1983) 86:7–28. doi: 10.1017/S0031182000050824
25. Sinden R. Sexual development of malarial parasites. *Adv Parasitol.* (1983) 22:153–216. doi: 10.1016/S0065-308X(08)60462-5
26. Vaughan JA. Population dynamics of *Plasmodium* sporogony. *Trends Parasitol.* (2007) 23:63–70. doi: 10.1016/j.pt.2006.12.009
27. Schneider P, Bousema JT, Gouagna LC, Otieno S, Van De Vegte-Bolmer M, Omar SA, et al. Submicroscopic *Plasmodium falciparum* gametocyte densities frequently result in mosquito infection. *Am J Trop Med Hyg.* (2007) 76:470–4. doi: 10.4269/ajtmh.2007.76.470
28. Targett G, Drakeley C, Jawara M, von Seidlein L, Coleman R, Deen J, et al. Artesunate reduces but does not prevent posttreatment transmission of *Plasmodium falciparum* to *Anopheles gambiae*. *J Infect Dis.* (2001) 183:1254–9. doi: 10.1086/319689
29. Bousema J, Drakeley C, Sauerwein R. Sexual-stage antibody responses to *P. falciparum* in endemic populations. *Curr Mol Med.* (2006) 6:223–9. doi: 10.2174/156652406776055140
30. Bousema T, Okell L, Shekalaghe S, Griffin JT, Omar S, Sawa P, et al. Revisiting the circulation time of *Plasmodium falciparum* gametocytes: molecular detection methods to estimate the duration of gametocyte carriage and the effect of gametocytocidal drugs. *Malar J.* (2010) 9:136. doi: 10.1186/1475-2875-9-136
31. Stone WJ, Dantzler KW, Nilsson SK, Drakeley CJ, Marti M, Bousema T, et al. Naturally acquired immunity to sexual stage *P. falciparum* parasites. *Parasitology* (2016) 143:187–98. doi: 10.1017/S0031182015001341
32. Gouagna LC, Mulder B, Noubissi E, Tchuinkam T, Verhave JP, Boudin C. The early sporogonic cycle of *Plasmodium falciparum* in laboratory-infected *Anopheles gambiae*: an estimation of parasite efficacy. *Trop Med Int Health* (1998) 3:21–8. doi: 10.1046/j.1365-3156.1998.00156.x
33. Smith RC, Vega-Rodríguez J, Jacobs-Lorena M. The *Plasmodium* bottleneck: malaria parasite losses in the mosquito vector. *Mem Inst Oswaldo Cruz.* (2014) 109:644–61. doi: 10.1590/0074-0276130597
34. Whitten MM, Shiao SH, Levashina EA. Mosquito midguts and malaria: cell biology, compartmentalization and immunology. *Parasite Immunol.* (2006) 28:121–30. doi: 10.1111/j.1365-3024.2006.00804.x
35. Mendis K, Munesinghe Y, De Silva Y, Keragalla I, Carter R. Malaria transmission-blocking immunity induced by natural infections of *Plasmodium vivax* in humans. *Infect Immun.* (1987) 55:369–72.
36. Alano P. *Plasmodium* sexual stage antigens. *Parasitol Today* (1991) 7:199–203. doi: 10.1016/0169-4758(91)90138-E
37. Sinden R. A biologist's perspective on malaria vaccine development. *Hum Vaccin.* (2010) 6:3–11. doi: 10.4161/hv.6.1.9604
38. Mendis KN, David PH, Carter R. Human immune responses against sexual stages of malaria parasites: considerations for malaria vaccines. *Int J Parasitol.* (1990) 20:497–502. doi: 10.1016/0020-7519(90)90197-U
39. Mendis KN, Munesinghe YD, de Silva YN, Keragalla I, Carter R. Malaria transmission-blocking immunity induced by natural infections of *Plasmodium vivax* in humans. *Infect Immun.* (1987) 55:369–72.
40. Drakeley C, Bousema J, Akim N, Teelen K, Roeffen W, Lensen A, et al. Transmission-reducing immunity is inversely related to age in *Plasmodium falciparum* gametocyte carriers. *Parasite Immunol.* (2006) 28:185–90. doi: 10.1111/j.1365-3024.2005.00818.x
41. Graves P, Wirtz R, Carter R, Burkot T, Looker M, Targett G. Naturally occurring antibodies to an epitope on *Plasmodium falciparum* gametes detected by monoclonal antibody-based competitive enzyme-linked immunosorbent assay. *Infect Immun.* (1988) 56:2818–21.
42. Mulder B, Lensen T, Tchuinkam T, Roeffen W, Verhave JP, Boudin C, et al. *Plasmodium falciparum*: membrane feeding assays and competition ELISAs for the measurement of transmission reduction in sera from Cameroon. *Exp Parasitol.* (1999) 92:81–6. doi: 10.1006/expr.1999.4398
43. van der Kolk M, de Vlas SJ, Sauerwein RW. Reduction and enhancement of *Plasmodium falciparum* transmission by endemic human sera. *Int J Parasitol.* (2006) 36:1091–5. doi: 10.1016/j.ijpara.2006.05.004
44. Sutherland CJ. Surface antigens of *Plasmodium falciparum* gametocytes—a new class of transmission-blocking vaccine targets? *Mol Biochem Parasitol.* (2009) 166:93–8. doi: 10.1016/j.molbiopara.2009.03.007
45. Bousema T, Sutherland CJ, Churcher TS, Mulder B, Gouagna LC, Riley EM, et al. Human immune responses that reduce the transmission of *Plasmodium falciparum* in African populations. *Int J Parasitol.* (2011) 41:293–300. doi: 10.1016/j.ijpara.2010.09.008
46. Graves PM, Carter R, Burkot TR, Quakyi IA, Kumar N. Antibodies to *Plasmodium falciparum* gamete surface antigens in Papua New Guinea sera. *Parasite Immunol.* (1988) 10:209–18. doi: 10.1111/j.1365-3024.1988.tb00215.x
47. Ouedraogo AL, Eckhoff PA, Luty AJF. Modeling the impact of *Plasmodium falciparum* sexual stage immunity on the composition and dynamics of the human infectious reservoir for malaria in natural settings. *PLoS Pathog.* (2018) 14:e1007034. doi: 10.1371/journal.ppat.1007034
48. Stone WJR, Campo JJ, Ouedraogo AL, Meerstein-Kessel L, Morlais I, Da D, et al. Unravelling the immune signature of *Plasmodium falciparum* transmission-reducing immunity. *Nat Commun.* (2018) 9:558. doi: 10.1038/s41467-017-02646-2
49. Jones S, Grignard L, Nebie I, Chilongola J, Dodoo D, Sauerwein R, et al. Naturally acquired antibody responses to recombinant Pfs230 and Pfs48/45 transmission blocking vaccine candidates. *J Infect.* (2015) 71:117–27. doi: 10.1016/j.jinf.2015.03.007
50. Ouédraogo AL, Roeffen W, Luty AJ, de Vlas SJ, Nebie I, Ilboudo-Sanogo E, et al. (2011). Naturally acquired immune responses to *Plasmodium*

falciparum sexual stage antigens Pfs48/45 and Pfs230 in an area of seasonal transmission. *Infect. Immun.* 79, 4957–64. doi: 10.1128/iai.05288-11
51. Nunes JK, Woods C, Carter T, Raphael T, Morin MJ, Diallo D, et al. Development of a transmission-blocking malaria vaccine: progress, challenges, and the path forward. *Vaccine* (2014) 32:5531–9. doi: 10.1016/j.vaccine.2014.07.030
52. Tonwong N, Sattabongkot J, Tsuboi T, Iriko H, Takeo S, Sirichaisinthop J, et al. Natural infection of *Plasmodium falciparum* induces inhibitory antibodies against gametocyte development in human hosts. *Jpn J Infect Dis.* (2012) 65:152–6. doi: 10.1186/1475-2875-9-S2-P53
53. Baird JK, Jones TR, Masbar PS, Ratiwayanto S, Leksana B. Evidence for specific suppression of gametocytemia by *Plasmodium falciparum* in residents of hyperendemic Irian Jaya. *Am J Trop Med Hyg.* (1991) 44:183–90. doi: 10.4269/ajtmh.1991.44.183
54. Saeed M, Roeffen W, Alexander N, Drakeley CJ, Targett GA, Sutherland CJ. *Plasmodium falciparum* antigens on the surface of the gametocyte-infected erythrocyte. *PLoS ONE* (2008) 3:e2280. doi: 10.1371/journal.pone.0002280
55. Silvestrini F, Tibúrcio M, Bertuccini L, Alano P. Differential adhesive properties of sequestered asexual and sexual stages of *Plasmodium falciparum* on human endothelial cells are tissue independent. *PLoS ONE* (2012) 7:e31567. doi: 10.1371/journal.pone.0031567
56. Alano P. *Plasmodium falciparum* gametocytes: still many secrets of a hidden life. *Mol Microbiol.* (2007) 66:291–302. doi: 10.1111/j.1365-2958.2007.05904.x
57. Day KP, Hayward RE, Smith D, Culvenor JG. CD36-dependent adhesion and knob expression of the transmission stages of *Plasmodium falciparum* is stage-specific. *Mol Biochem Parasitol.* (1998) 93:167–77. doi: 10.1016/S0166-6851(98)00040-1
58. Rogers NJ, Hall BS, Obiero J, Targett GA, Sutherland CJ. A model for sequestration of the transmission stages of *Plasmodium falciparum*: adhesion of gametocyte-infected erythrocytes to human bone marrow cells. *Infect Immun.* (2000) 68:3455–62. doi: 10.1128/IAI.68.6.3455-3462.2000
59. Bousema J, Drakeley C, Kihonda J, Hendriks J, Akim N, Roeffen W, et al. A longitudinal study of immune responses to *Plasmodium falciparum* sexual stage antigens in Tanzanian adults. *Parasite Immunol.* (2007) 29:309–17. doi: 10.1111/j.1365-3024.2007.00948.x
60. Harte PG, Rogers NC, Targett GA. Role of T cells in preventing transmission of rodent malaria. *Immunology* (1985) 56:1–7.
61. Good M, Quakyi I, Saul A, Berzofsky J, Carter R, Miller L. Human T clones reactive to the sexual stages of *Plasmodium falciparum* malaria. High frequency of gamete-reactive T cells in peripheral blood from nonexposed donors. *J Immunol.* (1987) 138:306–11.
62. Riley EM, Ong C, Olerup O, Eida S, Allen S, Bennett S, et al. Cellular and humoral immune responses to *Plasmodium falciparum* gametocyte antigens in malaria-immune individuals. Limited response to the 48/45-kilodalton surface antigen does not appear to be due to MHC restriction. *J Immunol.* (1990) 144:4810–6.
63. Goodier MR, Targett GA. Polyclonal T-cell responses to *Plasmodium falciparum* gametocytes in malaria nonexposed donors. *Parasite Immunol.* (1997) 19:419–25. doi: 10.1046/j.1365-3024.1997.d01-238.x
64. Ndungu FM, Sanni L, Urban B, Stephens R, Newbold CI, Marsh K, et al. CD4 T cells from malaria-nonexposed individuals respond to the CD36-binding domain of *Plasmodium falciparum* erythrocyte membrane protein-1 via an MHC class II-TCR-independent pathway. *J Immunol.* (2006) 176:5504–12. doi: 10.4049/jimmunol.176.9.5504
65. Karunaweera ND, Carter R, Grau G, Kwiatkowski D, Giudice G, Mendis K. Tumour necrosis factor-dependent parasite-killing effects during paroxysms in non-immune *Plasmodium vivax* malaria patients. *Clin Exp Immunol.* (1992) 88:499–505. doi: 10.1111/j.1365-2249.1992.tb06478.x
66. Naotunne TDS, Karunaweera ND, Del Giudice G, Kularatne M, Grau G, Carter R, et al. Cytokines kill malaria parasites during infection crisis: extracellular complementary factors are essential. *J Exp Med.* (1991) 173:523–9. doi: 10.1084/jem.173.3.523
67. Naotunne TS, Karunaweera ND, Mendis KN, Carter R. Cytokine-mediated inactivation of malarial gametocytes is dependent on the presence of white blood cells and involves reactive nitrogen intermediates. *Immunology* (1993) 78:555–62.
68. Motard A, Landau I, Nussler A, Grau G, Baccam D, Mazier D, et al. The role of reactive nitrogen intermediates in modulation of gametocyte infectivity of rodent malaria parasites. *Parasite Immunol.* (1993) 15:21–6. doi: 10.1111/j.1365-3024.1993.tb00568.x
69. Smith TG, Serghides L, Patel SN, Febbraio M, Silverstein RL, Kain KC. CD36-mediated nonopsonic phagocytosis of erythrocytes infected with stage I and IIA gametocytes of *Plasmodium falciparum*. *Infect Immun.* (2003) 71:393–400. doi: 10.1128/IAI.71.1.393-400.2003
70. Hayward RE, Tiwari B, Piper KP, Baruch DI, Day KP. Virulence and transmission success of the malarial parasite *Plasmodium falciparum*. *Proc Natl Acad Sci USA.* (1999) 96:4563–8. doi: 10.1073/pnas.96.8.4563
71. Jain V, Singh PP, Silawat N, Patel R, Saxena A, Bharti PK, et al. A preliminary study on pro- and anti-inflammatory cytokine profiles in *Plasmodium vivax* malaria patients from central zone of India. *Acta Trop.* (2010) 113:263–8. doi: 10.1016/j.actatropica.2009.11.009
72. Ramsey JM, Tello A, Contreras CO, Ordonez R, Chirino N, Rojo J, et al. *Plasmodium falciparum* and *P. vivax* gametocyte-specific exoantigens stimulate proliferation of TCR gammadelta+ lymphocytes. *J Parasitol.* (2002) 88:59–68. doi: 10.1645/0022-3395(2002)088[0059:PFAPVG]2.0.CO;2
73. Ho M, Webster HK, Tongtawe P, Pattanapanyasat K, Weidanz WP. Increased gamma delta T cells in acute *Plasmodium falciparum* malaria. *Immunol Lett.* (1990) 25:139–41. doi: 10.1016/0165-2478(90)90105-Y
74. Sinden RE, Billingsley PF. *Plasmodium* invasion of mosquito cells: hawk or dove? *Trends Parasitol.* (2001) 17:209–12. doi: 10.1016/S1471-4922(01)01928-6
75. Dinglasan RR, Devenport M, Florens L, Johnson JR, McHugh CA, Donnelly-Doman M, et al. The *Anopheles gambiae* adult midgut peritrophic matrix proteome. *Insect Biochem Mol Biol.* (2009) 39:125–34. doi: 10.1016/j.ibmb.2008.10.010
76. Shao L, Devenport M, Jacobs-Lorena M. The peritrophic matrix of hematophagous insects. *Arch Insect Biochem Physiol.* (2001) 47:119–25. doi: 10.1002/arch.1042
77. Vinetz JM, Dave SK, Specht CA, Brameld KA, Xu B, Hayward R, et al. The chitinase PfCHT1 from the human malaria parasite *Plasmodium falciparum* lacks proenzyme and chitin-binding domains and displays unique substrate preferences. *Proc Natl Acad Sci USA.* (1999) 96:14061–6. doi: 10.1073/pnas.96.24.14061
78. Garver LS, de Almeida Oliveira G, Barillas-Mury C. The JNK pathway is a key mediator of *Anopheles gambiae* antiplasmodial immunity. *PLoS Pathog.* (2013) 9:e1003622. doi: 10.1371/journal.ppat.1003622
79. Kumar S, Gupta L, Han YS, Barillas-Mury C. Inducible peroxidases mediate nitration of anopheles midgut cells undergoing apoptosis in response to *Plasmodium* invasion. *J Biol Chem.* (2004) 279:53475–82. doi: 10.1074/jbc.M409905200
80. Blandin S, Shiao SH, Moita LF, Janse CJ, Waters AP, Kafatos FC, et al. Complement-like protein TEP1 is a determinant of vectorial capacity in the malaria vector *Anopheles gambiae*. *Cell* (2004) 116:661–70. doi: 10.1016/S0092-8674(04)00173-4
81. Moita LF, Wang-Sattler R, Michel K, Zimmermann T, Blandin S, Levashina EA, et al. *In vivo* identification of novel regulators and conserved pathways of phagocytosis in *A. gambiae*. *Immunity* (2005) 23:65–73. doi: 10.1016/j.immuni.2005.05.006
82. Shokal U, Eleftherianos I. Evolution and function of thioester-containing proteins and the complement system in the innate immune response. *Front Immunol.* (2017) 8:759. doi: 10.3389/fimmu.2017.00759
83. Ukegbu CV, Giorgalli M, Yassine H, Ramirez JL, Taxiarchi C, Barillas-Mury C, et al. *Plasmodium berghei* P47 is essential for ookinete protection from the *Anopheles gambiae* complement-like response. *Sci Rep.* (2017) 7:6026. doi: 10.1038/s41598-017-05917-6
84. van Dijk MR, van Schaijk BC, Khan SM, van Dooren MW, Ramesar J, Kaczanowski S, et al. Three members of the 6-cys protein family of *Plasmodium* play a role in gamete fertility. *PLoS Pathog.* (2010) 6:e1000853. doi: 10.1371/journal.ppat.1000853
85. Richman AM, Dimopoulos G, Seeley D, Kafatos FC. *Plasmodium* activates the innate immune response of *Anopheles gambiae* mosquitoes. *EMBO J.* (1997) 16:6114–9. doi: 10.1093/emboj/16.20.6114

86. Smith RC, Eappen AG, Radtke AJ, Jacobs-Lorena M. Regulation of anti-Plasmodium immunity by a LITAF-like transcription factor in the malaria vector *Anopheles gambiae*. *PLoS Pathog.* (2012) 8:e1002965. doi: 10.1371/journal.ppat.1002965
87. Oduol F, Xu J, Niare O, Natarajan R, Vernick KD. Genes identified by an expression screen of the vector mosquito *Anopheles gambiae* display differential molecular immune response to malaria parasites and bacteria. *Proc Natl Acad Sci USA.* (2000) 97:11397–402. doi: 10.1073/pnas.180060997
88. Dong Y, Aguilar R, Xi Z, Warr E, Mongin E, Dimopoulos G. *Anopheles gambiae* immune responses to human and rodent *Plasmodium* parasite species. *PLoS Pathog.* (2006) 2:e52. doi: 10.1371/journal.ppat.0020052
89. Greenwood B. Malaria vaccines. Evaluation and implementation. *Acta Trop.* (2005) 95:298–304. doi: 10.1016/j.actatropica.2005.04.017
90. Webster D, Hill AV. Progress with new malaria vaccines. *Bull World Health Organ.* (2003) 81:902–9. Available online at: https://www.scielosp.org/article/bwho/2003.v81n12/902-909/#ModalArticles
91. Healer J, McGuinness D, Hopcroft P, Haley S, Carter R, Riley E. Complement-mediated lysis of *Plasmodium falciparum* gametes by malaria-immune human sera is associated with antibodies to the gamete surface antigen Pfs230. *Infect Immun.* (1997) 65:3017–23.
92. Kaslow DC. Transmission-blocking immunity against malaria and other vector-borne diseases. *Curr Opin Immunol.* (1993) 5:557–65. doi: 10.1016/0952-7915(93)90037-S
93. Ponnudurai T, Van Gemert G, Bensink T, Lensen A, Meuwissen JT. Transmission blockade of *Plasmodium falciparum*: its variability with gametocyte numbers and concentration of antibody. *Trans R Soc Trop Med Hyg.* (1987) 81:491–3. doi: 10.1016/0035-9203(87)90172-6
94. Kaslow DC. Immunogenicity of *Plasmodium falciparum* sexual stage antigens: implications for the design of a transmission blocking vaccine. *Immunol Lett.* (1990) 25:83–6. doi: 10.1016/0165-2478(90)90096-9
95. Stowers A, Carter R. Current developments in malaria transmission-blocking vaccines. *Expert Opin Biol Ther.* (2001) 1:619–28. doi: 10.1517/14712598.1.4.619
96. Tsuboi T, Tachibana M, Kaneko O, Torii M. Transmission-blocking vaccine of vivax malaria. *Parasitol Int.* (2003) 52:1–11. doi: 10.1016/S1383-5769(02)00037-5
97. Carter R, Graves PM, Keister DB, Quakyi IA. Properties of epitopes of Pfs 48/45, a target of transmission blocking monoclonal antibodies, on gametes of different isolates of *Plasmodium falciparum*. *Parasite Immunol.* (1990) 12:587–603. doi: 10.1111/j.1365-3024.1990.tb00990.x
98. Kaushal DC, Carter R, Howard RJ, McAuliffe FM. Characterization of antigens on mosquito midgut stages of *Plasmodium gallinaceum*. I Zygote surface antigens. *Mol Biochem Parasitol.* (1983) 8:53–69. doi: 10.1016/0166-6851(83)90034-8
99. Kapulu M, Da D, Miura K, Li Y, Blagborough A, Churcher T, et al. Comparative assessment of transmission-blocking vaccine candidates against *Plasmodium falciparum*. *Sci Rep.* (2015) 5:11193. doi: 10.1038/srep11193
100. Eksi S, Czesny B, van Gemert GJ, Sauerwein RW, Eling W, Williamson KC. Malaria transmission-blocking antigen, Pfs230, mediates human red blood cell binding to exflagellating male parasites and oocyst production. *Mol Microbiol.* (2006) 61:991–8. doi: 10.1111/j.1365-2958.2006.05284.x
101. Farrance CE, Rhee A, Jones RM, Musiychuk K, Shamloul M, Sharma S, et al. A plant-produced Pfs230 vaccine candidate blocks transmission of *Plasmodium falciparum*. *Clin Vaccine Immunol.* (2011) 18:1351–7. doi: 10.1128/CVI.05105-11
102. Amlabu E, Mensah-Brown H, Nyarko PB, Akuh OA, Opoku G, Ilani P, et al. Functional characterization of *Plasmodium falciparum* surface related antigen (PfSRA) as a potential blood-stage vaccine target. *J Infect Dis.* (2018) 218:778–90. doi: 10.1093/infdis/jiy222
103. Scholz SM, Simon N, Lavazec C, Dude M-A, Templeton TJ, Pradel G. PfCCp proteins of *Plasmodium falciparum*: gametocyte-specific expression and role in complement-mediated inhibition of exflagellation. *Int J Parasitol.* (2008) 38:327–40. doi: 10.1016/j.ijpara.2007.08.009
104. Hermand P, Cicéron L, Pionneau C, Vaquero C, Combadière C, Deterre P. *Plasmodium falciparum* proteins involved in cytoadherence of infected erythrocytes to chemokine CX3CL1. *Sci Rep.* (2016) 6:33786. doi: 10.1038/srep33786
105. Tibúrcio M, Dixon MW, Looker O, Younis SY, Tilley L, Alano P. Specific expression and export of the *Plasmodium falciparum* gametocyte exported protein-5 marks the gametocyte ring stage. *Malar J.* (2015) 14:334. doi: 10.1186/s12936-015-0853-6
106. Tsai YL, Hayward RE, Langer RC, Fidock DA, Vinetz JM. Disruption of *Plasmodium falciparum* chitinase markedly impairs parasite invasion of mosquito midgut. *Infect Immun.* (2001) 69:4048–54. doi: 10.1128/IAI.69.6.4048-4054.2001
107. Yuda M, Yano K, Tsuboi T, Torii M, Chinzei Y. von Willebrand Factor A domain-related protein, a novel microneme protein of the malaria ookinete highly conserved throughout *Plasmodium* parasites. *Mol Biochem Parasitol.* (2001) 116:65–72. doi: 10.1016/S0166-6851(01)00304-8
108. Ramakrishnan C, Dessens JT, Armson R, Pinto SB, Talman AM, Blagborough AM, et al. Vital functions of the malarial ookinete protein CTRP reside in the A domains. *Int J Parasitol.* (2011) 41:1029–39. doi: 10.1016/j.ijpara.2011.05.007
109. Kadota K, Ishino T, Matsuyama T, Chinzei Y, Yuda M. Essential role of membrane-attack protein in malarial transmission to mosquito host. *Proc Natl Acad Sci USA.* (2004) 101:16310–5. doi: 10.1073/pnas.0406187101
110. Dessens JT, Siden-Kiamos I, Mendoza J, Mahairaki V, Khater E, Vlachou D, et al. SOAP, a novel malaria ookinete protein involved in mosquito midgut invasion and oocyst development. *Mol Microbiol.* (2003) 49:319–29. doi: 10.1046/j.1365-2958.2003.03566.x
111. Espinosa DA, Vega-Rodriguez J, Flores-Garcia Y, Noe AR, Muñoz C, Coleman R, et al. The *Plasmodium falciparum* cell-traversal protein for ookinetes and sporozoites as a candidate for preerythrocytic and transmission-blocking vaccines. *Infect Immun.* (2017) 85:e00498–16. doi: 10.1128/IAI.00498-16
112. Armistead JS, Morlais I, Mathias DK, Jardim JG, Joy J, Fridman A, et al. Antibodies to a single, conserved epitope in *Anopheles* APN1 inhibit universal transmission of *Plasmodium falciparum* and *Plasmodium vivax* malaria. *Infect Immun.* (2014) 82:818–29. doi: 10.1128/IAI.01222-13
113. Dinglasan RR, Kalume DE, Kanzok SM, Ghosh AK, Muratova O, Pandey A, et al. Disruption of *Plasmodium falciparum* development by antibodies against a conserved mosquito midgut antigen. *Proc Natl Acad Sci USA.* (2007) 104:13461–6. doi: 10.1073/pnas.0702239104
114. Mathias DK, Jardim JG, Parish LA, Armistead JS, Trinh HV, Khumpitak C, et al. Differential roles of an Anopheline midgut GPI-anchored protein in mediating *Plasmodium falciparum* and *Plasmodium vivax* ookinete invasion. *Infect Genet Evol.* (2014) 28:635–47. doi: 10.1016/j.meegid.2014.05.025
115. Mathias DK, Plieskatt JL, Armistead JS, Bethony JM, Abdul-Majid KB, McMillan A, et al. Expression, immunogenicity, histopathology, and potency of a mosquito-based malaria transmission-blocking recombinant vaccine. *Infect Immun.* (2012) 80:1606–14. doi: 10.1128/IAI.06212-11
116. Lavazec C, Boudin C, Lacroix R, Bonnet S, Diop A, Thiberge S, et al. Carboxypeptidases B of *Anopheles gambiae* as targets for a *Plasmodium falciparum* transmission-blocking vaccine. *Infect Immun.* (2007) 75:1635–42. doi: 10.1128/IAI.00864-06
117. Raz A, Dinparast Djadid N, Zakeri S. Molecular characterization of the Carboxypeptidase B1 of *Anopheles stephensi* and its evaluation as a target for transmission-blocking vaccines. *Infect Immun.* (2013) 81:2206–16. doi: 10.1128/IAI.01331-12
118. Williams AR, Zakutansky SE, Miura K, Dicks MJD, Churcher TS, Jewell KE, et al. Immunization against a serine protease inhibitor reduces intensity of *Plasmodium berghei* infection in mosquitoes. *Int J Parasitol.* (2013) 43:869–74. doi: 10.1016/j.ijpara.2013.06.004
119. Ghosh AK, Devenport M, Jethwaney D, Kalume DE, Pandey A, Anderson VE, et al. Malaria parasite invasion of the mosquito salivary gland requires interaction between the *Plasmodium* TRAP and the *Anopheles* saglin proteins. *PLoS Pathog.* (2009) 5:e1000265. doi: 10.1371/journal.ppat.1000265
120. Okulate MA, Kalume DE, Reddy R, Kristiansen T, Bhattacharyya M, Chaerkady R, et al. Identification and molecular characterization of a novel protein Saglin as a target of monoclonal antibodies affecting salivary gland infectivity of *Plasmodium* sporozoites. *Insect Mol Biol.* (2007) 16:711–22. doi: 10.1111/j.1365-2583.2007.00765.x
121. Nikolaeva D, Illingworth JJ, Miura K, Alanine DG, Brian IJ, Li Y, et al. Functional characterization and comparison of *Plasmodium falciparum* proteins as targets of transmission-blocking antibodies. *Mol Cell Proteomics* (2017) doi: 10.1074/mcp.RA117.000036. [Epub ahead of print].
122. Chaturvedi N, Bharti PK, Tiwari A, Singh N. Strategies and recent development of transmission-blocking vaccines against

Plasmodium falciparum. *Indian J Med Res.* (2016) 143:696–711. doi: 10.4103/0971-5916.191927

123. Mahmoudi S, Keshavarz H. Efficacy of phase 3 trial of RTS, S/AS01 malaria vaccine: the need for an alternative development plan. *Hum Vaccin Immunother.* (2017) 13:2098–101. doi: 10.1080/21645515.2017.1295906
124. Drakeley CJ, Eling W, Teelen K, Bousema JT, Sauerwein R, Greenwood BM, et al. Parasite infectivity and immunity to *Plasmodium falciparum* gametocytes in Gambian children. *Parasite Immunol.* (2004) 26:159–65. doi: 10.1111/j.0141-9838.2004.00696.x
125. Shimp RLJr, Rowe C, Reiter K, Chen B, Nguyen V, Aebig J, et al. Development of a Pfs25-EPA malaria transmission blocking vaccine as a chemically conjugated nanoparticle. *Vaccine* (2013) 31:2954–62. doi: 10.1016/j.vaccine.2013.04.034
126. Jones RM, Chichester JA, Mett V, Jaje J, Tottey S, Manceva S, et al. A plant-produced Pfs25 VLP malaria vaccine candidate induces persistent transmission blocking antibodies against *Plasmodium falciparum* in immunized mice. *PLoS ONE* (2013) 8:e79538. doi: 10.1371/journal.pone.0079538
127. Chichester JA, Green BJ, Jones RM, Shoji Y, Miura K, Long CA, et al. Safety and immunogenicity of a plant-produced Pfs25 virus-like particle as a transmission blocking vaccine against malaria: A Phase 1 dose-escalation study in healthy adults. *Vaccine* (2018) 36:5865–71. doi: 10.1016/j.vaccine.2018.08.033
128. Talaat KR, Ellis RD, Hurd J, Hentrich A, Gabriel E, Hynes NA, et al. Safety and immunogenicity of Pfs25-EPA/Alhydrogel(R), a transmission blocking vaccine against *Plasmodium falciparum*: an open label study in malaria naive adults. *PLoS ONE* (2016) 11:e0163144. doi: 10.1371/journal.pone.0163144
129. Menon V, Kapulu MC, Taylor I, Jewell K, Li Y, Hill F, et al. Assessment of antibodies induced by multivalent transmission-blocking malaria vaccines. *Front Immunol.* (2018) 8:1998. doi: 10.3389/fimmu.2017.01998
130. Li Y, Leneghan DB, Miura K, Nikolaeva D, Brian IJ, Dicks MD, et al. Enhancing immunogenicity and transmission-blocking activity of malaria vaccines by fusing Pfs25 to IMX313 multimerization technology. *Sci Rep.* (2016) 6:18848. doi: 10.1038/srep18848
131. Malkin EM, Durbin AP, Diemert DJ, Sattabongkot J, Wu Y, Miura K, et al. Phase 1 vaccine trial of Pvs25H: a transmission blocking vaccine for *Plasmodium vivax* malaria. *Vaccine* (2005) 23:3131–8. doi: 10.1016/j.vaccine.2004.12.019
132. Pereira VB, Zurita-Turk M, Saraiva TDL, De Castro CP, Souza BM, Agresti PM, et al. DNA vaccines approach: from concepts to applications. *World J Vaccines* (2014) 4:50. doi: 10.4236/wjv.2014.42008
133. Ura T, Okuda K, Shimada M. Developments in viral vector-based vaccines. *Vaccines* (2014) 2:624–41. doi: 10.3390/vaccines2030624
134. Azmi F, Ahmad Fuaad AAH, Skwarczynski M, Toth I. Recent progress in adjuvant discovery for peptide-based subunit vaccines. *Hum Vaccin Immunother.* (2014) 10:778–96. doi: 10.4161/hv.27332
135. Wykes M, Good MF. A case for whole-parasite malaria vaccines. *Int J Parasitol.* (2007) 37:705–12. doi: 10.1016/j.ijpara.2007.02.007
136. An C, Budd A, Kanost MR, Michel K. Characterization of a regulatory unit that controls melanization and affects longevity of mosquitoes. *Cell Mol Life Sci.* (2011) 68:1929–39. doi: 10.1007/s00018-010-0543-z
137. Michel K, Budd A, Pinto S, Gibson TJ, Kafatos FC. *Anopheles gambiae* SRPN2 facilitates midgut invasion by the malaria parasite *Plasmodium berghei*. *EMBO Rep.* (2005) 6:891–7. doi: 10.1038/sj.embor.7400478
138. Tarlinton D, Good-Jacobson K. Diversity among memory B cells: origin, consequences, and utility. *Science* (2013) 341:1205–11. doi: 10.1126/science.1241146
139. Lasonder E, Rijpma SR, van Schaijk BC, Hoeijmakers WA, Kensche PR, Gresnigt MS, et al. Integrated transcriptomic and proteomic analyses of *P. falciparum* gametocytes: molecular insight into sex-specific processes and translational repression. *Nucleic Acids Res.* (2016) 44:6087–101. doi: 10.1093/nar/gkw536
140. Reid AJ, Talman AM, Bennett HM, Gomes AR, Sanders MJ, Illingworth CJR. Single-cell RNA-seq reveals hidden transcriptional variation in malaria parasites. *Elife* (2018) 7:e33105. doi: 10.7554/eLife.33105
141. Suarez-Cortes P, Sharma V, Bertuccini L, Costa G, Bannerman NL, Sannella AR, et al. Comparative proteomics and functional analysis reveal a role of *Plasmodium falciparum* osmiophilic bodies in malaria parasite transmission. *Mol Cell Proteomics* (2016) 15:3243–55. doi: 10.1074/mcp.M116.060681
142. Conway DJ. Paths to a malaria vaccine illuminated by parasite genomics. *Trends Genet.* (2015) 31:97–107. doi: 10.1016/j.tig.2014.12.005
143. He Y. Omics-based systems vaccinology for vaccine target identification. *Drug Dev Res.* (2012) 73:559–68. doi: 10.1002/ddr.21049
144. Bah SY, Morang'a CM, Kengne-Ouafo JA, Amenga–Etego L, Awandare GA. Highlights on the application of genomics and bioinformatics in the fight against infectious diseases: challenges and opportunities in Africa. *Front Genet.* (2018) 9:575. doi: 10.3389/fgene.2018.00575
145. Masignani V, Rappuoli R, Pizza M. Reverse vaccinology: a genome-based approach for vaccine development. *Expert Opin Biol Ther.* (2002) 2:895–905. doi: 10.1517/14712598.2.8.895
146. Rappuoli R. Reverse vaccinology, a genome-based approach to vaccine development. *Vaccine* (2001) 19:2688–91. doi: 10.1016/S0264-410X(00)00554-5
147. Rappuoli R. Bridging the knowledge gaps in vaccine design. *Nat Biotechnol.* (2007) 25:1361. doi: 10.1038/nbt1207-1361
148. Davies DH, Duffy P, Bodmer J-L, Felgner PL, Doolan DL. Large screen approaches to identify novel malaria vaccine candidates. *Vaccine* (2015) 33:7496–505. doi: 10.1016/j.vaccine.2015.09.059
149. Grubaugh D, Flechtner JB, Higgins DE. Proteins as T cell antigens: methods for high-throughput identification. *Vaccine* (2013) 31:3805–10. doi: 10.1016/j.vaccine.2013.06.046
150. Sidney J, Assarsson E, Moore C, Ngo S, Pinilla C, Sette A, et al. Quantitative peptide binding motifs for 19 human and mouse MHC class I molecules derived using positional scanning combinatorial peptide libraries. *Immunome Res.* (2008) 4:2. doi: 10.1186/1745-7580-4-2
151. Lavazec C, Sanyal S, Templeton TJ. Expression switching in the stevor and Pfmc-2TM superfamilies in *Plasmodium falciparum*. *Mol Microbiol.* (2007) 64:1621–34. doi: 10.1111/j.1365-2958.2007.05767.x
152. Chan J-A, Fowkes FJI, Beeson JG. Surface antigens of *Plasmodium falciparum*-infected erythrocytes as immune targets and malaria vaccine candidates. *Cell Mol Life Sci.* (2014) 71:3633–57. doi: 10.1007/s00018-014-1614-3
153. Goel S, Palmkvist M, Moll K, Joannin N, Lara P, Akhouri RR, et al. RIFINs are adhesins implicated in severe *Plasmodium falciparum* malaria. *Nat Med.* (2015) 21:314. doi: 10.1038/nm.3812
154. Khattab A, Bonow I, Schreiber N, Petter M, Schmetz C, Klinkert MQ. *Plasmodium falciparum* variant STEVOR antigens are expressed in merozoites and possibly associated with erythrocyte invasion. *Malar J.* (2008) 7:137. doi: 10.1186/1475-2875-7-137
155. Niang M, Bei AK, Madnani KG, Pelly S, Dankwa S, Kanjee U, et al. STEVOR is a *Plasmodium falciparum* erythrocyte binding protein that mediates merozoite invasion and rosetting. *Cell Host Microbe* (2014) 16:81–93. doi: 10.1016/j.chom.2014.06.004
156. Nunes-Alves C. RIFINs promote rosette formation during malaria. *Nat Rev Microbiol.* (2015) 13:250. doi: 10.1038/nrmicro3472
157. Yam XY, Niang M, Madnani KG, Preiser PR. Three is a crowd–new insights into rosetting in *Plasmodium falciparum*. *Trends Parasitol.* (2017) 33:309–20. doi: 10.1016/j.pt.2016.12.012
158. Schreiber N, Khattab A, Petter M, Marks F, Adjei S, Kobbe R, et al. Expression of *Plasmodium falciparum* 3D7 STEVOR proteins for evaluation of antibody responses following malaria infections in naive infants. *Parasitology* (2008) 135:155–67. doi: 10.1017/S0031182007003794

15

Parasite Recognition and Signaling Mechanisms in Innate Immune Responses to Malaria

D. Channe Gowda and Xianzhu Wu*

Department of Biochemistry and Molecular Biology, The Pennsylvania State University College of Medicine, Hershey, PA, United States

Correspondence:
D. Channe Gowda
gowda@psu.edu

Malaria caused by the *Plasmodium* family of parasites, especially *P.falciparum* and *P. vivax*, is a major health problem in many countries in the tropical and subtropical regions of the world. The disease presents a wide array of systemic clinical conditions and several life-threatening organ pathologies, including the dreaded cerebral malaria. Like many other infectious diseases, malaria is an inflammatory response-driven disease, and positive outcomes to infection depend on finely tuned regulation of immune responses that efficiently clear parasites and allow protective immunity to develop. Immune responses initiated by the innate immune system in response to parasites play key roles both in protective immunity development and pathogenesis. Initial pro-inflammatory responses are essential for clearing infection by promoting appropriate cell-mediated and humoral immunity. However, elevated and prolonged pro-inflammatory responses owing to inappropriate cellular programming contribute to disease conditions. A comprehensive knowledge of the molecular and cellular mechanisms that initiate immune responses and how these responses contribute to protective immunity development or pathogenesis is important for developing effective therapeutics and/or a vaccine. Historically, in efforts to develop a vaccine, immunity to malaria was extensively studied in the context of identifying protective humoral responses, targeting proteins involved in parasite invasion or clearance. The innate immune response was thought to be non-specific. However, during the past two decades, there has been a significant progress in understanding the molecular and cellular mechanisms of host-parasite interactions and the associated signaling in immune responses to malaria. Malaria infection occurs at two stages, initially in the liver through the bite of a mosquito, carrying sporozoites, and subsequently, in the blood through the invasion of red blood cells by merozoites released from the infected hepatocytes. Soon after infection, both the liver and blood stage parasites are sensed by various receptors of the host innate immune system resulting in the activation of signaling pathways and production of cytokines and chemokines. These immune responses play crucial roles in clearing parasites and regulating adaptive immunity. Here, we summarize the knowledge on molecular mechanisms that underlie the innate immune responses to malaria infection.

Keywords: malaria, immunostimulatory factors, host receptors, signaling mechanisms, innate immune responses, protective immunity, pathogenesis

BACKGROUND

Malaria is a widespread infectious disease that is prevalent in most tropical regions of the world (1–4). About half of the world population is at risk of contracting malaria. World Health Organization has reported an estimated 216 million malaria clinical cases and about 445,000 deaths during 2016 (1). Besides huge health burden and mortality, malaria morbidity is a substantial hindrance to socio-economic development in endemic areas due to the loss of man power (5, 6). The disease is caused by protozoan parasites of the genus *Plasmodium*. Five parasite species infect humans that include *Plasmodium falciparum*, *P. vivax*, *P. malariae*, *P. ovale*, and *P. knowlesi* (7–9). However, most malaria infections are caused by *P. falciparum* and *P. vivax*, and infections by the other three species are relatively rare. Several parasite species, including *P. berghei*, *P. yoelii*, *P. chabaudi*, and *P. vinckei*, infect rodents, but not humans (10). Different strains of rodent parasites used in laboratories show distinct growth rates, and infected mice exhibit a range of immunological and pathological conditions, resembling a wide spectrum of pathophysiologic conditions of human malaria infection. As such, mice infected with different parasite strains are useful models to study distinct systemic and organ-specific clinical conditions of human malaria.

Malaria is a highly complex disease that displays a wide variety of pathological conditions. At the early stages, malaria infection presents a number of systemic clinical conditions, including the characteristic periodic fever, chills, headache, dizziness, malaise, abdominal discomfort, nausea, and muscle and joint aches (11, 12). As the infection progresses and parasite biomass increases, pathogenic processes follow, resulting in severe anemia, blood acidosis, splenomegaly and hepatomegaly, acute respiratory distress syndrome, and several other clinical conditions. In the case of *P. falciparum*, the infected red blood cells (IRBCs) bind to certain cell surface proteins of vascular endothelia, including CD36, intracellular adhesion molecule 1 (ICAM-1), vascular adhesion molecule 1 (VCAM-1), and endothelial protein receptor (EPCR) (4, 13–20). These binding events allow parasites to sequester in organs, such as brain, lungs, liver, intestine, dermal tissues, and placenta, thereby avoiding splenic clearance. Parasite sequestration contributes to single and multiorgan fatal pathologic conditions, including cerebral malaria, and renal, liver and lung dysfunction and failure. In pregnant women, *P. falciparum* sequesters in the placenta through the binding of IRBCs to chondroitin 4-sulfate in the intervillous space and on the syncytiotrophoblast cell surface (21–23). This process contributes to pregnancy-associated malaria, characterized by a number of clinical conditions, including low birth weight, abortion, and death in the baby and the mother (24). The binding of IRBCs to the endothelial cell surface proteins in the microvasculature of vital organs and chondroitin 4-sulfate in the placenta is mediated by a family of antigenically variant parasite proteins encoded by about 60 *var* genes (15, 16, 25). These proteins are collectively called *P. falciparum* erythrocyte membrane protein 1 (PfEMP1). PfEMP1 confers virulence to *P. falciparum* through IRBC binding to endothelial cells in various organs contributing to microvascular plugging and hypoxia. In addition, IRBC-binding and parasite accumulation amplify inflammatory responses locally, leading to immune cell infiltration, endothelial damage, and organ dysfunction and failure. *P. vivax* lacks PfEMP1 ortholog (26) and thus, *P. vivax* is less virulent compared to *P. falciparum*. However, in recent years, *P. vivax* is becoming increasingly virulent, causing severe malaria in significant numbers (11, 27–30). Although, the underlying reasons in *P. vivax* causing severe illnesses remain unclear, drug resistance and changes in genetic makeup appear to be significant factors (31, 32).

Innate immune responses that are initiated in response to malaria infection play key roles both in the development of protective immunity and pathogenesis (14, 33–38). Early pro-inflammatory responses regulate antiparasitic Th1 development and promote effector cell function for efficiently clearing infections. Usually, as infection progresses, pro-inflammatory responses are gradually downregulated with parallel increase in anti-inflammatory responses (39). Generally, this leads to Th2 development, resulting in balanced pro-/anti-inflammatory and Th1/Th2 responses and resistance against pathogenesis (35, 39–42). However, this is not always the case. Depending upon the host-parasite interaction dynamics, factors such as parasite sequestration and alterations in host genetics, pro-inflammatory responses may be overly upregulated, resulting in systemic and organ-related severe illnesses.

During the past two decades, there has been a substantial progress in our understanding of the host receptors that sense parasite factors involved in inducing immune responses and the associated signaling pathways (43–47). A substantial progress has also been made in our understanding of parasite immunostimulatory factors that are the targets of host receptors (43–47). However, much remained to be learned on the spectrum of molecular and cellular processes and immune responses that are initiated upon parasite sensing. Development of protective immunity to malaria requires repetitive infection over a period of time (48, 49). Information is limited as to whether and how the innate immune responses contribute to the inefficient development of protective immunity to malaria. In addition to signaling initiated by specific sensing of parasite factors, signals

Abbreviations: IRBCs, infected red blood cells; DC, dendritic cell; Mφ, macrophage; NK cells, natural killer cells; NKT cells, NK T cells; GPI, glycosylphosphatidylinositol; PfEMP1, *P. falciparum* erythrocyte membrane protein 1; ICAM-1, intracellular adhesion molecule 1; VCAM-1, vascular adhesion molecule 1; LFA-1, lymphocyte function-associated antigen-1; EPCR, endothelial protein receptor; Th, helper T cells; IFNαR, type I IFN-α receptor; PAMPs, pathogen-associated molecular patterns; DAMPs, danger-associated molecular patterns; PRRs, pathogen recognition receptors; TLR, toll-like receptor; MyD88, myeloid differentiation factor 88; MAL, MyD88 adapter-like; IRAK, IL-1 receptor-associated kinase; TRAF6, tumor necrosis factor receptor-associated factor 6; TRIF, TIR (Toll/IL-1 receptor) domain-containing adaptor inducing IFN-β; TRAM, TRIF-related adaptor molecule; MAPK, mitogen-activated protein kinases; ERK, extracellular signal-regulated kinases; JNK, c-Jun N-terminal kinases; NF-κB, nuclear factor κB; TBK1, TRAF family member-associated NF-κB activator (TANK)-binding kinase 1; cGAS, cyclic GMP-AMP synthase; STING, stimulator of IFN genes; MDA5, melanoma differentiation-associated gene 5; MVAS, mitochondrial antiviral-signaling protein; IRF, IFN regulatory factor; AIM2, absent in melanoma 2; NOD, nucleotide-binding oligomerization domain; NLR, (NOD)-like receptor; LLR, leucine-rich repeat kinase-like protein; NLRP, NOD- LRR- and pyrin domain-containing protein.

TABLE 1 | Prevalence and features of human blood stage malaria parasites.

Parasite species	Prevalence	Erythrocyte stage life cycle duration	Merozoite numbers in matured IRBCs	Cytoadherence capacity and organs where adherence occurs	Frequency of causing severe illnesses and fatality	References
P. falciparum	Worldwide (high prevalence in Africa)	48 h	8–24	Strong; in most organs, including skin, intestine and placenta	Often causes severe illnesses, highly fatal	(53)
P. vivax	Asia, Latin America, some parts of Africa	48 h	12–18	Weak; mostly in lungs	Mostly uncomplicated malaria, occasionally fatal	(53)
P. ovale	Africa, Western pacific islands	48 h	8–16	Absent	Mostly uncomplicated malaria, fatality is rare	(53, 54)
P. malariae	Worldwide	72 h	6–12	Absent	Mostly uncomplicated malaria, fatality is rare	(53, 54)
P. knowlesi	Southeast Asia	24 h	Up to 16	Weak; in lungs, and likely brain and other organs	Uncomplicated to severe illnesses (60–70% of infected cases develop ARDS[a])	(8, 9, 55)

[a]*ARDS, acute respiratory distress syndrome.*

induced by processes such as phagocytosis and cytoadherence also contribute; information is also limited as to whether and to what extent these signaling contribute to the overall innate immune responses. In this review, we are providing an overview of the available information on the molecular and cellular mechanisms of parasite-host interactions that involved in innate immune responses to malaria.

MALARIA INFECTION

Malaria infection begins with the entry of sporozoite form of parasites when infected mosquitoes inject saliva during blood meal (7, 46, 50–52). A substantial number of injected sporozoites is unable to enter the blood stream and stuck in the dermis, and these parasites are removed likely by the resident macrophages (Mφs). Those sporozoites that enter the blood stream target liver, where they exclusively infect hepatocytes. In hepatocytes, parasites reside inside parasitophorous vacuole formed during invasion and develop into merozoites over a period of 7–10 days in humans and 2 days in rodents, vastly expanding hepatocyte size. Upon parasite maturation, each infected hepatocyte releases 10,000–30,000 merozoites into the blood stream (46, 50–52). This period of cell cycles represents the first stage of malaria infection, referred to as the liver stage or the tissue stage infection. The merozoites released from the matured infected hepatocytes are called exo-erythrocytic merozoites. These merozoites do not infect hepatocytes, but instead exclusively invade red blood cells, and reside inside parasitophorous vacuole. Soon after invasion, parasites appear morphologically like rings inside IRBCs. Parasites then develop into early and late trophozoites, and finally undergo schizogony to form differentiated merozoites, which are released into the blood stream. Each matured erythrocytic stage schizont releases 8–24 merozoites (53) (**Table 1**), which can invade red blood cells. The parasite developmental process inside red blood cells occurs over a period of 24–72 h, depending on the *Plasmodium* species (**Table 1**). This cycle of invading red blood cells and parasite growth is called the blood stage infection. The repetitive erythrocytic cell cycles result in the exponential growth of parasites and if the growth is unchecked, most red blood cells are consumed, resulting in severe anemia and pathologies, and death. However, soon after infection, the innate immune system detects parasites at both the liver and blood stages, and responds by inducing pro-inflammatory cytokines and chemokines. The cytokines prime phagocytes for an efficient uptake and clearance, while chemokines help recruit effector cells to sites, where parasites are sequestered or accumulated, for effective infection clearance.

PATHOGEN SENSING MECHANISMS

Hosts respond to various infections by sensing certain evolutionarily conserved molecules (signature structures) of pathogens called pathogen-associated molecular patterns (PAMPs); these include bacterial LPS and peptidoglycan, fungal glucans, and microbial DNA and RNA, and even self-DNA under certain pathologic conditions (56–61). Host detects PAMPs through receptors called pathogen-recognition receptors (PRRs). Host also detects certain endogenous factors released during infection and thus can induce danger signaling. These factors are called danger-associated molecular patterns (DAMPs). Examples of DAMPs include high mobility box 1 (HMGB1), HSP70, SP100 family of proteins, and degraded hyaluronic acid (62–65). The innate immune system is equipped with a wide range of PAMP- and DAMP-recognizing PRRs. After recognition of PAMPs and DAMPs by PRRs, the innate immune cells are activated through the initiation of specific signaling pathways, producing cytokines and chemokines. PRRs are present at various cellular locations, including outer surface of plasma membrane, luminal surface of endosomal membrane, outer membrane of mitochondria, and cytosol (59, 60, 66). Prominent among transmembrane PRRs are toll-like receptors (TLRs) (56–59, 61); others transmembrane PRRs include, c-type lectin receptors, such as mannose- and galactose-binding proteins, and scavenger receptors, such as CD36, CD204, and MARCO (67). Examples of cytosolic sensors include dectin-1 that binds fungal β-1,3-glucan, cyclic GMP-AMP synthase (cGAS, senses dsDNA), retinoic acid-inducible gene-I (RIG-I, respond to viral RNA), RIG-I-like receptors (RLRs), such as melanoma differentiation-associated gene 5 (MDA5) that respond to dsRNA, nucleotide-binding oligomerization domain (NOD)-like receptors (NLRs, senses bacterial peptidoglycan), and absent in melanoma 2 (AIM2, respond to dsDNA). Malaria parasites are sensed by several receptors, leading to cell activation and immune responses (see below). Several excellent reviewers that comprehensively discuss various host-pathogen interactions and signaling mechanisms are available (56–60, 62–66, 68–70).

MALARIAL PAMPs AND HOST PRRs

A notable feature of malaria infection is that the liver stage is clinically completely silent, that is, the host does not exhibit any symptoms of malaria (71–73). All the malaria clinical conditions and fatal illnesses are manifested during the blood stage infection (74). At both stages of infection, the host detects parasites immediately after infection and initiates innate immune responses. These responses are geared toward clearing the infection and shaping the development of protective adaptive immunity (14, 34, 44, 71–78). However, the complex parasite-host interaction dynamics are not always in favor of achieving this goal, but instead often result in dysregulated immune responses and uncontrolled parasite growth, leading to pathogenesis. Understanding the malaria parasite-host interaction dynamics that shape the parasite-specific immunity and the molecular and cellular processes that contribute to pathogenesis is important for developing suitable treatment strategies. Below, we summarize the advancements that have been made in identifying the malaria PAMPs, the cognate host PRRs, and the signaling events that lead to innate immune responses.

LIVER STAGE PARASITE SENSING

Since the liver stage malaria infection is clinically silent, it has long been thought that parasites inside hepatocytes grow undetected by the innate immune system. However, recent studies in *P. berghei-* and *P. yoelii*-infected mice show that, although parasites inside hepatocytes are shielded from recognition by Mφs and dendritic cells (DCs), the growing parasites are recognized by the cytosolic PRRs of hepatocytes,

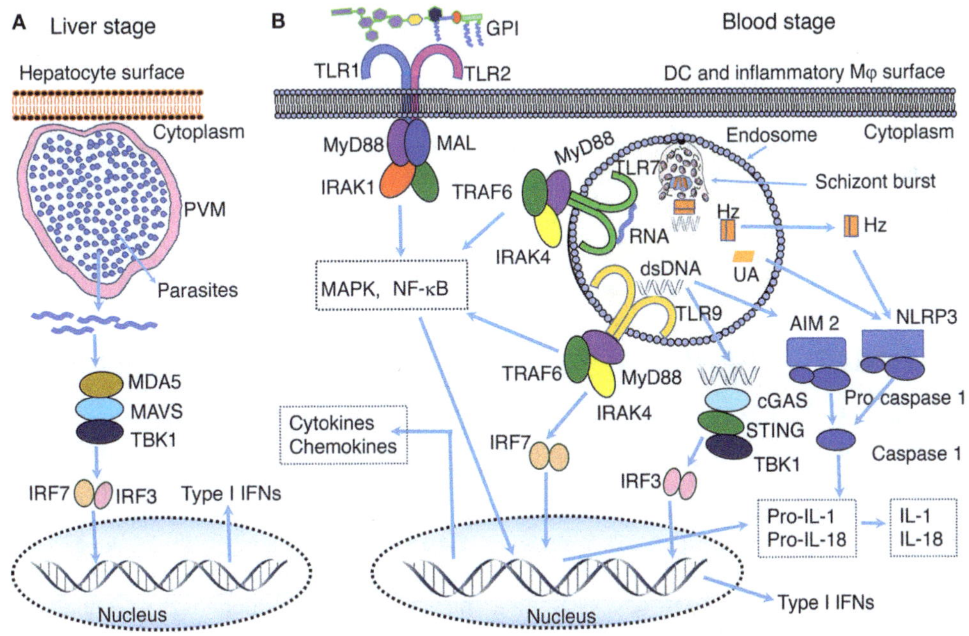

FIGURE 1 | PAMP-PRR interaction-induced signaling pathways. **(A)** RNA of the liver stage parasites growing inside hepatocytes is recognized by MDA5 leading to the activation of MAVS-TBK1-IRF3/IRF7 signaling and downstream production of type I IFNs. **(B)** At the blood stage infection, parasite DNA, RNA and GPI interact with, respectively, TLR9, TLR7, and TLR2, leading to the activation of primarily MAPK and NF-κB signaling pathways and downstream cytokine and chemokine responses. In the cytosol, similar to the liver stage parasite RNA, the blood stage parasite RNA is sensed by MDA5 leading to the activation of MAVS-TBK1-IRF3/IRF7 signaling (see **A**). However, this signaling seems induce the expression of SOCS1, which downregulate RNA-TLR7-induced type I IFN production (81). Parasite DNA in the cytosol is sensed by cGAS, resulting in the activation of STING-TBK1-IRF3 signaling and type I IFN response. Parasite DNA also activates AIM2 inflammasome, which cleaves pro-caspase 1 to activate caspase 1. Hemozoin (Hz) and uric acid (UA) induce danger signaling, activating NLRP3 inflammasome and the cleavage of pro-caspase 1 to activate caspase 1. Parasites have also been reported to activate NLRP12 inflammasome through unidentified interaction, leading to the cleavage of pro-caspase 1 to activate caspase 1 (44, 82). It appears that microparticles released from IRBCs and heme produced during infection activate TLR4 signaling (83, 84). Ligands bind to TLR4 homodimer through the cooperation of accessory proteins CD14 and MD2, leading to MAPK, NF-κB and TRIF-TBK1-IRF3 signaling. Note: the diagram depicts a simplified version of indicated signaling pathways and additional details can be found in review articles (44, 56–70). The abbreviations are defined in footnote in page 1.

initiating antiparasitic type I IFN response (79, 80). The parasites in infected hepatocytes are detected through the interaction of parasite RNA with RIG-I family of proteins homolog called melanoma differentiation-associated protein 5 (MDA5), but not by RIG-I, leading to the activation of MDA5-MAVS-IRF3/IRF7 signaling axis and downstream production of type I IFN (79, 80) (**Figure 1**). This signaling event results in an array of type I IFN receptor (IFNαR)-mediated innate immune responses, which include: (i) expression of interferon-stimulated genes by hepatocytes; (ii) production of chemokines by hepatocytes, and chemotaxis-mediated recruitment of Mφs, neutrophils and lymphocytes to the proximity of infected hepatocytes; (iii) production of IFN-γ and chemokines by NK and NKT cells, which are abundantly present in the liver; (iv) infiltration of NK and NKT cells to the liver; (v) CD1d-resitrcted elimination of infected hepatocytes by NKT cells (79, 80). Since parasites reside inside parasitophorous vacuole, it appears that parasite RNA is exported to the cytosol, but not to phagolysosomes. It is unlikely that cytosolic RNA can enter endosomes and moreover hepatocytes may not express significant levels of TLR7. Thus, it appears that cytosolic sensors are the only PRRs that interact with parasite factors in infected hepatocytes. These findings represent a significant advancement in our understanding of parasite recognition mechanisms involved in innate immune responses to the liver stage malaria infection. However, it remains unclear if parasite DNA is exported to the cytosol, where it can be sensed by cytosolic nucleic acid sensors. DNA is a prominent immunostimulatory PAMP of the blood stage malaria parasites and the AT-rich stem loops of parasite DNA can induce the production of type I IFN through sensing in the cytosol (44, 60). If the liver stage parasite DNA has no role in type I IFN response, then DNA is either not exported to the cytosol of hepatocytes or non-stimulatory.

BLOOD STAGE PARASITE SENSING

As mentioned earlier, the blood stage infection accounts for all the pathological conditions of malaria (74). In infected non-immune people, *P. falciparum* parasites multiply rapidly through the release of large numbers of merozoites by matured schizonts to the blood circulation every 48 h (53, 85). Some of the released merozoites invade erythrocytes and the reminders become dead and are likely targeted by Mφs and DCs. In addition, the burst of schizont stage erythrocytes releases large amounts of parasite's digestive vacuoles containing hemozoin and other waste products. The blood stage parasites grow synchronously by adapting to daily rhythm of systemic TNF-α production and the level of glucose in the blood (86). Thus, parasites develop at similar rates, releasing merozoites, digestive vacuoles and other contents more or less at the same time point (86). This leads to peak concentrations of parasite stimulatory components, to which the innate immune system potently responds and induces the production of pro-inflammatory cytokines and chemokines at high levels. This periodic elicitation of strong inflammatory responses within a narrow window of time period after each erythrocytic cell cycle is responsible for the characteristic periodicity of malaria paroxysms, including periodic recurrent of peak levels of fever, chills, headache, shock, and malaise. Several malaria parasite PAMPs have been identified, and the mechanisms by which they are sensed and the associated signaling pathways and immune responses have been delineated (44, 46, 73, 87). This body of information represents a substantial progress in our understanding of malaria innate immunity. Below we describe the current knowledge on malaria parasite PAMP and host PRR interaction mechanisms involved in innate immune responses.

MALARIAL PAMPs

GPI

P. falciparum glycosylphosphatidylinositol (GPI) is the first factor that was identified as a malaria parasite PAMP (88). Structurally, parasite GPI comprises a heterogenous group of molecules consisting of triacylated phosphatidylinositol linked to the glucosamine moiety of glycan having four mannose residues and a glucosamine residue (89–91). The structural heterogeneity of malaria GPI is due to the variation in length and level of unsaturation in acyl residues present at different positions of the phosphatidylinositol moiety. This structural heterogeneity in the lipid moieties has no bearing on immune response-inducing activity of GPI. This is evident from the fact that the *sn-2 lyso* GPI, obtained by the removal of acyl moiety at the *sn-2* position of parasite GPI, could efficiently induce cytokine responses similar to the unmodified parasite GPI. The biosynthesis of GPI is essential for the survival of parasites as GPI anchors several proteins of merozoites to the plasma membrane that are involved in erythrocyte invasion (92–94). In the absence of GPI anchoring, these proteins are not expressed on the surface and hence merozoites cannot invade erythrocytes. Malaria parasites synthesize GPI in several folds excess over the actual amounts needed for anchoring proteins to the surface of merozoites and thus, significant amounts of GPI remain not linked to proteins (90). The GPI molecules that are not linked to proteins are exposed on the cell surface and thus are likely targeted by the innate immune system.

The identification that parasite GPI is a malaria inflammatory response-inducing pathogenicity factor was based on the observation that the purified parasite GPI could induce strong pro-inflammatory responses by Mφs (88). When administered to mice, GPI induced symptoms that resembled the systemic clinical conditions of malaria, including pyrexia, cachexia, hypoglycemia, and TNF-α-induced sepsis. In several subsequent studies, GPI was shown to induce a wide range of immune responses, including the production of TNF-α and IL-1 by Mφs, expression of nitric oxide synthase by Mφs and endothelial cells, and the expression of ICAM-1, VCAM-1, and E-selectin by leukocytes and endothelial cells through the activation of several signaling events (95–97). Consistent with the property of GPI in inducing malaria-like symptoms, immunization of mice with a synthetic glycan portion of GPI produced anti-GPI antibodies, and immunized mice infected with *P. berghei* ANKA, an experimental cerebral malaria model, were protected from cerebral malaria

(98). Further, the presence of anti-GPI antibodies in people in malaria endemic was associated with a significant protective immunity against malaria illnesses (99, 100).

Subsequent studies have shown that *P. falciparum* GPI activates Mφs through the induction of an outside-in signaling, without binding to plasma membrane or being internalized by the cells, but instead by recognition through weak interactions on the cell surface (101). The intact structure of GPI is essential for bioactivity as neither the carbohydrate moiety nor the triacylated phosphatidylinositol lipid portion can induce immune responses. Further studies have shown that the parasite GPI induced production of pro-inflammatory cytokines by Mφs occurs through recognition mainly by TLR2-TLR1 heterodimer and to a much lesser extent by TLR4 (102–105); **Figure 1** and **Table 2**. Sensing of GPI by TLR2-TLR1 leads to the activation of ERK, p38, JNK MAPK, and NF-κB signaling pathways, which differentially contribute to the production of various inflammatory mediators (103). Thus, malaria parasite GPI is mainly a TLR2-activating PAMP.

DNA

A large body of accumulated data over the past two decades demonstrates that microbial (bacteria, viruses, and parasites) DNA, and self-DNA in some pathological situations, function as PAMP and are recognized by TLR9 in endosomes and by DNA sensors in the cytosol (56–60). In the case of malaria, the first demonstration that TLR9 senses malaria parasites and induces immune responses was by Pinchyangukul et al. (123). They showed that a soluble component in the schizont extract of *P. falciparum* that was heat labile and precipitable with ammonium sulfate (the description agrees with the active component being protein-DNA complex) induces cytokine and chemokine responses by human plasmacytoid DCs (pDCs) and mouse DCs through the activation of TLR9-MyD88 signaling pathway. Subsequently, it was shown that the TLR9 signaling-inducing malaria factor is DNA (107, 108, 124). TLR9 specifically recognizes the unmethylated CpG motifs of DNA (68, 69). The genomic DNA of *P. falciparum* and *P. vivax* contain, respectively, ~300 and ~2,000 CpG motifs (109). The higher content of CpG motifs is likely responsible for the strong fever-inducing ability of *P. vivax* compared to *P. falciparum* (125).

Malaria parasite DNA enters the endosomes of the innate immune cells, such as Mφs and DCs, through phagocytic uptake of IRBCs, merozoites, the nuclear material of parasites, DNA-protein-hemozoin complex, and DNA-containing immune complexes (107, 108, 124, 126). The endosomes are then fused to lysosomes to form phagolysosomes. In the acidic environment of phagolysosomes, DNA is released and recognized by TLR9, leading to the activation of MAPK and NF-κB signaling pathways and cytokine and chemokine responses (**Figure 1** and **Table 2**). In addition to TLR9, parasite DNA is recognized by cytosolic DNA sensors upon the release of phagolysosomal contents into the cytosol. In the cytosol, several distinct cytosolic sensors can potentially recognize DNA (**Figure 1**). Thus far, it has been demonstrated that two cytosolic PRRs sense parasite DNA: (i) cGAS sensing dsDNA and inducing the activation of STING-TBK1-IRF3 signaling and downstream production of type I IFNs (44, 110), and (ii) AIM2 recognizing dsDNA, resulting in the activation of inflammasome and caspase 1. The activated caspase 1 converts pro forms of IL-1 and IL-18 into active IL-1 and IL-18. Robust production of IL-1 and IL-18 in response to malaria infection requires, in addition to inflammasome signaling, TLR (mainly TLR9 and TLR7) mediated production of pro-IL-1 and pro-IL-18. *P. falciparum* genomic DNA contains >80% AT nucleotides. The AT-rich motifs of parasite DNA form loop structures, which have been shown to induce type I IFN response through STING-TBK1-IRF3 signaling (109). In some viruses, the AT-rich loop motifs of DNA are transcribed by RNA polymerase III to form double-stranded RNA containing 5′-triphosphate that induces type I IFNs through RIG-I-MAVS-IRF3 signaling (110). However, in the case of *P. falciparum* DNA, pol III-dependent recognition of AT-rich motifs of DNA seems to be not involved in cytosolic sensing as deficiency in pol III had no effect on immune responses to the parasite DNA (109).

RNA

The innate immune system senses RNA of both the liver and the blood stage parasites. In the liver stage, as described in the section Liver Stage Parasite Sensing above, RNA is recognized exclusively in the cytosol by MDA5 (**Figure 1**) (79, 80). In contrast, in the blood stage infection, mouse parasite RNA is recognized by TLR7 in phagolysosomes of DCs, leading to type I IFN production (**Figure 1**). In fact, studies in a mouse model of *P. chabaudi*-infection showed that type I IFN production is the earliest cytokine response (24 h postinfection) during the blood stage malaria infection (127). Parasite RNA enters endosomes of Mφs and DCs upon the uptake of parasites/parasite components, inducing type I IFN response through TLR7 signaling (81, 106, 128). Type I IFNs thus produced prominently contribute to the upregulation of pro-inflammatory cytokines, such as IFN-γ and IL-12, during the early stages of infection (106). RNA of the blood stage mouse parasites is also sensed by cytosolic MDA5, leading to type I IFN production (81).

While it is clear that RNA induced TLR7 signaling plays an important role in early type I IFN production in mouse malaria, it remains unclear whether or to what extent RNA of human parasites is able to induce type I IFN response. This is because, although RNA of human malaria parasite *P. falciparum* has been reported to induce cytokine responses through TLR7 recognition, the reported activity appears to be very low (106). Further studies are needed to determine whether or to what extent *P. falciparum* RNA is immunostimulatory.

MALARIAL DANGER-ASSOCIATED MOLECULAR PATTERNS (DAMPs)

Hemozoin

Hemozoin is a hydrophobic, crystalline insoluble polymer of heme formed during the digestion of hemoglobin by parasites in the digestive vacuoles to use the released amino acid as a food source (45, 129–131). In parasites, hemozoin is associated with lipids and proteins, and is released into the blood circulation when merozoites are egressed from matured schizonts. Hemozoin by itself is an inert material and appears

TABLE 2 | Innate sensing of malaria parasites and signaling mechanisms.

PRRs (host receptors)	PRR cellular location	PAMPs and DAPMs	Signaling pathway	References
TLRs				
TLR1,2 dimer	Cell surface	GPI	MAPK, NF-κB	(43, 89, 103, 104)
TLR4	Cell surface	GPI, heme, IRBC micro-particles	MAPK, TRIF, NF-κB	(43, 44, 83, 84)
TLR7	Endosome	RNA	MAPK, NF-κB	(106)
TLR9	Endosome	DNA	MAPK, NF-κB	(44, 107, 108)
CYTOSOLIC NUCLEIC ACID SENSORS				
MDA5	Cytosol	RNA	MAVS-TBK1-IRF3/IRF7	(79–81)
cGAS	Cytosol	DNA	STING-TBK1-IRF3/IRF7	(44, 109, 110)
AIM2	Cytosol	DNA	NLRP3 inflammasome	(44, 109, 111)
DANGER SIGNALING				
-	Cytosol	Hemozoin	NLRP3 inflammasome	(45, 111–114)
-	Cytosol	Uric acid	NLRP3 inflammasome	(114–116)
-	Cytosol	Unidentified factor	NLRP12 and NLRP4 inflammasome	(44, 82)
PHAGOCYTIC RECEPTORS				
CD36	Cell surface	PfEMP1, and unidentified ligand(s)	Src/Syk, MAPK	(117–120)
ADHESION RECEPTOR				
ICAM-1	Cell surface	PfEMP1	Src-PI3K-Akt, Rho, MAPK?	(121, 122)
EPCR	Cell surface	PfEMP1	Not known	

to have no specific receptor for recognition, but it influences the innate immune responses to malaria parasites in several ways; reviewed in Olivier et al. (45). Studies have reported that hemozoin is a carrier of malaria parasite DNA into endosomes for TLR9 recognition (107). Although how and where parasite DNA associates with hemozoin have not been specifically studied *in vivo*, there exist several possibilities. Malaria merozoites egressed from the matured schizonts have a half-life of <5 min (132), and many merozoites cannot invade red blood cells within this short period time. These uninvaded merozoites are likely to be lysed, releasing DNA that may complex with hemozoin *via* the associated proteins. Additionally, Mφs and neutrophils undergo apoptotic death after ingesting IRBCs (133), releasing the degraded parasite materials, including DNA, RNA, hemozoin and other components. The released DNA can complex with hemozoin. However, hemozoin is not obligatory for the entry of parasite DNA into endosomes. The parasite nuclear material, DNA containing immune complexes, merozoites, and IRBCs are also taken up by phagocytic cells (107, 108, 124, 126). It is difficult to quantify *in vivo* the extent to which DNA enters endosomes through phagocytic uptake of infected erythrocytes, merozoites and nuclear materials compared to hemozoin-bound DNA in inducing immune responses.

Since hemozoin is an inert, indigestible material, it curtails the ability of Mφs to induce innate immune responses to malaria. Upon uptake of IRBCs or hemozoin, Mφs become immunosuppressive and dysfunctional due to damages caused by oxidative burst (134). Monocytes and Mφs that ingest parasite IRBCs undergo apoptotic death with little or negligible release of cytokines, although cytokines are expressed to certain extent (133). Phagocytic internalization of large amounts of whole parasites and non-digestible hemozoin renders Mφs nonfunctional because of phagolysosomal acidification and apoptotic death (133, 135). Hemozoin is known to inhibit the differentiation and maturation of human monocyte-derived DCs as well (136, 137). However, certain subsets of inflammatory Mφs, such as spleen red pulp Mφs, CD169$^+$ Mφs, and CD16$^+$ monocytes produce cytokines in response to malaria parasites (126–128). It is not known whether hemozoin significantly alters the capacity of these cells to produce cytokines and chemokines.

The effect of hemozoin on DC function remains unclear, reviewed in Wykes and Good (138). A previous study has shown that hemozoin-internalized DCs localized in T cell areas of the spleen in *P. chabaudi*-infected mice and that T cell activated by these DCs lacked effector function (139). These results suggest that hemozoin considerably compromises DC function. However, in a later study, DCs efficiently produced DNA-TLR9 signaling-induced cytokines in response to DNA bound to natural hemozoin and thus it was suggested that hemozoin enhances the activity of DNA by facilitating its entry to endosomes (107). It remains unclear whether this is the case in infected host. On the other hand, it has been shown that subsequent to the uptake of parasite components and the activation of TLR7 and TLR9 signaling, hemozoin destabilizes phagolysosomal membrane, leading to the release of nucleic acid and hemozoin into the cytosol (111). The released parasite components are sensed by cytosolic PRRs, leading to several signaling pathways (44, 81, 111–113), including: (i) cGAS-STING-TBK1-IRF3 signaling by dsDNA; (ii) MDA5-MAVS-TBK1-IRF3 signaling by RNA; (iii) STING signaling mediated by AT-rich motifs through sensing by an unidentified receptor; (iv) AIM2 inflammasome signaling induced by parasite DNA, and (v) NLRP12 inflammasome activation *via* an unidentified mechanism (82). In addition, hemozoin also activates NLRP3 inflammasome (45, 111–113); **Figure 1** and **Table 2**. The activation of NLRP3 inflammasome by malarial hemozoin is mediated through the activation of Lyn and Syk tyrosine kinases (45). Synthetic hemozoin also activates Lyn and Syk signaling and, depending on the morphology and particle size, induces distinct immune response. It appears that hemozoin has no specific PRR, but it induces a danger signal (112, 113); hence, hemozoin is a DAPM. While nucleic acid-TLR-mediated signaling results in the synthesis of large amounts of pro-IL-1, inflammasome signaling and activation of caspase 1 lead to the cleavage of pro-IL-1 to the active, fever-inducing IL-1. Thus, hemozoin plays a significant role in the production of IL-1, contributing to fever induction in infected people. Besides hemozoin, parasite biomass, and purified merozoites that are devoid of hemozoin can potentially activate inflammasome and caspase 1 as it is known that even inert materials such as alum, asbestos, silica, uric acid crystals and cholesterol particles, activate NLRP3 inflammasome (45).

Uric Acid

Uric acid is the final oxidation product of purine metabolism and is released in large amounts by dying cells. Under physiological conditions, uric acid exists as a monoionic urate and forms insoluble monourate crystal (140). Uric acid is an important antioxidant in plasma and can induce protective anti-inflammatory responses in vascular and other diseases (141, 142). However, excessive formation of uric acid promotes pathogenic conditions, such as severe and chronic inflammatory arthritis, gout, and certain metabolic syndromes (141, 142). The pathogenic role of uric acid is due to the activation of NLRP3 inflammasome, which results in caspase 1 activation and conversion of pro-IL-1 into active IL-1 (114–116); **Figure 1** and **Table 2**. During malaria, a large number of parasite-ingested Mφs, neutrophils and other immune cells die, which likely release high levels of uric acid. Importantly, a significant amount of uric acid is formed during purine nucleotide metabolism by parasites and accumulates as a precipitate in IRBCs (143). Large amounts of hypoxanthine also accumulate in parasite IRBCs. The uric acid precipitate and hypoxanthine are released to the blood upon schizont burst. In the blood stream, hypoxanthine is oxidized to uric acid. In agreement with its pathogenic role, high levels of uric acid are found in the blood circulation of patients having severe malaria (144).

PHAGOCYTOSIS- AND ADHERENCE-INDUCED SIGNALING

Phagocytic uptake of parasite IRBCs, merozoites, hemozoin, and immune complexes by Mφs, neutrophils and DCs is an important process during malaria infection. Studies have shown that phagocytosis generally activates Src/Syk family of nonreceptor kinases, leading to the activation of a wide range of signaling pathways, including PKC, RAS-ERK, Ca_2^+, NF-κB signaling (145–147). These signaling events can integrate into TLR and inflammasome signaling, thereby modulating immune responses (148). Phagocytosis of malaria parasites and hemozoin suppresses immune function of Mφs and monocytes due to phagolysosomal acidification (133, 135). However, phagocytosis by DCs and inflammatory Mφs likely induces Src/Syk-mediated signaling, contributing to immune responses. The signaling induced by CD36-mediated phagocytosis and IRBC adherence in malaria immune responses are described below.

CD36 Signaling

CD36 is a multifunctional class B scavenger receptor that binds diverse types of ligands and pathogens, facilitating internalization by cells (67, 118, 149). Many cell types, including Mφs, DCs, platelets, and endothelial cells, express CD36. CD36-mediated phagocytosis of pathogens and pathogenic molecules activates Src/Syk kinases, leading to the activation of ERK, p38 and Jun members of the MAPK signaling pathways and NF-κB (67, 118, 119, 150) (**Figure 2**). Signals of these pathways synergize with TLR and inflammasome signaling, contributing to innate immune responses (119, 156). In malaria, CD36 plays several roles, including (i) mediating the sequestration of *P. falciparum* in vascular capillaries through the binding of adhesive PfEMP1 expressed on the surface of IRBCs, (ii) phagocytic uptake of parasites, and (iii) enhancing innate immune responses (120, 157–162). Studies have shown that CD36-induced MAPK signaling contributes to the production of TNF-α in mouse malaria infection and modulates parasite GPI-induced cytokine responses in mouse Mφs and human blood DCs (120, 161, 163). In *P. falciparum* endemic regions, single nucleotide polymorphisms in the *Cd36* gene have been linked to protection from cerebral and other severe malaria (164, 165). A more recent study in *P. yoelii*-infected mice demonstrated that CD36 significantly contributes to cytokine responses by innate immune cells, and the upregulation of MHCII expression, phagocytic activity, Th1 responses and expression of complement and Fc receptors (117). Overall, these responses lead to decreased parasite burden in infected host. It is possible that, similar to CD36, other scavenger receptors, such as MARCO modulate innate immunity to malaria to a certain extent.

EPCR Signaling

Endothelial protein C receptor (EPCR), which is also known as activated protein C (APC) receptor, is a transmembrane glycoprotein in vasculatures that binds protein C and promotes thrombin-thrombomodulin complex-mediated protein C activation (166). Under normal conditions, thrombomodulin on the endothelial surface binds thrombin and activates protein C to APC; this process is strongly promoted by EPCR. APC is detached from EPCR and inactivates blood coagulation factors Va and VIIIa, thereby exerting anticoagulant effect. APC binding to EPCR confers cytoprotective roles, such as antiapoptotic, anti-inflammatory and barrier stabilization responses (153–155). In malaria, EPCR binds certain members of PfEMP1 expressed on the surface of IRBCs and contributes to severe malaria (17, 167–169). Although the downstream

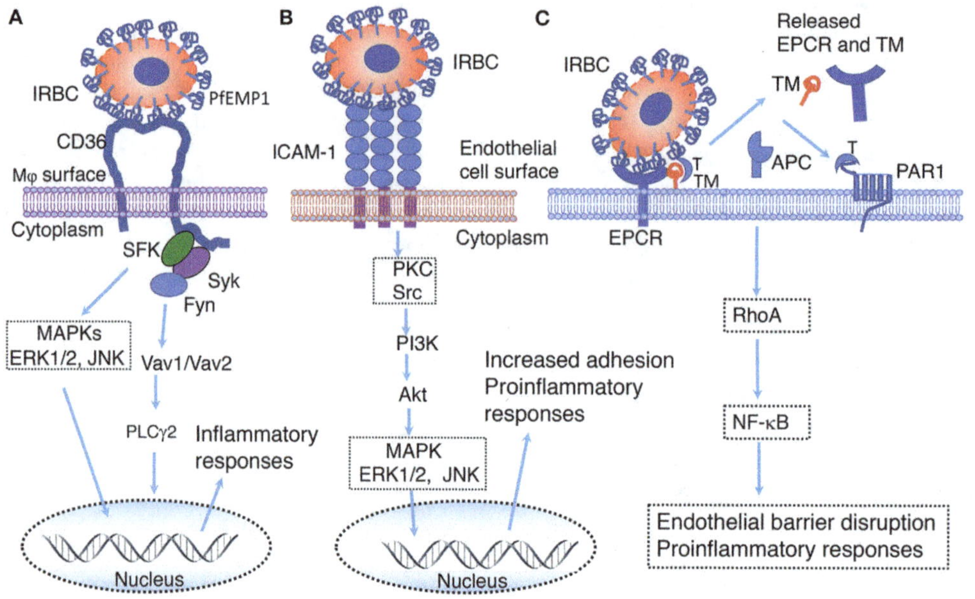

FIGURE 2 | Illustration of predicted pathways activated by the binding of PfEMP 1 expressed on the IRBC surface to CD36 **(A)**, ICAM-1 **(B)** and EPCR **(C)**. **(A)** Interaction of PfEMP1 on the surface of IRBC with CD36 on the surface of macrophages. SFK, Src family of protein tyrosine kinases; Syk, spleen tyrosine kinase; Fyn, proto-oncogene tyrosine protein kinase Fyn; MAPK, mitogen-activated protein kinase; ERK1/2, extracellular signal-regulated kinase 1 and 2; JNK, c-Jun N-terminal kinase; Vav1/Vav2, Vav family of guanine nucleotide exchange factors; PLCγ2, phospholipase Cγ2 (151). **(B)** Interaction of PfEMP1 on the surface of IRBC with ICAM-1 on the surface of endothelial cells surface. PKC, protein kinase C; Src, proto-oncogene tyrosine-protein kinase Src; PI3K, Phosphatidyl inositol 3-kinase; Akt, RAC-alpha serine/threonine-protein kinase (152). **(C)** Interaction of EPCR on the surface of endothelial cells with PfEMP1 on the surface of IRBCs (153–155). EPCR, endothelial protein C receptor; TM, thrombomodulin; T, thrombin; APC, Activated protein C; PAR1, protease-activated receptor 1; RhoA, Ras homolog gene family, member A GTAase.

events of EPCR-PfEMP1 binding-mediated signaling remain to be understood, it appears that the binding results in the loss of EPCR and thrombomodulin from the endothelial cell surface by shedding, leading to decreased protein C activation and compromised EPCR-mediated protection (**Figure 2**). This may reduce anti-inflammatory responses and increase thrombin production, blood coagulation, pro-inflammatory responses, endothelial cell apoptosis, leading to the loss of barrier function. The cumulative effects of these responses may contribute to endothelial cell damage, promoting cerebral and other severe malaria illnesses.

ICAM-1 Signaling

ICAM-1 mediates the sequestration of *P. falciparum* in the brain through the binding of PfEMP1 on the surface of IRBCs to endothelial cells (15, 16, 25). The sequestration of parasites in vascular capillaries of the brain induces inflammatory responses, resulting in the infiltration of cytotoxic effector cells and endothelial barrier damage. These processes have been implicated in the development of cerebral malaria, but the experimental evidence is controversial. An earlier study has reported that interaction with ICAM-1 contributes to increased serum TNF-α in cerebral malaria model of *P. berghei* ANKA-infected mice and that ICAM-1 deficient mice survive >15 days compared to 6–8 days in wild type (WT) mice (170). However, a later study reported that ICAM-1 is dispensable for cerebral malaria pathogenesis (171). NK cells cross-talk with myeloid cells through LFA-1 binding to ICAM-1, producing IFN-γ (172). Similarly, T cells are also known to interact with endothelial cells through LFA-1 mediated binding to ICAM-1, producing IFN-γ. Studies have shown that, upon binding to its ligands, ICAM-1 is activated by phosphorylation, inducing Src-PI3K-Akt, Ca_2^+, Rho and MAPK signaling (121, 122) (**Figure 2**). It is likely that these signals contribute to immune responses to malaria; thus far this aspect has not been examined.

INNATE IMMUNE RESPONSES TO MALARIA

Innate Immune Responses at the Liver Stage Infection

In malaria, like in most pathogenic infections, the innate immune system functions as the first line of defense by controlling parasite growth and regulating the development of adaptive immunity (14, 75–77). As discussed in section Liver Stage Parasite Sensing, during the liver stage malaria infection, parasite-infected hepatocytes produce type I IFNs through cytosolic sensing of RNA. This cytokine response contributes to the killing of parasite-infected hepatocytes by NKT cells, exposing parasite components. The antigen-presenting cells, primarily DCs and inflammatory Mφs, can potentially recognize the exposed parasite factors. In addition, sporozoites injected by infected mosquitoes that could not enter the blood circulation remain in dermis and die. In addition, some sporozoites that enter blood circulation may not invade hepatocytes and die. These dead parasites are likely sampled by DCs and inflammatory Mφs, leading to TLR- and inflammasome-mediated immune responses. The activated antigen-presenting cells have potential to modulate immune responses to the blood stage infection. However, because the parasite load in liver in natural infections is very low, the innate immune responses are likely to be also very low. Thus, the responses produced by antigen presenting cells against liver stage parasites may not exert a significant influence on immune responses induced by the blood stage parasites. However, in hyper endemic areas, repetitive infections in humans may induce immune tolerance in antigen-presenting cells that may modulate immunity to the blood stage infection to a certain extent.

Innate Immune Responses at the Blood Stage Infection

During the blood stage infection, unlike the liver stage, parasites grow exponentially through repetitive erythrocytic cycles, rapidly accumulating the biomass. This leads to an efficient induction of innate immune responses. Early during the blood stage infection, DCs and Mφs are key first responders of the innate immune system. However, as noted above, Mφs upon internalization of infected erythrocytes, merozoites or hemozoin become immunosuppressive and dysfunctional (133–137); unable to secrete cytokines and chemokines. It appears that the primary role of Mφs during the early stages of blood stage malaria infection is to control parasite growth through phagocytic clearance. In contrast to Mφs, DCs efficiently produce cytokines and chemokines in response malaria parasites, and effectively interact with cells of the innate and adaptive immune system. Thus, DCs play key roles in the initiation and regulation of innate and adaptive immunity to malaria. Also, it should be noted that some subsets of Mφs having certain features of DCs, such as $CD11c^+$ spleen red pulp Mφs and $CD169^+$ inflammatory Mφs, produce cytokines (127, 133, 173).

As noted in section RNA, during the blood stage malaria infection, type I IFNs are the earliest (24 h postinfection) cytokines produced through the activation of TLR7-MyD88 and IRF7 signaling (174). Early type I IFN response is produced primarily by the spleen red pulp Mφs and pDCs in *P. chabaudi*-infected mice (106, 127). Two recent studies by using lethal malaria model of *P. yoelii* YM infection, in which parasites grow rapidly to attain peak parasitemia of ~80% by 6 days postinfection, have also showed TLR7-dependent peak levels of type I IFN production at 24–36 h postinfection (81, 128). This early cytokine response is mediated through the coordination of TLR7- and cytosolic sensing mechanisms: TLR7-MyD88-IRF7 signaling in endosomes, and DNA-cGAS-STING-TBK1-IRF3/IRF7 and RNA-MDA5-MAVS-TBK1-IRF3 signaling in the cytosol (81). It has been found that SOCS1 expressed in response to cytosolic nucleic acid sensor-mediated signaling significantly downregulates TLR7-mediated type I IFN response. As such, deficiency in SOCS1 results in markedly high levels of type I IFNs, providing resistance against high parasite burden-dependent lethality (81). Additionally, it has been shown that $CD169^+$ Mφs activated through STING-mediated signaling migrate to bone marrow, where they interact with pDCs to induce type I IFN production through TLR7-MyD88 signaling (128). Interaction of classical DCs with pDCs is also important in pDCs producing cytokine responses to malaria parasites (38, 108). It appears that Mφs and neutrophils that internalize parasites undergo pyroptosis (111), exposing parasite components, which are taken up by classical DCs and $CD169^+$ Mφs, and activated through STING-mediated cytosolic signaling. The early type I IFN response triggers the infiltration of immune cells to the blood that may subsequently localize to the spleen. In contrast, in *P. berghei* ANKA-infected mice, relatively high level of IFN-α was seen at 4 days postinfection with low or negligible IFN-α production during 1–3 days postinfection (175). Collectively, the above results indicate that different strains of malaria parasites differentially induce type I IFN. That is, the earliest type I IFN production (24–36 h postinfection) by *P. chabaudi* and *P. yoelii* is mediated mainly through parasite RNA-induced TLR7 signaling (81, 106, 128), whereas such RNA-mediated early type I IFN response is not readily apparent in *P. berghei* ANKA (175). The production of type I IFNs at later stages of *P. berghei* ANKA infection likely involves a different mechanism. In other studies, cGAS sensing of the AT-rich motifs of *P. falciparum* DNA in the cytosol could induce type I IFN production through the STING-TBK1-IRF3/IRF7 signaling pathway, independent of TLR9-MyD88 signaling (109, 110). This could be the mechanism through which *P. berghei* ANKA induces significant levels of type I IFN at 4 days pi (175).

Early type I IFN response to malaria infection contributes to the suppression of antiparasitic immunity and promotes cerebral and other severe malaria illnesses under certain situations. This is evident from the observations that deficiency in IFNαR in *P. yoelii* YM infection resulted in increased IFN-γ levels, significantly decreased parasitemia and resistant to parasite burden-dependent death (128). Also, in *P. berghei* ANKA-infected mice, which produce low levels of early type I IFN response but produce a significant amount at a somewhat later stage (4 days postinfection), deficiency in IFNαR or treatment with anti-IFNαR1 antibody resulted in increased IFN-γ production, increased number of IFN-γ-positive NK and $CD4^+$ T cells in the spleen, and significantly decreased parasitemia and protection from cerebral malaria (175, 176). From these results, it is evident that type I IFNs suppress the production of IFN-γ and thus anti-parasitic function under certain conditions. By contrast, in a different situation, high levels of type I IFN production at early stages of *P. yoelii* YM infection promoted antiparasitic immunity. In this case, blocking of SOCS1, a suppressor of cytokine signaling 1, expression resulted in high levels of type I IFN production, leading to increased IFN-γ production and reduced parasitemia, protecting mice from parasite burden-dependent death (81). Consistent with the observations of the latter study (81), daily treatment of *P. berghei* ANKA-infected mice with recombinant IFN-α, which to a certain extent resembles a situation of high levels of type I IFN production at early stage of infection, also significantly increased IFN-γ production by splenic $CD8^+$ T cells, markedly reducing parasitemia and preventing cerebral malaria (177). The results of these two studies suggest that type I IFNs promote IFN-γ-dependent anti-parasitic immunity, providing resistance against severe malaria. On the other hand, treatment of *P. berghei* ANKA-infected mice with recombinant IFN-β resulted in reduced TNF-α and IFN-γ production, decreased expression of ICAM-1 and CXCL9 in the brain, reduced CXCR3 expression by T cells and T cell infiltration to the brain, thereby significantly preventing cerebral malaria and increasing mice survival (178). Thus, type I IFNs play contrasting roles in malaria in a context-dependent manner and also dependent on type I IFN isomeric composition.

Compared to the results of two studies outlined above (175, 176), wherein deficiency in IFNαR contributed to increased IFN-γ response and decreased parasitemia in *P. berghei* ANKA-infected mice, Palomo *et al.* observed contrasting immune responses (179), although in all these studies mice were protected from cerebral malaria. Palomo et al. found that, compared to infected WT mice, *P. berghei* ANKA-infected mice deficient in IFNαR had similar parasitemia, reduced expression of IFN-γ and granzyme B by T cells, decreased expression of T cell-attracting chemokine CXCL9, and low infiltration of $CXCR3^{+}$-expressing CD8 T cells to the brain. A notable difference in these studies is that the latter study used GFP knock-in transgenic parasite clone, which appeared to have slower growth rate than the WT parasites used in the former study. These differences may alter the dynamics of immune responses. Nevertheless, the results agree with the notion that type I IFNs play distinct roles under different malaria conditions.

Overall, the available data indicate that type I IFNs play disparate roles in malaria infection depending on the timing and amount of production, relative levels of IFN-α, IFN-β and perhaps other isomers, and compositions of cellular and cytokine milieu during the progression of infection, and parasite strains. A recent review provides a comprehensive and up-to-date account on the role and contrasting effects of type I IFNs in malaria (180). Type I IFNs are pleiotropic cytokines and as such, they induce a wide range of effects on innate and adaptive immune cells during various pathogenic infections, contributing to either protection against infection or pathogenesis (181–183). These differential effects are likely dependent on the levels of type I IFNs; low levels at early stages of infection mediate cell-mediated immunity, but high levels cause immunosuppression (182). Thus, it is not surprising that type I IFNs produced during malaria infection also induce a wide range of cellular effects involving a complex interplay between various cell types.

In addition to producing type I IFNs, DCs produce a wide range of pro-inflammatory cytokines, including TNF-α, IL-12, and IL-6, and chemokines, such as CXCL1, CXCL2, CCL2, CCL5, CXCL9, and CXCL10 in response to malaria parasites, and play crucial roles in malaria immunity and pathogenesis (34, 38, 108, 184–186). Type I IFNs prime DCs for efficient cytokine and chemokine production and activate NK, NKT, γδ T, and T cells to induce IFN-γ and other inflammatory responses (182). IL-12 produced by DCs activates NK cells to induce the production of IFN-γ, which promotes Th1 and effector T cell responses (187). The augmented production of IFN-γ contributes to an efficient parasitemia control by priming Mφs and neutrophils for increased phagocytic activity and thus parasite clearance (188, 189). IFN-γ also contributes to cerebral and other severe malaria clinical conditions under certain situations, such as parasite sequestering in vital organs (187, 188, 190). Chemokines, on the other hand, promote the recruitment of immune cells to mount effective cell-mediated anti-parasitic effects (191). However, these responses also contribute to severe pathology (37, 192, 193). By and large, the initial innate immune responses are mainly aimed at controlling parasite growth by potentiating antiparasitic cell-mediated immunity. However, since pro-inflammatory responses contribute to pathogenesis (14, 33–38), as infection progresses, the function of DCs switches from pro-inflammatory and Th1-inducing to anti-inflammatory and Th2-inducing phenotypes (39, 40, 194). Eventually, balanced pro- and anti-inflammatory and Th1/Th2 responses prevent pathogenesis and promote protective humoral immunity to malaria (39–42); imbalanced responses contribute to pathogenesis. Thus, innate immune responses contribute to either protective immunity or pathogenesis in a context dependent manner.

TLR-MYD88 Signaling Prominently Contributes to Protective Immunity and Pathogenesis

DNA and RNA play prominent roles in mouse malaria immunity and pathogenesis; under certain conditions TLR2 and TLR4 also play important roles. As such, studies in various mouse models have demonstrated that TLR9, TLR7, TLR4, and TLR2 play important roles in malaria immunity and cerebral, placental and other severe malaria pathology (43, 44, 81, 102, 103, 106–108, 124, 128, 174, 195–201). Gene polymorphism studies in endemic areas that assessed the role of TLRs in malaria have linked TLR9, TLR4, and TLR2 to either susceptibility or resistance to malaria (202–214). While the involvement of TLR9, TLR4, and TLR2 in malaria immunity/pathology is evident from studies in both mouse malaria models and in humans (43, 106, 195, 197, 198, 200–203, 205, 210), thus far none of the studies in endemic areas have revealed the association of TLR7 with human malaria immunity/pathology. It is unclear whether studies in endemic areas that have assessed association of TLRs have investigated the role of TLR7 in malaria susceptibility/resistance. However, since *P. falciparum* RNA appears to have very low immunostimulatory activity, it is possible that TLR7 has either minor or no role in human malaria. Accumulated evidence indicates that TLRs prominently contribute malaria immunity and pathology, whereas other signaling mechanisms such as inflammasome and adherence-mediated signaling may play minor roles (172, 215).

The contribution of pro-inflammatory responses produced by the innate immune system to protective immunity and pathogenesis is primarily context dependent. In non-cytoadherent parasites, such as *P. yoelii* 17XNL strain and *P. chabaudi* that exhibit slow growth rates during the initial phase of infection, pro-inflammatory responses are protective by facilitating anti-parasitic effector function and cell-mediated immunity. In contrast, in the case of cytoadherent parasites, such as *P. berghei* ANKA that sequesters in brain, lungs, liver and adipose tissues, and *P. berghei* NK65 that sequesters in lungs and liver, pro-inflammatory responses are pathogenic by promoting cytotoxicity in effector cells, which cause organ damage. In this regard, the observations made in mouse models parallel those of vivax and falciparum malaria in humans. In *P. falciparum* infection, strong pro-inflammatory responses contribute to an effective control of parasitemia which otherwise results in fulminant infection (41, 42). However, despite this beneficial effect, pro-inflammatory responses promote effector cell function, which contributes to organ damage and severe illnesses. In contrast, in the case of *P. vivax*, which is relatively slow growing and does not cytoadhere except at low levels in lungs and the placenta (125), despite causing a number of clinical conditions, fatal illnesses are relatively rare compared to *P. falciparum*.

CONCLUDING REMARKS

Malaria continues to be a major global health problem. In many endemic areas, parasites are becoming increasingly resistant to the currently widely used artemisinin-based combination drugs, which have been very effective in treating infection. Therefore, new drugs or other treatment strategies are urgently needed. Mass vaccination is the best strategy to prevent malaria. However, despite huge efforts during the past decades in many laboratories around the world, obtaining an efficacious vaccine suitable for mass vaccination remains challenging. It is thought that better understanding of molecular and cellular processes involved in the development of protective immunity and those that contribute to severe pathogenesis will be useful in designing an effective vaccine. During the past decades, a significant progress has been made in identifying the parasite factors and host receptors involved in the activation of the innate immune system and the associated cell signaling pathways. Significant progress has also been made in understanding how cellular activation and immune responses initiated upon parasite-host interactions influence subsequent development of antiparasitic immunity and contribute to severe pathogenesis.

AUTHOR CONTRIBUTIONS

All authors listed have made a substantial, direct and intellectual contribution to the work, and approved it for publication.

ACKNOWLEDGMENTS

This work was supported by grants AI41139 and AI104844 from the National Institute of Allergy and Infectious Diseases, National Institutes of Health, and by the financial support from the Department of Biochemistry and Molecular Biology, The Penn State University College of Medicine.

REFERENCES

1. World Health Organization. *World Malaria Report Geneva*. (2017). Available online at: http://www.who.int/malaria/publications/world-malaria-report-2017/en/
2. Battle KE, Guerra CA, Golding N, Duda KA, Cameron E, Howes RE, et al. Global database of matched *Plasmodium falciparum* and *P. vivax* incidence and prevalence records from 1985-2013. *Sci Data* (2015) 2:150012. doi: 10.1038/sdata.2015.12
3. Howes RE, Battle KE, Mendis KN, Smith DL, Cibulskis RE, Baird JK, et al. Global epidemiology of *Plasmodium vivax*. *Am J Trop Med Hyg.* (2016) 95(Suppl. 6):15–34. doi: 10.4269/ajtmh.16-0141
4. Rogerson SJ, Desai M, Mayor A, Sicuri E, Taylor SM, van Eijk AM. Burden, pathology, and costs of malaria in pregnancy: new developments for an old problem. *Lancet Infect Dis.* (2018) 18:e107–18. doi: 10.1016/S1473-3099(18)30066-5
5. Gallup JL, Sachs JD. The economic burden of malaria. *Am J Trop Med Hyg.* (2001) 64(Suppl. 1-2):85–96. doi: 10.4269/ajtmh.2001.64.85
6. Chima RI, Goodman CA, Mills A. The economic impact of malaria in Africa: a critical review of the evidence. *Health Policy* (2003) 63:17–36. doi: 10.1016/S0168-8510(02)00036-2
7. Phillips MA, Burrows JN, Manyando C, van Huijsduijnen RH, Van Voorhis WC, Wells TNC. Malaria. *Nat Rev Dis Primers* (2017) 3:17050. doi: 10.1038/nrdp.2017.50
8. Singh B, Daneshvar C. Human infections and detection of *Plasmodium knowlesi*. *Clinical Microbiol Rev.* (2013) 26:165–84. doi: 10.1128/CMR.00079-12
9. Lee K-S, Cox-Singh J, Singh B. Morphological features and differential counts of *Plasmodium knowlesi* parasites in naturally acquired human infections. *Malaria J.* (2009) 8:73. doi: 10.1186/1475-2875-8-73
10. Otto TD, Bohme U, Jackson AP, Hunt M, Franke-Fayard B, Hoeijmakers WA, et al. A comprehensive evaluation of rodent malaria parasite genomes and gene expression. *BMC Biol.* (2014) 12:86. doi: 10.1186/s12915-014-0086-0
11. Anstey NM, Russell B, Yeo TW, Price RN. The pathophysiology of vivax malaria. *Trends Parasitol.* (2009) 25:220–7. doi: 10.1016/j.pt.2009.02.003
12. Autino B, Corbett Y, Castelli F, Taramelli D. Pathogenesis of malaria in tissues and blood. *Mediterr J Hematol Infect Dis.* (2012) 4:e2012061. doi: 10.4084/mjhid.2012.061
13. Storm J, Craig AG. Pathogenesis of cerebral malaria–inflammation and cytoadherence. *Front Cellular Infect Microbiol.* (2014) 4:100. doi: 10.3389/fcimb.2014.00100
14. Deroost K, Pham T-T, Opdenakker G, Van den Steen PE. The immunological balance between host and parasite in malaria. *FEMS Microbiol Rev.* (2015) 40:208–57. doi: 10.1093/femsre/fuv046
15. Wahlgren M, Goel S, Akhouri RR. Variant surface antigens of *Plasmodium falciparum* and their roles in severe malaria. *Nat Rev Microbiol.* (2017) 15:479–91. doi: 10.1038/nrmicro.2017.47
16. Smith JD, Rowe JA, Higgins MK, Lavstsen T. Malaria's deadly grip: cytoadhesion of *Plasmodium falciparum*-infected erythrocytes. *Cellular Microbiol.* (2013) 15:1976–83. doi: 10.1111/cmi.12183
17. Bernabeu M, Smith JD. EPCR and malaria severity: the center of a perfect storm. *Trends Parasitol.* (2017) 33:295–308. doi: 10.1016/j.pt.2016.11.004
18. Sharma L, Shukla G. Placental malaria: a new insight into the pathophysiology. *Front Med.* (2017) 4:117. doi: 10.3389/fmed.2017.00117
19. Coban C, Lee MSJ, Ishii KJ. Tissue-specific immunopathology during malaria infection. *Nat Rev Immunol.* (2018) 18:266–78. doi: 10.1038/nri.2017.138
20. Lee MSJ, Coban C. Unforeseen pathologies caused by malaria. *Int Immunol.* (2018) 30:121–9. doi: 10.1093/intimm/dxx076
21. Fried M, Duffy PE. Adherence of *Plasmodium falciparum* to chondroitin sulfate A in the human placenta. *Science* (1996) 272:1502–4. doi: 10.1126/science.272.5267.1502
22. Nunes MC, Scherf A. *Plasmodium falciparum* during pregnancy: a puzzling parasite tissue adhesion tropism. *Parasitology* (2007) 134(Pt 13):1863–9. doi: 10.1017/S0031182007000133

23. Goel S, Gowda DC. How specific is *Plasmodium falciparum* adherence to chondroitin 4-sulfate? *Trends Parasitol.* (2011) 27:375–81. doi: 10.1016/j.pt.2011.03.005
24. Fried M, Duffy PE. Malaria during pregnancy. *Cold Spring Harb Perspect Med.* (2017) 7:a025551. doi: 10.1101/cshperspect.a025551
25. Hviid L, Jensen AT. PfEMP1 - a parasite protein family of key importance in *Plasmodium falciparum* malaria immunity and pathogenesis. *Adv Parasitol.* (2015) 88:51–84. doi: 10.1016/bs.apar.2015.02.004
26. Totino PR, Lopes SC. Insights into the cytoadherence phenomenon of *Plasmodium vivax*: the putative role of phosphatidylserine. *Front Immunol.* (2017) 8:1148. doi: 10.3389/fimmu.2017.01148
27. Kochar DK, Saxena V, Singh N, Kochar SK, Kumar SV, Das A. *Plasmodium vivax* malaria. *Emerg Infect Dis.* (2005) 11:132–4. doi: 10.3201/eid1101.040519
28. Genton B, D'Acremont V, Rare L, Baea K, Reeder JC, Alpers MP, et al. *Plasmodium vivax* and mixed infections are associated with severe malaria in children: a prospective cohort study from Papua New Guinea. *PLoS Med.* (2008) 5:e127. doi: 10.1371/journal.pmed.0050127
29. Baird JK. Evidence and implications of mortality associated with acute *Plasmodium vivax* malaria. *Clin Microbiol Rev.* (2013) 26:36–57. doi: 10.1128/CMR.00074-12
30. Naing C, Whittaker MA, Wai VN, Mak JW. Is *Plasmodium vivax* malaria a severe malaria?: a systematic review and meta-analysis. *PLoS Neglect Trop Dis.* (2014) 8:e3071. doi: 10.1371/journal.pntd.0003071
31. Price RN, Douglas NM, Anstey NM. New developments in *Plasmodium vivax* malaria: severe disease and the rise of chloroquine resistance. *Curr Opin Infect Dis.* (2009) 22:430–5. doi: 10.1097/QCO.0b013e32832f14c1
32. Lima-Junior Jda C, Pratt-Riccio LR. Major histocompatibility complex and malaria: focus on *Plasmodium vivax* infection. *Front Immunol.* (2016) 7:13. doi: 10.3389/fimmu.2016.00013
33. Angulo I, Fresno M. Cytokines in the pathogenesis of and protection against malaria. *Clin Diagn Lab Immunol.* (2002) 9:1145–52. doi: 10.1128/CDLI.9.6.1145-1152.2002
34. Stevenson MM, Riley EM. Innate immunity to malaria. *Nat Rev Immunol.* (2004) 4:169–80. doi: 10.1038/nri1311
35. Schofield L, Grau GE. Immunological processes in malaria pathogenesis. *Nat Rev Immunol.* (2005) 5:722–35. doi: 10.1038/nri1686
36. Clark IA, Alleva LM, Budd AC, Cowden WB. Understanding the role of inflammatory cytokines in malaria and related diseases. *Travel Med Infect Dis.* (2008) 6:67–81. doi: 10.1016/j.tmaid.2007.07.002
37. Dunst J, Kamena F, Matuschewski K. Cytokines and chemokines in cerebral malaria pathogenesis. *Front Cellular Infect Microbiol.* (2017) 7:324. doi: 10.3389/fcimb.2017.00324
38. Gotz A, Tang MS, Ty MC, Arama C, Ongoiba A, Doumtabe D, et al. Atypical activation of dendritic cells by *Plasmodium falciparum*. *Proc Natl Acad Sci USA.* (2017) 114:E10568–77. doi: 10.1073/pnas.1708383114
39. Perry JA, Olver CS, Burnett RC, Avery AC. Cutting edge: the acquisition of TLR tolerance during malaria infection impacts T cell activation. *J Immunol.* (2005) 174:5921–5. doi: 10.4049/jimmunol.174.10.5921
40. Riley EM, Wahl S, Perkins DJ, Schofield L. Regulating immunity to malaria. *Parasite Immunol.* (2006) 28:35–49. doi: 10.1111/j.1365-3024.2006.00775.x
41. Goncalves RM, Scopel KK, Bastos MS, Ferreira MU. Cytokine balance in human malaria: does *Plasmodium vivax* elicit more inflammatory responses than *Plasmodium falciparum*? *PLoS ONE* (2012) 7:e44394. doi: 10.1371/journal.pone.0044394
42. Goncalves RM, Lima NF, Ferreira MU. Parasite virulence, co-infections and cytokine balance in malaria. *Pathogens Global Health* (2014) 108:173–8. doi: 10.1179/2047773214Y.0000000139
43. Eriksson E, Sampaio N, Schofield L. Toll-like receptors and malaria–sensing and susceptibility. *J Trop Dis.* (2013) 2:126. doi: 10.4172/2329-891X.1000126
44. Gazzinelli RT, Kalantari P, Fitzgerald KA, Golenbock DT. Innate sensing of malaria parasites. *Nat Rev Immunol.* (2014) 14:744–57. doi: 10.1038/nri3742
45. Olivier M, Van Den Ham K, Shio MT, Kassa FA, Fougeray S. Malarial pigment hemozoin and the innate inflammatory response. *Front Immunol.* (2014) 5:25. doi: 10.3389/fimmu.2014.00025
46. Liehl P, Meireles P, Albuquerque IS, Pinkevych M, Baptista F, Mota MM, et al. Innate immunity induced by *Plasmodium* liver infection inhibits malaria reinfections. *Infect Immun.* (2015) 83:1172–80. doi: 10.1128/IAI.02796-14
47. Kalantari P. The emerging role of pattern recognition receptors in the pathogenesis of malaria. *Vaccines* (2018) 6:1–15. doi: 10.3390/vaccines6010013
48. Struik SS, Riley EM. Does malaria suffer from lack of memory? *Immunol Rev.* (2004) 201:268–90. doi: 10.1111/j.0105-2896.2004.00181.x
49. Langhorne J, Ndungu FM, Sponaas AM, Marsh K. Immunity to malaria: more questions than answers. *Nat Immunol.* (2008) 9:725–32. doi: 10.1038/ni.f.205
50. Aly AS, Vaughan AM, Kappe SH. Malaria parasite development in the mosquito and infection of the mammalian host. *Ann Rev Microbiol.* (2009) 63:195–221. doi: 10.1146/annurev.micro.091208.073403
51. Vaughan AM, Aly AS, Kappe SH. Malaria parasite pre-erythrocytic stage infection: gliding and hiding. *Cell Host Microbe* (2008) 4:209–18. doi: 10.1016/j.chom.2008.08.010
52. Bertolino P, Bowen DG. Malaria and the liver: immunological hide-and-seek or subversion of immunity from within? *Front Microbiol.* (2015) 6:41. doi: 10.3389/fmicb.2015.00041
53. Bruce-Chwatt LJ. *Essential Malariology*. London, UK: William Heinemann Medical Books Ltd. (1985).
54. Roucher C, Rogier C, Sokhna C, Tall A, Trape JF. A 20-year longitudinal study of *Plasmodium ovale* and *Plasmodium malariae* prevalence and morbidity in a West African population. *PLoS ONE* (2014) 9:e87169. doi: 10.1371/journal.pone.0087169
55. Van den Steen PE, Deroost K, Deckers J, Van Herck E, Struyf, Opdenakker G. Pathogenesis of malaria-associated acute respiratory distress syndrome. *Trends Parasitol.* (2013) 29:346–58. doi: 10.1016/j.pt.2013.04.006
56. Beutler BA. TLRs and innate immunity. *Blood* (2009) 113:1399–407. doi: 10.1182/blood-2008-07-019307
57. Takeuchi O, Akira S. Pattern recognition receptors and inflammation. *Cell* (2010) 140:805–20. doi: 10.1016/j.cell.2010.01.022
58. Brubaker SW, Bonham KS, Zanoni I, Kagan JC. Innate immune pattern recognition: a cell biological perspective. *Ann Rev Immunol.* (2015) 33:257–90. doi: 10.1146/annurev-immunol-032414-112240
59. Kawasaki T, Kawai T. Toll-like receptor signaling pathways. *Front Immunol.* (2014) 5:461. doi: 10.3389/fimmu.2014.00461
60. Wu J, Chen ZJ. Innate immune sensing and signaling of cytosolic nucleic acids. *Ann Rev Immunol.* (2014) 32:461–88. doi: 10.1146/annurev-immunol-032713-120156
61. Vijay K. Toll-like receptors in immunity and inflammatory diseases: past, present, and future. *Intl Immunopharmacol.* (2018) 59:391–412. doi: 10.1016/j.intimp.2018.03.002
62. Rubartelli A, Lotze MT. Inside, outside, upside down: damage-associated molecular-pattern molecules (DAMPs) and redox. *Trends Immunol.* (2007) 28:429–36. doi: 10.1016/j.it.2007.08.004
63. Tang D, Kang R, Coyne CB, Zeh HJ, Lotze MT. PAMPs and DAMPs: signal 0s that spur autophagy and immunity. *Immunol Rev.* (2012) 249:158–75. doi: 10.1111/j.1600-065X.2012.01146.x
64. Kaczmarek A, Vandenabeele P, Krysko DV. Necroptosis: the release of damage-associated molecular patterns and its physiological relevance. *Immunity* (2013) 38:209–23. doi: 10.1016/j.immuni.2013.02.003
65. Venereau E, Ceriotti C, Bianchi ME. DAMPs from cell death to new life. *Front Immunol.* (2015) 6:422. doi: 10.3389/fimmu.2015.00422
66. Kawai T, Akira S. Toll-like receptors and their crosstalk with other innate receptors in infection and immunity. *Immunity* (2011) 34:637–50. doi: 10.1016/j.immuni.2011.05.006
67. Freeman SA, Grinstein S. Phagocytosis: receptors, signal integration, and the cytoskeleton. *Immunol Rev.* (2014) 262:193–215. doi: 10.1111/imr.12212
68. Lamphier MS, Sirois CM, Verma A, Golenbock DT, Latz E. TLR9 and the recognition of self and non-self nucleic acids. *Ann N Y Acad Sci.* (2006) 1082:31–43. doi: 10.1196/annals.1348.005
69. Ohto U, Shimizu T. Structural aspects of nucleic acid-sensing Toll-like receptors. *Biophys Rev.* (2016) 8:33–43. doi: 10.1007/s12551-015-0187-1
70. Franchi L, McDonald C, Kanneganti TD, Amer A, Núñez G. Nucleotide-binding oligomerization domain-like receptors: intracellular pattern

recognition molecules for pathogen detection and host defense. *J Immunol.* (2006) 177:3507–13. doi: 10.4049/jimmunol.177.6.3507
71. Silvie O, Amino R, Hafalla JC. Tissue-specific cellular immune responses to malaria pre-erythrocytic stages. *Curr Opin Microbiol.* (2017) 40:160–7. doi: 10.1016/j.mib.2017.12.001
72. Holz LE, Fernandez-Ruiz D, Heath WR. Protective immunity to liver-stage malaria. *Clin Transl Immunol.* (2016) 5:e105. doi: 10.1038/cti.2016.60
73. Gätz A, Ty M, Chora AF, Zuzarte-Luís V, Mota MM, Rodriguez A. Innate immunity to malaria. In: *Malaria: Immune Response to Infection and Vaccination*, eds Mota MM and Rodriguez A (Cham: Springer International Publishing AG) (2017). p. 3–25.
74. Yazdani SS, Mukherjee P, Chauhan VS, Chitnis CE. Immune responses to asexual blood-stages of malaria parasites. *Curr Mol Med.* (2006) 6:187–203. doi: 10.2174/156652406776055212
75. Smith TG, Ayi K, Serghides L, McAllister CD, Kain KC. Innate immunity to malaria caused by *Plasmodium falciparum*. *Clin Invest Med.* (2002) 25:262–72.
76. Urban BC, Ing R, Stevenson MM. Early interactions between blood-stage *Plasmodium* parasites and the immune system. *Curr Top Microbiol Immunol.* (2005) 297:25–70. doi: 10.1007/3-540-29967-X_2
77. Walther M, Woodruff J, Edele F, Jeffries D, Tongren JE, King E, et al. Innate immune responses to human malaria: heterogeneous cytokine responses to blood-stage *Plasmodium falciparum* correlate with parasitological and clinical outcomes. *J Immunol.* (2006) 177:5736–45. doi: 10.4049/jimmunol.177.8.5736
78. Stevenson MM, Ing R, Berretta F, Miu J. Regulating the adaptive immune response to blood-stage malaria: role of dendritic cells and $CD4^{+}Foxp3^{+}$ regulatory T cells. *Int J Biol Sci.* (2011) 7:1311–22. doi: 10.7150/ijbs.7.1311
79. Liehl P, Zuzarte-Luis V, Chan J, Zillinger T, Baptista F, Carapau D, et al. Host-cell sensors for *Plasmodium* activate innate immunity against liver-stage infection. *Nat Med.* (2014) 20:47–53. doi: 10.1038/nm.3424
80. Miller JL, Sack BK, Baldwin M, Vaughan AM, Kappe SH. Interferon-mediated innate immune responses against malaria parasite liver stages. *Cell Rep.* (2014) 7:436–47. doi: 10.1016/j.celrep.2014.03.018
81. Yu X, Cai B, Wang M, Tan P, Ding X, Wu J, et al. Cross-regulation of two type I interferon signaling pathways in plasmacytoid dendritic cells controls anti-malaria immunity and host mortality. *Immunity* (2016) 45:1093–107. doi: 10.1016/j.immuni.2016.10.001
82. Ataide MA, Andrade WA, Zamboni DS, Wang D, do Carmo Souza M, Franklin BS, et al. Malaria-induced NLRP12/NLRP3-dependent caspase-1 activation mediates inflammation and hypersensitivity to bacterial superinfection. *PLoS Pathog.* (2014) 10:e1003885. doi: 10.1371/journal.ppat.1003885
83. Couper KN, Barnes T, Hafalla JC, Combes V, Ryffel B, Secher T, et al. Parasite-derived plasma microparticles contribute significantly to malaria infection-induced inflammation through potent macrophage stimulation. *PLoS Pathog.* (2010) 6:e1000744 . doi: 10.1371/journal.ppat.1000744
84. Figueiredo RT, Fernandez PL, Mourao-Sa DS, Porto BN, Dutra FF, Alves LS, et al. Characterization of heme as activator of Toll-like receptor 4. *J Biol Chem.* (2007) 282:20221–9. doi: 10.1074/jbc.M6107 37200
85. Cowman AF, Healer J, Marapana D, Marsh K. Malaria: biology and disease. *Cell* (2016) 167:610–24. doi: 10.1016/j.cell.2016.07.055
86. Hirako IC, Assis PA, Hojo-Souza NS, Reed G, Nakaya H, Golenbock DT, et al. Daily rhythms of TNF-α expression and food intake regulate synchrony of *Plasmodium* stages with the host circadian cycle. *Cell Host Microbe* (2018) 23:796–808.e6. doi: 10.1016/j.chom.2018.04.016
87. Schreibelt G, Tel J, Sliepen KH, Benitez-Ribas D, Figdor CG, Adema GJ, et al. Toll-like receptor expression and function in human dendritic cell subsets: implications for dendritic cell-based anti-cancer immunotherapy. *Cancer Immunol Immunother.* (2010) 59:1573–82. doi: 10.1007/s00262-010-0833-1
88. Schofield L, Hackett F. Signal transduction in host cells by a glycosylphosphatidylinositol toxin of malaria parasites. *J Exp Med.* (1993)177:145–53. doi: 10.1084/jem.177.1.145
89. Gowda DC. TLR-mediated cell signaling by malaria GPIs. *Trends Parasitol.* (2007) 23:596–604. doi: 10.1016/j.pt.2007.09.003
90. Naik RS, Branch OH, Woods AS, Vijaykumar M, Perkins DJ, Nahlen BL, et al. Glycosylphosphatidylinositol anchors of *Plasmodium falciparum*: molecular characterization and naturally elicited antibody response that may provide immunity to malaria pathogenesis. *J Exp Med.* (2000) 192:1563–76. doi: 10.1084/jem.192.11.1563
91. Gerold P, Jung N, Azzouz N, Freiberg N, Kobe S, Schwarz RT. Biosynthesis of glycosylphosphatidylinositols of *Plasmodium falciparum* in a cell-free incubation system: inositol acylation is needed for mannosylation of glycosylphosphatidylinositols. *Biochem J.* (1999) 344(Pt 3):731–8. doi: 10.1042/bj3440731
92. Gowda DC, Gupta P, Davidson EA. Glycosylphosphatidylinositol anchors represent the major carbohydrate modification in proteins of intraerythrocytic stage *Plasmodium falciparum*. *J Biol Chem.* (1997) 272:6428–39. doi: 10.1074/jbc.272.10.6428
93. Gilson PR, Nebl T, Vukcevic D, Moritz RL, Sargeant T, Speed TP, et al. Identification and stoichiometry of glycosylphosphatidylinositol-anchored membrane proteins of the human malaria parasite *Plasmodium falciparum*. *Mol Cell Proteomics* (2006) 5:1286–99. doi: 10.1074/mcp.M600035-MCP200
94. Sanders PR, Gilson PR, Cantin GT, Greenbaum DC, Nebl T, Carucci DJ, et al. Distinct protein classes including novel merozoite surface antigens in Raft-like membranes of *Plasmodium falciparum*. *J Biol Chem.* (2005) 280:40169–76. doi: 10.1074/jbc.M509631200
95. Schofield L, Novakovic S, Gerold P, Schwarz RT, McConville MJ, Tachado SD. Glycosylphosphatidylinositol toxin of *Plasmodium* up-regulates intercellular adhesion molecule-1, vascular cell adhesion molecule-1, and E-selectin expression in vascular endothelial cells and increases leukocyte and parasite cytoadherence via tyrosine kinase-dependent signal transduction. *J Immunol.* (1996) 156:1886–96.
96. Tachado SD, Gerold P, McConville MJ, Baldwin T, Quilici D, Schwarz RT, et al. Glycosylphosphatidylinositol toxin of *Plasmodium* induces nitric oxide synthase expression in macrophages and vascular endothelial cells by a protein tyrosine kinase-dependent and protein kinase C-dependent signaling pathway. *J Immunol.* (1996) 156:1897–907.
97. Tachado SD, Gerold P, Schwarz R, Novakovic S, McConville M, Schofield L. Signal transduction in macrophages by glycosylphosphatidylinositols of *Plasmodium*, *Trypanosoma*, and *Leishmania*: activation of protein tyrosine kinases and protein kinase C by inositolglycan and diacylglycerol moieties. *Proc Natl Acad Sci USA.* (1997) 94:4022–7. doi: 10.1073/pnas.94.8.4022
98. Schofield L, Hewitt MC, Evans K, Siomos MA, Seeberger PH. Synthetic GPI as a candidate anti-toxic vaccine in a model of malaria. *Nature* (2002) 418:785–9. doi: 10.1038/nature00937
99. Naik RS, Krishnegowda G, Gowda DC. Glucosamine inhibits inositol acylation of the glycosylphosphatidylinositol anchors in intraerythrocytic *Plasmodium falciparum*. *J Biol Chem.* (2003) 278:2036–42. doi: 10.1074/jbc.M208976200
100. Franca CT, Li Wai Suen CSN, Carmagnac A, Lin E, Kiniboro B, Siba P, et al. IgG antibodies to synthetic GPI are biomarkers of immune-status to both *Plasmodium falciparum* and *Plasmodium vivax* malaria in young children. *Malar J.* (2017) 16:386. doi: 10.1186/s12936-017-2042-2
101. Vijaykumar M, Naik RS, Gowda DC. *Plasmodium falciparum* glycosylphosphatidylinositol-induced TNF-α secretion by macrophages is mediated without membrane insertion or endocytosis. *J Biol Chem.* (2001) 276:6909–12. doi: 10.1074/jbc.C100007200
102. Krishnegowda G, Hajjar AM, Zhu J, Douglass EJ, Uematsu S, Akira S, et al. Induction of proinflammatory responses in macrophages by the glycosylphosphatidylinositols of *Plasmodium falciparum*: cell signaling receptors, glycosylphosphatidylinositol (GPI) structural requirement, and regulation of GPI activity. *J Biol Chem.* (2005) 280:8606–16. doi: 10.1074/jbc.M413541200
103. Zhu J, Krishnegowda G, Gowda DC. Induction of proinflammatory responses in macrophages by the glycosylphosphatidylinositols of *Plasmodium falciparum*: the requirement of extracellular signal-regulated kinase, p38, c-Jun N-terminal kinase and NF-κB pathways for the expression of proinflammatory cytokines and nitric oxide. *J Biol Chem.* (2005) 280:8617–27. doi: 10.1074/jbc.M413539200
104. Lu Z, Serghides L, Patel SN, Degousee N, Rubin BB, Krishnegowda G, et al. Disruption of JNK2 decreases the cytokine response to *Plasmodium falciparum* glycosylphosphatidylinositol *in vitro* and confers protection in a cerebral malaria model. *J Immunol.* (2006) 177:6344–52. doi: 10.4049/jimmunol.177.9.6344

105. Zhu J, Wu X, Goel S, Gowda NM, Kumar S, Krishnegowda G, et al. MAPK-activated protein kinase 2 differentially regulates *Plasmodium falciparum* glycosylphosphatidylinositol-induced production of tumor necrosis factor-α and interleukin-12 in macrophages. *J Biol Chem.* (2009) 284:15750–61. doi: 10.1074/jbc.M901111200
106. Baccarella A, Fontana MF, Chen EC, Kim CC. Toll-like receptor 7 mediates early innate immune responses to malaria. *Infect Immun.* (2013) 81:4431–42. doi: 10.1128/IAI.00923-13
107. Parroche P, Lauw FN, Goutagny N, Latz E, Monks BG, Visintin A, et al. Malaria hemozoin is immunologically inert but radically enhances innate responses by presenting malaria DNA to Toll-like receptor 9. *Proc Natl Acad Sci USA.* (2007) 104:1919–24. doi: 10.1073/pnas.0608745104
108. Wu X, Gowda NM, Kumar S, Gowda DC. Protein-DNA complex is the exclusive malaria parasite component that activates dendritic cells and triggers innate immune responses. *J Immunol.* (2010) 184:4338–48. doi: 10.4049/jimmunol.0903824
109. Sharma S, DeOliveira RB, Kalantari P, Parroche P, Goutagny N, Jiang Z, et al. Innate immune recognition of an AT-rich stem-loop DNA motif in the *Plasmodium falciparum* genome. *Immunity* (2011) 35:194–207. doi: 10.1016/j.immuni.2011.05.016
110. Gallego-Marin C, Schrum JE, Andrade WA, Shaffer SA, Giraldo LF, Lasso AM, et al. Cyclic GMP-AMP synthase is the cytosolic sensor of *Plasmodium falciparum* genomic DNA and activates type I IFN in malaria. *J Immunol.* (2018) 200:768–74. doi: 10.4049/jimmunol.1701048
111. Kalantari P, DeOliveira RB, Chan J, Corbett Y, Rathinam V, Stutz A, et al. Dual engagement of the NLRP3 and AIM2 inflammasomes by plasmodium-derived hemozoin and DNA during malaria. *Cell Rep.* (2014) 6:196–210. doi: 10.1016/j.celrep.2013.12.014
112. Shio MT, Eisenbarth SC, Savaria M, Vinet AF, Bellemare MJ, Harder KW, et al. Malarial hemozoin activates the NLRP3 inflammasome through Lyn and Syk kinases. *PLoS Pathog.* (2009) 5:e1000559. doi: 10.1371/annotation/abca067d-b82b-4de6-93c5-0fcc38e3df05
113. Dostert C, Guarda G, Romero JF, Menu P, Gross O, Tardivel A, et al. Malarial hemozoin is a Nalp3 inflammasome activating danger signal. *PLoS ONE* (2009) 4:e6510. doi: 10.1371/journal.pone.0006510
114. Griffith JW, Sun T, McIntosh MT, Bucala R. Pure Hemozoin is inflammatory *in vivo* and activates the NALP3 inflammasome via release of uric acid. *J Immunol.* (2009) 183:5208–20. doi: 10.4049/jimmunol.0713552
115. Braga TT, Forni MF, Correa-Costa M, Ramos RN, Barbuto JA, Branco P, et al. Soluble uric acid activates the NLRP3 inflammasome. *Sci Rep.* (2017) 7:39884. doi: 10.1038/srep39884
116. Romero CA, Remor A, Latini A, De Paul AL, Torres AI, Mukdsi JH. Uric acid activates NRLP3 inflammasome in an *in-vivo* model of epithelial to mesenchymal transition in the kidney. *J Mol Histol.* (2017) 48:209–18. doi: 10.1007/s10735-017-9720-9
117. Thylur RP, Wu X, Gowda NM, Punnath K, Neelgund SE, Febbraio M, et al. CD36 receptor regulates malaria-induced immune responses primarily at early blood stage infection contributing to parasitemia control and resistance to mortality. *J Biol Chem.* (2017) 292:9394–408. doi: 10.1074/jbc.M117.781294
118. Silverstein RL, Febbraio M. CD36, a scavenger receptor involved in immunity, metabolism, angiogenesis, and behavior. *Sci Signal.* (2009) 2:re3. doi: 10.1126/scisignal.272re3
119. Stewart CR, Stuart LM, Wilkinson K, van Gils JM, Deng J, Halle A, et al. CD36 ligands promote sterile inflammation through assembly of a Toll-like receptor 4 and 6 heterodimer. *Nat Immunol.* (2010) 11:155–61. doi: 10.1038/ni.1836
120. Erdman LK, Cosio G, Helmers AJ, Gowda DC, Grinstein S, Kain KC. CD36 and TLR interactions in inflammation and phagocytosis: implications for malaria. *J Immunol.* (2009) 183:6452–9. doi: 10.4049/jimmunol.0901374
121. Liu G, Place AT, Chen Z, Brovkovych VM, Vogel SM, Muller WA, et al. ICAM-1-activated Src and eNOS signaling increase endothelial cell surface PECAM-1 adhesivity and neutrophil transmigration. *Blood* (2012) 120:1942–52. doi: 10.1182/blood-2011-12-397430
122. Ramos TN, Bullard DC, Barnum SR. ICAM-1: isoforms and phenotypes. *J Immunol.* (2014) 192:4469–74. doi: 10.4049/jimmunol.1400135
123. Pichyangkul S, Yongvanitchit K, Kum-arb U, Hemmi H, Akira S, Krieg AM, et al. Malaria blood stage parasites activate human plasmacytoid dendritic cells and murine dendritic cells through a Toll-like receptor 9-dependent pathway. *J Immunol.* (2004) 172:4926–33. doi: 10.4049/jimmunol.172.8.4926
124. Gowda NM, Wu X, Gowda DC. The nucleosome (histone-DNA complex) is the TLR9-specific immunostimulatory component of *Plasmodium falciparum* that activates DCs. *PLoS ONE* (2011) 6:e20398. doi: 10.1371/journal.pone.0020398
125. Anstey NM, Douglas NM, Poespoprodjo JR, Price RN. *Plasmodium vivax*: clinical spectrum, risk factors and pathogenesis. *Adv Parasitol.* (2012) 80:151–201. doi: 10.1016/B978-0-12-397900-1.00003-7
126. Hirako IC, Gallego-Marin C, Ataide MA, Andrade WA, Gravina H, Rocha BC, et al. DNA-containing immunocomplexes promote inflammasome assembly and release of pyrogenic cytokines by $CD14^{+}CD16^{+}CD64^{high}CD32^{low}$ inflammatory monocytes from malaria patients. *MBio* (2015) 6:e01605–15. doi: 10.1128/mBio.01605-15
127. Kim CC, Nelson CS, Wilson EB, Hou B, DeFranco AL, DeRisi JL. Splenic red pulp macrophages produce type I interferons as early sentinels of malaria infection but are dispensable for control. *PloS ONE* (2012) 7:e48126. doi: 10.1371/journal.pone.0048126
128. Spaulding E, Fooksman D, Moore JM, Saidi A, Feintuch CM, Reizis B, et al. STING-licensed macrophages prime type I IFN production by plasmacytoid dendritic cells in the bone marrow during severe *Plasmodium yoelii* malaria. *PLoS Pathog.* (2016) 12:e1005975. doi: 10.1371/journal.ppat.1005975
129. Pagola S, Stephens PW, Bohle DS, Kosar AD, Madsen SK. The structure of malaria pigment β-haematin. *Nature* (2000) 404:307–10. doi: 10.1038/35005132
130. Jani D, Nagarkatti R, Beatty W, Angel R, Slebodnick C, Andersen J, et al. HDP—a novel heme detoxification protein from the malaria parasite. *PLoS Pathog.* (2008) 4:e1000053. doi: 10.1371/journal.ppat.1000053
131. Arese P, Schwarzer E. Malarial pigment (haemozoin): a very active 'inert' substance. *Ann Trop Med Parasitol.* (1997) 91:501–16. doi: 10.1080/00034983.1997.11813168
132. Boyle MJ, Wilson DW, Richards JS, Riglar DT, Tetteh KK, Conway DJ, et al. Isolation of viable *Plasmodium falciparum* merozoites to define erythrocyte invasion events and advance vaccine and drug development. *Proc Natl Acad Sci USA.* (2010) 107:14378–83. doi: 10.1073/pnas.1009198107
133. Wu X, Gowda NM, Gowda DC. Phagosomal acidification prevents macrophage inflammatory cytokine production to malaria, and dendritic cells are the major source at the early stages of infection: IMPLICATION FOR MALARIA PROTECTIVE IMMUNITY DEVELOPMENT. *J Biol Chem.* (2015) 290:23135–47. doi: 10.1074/jbc.M115.671065
134. Schwarzer E, Turrini F, Ulliers D, Giribaldi G, Ginsburg H, Arese P. Impairment of macrophage functions after ingestion of *Plasmodium falciparum*-infected erythrocytes or isolated malarial pigment. *J Exp Med.* (1992) 176:1033–41. doi: 10.1084/jem.176.4.1033
135. Schwarzer E, Bellomo G, Giribaldi G, Ulliers D, Arese P. Phagocytosis of malarial pigment haemozoin by human monocytes: a confocal microscopy study. *Parasitology* (2001) 123(Pt 2):125–31. doi: 10.1017/S0031182001008216
136. Skorokhod OA, Alessio M, Mordmuller B, Arese P, Schwarzer E. Hemozoin (malarial pigment) inhibits differentiation and maturation of human monocyte-derived dendritic cells: a peroxisome proliferator-activated receptor-gamma-mediated effect. *J Immunol.* (2004) 173:4066–74. doi: 10.4049/jimmunol.173.6.4066
137. Schwarzer E, Alessio M, Ulliers D, Arese P. Phagocytosis of the malarial pigment, hemozoin, impairs expression of major histocompatibility complex class II antigen, CD54, and CD11c in human monocytes. *Infect Immun.* (1998) 66:1601–6.
138. Wykes MN, Good MF. What really happens to dendritic cells during malaria? *Nat Rev Microbiol.* (2008) 6:864–70. doi: 10.1038/nrmicro1988
139. Millington OR, Di Lorenzo C, Phillips RS, Garside P, Brewer JM. Suppression of adaptive immunity to heterologous antigens during *Plasmodium* infection through hemozoin-induced failure of dendritic cell function. *J Biol.* (2006) 5:5. doi: 10.1186/jbiol34
140. Martillo MA, Nazzal L, Crittenden DB. The crystallization of monosodium urate. *Curr Rheumatol Rep.* (2014) 16:400. doi: 10.1007/s11926-013-0400-9

141. Jin M, Yang F, Yang I, Yin Y, Luo JJ, Wang H, et al. Uric acid, hyperuricemia and vascular diseases. *Front Biosci.* (2012) 17:656–69. doi: 10.2741/3950
142. El Ridi R, Tallima H. Physiological functions and pathogenic potential of uric acid: a review. *J Adv Res.* (2017) 8:487–93. doi: 10.1016/j.jare.2017.03.003
143. Gallego-Delgado J, Ty M, Orengo JM, van de Hoef D, Rodriguez A. A surprising role for uric acid: the inflammatory malaria response. *Curr Rheumatol Rep.* (2014)16:401. doi: 10.1007/s11926-013-0401-8
144. Lopera-Mesa TM, Mita-Mendoza NK, van de Hoef DL, Doumbia S, Konate D, Doumbouya M, et al. Plasma uric acid levels correlate with inflammation and disease severity in Malian children with *Plasmodium falciparum* malaria. *PLoS ONE* (2012) 7:e46424. doi: 10.1371/journal.pone.0046424
145. Underhill DM, Ozinsky A. Phagocytosis of microbes: complexity in action. *Annu Rev Immunol.* (2002) 20:825–52. doi: 10.1146/annurev.immunol.20.103001.114744
146. Mocsai A, Ruland J, Tybulewicz VL. The SYK tyrosine kinase: a crucial player in diverse biological functions. *Nat Rev Immunol.* (2010) 10:387–402. doi: 10.1038/nri2765
147. Lowell CA. Src-family and Syk kinases in activating and inhibitory pathways in innate immune cells: signaling cross talk. *Cold Spring Harb Perspect Biol.* (2011) 3:a002352. doi: 10.1101/cshperspect.a002352
148. Underhill DM, Gantner B. Integration of Toll-like receptor and phagocytic signaling for tailored immunity. *Microbes Infect.* (2004) 6:1368–73. doi: 10.1016/j.micinf.2004.08.016
149. Febbraio M, Hajjar DP, Silverstein RL. CD36: a class B scavenger receptor involved in angiogenesis, atherosclerosis, inflammation, and lipid metabolism. *J Clin Invest.* (2001) 108:785–91. doi: 10.1172/JCI14006
150. Cabrera A, Neculai D, Kain KC. CD36 and malaria: friends or foes? A decade of data provides some answers. *Trends Parasitol.* (2014) 30:436–44. doi: 10.1016/j.pt.2014.07.006
151. Silverstein RL. Disabling the platelet's brakes to promote thrombosis. *Blood* (2015) 125:2591–3. doi: 10.1182/blood-2015-03-630822
152. Dragoni S, Hudson N, Kenny BA, Burgoyne T, McKenzie JA, Gill Y et al. Endothelial MAPKs direct ICAM-1 signaling to divergent inflammatory functions. *J Immunol.* (2017) 198:4074–85. doi: 10.4049/jimmunol.1600823
153. Mohan Rao LV, Esmon CT, Pendurthi UR. Endothelial cell protein C receptor: a multi-liganded and multi-functional receptor. *Blood* (2014) 124:1553–62. doi: 10.1182/blood-2014-05-578328
154. Pendurthi UR, Rao LVM. Endothelial cell protein C receptor-dependent signaling. *Curr Opin Hematol.* (2018) 25:219–26. doi: 10.1097/MOH.0000000000000416
155. van der Poll T. The endothelial protein C receptor and malaria. *Blood* (2013) 122:624–5. doi: 10.1182/blood-2013-06-508531
156. Sheedy FJ, Grebe A, Rayner KJ, Kalantari P, Ramkhelawon B, Carpenter SB, et al. CD36 coordinates NLRP3 inflammasome activation by facilitating intracellular nucleation of soluble ligands into particulate ligands in sterile inflammation. *Nat Immunol.* (2013) 14:812–20. doi: 10.1038/ni.2639
157. Pasloske BL, Howard RJ. Malaria, the red cell, and the endothelium. *Annu Rev Med.* (1994) 45:283–95. doi: 10.1146/annurev.med.45.1.283
158. Day KP, Hayward RE, Smith D, Culvenor JG. CD36-dependent adhesion and knob expression of the transmission stages of *Plasmodium falciparum* is stage specific. *Mol Biochem Parasitol.* (1998) 93:167–77. doi: 10.1016/S0166-6851(98)00040-1
159. Weatherall DJ, Miller LH, Baruch DI, Marsh K, Doumbo OK, Casals-Pascual C, et al. Malaria and the red cell. *Hematol Am Soc Hematol Educ Program* (2002) 2002:35–57. doi: 10.1182/asheducation-2002.1.35
160. Hoebe K, Georgel P, Rutschmann S, Du X, Mudd S, Crozat K, et al. CD36 is a sensor of diacylglycerides. *Nature* (2005) 433:523–7. doi: 10.1038/nature03253
161. Patel SN, Lu Z, Ayi K, Serghides L, Gowda DC, Kain KC. Disruption of CD36 impairs cytokine response to *Plasmodium falciparum* glycosylphosphatidylinositol and confers susceptibility to severe and fatal malaria *in vivo*. *J Immunol.* (2007) 178:3954–61. doi: 10.4049/jimmunol.178.6.3954
162. Urban BC, Willcox N, Roberts DJ. A role for CD36 in the regulation of dendritic cell function. *Proc Natl Acad Sci USA.* (2001) 98:8750–5. doi: 10.1073/pnas.151028698
163. Gowda NM, Wu X, Kumar S, Febbraio M, Gowda DC. CD36 contributes to malaria parasite-induced pro-inflammatory cytokine production and NK and T cell activation by dendritic cells. *PLoS ONE* (2013) 8:e77604. doi: 10.1371/journal.pone.0077604
164. Pain A, Urban BC, Kai O, Casals-Pascual C, Shafi J, Marsh K, et al. A non-sense mutation in Cd36 gene is associated with protection from severe malaria. *Lancet* (2001) 357:1502–3. doi: 10.1016/S0140-6736(00)04662-6
165. Omi K, Ohashi J, Patarapotikul J, Hananantachai H, Naka I, Looareesuwan S, et al. CD36 polymorphism is associated with protection from cerebral malaria. *Am J Hum Genet.* (2003) 72:364–74. doi: 10.1086/346091
166. Van de Wouwer MV, Collen D, Conway EM. Thrombomodulin-protein C-EPCR system: integrated to regulate coagulation and inflammation. *Arterioscler Thromb Vasc Biol.* (2004) 24:1374–83. doi: 10.1161/01.ATV.0000134298.25489.92
167. Turner L, Lavstsen T, Berger SS, Wang CW, Petersen JE, Avril M, et al. Severe malaria is associated with parasite binding to endothelial protein C receptor. *Nature* (2013) 498:502–5. doi: 10.1038/nature12216
168. Avril M, Bernabeu M, Benjamin M, Brazier AJ, Smith JD. Interaction between endothelial protein C receptor and intercellular adhesion molecule 1 to mediate binding of *Plasmodium falciparum*-infected erythrocytes to endothelial cells. *MBio* (2016) 7:e00615–16. doi: 10.1128/mBio.00615-16
169. Tuikue Ndam N, Moussiliou A, Lavstsen T, Kamaliddin C, Jensen AT, Mama A, et al. Parasites causing cerebral falciparum malaria bind multiple endothelial receptors and express EPCR and ICAM-1-binding PfEMP1. *J Infect Dis.* (2017) 215:1918–25. doi: 10.1093/infdis/jix230
170. Favre N, Da Laperousaz C, Ryffel B, Weiss NA, Imhof BA, Rudin W, et al. Role of ICAM-1 (CD54) in the development of murine cerebral malaria. *Microbes Infect.* (1999) 1:961–8. doi: 10.1016/S1286-4579(99)80513-9
171. Ramos TN, Bullard DC, Darley MM, McDonald K, Crawford DF, Barnum SR. Experimental cerebral malaria develops independently of endothelial expression of intercellular adhesion molecule-1 (icam-1). *J Biol Chem.* (2013) 288:10962–6. doi: 10.1074/jbc.C113.457028
172. Baratin M, Roetynck S, Pouvelle B, Lemmers C, Viebig NK, Johansson S, et al. Dissection of the role of PfEMP1 and ICAM-1 in the sensing of *Plasmodium falciparum*-infected erythrocytes by natural killer cells. *PLoS ONE* (2007) 2:e228. doi: 10.1371/journal.pone.0000228
173. Gupta P, Lai SM, Sheng J, Tetlak P, Balachander A, Claser C, et al. Tissue-resident $CD169^+$ macrophages form a crucial front line against *Plasmodium* infection. *Cell Rep.* (2016) 16:1749–61. doi: 10.1016/j.celrep.2016.07.010
174. Baccarella A, Huang BW, Fontana MF, Kim CC. Loss of Toll-like receptor 7 alters cytokine production and protects against experimental cerebral malaria. *Malar J.* (2014) 13:354. doi: 10.1186/1475-2875-13-354
175. Haque A, Best SE, Montes de Oca M, James KR, Ammerdorffer A, Edwards CL, et al. Type I IFN signaling in $CD8^-$ DCs impairs Th1-dependent malaria immunity. *J Clin Invest.* (2014) 124:2483–96. doi: 10.1172/JCI70698
176. Haque A, Best SE, Ammerdorffer A, Desbarrieres L, de Oca MM, Amante FH, et al. Type I interferons suppress $CD4^+$ T-cell-dependent parasite control during blood-stage Plasmodium infection. *Eur J Immunol.* (2011) 41:2688–98. doi: 10.1002/eji.201141539
177. Vigario AM, Belnoue E, Gruner AC, Mauduit M, Kayibanda M, Deschemin JC, et al. Recombinant human IFN-α inhibits cerebral malaria and reduces parasite burden in mice. *J Immunol.* (2007) 178:6416–25. doi: 10.4049/jimmunol.178.10.6416
178. Morrell CN, Srivastava K, Swaim A, Lee MT, Chen J, Nagineni C, et al. Beta interferon suppresses the development of experimental cerebral malaria. *Infect Immun.* (2011) 79:1750–8. doi: 10.1128/IAI.00810-10
179. Palomo J, Fauconnier M, Coquard L, Gilles M, Meme S, Szeremeta F, et al. Type I interferons contribute to experimental cerebral malaria development in response to sporozoite or blood-stage *Plasmodium berghei* ANKA. *Eur J Immunol.* (2013) 43:2683–95. doi: 10.1002/eji.201343327
180. Sebina I, Haque A. Effects of type I interferons in malaria. *Immunology* (2018). 155:176–85. doi: 10.1111/imm.12971
181. Trinchieri G. Type I interferon: friend or foe? *J Exp Med.* (2010) 207:2053–63. doi: 10.1084/jem.20101664

182. McNab F, Mayer-Barber K, Sher A, Wack A, O'Garra A. Type I interferons in infectious disease. *Nat Rev Immunol.* (2015) 15:87–103. doi: 10.1038/nri3787
183. Moreira-Teixeira L, Mayer-Barber K, Sher A, O'Garra A. Type I interferons in tuberculosis: foe and occasionally friend. *J Exp Med.* (2018) 215:1273–85. doi: 10.1084/jem.20180325
184. Stevenson MM, Urban BC. Antigen presentation and dendritic cell biology in malaria. *Parasite Immunol.* (2006) 28:5–14. doi: 10.1111/j.1365-3024.2006.00772.x
185. Todryk SM, Urban BC. Dendritic cells in *Plasmodium* infection. *Future Microbiol.* (2008) 3:279–86. doi: 10.2217/17460913.3.3.279
186. Amorim KN, Chagas DC, Sulczewski FB, Boscardin SB. Dendritic cells and their multiple roles during malaria infection. *J Immunol Res.* (2016) 2016:2926436. doi: 10.1155/2016/2926436
187. Walsh KP, Mills KH. Dendritic cells and other innate determinants of T helper cell polarisation. *Trends Immunol.* (2013) 34:521–30. doi: 10.1016/j.it.2013.07.006
188. King T, Lamb T. Interferon-γ: the Jekyll and Hyde of malaria. *PLoS Pathog.* (2015) 11:e1005118. doi: 10.1371/journal.ppat.1005118
189. Ing R, Stevenson MM. Dendritic cell and NK cell reciprocal cross talk promotes gamma interferon-dependent immunity to blood-stage *Plasmodium chabaudi* AS infection in mice. *Infect Immun.* (2009) 77:770–82. doi: 10.1128/IAI.00994-08
190. D'ombrain MC, Robinson LJ, Stanisic DI, Taraika J, Bernard N, Michon P, et al. Association of early interferon-γ production with immunity to clinical malaria: a longitudinal study among Papua New Guinean children. *Clin Infect Dis.* (2008) 47:1380–7. doi: 10.1086/592971
191. McGovern KE, Wilson EH. Role of chemokines and trafficking of immune cells in parasitic infections. *Curr Immunol Rev.* (2013) 9:157–68. doi: 10.2174/15733955096661312170 00000
192. Rocha BC, Marques PE, Leoratti FMS, Junqueira C, Pereira DB, Antonelli L, et al. Type I interferon transcriptional signature in neutrophils and low-density granulocytes are associated with tissue damage in malaria. *Cell Rep.* (2015) 13:2829–41. doi: 10.1016/j.celrep.2015.11.055
193. Ioannidis LJ, Nie CQ, Hansen DS. The role of chemokines in severe malaria: more than meets the eye. *Parasitology* (2014) 141:602–13. doi: 10.1017/S0031182013001984
194. Sponaas AM, Cadman ET, Voisine C, Harrison V, Boonstra A, O'Garra A, et al. Malaria infection changes the ability of splenic dendritic cell populations to stimulate antigen-specific T cells. *J Exp Med.* (2006) 203:1427–33. doi: 10.1084/jem.20052450
195. Gowda NM, Wu X, Gowda DC. TLR9 and MyD88 are crucial for the development of protective immunity to malaria. *J Immunol.* (2012) 188:5073–85. doi: 10.4049/jimmunol.1102143
196. Coban C, Ishii KJ, Kawai T, Hemmi H, Sato S, Uematsu S, et al. Toll-like receptor 9 mediates innate immune activation by the malaria pigment hemozoin. *J Exp Med.* (2005) 201:19–25. doi: 10.1084/jem.20041836
197. Coban C, Ishii KJ, Uematsu S, Arisue N, Sato S, Yamamoto M, et al. Pathological role of Toll-like receptor signaling in cerebral malaria. *Int Immunol.* (2007) 19:67–79. doi: 10.1093/intimm/dxl123
198. Franklin BS, Ishizaka ST, Lamphier M, Gusovsky F, Hansen H, Rose J, et al. Therapeutical targeting of nucleic acid-sensing Toll-like receptors prevents experimental cerebral malaria. *Proc Natl Acad Sci USA.* (2011) 108:3689–94. doi: 10.1073/pnas.1015406108
199. Zhang Y, Zhu X, Feng Y, Pang W, Qi Z, Cui L, et al. TLR4 and TLR9 signals stimulate protective immunity against blood-stage *Plasmodium yoelii* infection in mice. *Exp Parasitol.* (2016) 170:73–81. doi: 10.1016/j.exppara.2016.09.003
200. Griffith JW, O'Connor C, Bernard K, Town T, Goldstein DR, Bucala R. Toll-like receptor modulation of murine cerebral malaria is dependent on the genetic background of the host. *J Infect Dis.* (2007) 196:1553–64. doi: 10.1086/522865
201. Barboza R, Lima FA, Reis AS, Murillo OJ, Peixoto EPM, Bandeira CL, et al. TLR4-mediated placental pathology and pregnancy outcome in experimental malaria. *Sci Rep.* (2017) 7:8623. doi: 10.1038/s41598-017-08299-x
202. Mockenhaupt FP, Cramer JP, Hamann L, Stegemann MS, Eckert J, Oh NR, et al. Toll-like receptor (TLR) polymorphisms in African children: common TLR-4 variants predispose to severe malaria. *Proc Natl Acad Sci USA.* (2006) 103:177–82. doi: 10.1073/pnas.0506803102
203. Esposito S, Molteni CG, Zampiero A, Baggi E, Lavizzari A, Semino M, et al. Role of polymorphisms of toll-like receptor (TLR) 4, TLR9, toll-interleukin 1 receptor domain containing adaptor protein (TIRAP) and FCGR2A genes in malaria susceptibility and severity in Burundian children. *Malar J.* (2012) 11:196. doi: 10.1186/1475-2875-11-196
204. Mockenhaupt FP, Hamann L, von Gaertner C, Bedu-Addo G, von Kleinsorgen C, Schumann RR, et al. Common polymorphisms of toll-like receptors 4 and 9 are associated with the clinical manifestation of malaria during pregnancy. *J Infect Dis.* (2006) 194:184–8. doi: 10.1086/505152
205. Leoratti FM, Farias L, Alves FP, Suarez-Mutis MC, Coura JR, Kalil J, et al. Variants in the toll-like receptor signaling pathway and clinical outcomes of malaria. *J Infect Dis.* (2008) 198:772–80. doi: 10.1086/590440
206. Khor CC, Chapman SJ, Vannberg FO, Dunne A, Murphy C, Ling EY, et al. A Mal functional variant is associated with protection against invasive pneumococcal disease, bacteremia, malaria and tuberculosis. *Nat Genet.* (2007) 39:523–8. doi: 10.1038/ng1976
207. Crompton PD, Mircetic M, Weiss G, Baughman A, Huang CY, Topham DJ, et al. The TLR9 ligand CpG promotes the acquisition of *Plasmodium falciparum*-specific memory B cells in malaria-naive individuals. *J Immunol.* (2009) 82:3318–26. doi: 10.4049/jimmunol.0803596
208. Munde EO, Okeyo WA, Anyona SB, Raballah E, Konah S, Okumu W, et al. Polymorphisms in Fc gamma receptor (FcγRIIIA-176 F/V) and Toll-like receptor (TLR9 [-1237 T/C]) are associated with protection against severe malarial anemia and changes in circulating IFN-γ. *Infect Immun.* (2012) 80:4435–43. doi: 10.1128/IAI.00945-12
209. Sawian CE, Lourembam SD, Banerjee A, Baruah S. Polymorphisms and expression of TLR4 and 9 in malaria in two ethnic groups of Assam, northeast India. *Innate Immun.* (2013) 19:174–83. doi: 10.1177/1753425912455675
210. Greene JA, Moormann AM, Vulule J, Bockarie MJ, Zimmerman PA, Kazura JW. Toll-like receptor polymorphisms in malaria-endemic populations. *Malar J.* (2009) 8:50. doi: 10.1186/1475-2875-8-50
211. Greene JA, Sam-Agudu N, John CC, Opoka RO, Zimmerman PA, Kazura JW. Toll-like receptor polymorphisms and cerebral malaria: TLR2 Δ22 polymorphism is associated with protection from cerebral malaria in a case control study. *Malar J.* (2012) 11:47. doi: 10.1186/1475-2875-11-47
212. Omar AH, Yasunami M, Yamazaki A, Shibata H, Ofori MF, Akanmori BD, et al. Toll-like receptor 9 (TLR9) polymorphism associated with symptomatic malaria: a cohort study. *Malar J.* (2012) 11:168. doi: 10.1186/1475-2875-11-168
213. Sam-Agudu NA, Greene JA, Opoka RO, Kazura JW, Boivin MJ, Zimmerman PA, et al. TLR9 polymorphisms are associated with altered IFN-γ levels in children with cerebral malaria. *Am J Trop Med Hyg.* (2010) 82:548–55. doi: 10.4269/ajtmh.2010.09-0467
214. Manning L, Cutts J, Stanisic DI, Laman M, Carmagnac A, Allen S. et al. A Toll-like receptor-1 variant and its characteristic cellular phenotype is associated with severe malaria in Papua New Guinean children. *Genes Immun.* (2016) 17:52–9. doi: 10.1038/gene.2015.50
215. Reimer T, Shaw MH, Franchi L, Coban C, Ishii KJ, Akira S, et al. Experimental cerebral malaria progresses independently of the Nlrp3 inflammasome. *Eur J Immunol.* (2010) 40:764–9. doi: 10.1002/eji.200939996

16

Functional Comparison of Blood-Stage *Plasmodium falciparum* Malaria Vaccine Candidate Antigens

Joseph J. Illingworth[1*], *Daniel G. Alanine*[1], *Rebecca Brown*[1], *Jennifer M. Marshall*[1], *Helen E. Bartlett*[1], *Sarah E. Silk*[1], *Geneviève M. Labbé*[1], *Doris Quinkert*[1], *Jee Sun Cho*[1], *Jason P. Wendler*[2], *David J. Pattinson*[1], *Lea Barfod*[1], *Alexander D. Douglas*[1], *Michael W. Shea*[1], *Katherine E. Wright*[3], *Simone C. de Cassan*[1], *Matthew K. Higgins*[3] and *Simon J. Draper*[1*]

[1] Jenner Institute, University of Oxford, Oxford, United Kingdom, [2] Wellcome Trust Centre for Human Genetics, University of Oxford, Oxford, United Kingdom, [3] Department of Biochemistry, University of Oxford, Oxford, United Kingdom

***Correspondence:**
Joseph J. Illingworth
joejamesillingworth@gmail.com
Simon J. Draper
simon.draper@ndm.ox.ac.uk

The malaria genome encodes over 5,000 proteins and many of these have also been proposed to be potential vaccine candidates, although few of these have been tested clinically. RH5 is one of the leading blood-stage *Plasmodium falciparum* malaria vaccine antigens and Phase I/II clinical trials of vaccines containing this antigen are currently underway. Its likely mechanism of action is to elicit antibodies that can neutralize merozoites by blocking their invasion of red blood cells (RBC). However, many other antigens could also elicit neutralizing antibodies against the merozoite, and most of these have never been compared directly to RH5. The objective of this study was to compare a range of blood-stage antigens to RH5, to identify any antigens that outperform or synergize with anti-RH5 antibodies. We selected 55 gene products, covering 15 candidate antigens that have been described in the literature and 40 genes selected on the basis of bioinformatics functional prediction. We were able to make 20 protein-in-adjuvant vaccines from the original selection. Of these, S-antigen and CyRPA robustly elicited antibodies with neutralizing properties. Anti-CyRPA IgG generally showed additive GIA with anti-RH5 IgG, although high levels of anti-CyRPA-specific rabbit polyclonal IgG were required to achieve 50% GIA. Our data suggest that further vaccine antigen screening efforts are required to identify a second merozoite target with similar antibody-susceptibility to RH5.

Keywords: malaria, vaccine, blood-stage malaria, antigen, merozoite, RH5, S-antigen, AARP

INTRODUCTION

Development of a vaccine against *Plasmodium falciparum* malaria is a key global health priority (1). RTS,S/AS01, the leading subunit malaria vaccine, targets the pre-erythrocytic stage of the *P. falciparum* parasite's lifecycle to deliver a short interval of moderate protection against malaria (2), which then wanes to yield 7 year efficacy of < 10% (3). Blood-stage vaccines aim to target the subsequent disease-causing stage of the *Plasmodium* life cycle and have the possibility of protecting against disease severity, reducing blood-stage asexual parasitemia as well as transmission, while allowing exposure to the parasite and the development of naturally-acquired immunity.

Blood-stage vaccines can be divided into those that aim to target the infected red blood cell (iRBC), and those that target the merozoite (1). Most anti-merozoite vaccines aim to elicit antibodies that bind to proteins involved in the process of red blood cell (RBC) entry thus leading to a block in RBC invasion. This antibody functionality can be routinely tested using the standardized *in vitro* assay of growth inhibitory activity (GIA) (4). A key challenge has been to identify antigens that are both well-conserved between disparate strains of *P. falciparum*, and sufficiently susceptible to antibody neutralization in the minute or so between schizont egress and RBC re-invasion (5) in a way to meaningfully impact the *in vivo* parasite multiplication rate. *P. falciparum* reticulocyte-binding protein homolog 5 (RH5) is the only protein to-date which has been demonstrated by multiple independent research groups to possess these properties (6–9). Notably, RH5 binds basigin on the surface of RBCs, forming an interaction that is essential for productive invasion of the RBC (10).

Phase I/II clinical trials are now underway to test the safety, immunogenicity and efficacy of first-generation vaccines containing the RH5 antigen (11, 12). The outcomes of these trials will serve as an important benchmark for the field of merozoite neutralizing vaccines. When interpreting the results of these clinical trials and deciding how to prioritize further research avenues, a critical question will be whether there are additional antigens (or combinations of antigens) encoded in the *P. falciparum* genome which could deliver higher efficacy than the vaccines currently being trialed that target RH5 alone.

To address this question, we generated a list of candidate antigens for a merozoite-neutralizing vaccine and tested their ability to elicit functional antibodies, comparing to RH5 as the "gold-standard" antigen. We aimed to minimize false-negatives by adopting the following approaches. First, we used protein-based vaccine immunization which, in contrast to genetic/nucleic acid-based immunization approaches such as recombinant viral vectors (7), allows for controlled administration of a fixed dose of antigen. Second, we produced recombinant protein which, wherever possible, represented the full-length ectodomain of the *P. falciparum* protein, to minimize the possibility of producing non-conformationally relevant protein fragments as initially occurred with RH5 (13–15). Third, wherever possible, rather than use Freund's adjuvant [a strong immunopotentiator that elicits extremely high titers of antibodies but which can also disrupt the fold of even the most stable proteins (16, 17)], we used AddaVax™, a squalene-based adjuvant similar in composition to the clinically-approved adjuvant MF59®.

Testing all 5,000 proteins encoded in the *P. falciparum* genome is not feasible and so in our first panel we aimed to test all of the proteins that have been the subject of promising vaccine antigen reports in the literature. We then selected a second panel, drawn from a list of 435 proteins that have been bioinformatically predicted (18) to have a role in merozoite invasion. This was 55 proteins in all. Proteins were generated for 20 of these, and then formulated in adjuvant for immunization into mice. The post-immunization mouse antibodies were harvested and then tested for activity in the GIA assay.

MATERIALS AND METHODS

Analysis of Polymorphism of Merozoite Proteins

The raw material for this polymorphism analysis was gathered from a range of sources [(19–22), Pf3K, 2012[1]]. We used sequence coverage of a gene as an initial indicator of vaccinological suitability. In a given dataset, sequence coverage is as defined by the number of Illumina reads that align to a given region of the *P. falciparum* clone 3D7 reference genome. Local drops in coverage can indicate divergence of an allele from the 3D7 reference, an A-T rich region (i.e., low complexity) or the presence of insertions/deletions. Therefore, genes with low sequence coverage, or spikes or drops in sequence coverage, were excluded from study. When counting single nucleotide polymorphisms (SNPs), we only considered non-synonymous SNPs with uniform sequence coverage and a prevalence of over 10%. This cut-off was chosen as a plausible indicator that a SNP is under some element of balancing selection. Polymorphism was assessed by counting the total number of non-synonymous SNPs along the gene, as opposed to measuring SNP density. This is because antigenic escape mutations may cluster around regions of a protein that are proximal in the tertiary, three-dimensional structure, but distant in the primary sequence. This simple counting analysis is unlikely to be confounded by the underlying base-rate SNP density across the genome, because the base rate of non-synonymous SNPs with prevalence of $>10\%$ is extremely low across the *P. falciparum* genome [(19–22), Pf3K, 2012[1]]. Genes with more than 4,000 bp (corresponding to 1,333 amino acids) were excluded due to the cost of producing synthetic genes longer than 4,000 bp.

Protein Expression and Purification

Protein sequences were uploaded to the TMHMM server (23) to predict the ectodomains of transmembrane proteins of interest (for proteins with no transmembrane region, the entire soluble protein sequence was used). Synthetized genes encoding these ectodomains (GeneArt, Germany) were cloned into a modified pENTR4 plasmid. This plasmid contains an extended version of the cytomegalovirus promoter (24) downstream of an N-terminal human tissue plasminogen activator (tPA) leader sequence and cloning site encoding "GTK" (MDAMKRGLCCVLLLCGAVFVSPSQEIHARFRRGTK) and upstream of a sequence encoding a C-terminal affinity construct consisting of a biotin acceptor peptide (BAP) and either a hexa-histidine tag ("BAP-6His," final C-terminal amino acid sequence GLNDIFEAQKIEWHEHHHHHH) or a Strep tag ("BAP-Strep," final C-terminal amino acid sequence GLNDIFEAQKIEWHEWSHPQFEK) or simply a C-tag (25) with no biotin acceptor peptide, so final C-terminal amino acid sequence: EPEA. All genes were codon-optimized for *Homo sapiens*. The only exception to the above details was the "CyRPA (Gly KO)" construct (**Figure S6**), where a complete expression plasmid using a different backbone with different signal peptide and C-terminal tags was kindly gifted by the laboratory of G.

[1] Pf3K (2012). *The Pf3K Project – 1.0 pilot data* release.

Wright, who had produced this plasmid [Add gene plasmid number: 50823 (26)]. Plasmids were transiently transfected into suspension HEK293E cells (250 mL typical culture volume) using a transfection method based on that described by Durocher et al. (27). Briefly, cells were grown in Expi293 Expression Medium (Thermo Fisher Scientific, USA) in a rotary shaking, 37°C and 8% CO_2, and passaged to 1×10^6 cells/mL 24 h prior to transfection. On the day of transfection, plasmid DNA was mixed with linear 25 kDa average molecular weight polyethylenimine (PEI) at a 1:2 mass ratio (Alfa Aesar, USA), and incubated for 20 min, before being added to the HEK293E cell culture. 4 days after transfection, supernatants were harvested by spinning at 500 *xg* for 10 min and supernatants clarified with a 0.22 μm filter. Proteins were purified by single-step affinity chromatography using either a HisTrap Excel Ni-Sepharose column (GE Healthcare, USA) and eluting in 400 mM imidazole; using a C-tag with elution into 2 M $MgCl_2$ (25); or dialysed extensively into phosphate-buffered saline (PBS) before application to a Streptactin Sepharose resin and elution into the supplied elution buffer (IBA, Germany). Purified proteins were exchanged into PBS using a 10 K MWCO centrifugal filter (Millipore, UK) and adjusted to 0.4 mg/mL. Proteins were resolved using 4–20% SDS-PAGE gels with reduction by 2-mercaptoethanol and visualized directly using Coomassie brilliant blue R-250 (Bio-Rad, USA), using Precision Plus protein Unstained Standards by BioRad (USA), or visualized by Western blot onto nitrocellulose membranes using streptactin-HRP conjugate (IBA, Germany) as detection reagent. PNGase treatment (NEB, USA) was performed as per manufacturer's instructions.

For the N-terminal apical asparagine-rich protein (AARP) construct in **Figure S3F**, a construct encoding I20 to D95 was cloned into an *Escherichia coli* expression plasmid with an N-terminal 6His tag followed by a tobacco etch virus cleavage site (amino-acid sequence ENLYFQGS). This construct was cloned into an *E. coli* expression host (BL21(DE3)Star, Thermo Fisher Scientific) and protein induced with 1 mM IPTG at 37°C for 4 h. Clarified soluble cell lysate was subject to Nickel-ion affinity purification (HisTrap™ Excel, GE Healthcare) following the manufacturer's instructions. This was followed by protease cleavage for removal of the 6His-tag and further size-exclusion chromatography, yielding a protein of apparent molecular weight 12 kDa.

Animal Immunization

All mouse experiments used female 6 week old BALB/c mice (n = 4 per group). Experiments and procedures were performed in accordance with the UK Animals (Scientific Procedures) Act Project License (PPLs 30/2889 and PA7D20B85) and were approved by the University of Oxford Local Ethical Review Body. Protein (20 μg/dose) was formulated with AddaVax™ (Invivogen, France) or Abisco®-100 (Isconova, Sweden) adjuvant, and injected intramuscularly on days 0, 21, and 42. Final serum harvest was performed on day 49. Each 100 μL dose of vaccine consisted of 50 μL protein solution at 0.4 mg/mL mixed with an equal volume of AddaVax™ or Abisco®-100 adjuvant (28), and was split across both quadriceps. For Poly (I:C), we added 50 μL of Poly(I:C) adjuvant (Invivogen, USA) at 1 mg/mL to each dose of 20 μg protein and split doses across both quadriceps. In the comparative assessment of Addavax™ and Abisco®-100, in addition to the GIA negative control groups in screening, we used chicken egg ovalbumin (OVA) (Sigma Aldrich, UK). RH5 protein, used as a functional antibody immunization control was prepared as described previously (29). When RH5 viral vectors (7) were used as a functional antibody immunization control, 10^{10} viral particles (vp) of recombinant human adenovirus serotype 5 (AdHu5) were administered intramuscularly on day 1 followed by 10^8 plaque-forming units (pfu) of recombinant modified vaccinia virus Ankara (MVA) intramuscularly on day 56, with serum harvested on day 70.

For rabbit and rat immunization, Freund's adjuvant was used to allow comparison with other studies. For S-Antigen-BAP-Strep and AARP-BAP-Strep rabbit immunization, Zika rabbits were injected intramuscularly by Biogenes (Germany). For Zika rabbits, each 400 μL dose consisted of 200 μL of protein solution at 0.5 mg/mL (100 μg dose) and 200 μL of complete Freund's adjuvant (day 1) or incomplete Freund's adjuvant (days 28 and 56). For CyRPA rabbit immunization, New Zealand White rabbits were immunized by Cambridge Research Biochemicals (UK). For these rabbits, each 400 μL dose consisted of 200 μL of protein solution at 0.5 mg/mL (100 μg dose) and 200 μL AddaVax™ adjuvant (Invivogen, France), on days 1, 28, and 56. For all rabbits the final bleed was day 63, 1 week after the final immunization. For CyRPA rat immunization, 2 Sprague-Dawley, and 2 Wistar rats were immunized intramuscularly by GenScript (Hong Kong) with 50 μg of protein formulated with complete Freund's adjuvant (day 1) and incomplete Freund's adjuvant (days 28 and 56). Rat serum was harvested on day 70 and IgG purified.

IgG Purification

Serum from immunized mice or rabbits was diluted 2:1 in protein G binding buffer (Pierce, UK) and applied to protein G sepharose columns. After washing twice with 3x serum volume of binding buffer, IgG was eluted in 10 mL protein G elution buffer (Pierce, UK) and restored to neutral pH by the addition of 300 μL Trizma pH 9.0 (Sigma Aldrich, USA). Where RBC pre-depletion was performed, 1 μg of packed 100% hematocrit RBC per 1 μg IgG was applied to sample, incubated at room temperature (RT) with agitation for 1 h. RBC were then pelleted by centrifugation at 1,000 *xg* for 5 min and the supernatant removed.

Immunofluorescence Assay

Cultures of 3D7 clone *P. falciparum*, synchronized to contain mainly late schizonts, were smeared onto glass slides to make thin films. Slides were fixed in 4% paraformaldehyde, blocked with 3% bovine serum albumin (BSA), and then probed with protein G purified serum IgG at 20 μg/mL. Secondary antibody was Alexa Fluor™ 488 goat anti-mouse IgG (H+L) at a dilution of 1:800 (Invitrogen, UK). Slides were mounted in ProLong Gold antifade reagent with DAPI (Life Technologies, USA). Images were acquired using a x100 oil-immersion objective and a cooled QICAM Fast 1,394 camera, each using the same exposure period.

Assay of Growth Inhibition Activity (GIA)

These were performed to the protocol of the GIA Reference Center, NIH, USA (4). Parasites were cultured in medium consisting of RPMI-1640 supplemented with 10% heat-inactivated human serum, 5.94 g/L HEPES, 0.05 g/L hypoxanthine, and 20 mg/L gentamycin. Synchronized parasites at 0.2–0.4% parasitemia in the trophozoite stage were grown in medium containing 20% human serum and 40 mg/L gentamycin, and then mixed with test antibody and cultured for 40 h at 1% hematocrit. Test samples were prepared by taking protein G eluate (see "IgG purification") or protein samples (see "Protein expression and purification"), and buffer exchanging three times into incomplete culture medium (lacking serum and gentamycin) using Amicon 10K MWCO centrifugal filtration devices. To deplete RBC-reactive antibodies, some samples were then incubated for 1 h with 100 μL O+ RBC at 100% hematocrit per mL of serum before centrifugation and removal of supernatant. Dialysis to exclude possibility of azide contamination was performed with Pierce MINI dialysis devices into incomplete culture medium.

Detection of parasite and inference of growth was performed using the lactate dehydrogenase method. BG98 is a rabbit anti-AMA1 purified immunoglobulin antibody pool (provided by Edmond Remarque, BPRC, Netherlands). It typically gives 80–90% GIA at 6 mg/mL and was used for quality control on assay runs.

Prediction of the GIA of an antibody mixture, GIA_{A+B}, given knowledge of the GIA of individual components (GIA_A and GIA_B), assuming Bliss Additivity between components, followed the equation (30):

$$GIA_{A+B} = [1 - \left(1 - \frac{GIA_A}{100}\right) \times \left(1 - \frac{GIA_B}{100}\right)] \times 100$$

Schizont Extract Western Blot

For **Figure S3E**, schizont and RBC extract were prepared by taking synchronized cultures of 3D7 clone schizonts or uninfected RBC, then pelleting and resuspending in a 10x volume of Laemmli buffer containing 2-mercaptoethanol, then subjecting to three cycles of freezing and thawing. Extracts were separated on 4–20% polyacrylamide gels along with Prestained Protein Marker, Broad Range (New England Biolabs, USA) and then blotted onto nitrocellulose membrane. Membranes were probed with total IgG from immunized mice at 20 μg/mL as primary antibody, then detected with alkaline phosphatase-conjugated anti-mouse IgG secondary antibody (Jackson, USA), using p-nitrophenylphosphate (pNPP) (Sigma Aldrich, USA) dissolved in water for detection.

Antigen-Specific Antibody Affinity Purification

CyRPA-specific rabbit IgG samples were generated in two stages. Total IgG was purified as above using protein G-sepharose. CyRPA-specific IgG was then purified from the total IgG using CyRPA-conjugated sepharose columns. These were generated using CyRPA (GlyKO)-C-tag protein and NHS-activated Sepharose 4 Fast Flow (GE Healthcare) according to the manufacturer's instructions. Total IgG was diluted 1:10 in 50 mM Na_2HPO_4 and applied to CyRPA-treated sepharose columns five times. After washing with 10 column volumes of 50 mM Na_2HPO_4 to remove the non-specific antibody, CyRPA-specific IgG was eluted with 0.1 M glycine and restored to neutral pH by addition of Trizma pH 9.0, before three rounds of buffer exchange into PBS using an Amicon 10K MWCO centrifugal filtration device.

ELISA

96-well Maxisorp plates were coated overnight with 100 ng/well CyRPA (GlyKO)-C-tag protein (glycan sites ablated) in PBS and then blocked with 10% milk powder. Test samples and secondary antibody (anti-mouse IgG (whole molecule) produced in goat and conjugated to alkaline phosphatase, Sigma, UK) were diluted in PBS plus 0.05% Tween-20. Alkaline phosphatase activity was measured by breakdown of pNPP using optical density at 405 nm (OD_{405}). Anti-OVA and anti-AARP titer was measured by defining the dilution factor required for a sample to yield a negative OD_{405}, defined as 0.15 using a pre-immune negative reference. For CyRPA, a standardized ELISA was also established according to principles outlined in (31) and automated by Gen5 software (BioTek, USA). Briefly, serum from the six rabbits shown in **Figures 5, 6** was pooled to make a standard sample whose concentration of anti-CyRPA IgG antibody was defined as 8,000 arbitrary units (AU). This sample was used to construct standard curves on assay plates. Samples were diluted such that they gave an OD_{405} lying on the linear region of the standard curve (generally between OD_{405} 0.3 and 2). The AU of the starting sample was then back-calculated based on the dilution of the sample and its position on the standard curve.

Anti-CyRPA Antibody Quantification by Concentration-Free Calibration Analysis (CFCA)

Our approach to CFCA has been described previously (30). To generate a source of mono-biotinylated CyRPA for use on a streptavidin Biacore capture chip, HEK293 cell cultures were co-transfected with a plasmid encoding CyRPA (GlyKO) (**Figure S6**) and a second plasmid encoding the BirA biotin ligase, and after 4 days centrifuged and filtered to remove cell debris prior to extensive dialysis into PBS. Total IgG samples were assayed at a 1:1,000 dilution of the concentrations shown in **Figure 6C**.

Statistics

Analysis was performed using GraphPad Prism version 5.04 (GraphPad Software Inc., USA). Tests and statistics are described in Figure Legends. To determine EC_{50} values from **Figures 5E,F**, for each individual rabbit a four-parameter sigmoidal dose-response curve was fitted to the relationship between $\log_{10}$(antibody concentration) and GIA, and then used to interpolate EC_{50}s for each rabbit. To generate conversion factors for ELISA AU into μg/mL of affinity purified CyRPA-specific IgG for each individual rabbit, linear interpolation was performed between individual data points for immune rabbits and the pre-immune data point in **Figure 6A**.

RESULTS

Protein-In-AddaVax™ Immunization Induces High-Titer Antibodies in BALB/c Mice

Freund's adjuvant has been widely used in the generation of high-titer polyclonal antibodies against proteins of interest. However, its suitability for the testing of potential vaccine antigens in animal models is questionable. Evidence that it can disrupt the tertiary structure of proteins (16), along with ethical issues concerning the adverse reactions associated with its use, persuaded us to consider alternatives for an antigen screening programme in mice. A previous study in our laboratory reported AbISCO®-100 as a potent, alternative preclinical adjuvant (28) and a more refined replacement for the Freund's adjuvant system. However, the promising and on-going clinical development of Matrix-M (32) (the successor formulation of AbISCO®-100), made acquiring this adjuvant difficult at the time of performing the study and so we examined instead AddaVax™, a preclinical analog of the licensed human adjuvant MF-59 which is a squalene-based oil-in-water emulsion (33, 34). Mice immunized with chicken egg ovalbumin (OVA) formulated with AbISCO®-100 and AddaVax™ produced comparable titers of anti-OVA serum IgG antibodies (**Figure S1**) and so we proceeded with AddaVax™ adjuvant for subsequent experiments.

Production of a Panel of Protein-In-Adjuvant Pre-clinical Vaccines

Fifty-five proteins of interest were selected, falling into two categories:

The first category consisted of 15 proteins, described in the literature as having properties that are desirable in a merozoite-blocking vaccine. These proteins met at least one of the following criteria: (i) susceptibility to vaccine-induced antibody, *in vitro* or *in vivo*; (ii) established involvement in the process of merozoite egress from schizonts or invasion into new RBC; (iii) essential to parasite viability, generally defined by reported failures to disrupt the relevant gene; or (iv) strong association with protection from clinical malaria in sero-epidemiological studies (**Table S1**). Candidate antigens which have already been characterized in our laboratory such as merozoite surface protein 1 (MSP1), erythrocyte-binding antigen-175 (EBA175), RH2, and RH4 were excluded [see (7) for full list]. We have previously attempted to produce viral vectors expressing MSP2 which were not immunogenic and which were subsequently found not to express MSP2 in mammalian cells (unpublished data). We therefore also excluded this protein from the literature-selected list.

The second category contained forty proteins selected from a pool of 435 genes whose protein products are implicated bioinformatically in merozoite invasion of RBC (18). A schematic for the selection of these 40 proteins is shown in **Figure S2**. Of these 435 genes, 104 are predicted to encode a signal peptide (35). A signal peptide is likely to be an essential property for traffic to the parasite surface, potentially via invasion-associated organelles, and is also true of all validated targets of merozoite-neutralizing antibody including MSP1, apical membrane antigen 1 (AMA1), RH5, RH4, and EBA175. Eliminating 18 proteins longer than 1,333 amino acids (due to challenges in synthesizing genes more than 4,000 bp in length), and 16 proteins which have previously been tested in our laboratory as vaccine antigens left a total of 70.

To select the final 40 from this list of 70 we ranked proteins according to polymorphism, with the intention of selecting the least polymorphic (see Methods)—it should be noted that subsequent and ongoing consolidation of genomic data into the MalariaGen portal (www.malariagen.net) means that the numbers of SNPs, and especially the frequencies within the population, have changed since our accessing these data in mid-2012. However, using AMA1, RH5, and RH4 as benchmark proteins we found that polymorphism across the list of 70 was much lower than expected. AMA1, a protein affected by strain-specific neutralization, has 34 SNPs, making it substantially more polymorphic than any protein in the set of 70. However, even proteins likely unaffected by strain-specific neutralization such as RH5 (4 non-synonymous SNPs) and RH4 (3 non-synonymous SNPs) also ranked among the top third most polymorphic proteins in the set. In fact, 33 of 70 proteins were found to contain zero non-synonymous SNPs of >10% prevalence. Presumably, RH4, and RH5 are still under a minimal degree of immune pressure which is absent for the proteins with no SNPs. This result meant that our original plan to select the 40 least polymorphic proteins from the list of 70 would have resulted in the exclusion of RH5 and RH4, which was counter to our overall strategy of selecting proteins with a similar profile to RH5.

We therefore changed our strategy for triage by polymorphism, aiming to select proteins with evidence of immune pressure, but without so many polymorphisms as to risk strain-specific immunity, i.e., a panel of minimally polymorphic proteins. Excluding 30 of the proteins with no SNPs of >10% prevalence left 40 proteins that, on the level of SNPs, resembled RH5 far more than they resembled AMA1 (see **Table S2**). The final selection contained 27 proteins with 0–5 SNPs, 8 proteins with 6–15 SNPs, and 5 with 15–25 SNPs. Of the literature-selected panel of 15 proteins, 8 would also have been identified using the final bioinformatic selection algorithm (**Table S1**).

We also aimed to minimize the probability of producing small polypeptide fragments that do not fold correctly and hence fail to elicit a functional antibody response, as occurred with RH5 in early studies of this target (7, 13, 14). Therefore, where possible, we aimed to express the entire ectodomain of the 55 shortlisted proteins. An important decision when using mammalian expression systems is whether to retain or ablate predicted sites of N-linked glycosylation (defined as N-X-S/T, where X is any animo acid residue except proline). As various *Plasmodium* antigens have been shown to elicit functional anti-parasitic antibody responses without modification to the primary amino acid sequence after expression *in situ* from mammalian cells (36–38), we obtained constructs that encoded the amino acid sequence exactly as predicted from the 3D7 clone parasite reference genome for all but one antigen candidate [P113 being the exception, the synthetic gene was the same as that used in a previous study and already had N-linked glycan sequons ablated (39)]. For SEA-1 and CyRPA, for which particularly promising vaccine antigen characteristics have been reported in the literature (40, 41), in addition to the native amino acid sequence, we also obtained constructs encoding versions of the protein with N-linked glycan sequons ablated (comparison shown in **Table S1**), in order to minimize the probability of a false-negative result in screening.

Mammalian expression plasmids encoding the 55 proteins of interest were successfully cloned and subsequently transfected into 500 mL cultures of HEK293E cells. Of the 55 different *P. falciparum* proteins, sufficient protein for a small scale mouse immunization campaign (approx. 300 μg, requiring expression at >0.6 μg/mL of cell culture supernatant) was obtained for 20 (**Figure 1**). This equates to a success rate 36.4% and is roughly in line with a previous attempt to produce a protein library using suspension HEK293 cells (42). We had significantly more success with the literature-selected panel than the bioinformatic panel (9/15 vs. 11/40, Fisher's exact test $P = 0.0329$), presumably reflecting publication bias toward proteins that can be expressed recombinantly. In a logistical regression analysis, neither protein length (OR = 0.9965, 95% CL 0.9914–1.0015) nor number of SNPs (OR = 0.8705, 95% CL 0.7125-1.0636) were predictive of expression in a statistically significant manner. Most proteins ran at a higher molecular weight than that predicted by the primary structure. Both variants of SEA-1 and CyRPA could also be expressed (**Figures 1A,B**). For SEA-1, no obvious difference in banding pattern was observed between the native version and the glycan-ablated version, and both constructs contained an additional band at approximately 75 kDa, which may represent the presence of a contaminant of SEA-1 dimer (**Figure 1A**). SEA-1 contains only two N-glycan sequons, both of which are judged unlikely to be glycosylated by the NetNGly server (http://www.cbs.dtu.dk/services/NetNGlyc/). The glycan-ablated version of CyRPA ran as a sharper band than the native version, presumably due to the presence of multiple glycoforms in the native version as CyRPA (native) contains 3 potential N-glycosylation sequons (**Figure 1B** and **Figure S6**). For many proteins, multiple smaller bands were observed, probably arising from proteolytic cleavage of the full-length construct. Given that the full-length protein was likely to be present, the presence of these smaller bands was deemed acceptable for screening purposes. Purified proteins were subsequently formulated with AddaVax™ adjuvant to produce pre-clinical protein-in-adjuvant vaccines.

Vaccines Induced Antigen-Specific IgG With Variable Neutralizing Activity

Groups of 4 mice were immunized with the vaccines over several independent experiments. Each experiment contained mice immunized with RH5 (7) as a functional antibody positive control and mice immunized with OVA as a negative control. Because production of RH5 protein at the time of vaccine preparation was not yet optimized, yield was low and therefore only the first experimental group received RH5 protein-in-adjuvant vaccine (**Figure 1A**) while subsequent groups received RH5 viral vectors. Gels in **Figure 1** show proteins immediately prior to formulation with AddaVax™ adjuvant. Following completion of the immunization phase, serum was harvested by terminal cardiac bleed. IgG was purified from the pooled sera of each group of mice and tested for binding to late schizonts by immunofluorescence (**Figure 2**). Total IgG from mice immunized with RH5 reacted strongly to schizonts whereas IgG from OVA-immunized mice did not. Of the remaining protein constructs tested, all but AARP-BAP-Strep and MSP11-BAP-Strep elicited IgG that reacted with schizonts. Although this experiment was not designed to assess localization, we did compare our results with previous studies to confirm similar staining patterns (**Table S3**). Most antibody samples showed staining consistent with previous reports, but for three proteins it was unclear whether our findings were in agreement with published work. Anti-ASP antibodies showed a punctate pattern as expected (43, 44), but additionally stained the external perimeter of the schizont. Pf92 was found to stain in a punctate manner, in contrast to a previous study using GFP-tagged Pf92 that localized to the merozoite surface (45). The GFP construct used in this study may have had non-natural trafficking, explaining the difference seen with our antibodies against native 3D7 parasite. Finally, a previous report has identified P113 as an interaction partner with RH5, and localized it to the surface of merozoites (39); however we were unable to identify any schizonts exhibiting merozoite surface staining with P113 (**Figure 2**), with staining more characteristic of the parasitophorous vacuole or iRBC surface, consistent with previous proteomics work (46).

Purified serum IgG was next screened for neutralizing activity in the *in vitro* assay of GIA at 1 mg/mL (**Figures 3A–D**). Anti-RH5 antibodies, whether raised using protein-in-adjuvant or virus vectors, had GIA ranging from 48 to 67%, whereas antibodies raised against OVA had < 5% GIA. In this initial screening, three vaccines appeared to have elicited functional antibodies which merited further study: CyRPA (**Figure 3A**), S-antigen and AARP (**Figure 3B**). All other IgG samples showed < 10% GIA at 1 mg/mL, which is indistinguishable from background GIA with anti-OVA antibodies.

Investigation of Antibodies Against AARP and S-Antigen

Given the screening results above, we next sought to further analyse the antibodies against S-antigen and AARP. Murine polyclonal IgG antibodies to AARP showed high-level GIA against both 3D7 and FVO parasites (**Figure 4A**). However, given that the murine anti-AARP antibodies showed no discernible binding to schizonts in the IFA assay (**Figure 2**), their ability to neutralize parasites in the assay of GIA raised concerns about their mechanism of action and the validity of this result. We first aimed to rule out contamination of the sample with sodium azide, which is present in small amounts in the protein G binding buffer used for IgG purification. Dialysis of the small amount of remaining antibody sample showed that small molecule contamination was unlikely (**Figure S3A**). These experiments depleted the remaining sample of IgG from the screening experiment, however a subsequent attempt to immunize rabbits with AARP-BAP-Strep did not yield functional antibodies (**Figure S3B**). Therefore, a further 10 mice were

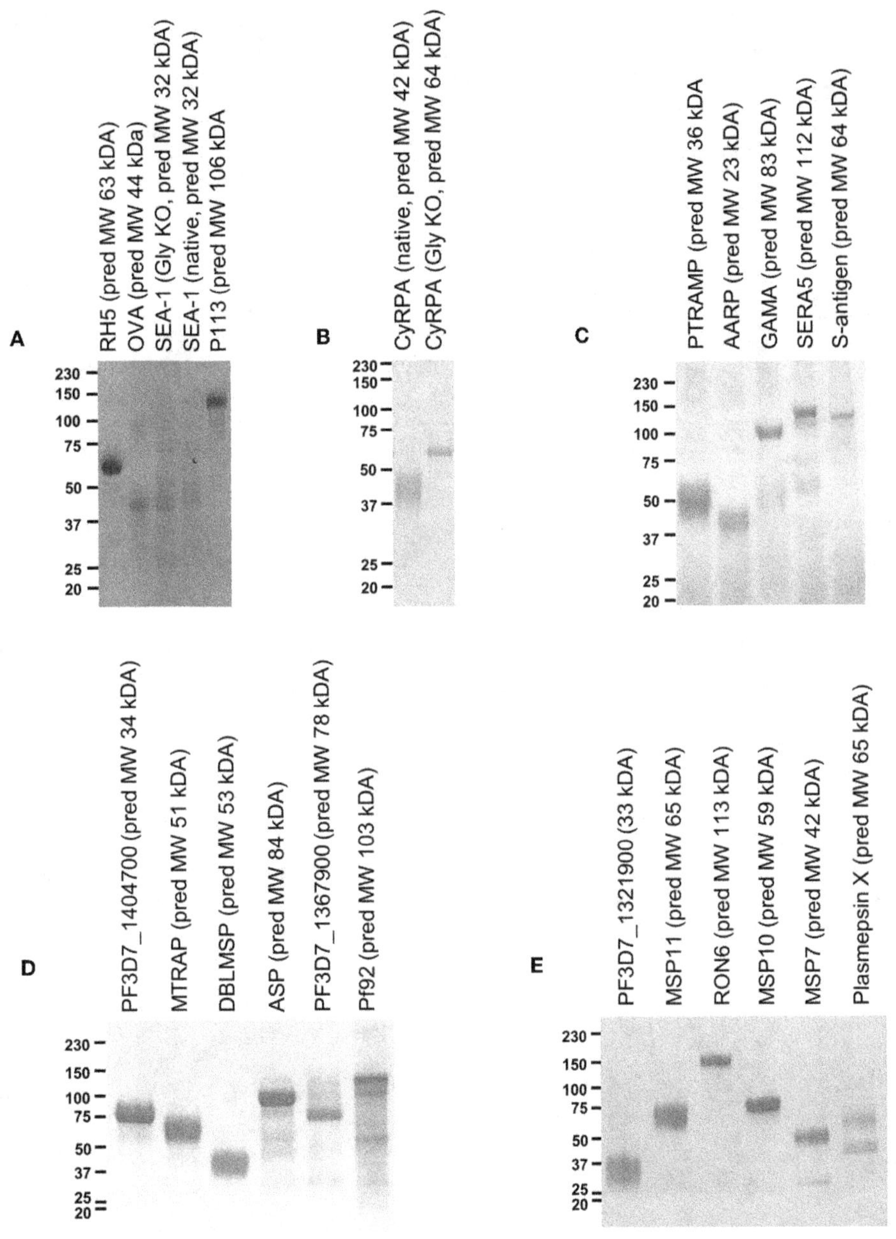

FIGURE 1 | Twenty-two protein antigens representing 20 different *P. falciparum* proteins. Just prior to formulation with AddaVax^{TM} and immunization into mice, approximately 2 μg protein was analyzed by reducing SDS-PAGE. Four immunization campaigns were run in total, with **(A,B)** combined into one campaign, and **(C–E)** each having their own campaign. **(A)** also includes analysis of "GIA positive" and "negative" control proteins, RH5, and OVA.

immunized again exactly as for the screening study with AARP-BAP-Strep protein, and serum from pairs of mice was pooled to give five samples. Interestingly, three of the five samples showed high GIA whereas the remaining two samples showed no GIA (**Figure S3C**). To test whether the functional antibodies in the samples cross-reacted with the RBC surface, we pooled the five samples and assessed GIA after an RBC pre-incubation step (**Figure 4B**). RBC pre-treatment totally ablated all GIA of the anti-AARP antibodies in a manner comparable to the anti-basigin mAb TRA-1-85 (10) (a mAb against the RH5 receptor, used here as an anti-RBC control). Notably, these results with anti-AARP IgG contrasted with anti-AMA1 antibodies where no effect of RBC pre-incubation was seen (**Figure 4B**). These data suggested that the mechanism of GIA of IgG from mice immunized with AARP was through binding to a molecule on the RBC surface. Alternatively, the inhibitory antibodies raised by vaccination with this protein preparation may function by neutralizing the parasite, but also cross-react to a non-inhibitory epitope on RBCs. The negative anti-schizont IFA (**Figure 2**) points away from this latter conclusion.

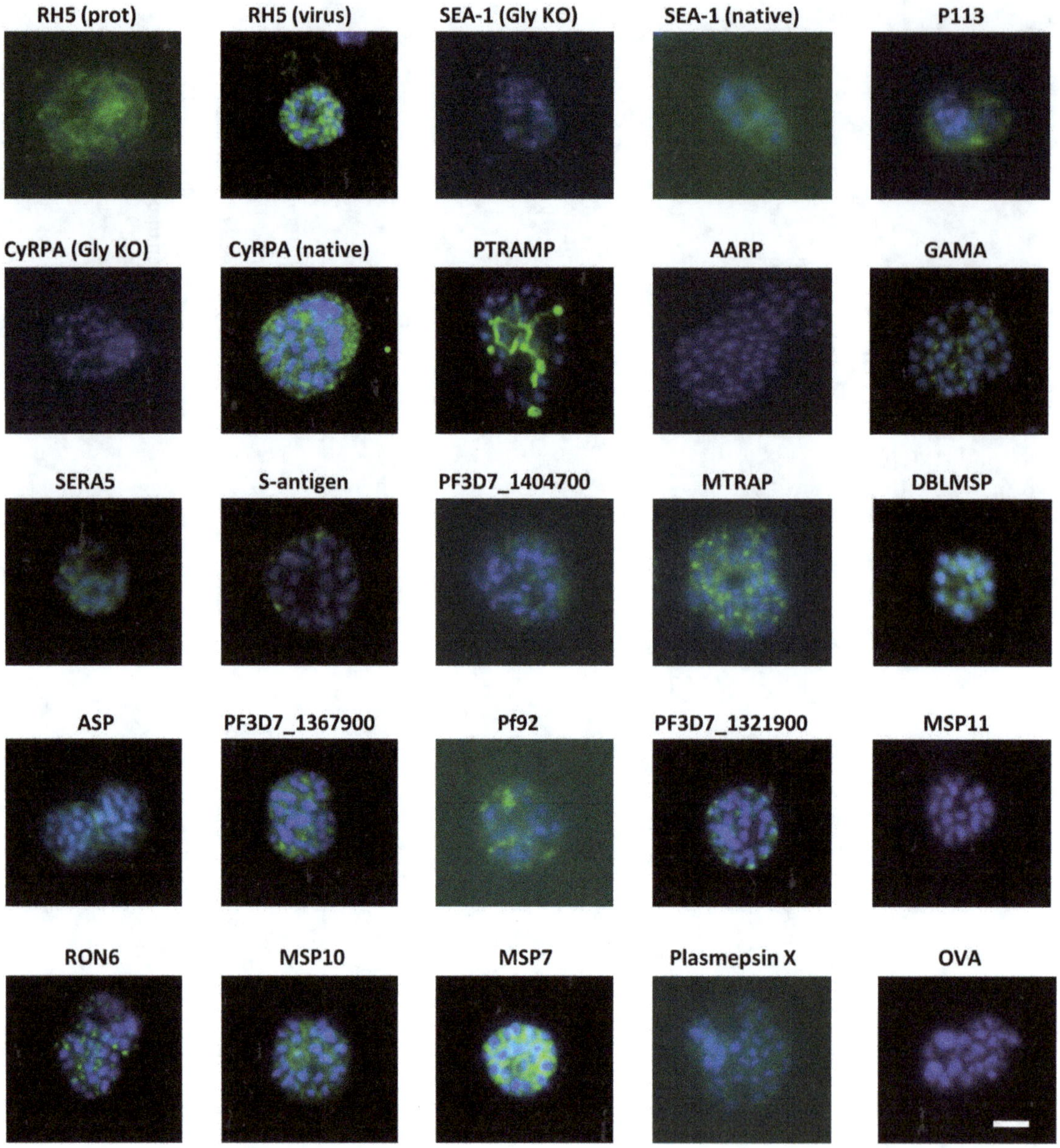

FIGURE 2 | Eighteen of twenty antigens elicit antibodies that react with *P. falciparum* schizonts. Groups of 4 mice were immunized with the proteins in adjuvants as shown in **Figure 1**. Seven days after the final injection, serum was harvested and pooled for each group before purification of IgG using protein G. The IgG was then probed for reactivity to paraformaldehyde-fixed schizonts in an immunofluorescence assay at a total IgG concentration of 20 μg/mL. All images were captured using the same microscope settings on the same day. Scale bar = 5 μm.

To further interrogate this, we prepared a new batch of AARP-BAP-Strep protein and tested its ability to reverse the GIA of the murine anti-AARP IgG antibodies. GIA from the anti-AARP antibodies could not be reversed by the addition of 2.5 mg/mL of the new batch of AARP-BAP-Strep protein, whereas 2.5 mg/mL AMA1-BAP-His protein was sufficient to fully deplete the GIA activity of anti-AMA1 IgG antibodies in the assay (**Figure 4C**). Taken together these results did not support neutralization of parasite AARP by IgG raised in our screen as a mechanism of GIA; they also suggested that antibodies against a HEK293 cell contaminant protein in the AARP vaccine were the most likely cause of the GIA. We could also not ascertain as to why this only occurred with the AARP protein vaccine in mice (noting we failed to induce growth inhibitory IgG in rabbits immunized with the same protein), and therefore we could not exclude the possibility of murine antibodies binding to a cryptic epitope such as a transient conformer of AARP or a rare glycoform, which cross-reacted with human RBC. Of note, AARP does carry two glycosylation sequons and AARP-BAP-Strep as expressed did contain PNGase-sensitive glycans (**Figure S3G**). Attempts to express AARP using a construct with glycan sequons ablated were not successful in the HEK293 system (data not shown).

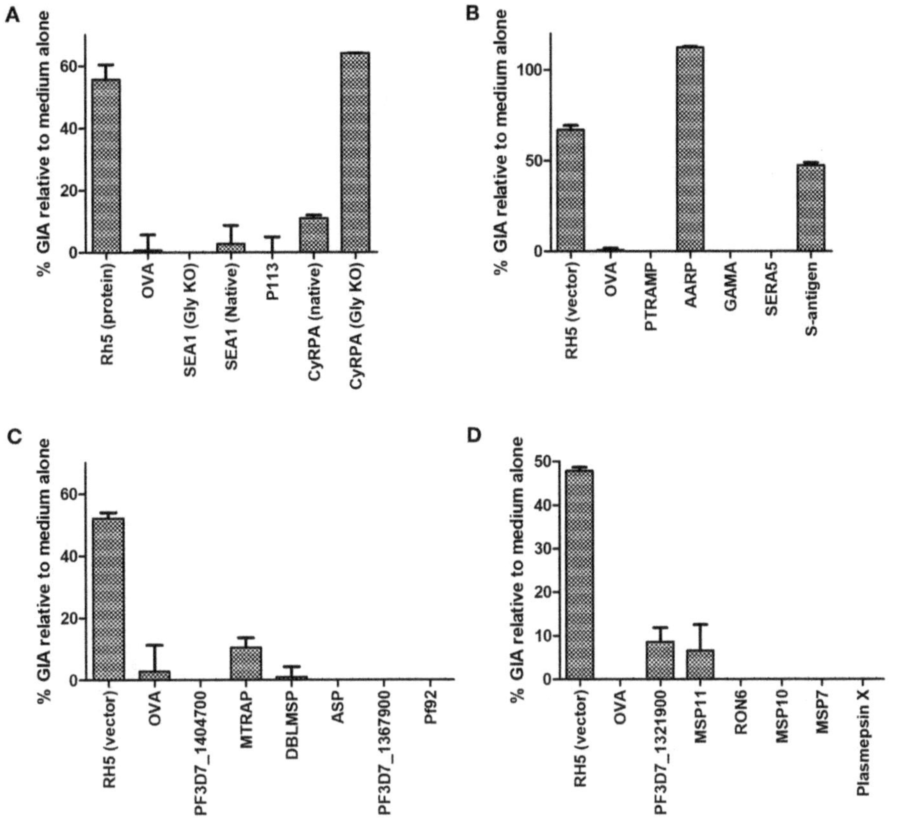

FIGURE 3 | Growth inhibitory activity of antibody specificities. The protein-G purified total IgG samples tested for schizont reactivity as shown in **Figure 2** were screened for activity in the standardized assay of GIA at 1 mg/mL. Each of panels **(A–D)** represents IgG from one independent mouse immunization campaign. Samples were not subjected to pre-incubation with RBC prior to GIA testing. Data is shown as mean of triplicate wells of a single GIA assay, and are representative of two independent assays.

Given the high level of neutralization of the antibodies, and their ability to strongly inhibit the growth of two divergent *P. falciparum* strains (**Figure 4A**) we attempted to further characterize the mechanism of neutralization by comparing the properties of the three pools shown in **Figure S3C** that did have GIA with the 2 pools that did not. However, we were hampered by the relatively small sample volume that can be obtained from mouse serum and an inability to produce functional rabbit antibodies (**Figure S3B**). The five samples shown in **Figure S3C** showed no difference in anti-immunogen ELISA (**Figure S3D**), and no consistent difference in binding to either schizont lysate or RBC lysate as measured by Western blot (**Figure S3E**). Notably, previous reports of AARP as a candidate vaccine antigen have expressed a short construct of AARP from *E. coli* [amino acids I20-D107 (9, 47)]. We therefore tested a construct mirroring this published version as closely as possible. We were only able to produce a construct encoding residues I20-D95 in *E. coli* (**Figure S3F**). We found that when formulated in AddaVax^{TM} and immunized into mice, antibodies elicited by this construct did not have any GIA, in contrast to AMA1 (**Figure S3H**).

In light of these data, we elected to not pursue this candidate antigen any further and processed to assess antibodies against the second hit in our screen—S-antigen. Here results were more promising. Murine polyclonal IgG antibodies to S-antigen showed GIA against both 3D7 clone and FVO strain parasites (**Figure 4D**), an effect that was reproduced against the 3D7 clone using immunized rabbit polyclonal IgG antibodies pre-depleted with RBC (**Figure 4E**). Importantly, mixing of purified S-antigen protein with rabbit total IgG could reverse the GIA of S-antigen antibodies, but not RH5 antibodies (**Figure 4F**). The antibodies isolated from mice immunized with S-antigen were probed against schizont extract by Western blot (**Figure S5**) and found to react to a single band of similar size to the recombinant S-antigen in **Figure 1**. These results suggest that S-antigen can be a target of neutralizing vaccine-induced antibodies. The ability of antibodies to neutralize 3D7 and FVO parasite was surprising because S-antigen is polymorphic (**Figure S4**), with 3D7 and FVO varying substantially: even among the relatively conserved 97-amino acid N-terminus of S-antigen, there are 41 sites of amino-acid divergence, with FVO and 3D7 diverging at 27 of these (**Figure S4**).

Investigation of Antibodies Against CyRPA

In our initial antigen screen, we found a striking difference in the potency of the polyclonal IgG mouse antibodies elicited to CyRPA (Gly KO) compared to CyRPA (native), both

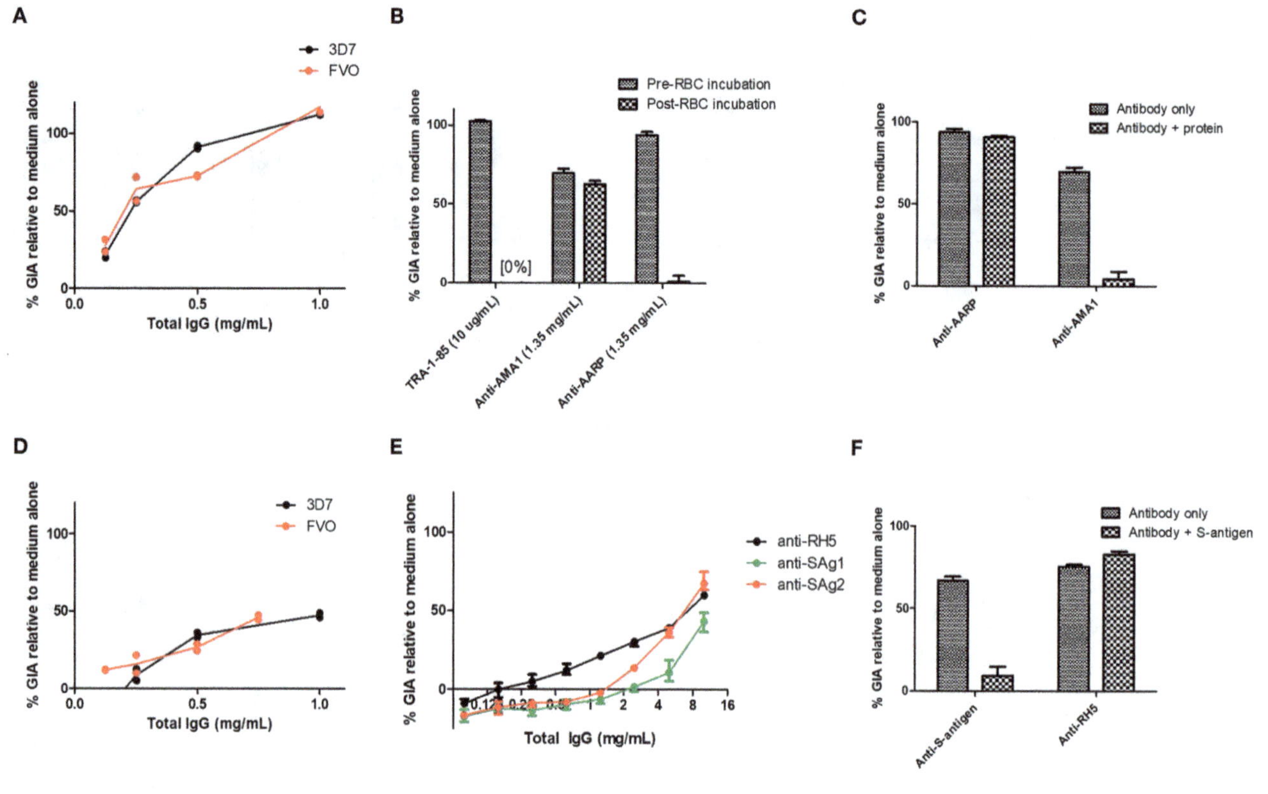

FIGURE 4 | Functional activity of anti-S-antigen and anti-AARP antibodies in the assay of GIA. **(A)** Titration of the same anti-AARP-BAP-Strep sample shown in **Figure 3B** against the 3D7 clone and FVO strain. **(B)** Effect of RBC pre-incubation on a range of mouse antibody specificities. TRA-1-85 is a mouse anti-basigin monoclonal antibody. Other samples are total IgG from immunized mice (see **Figure S3** for further details). **(C)** Pre-mixing of the relevant immunizing antigen with mouse total IgG. Final antigen concentration was 1.35 mg/mL, IgG concentration was 1 mg/mL. **(D)** Titration of the same anti-S-antigen-BAP-Strep sample shown in **Figure 3B** against the 3D7 clone and FVO strain. **(E)** Total IgG from two Zika rabbits immunized with S-antigen-BAP-Strep formulated with Freund's adjuvant system. Samples were subjected to pre-depletion with RBCs. **(A–D)** are each from a single GIA assay run due to sample volume constraints. **(A,D)**, lines are connected mean and points individual replicate wells (two per concentration). **(F)** Pre-mixing of S-antigen protein with pooled rabbit total IgG from **(E)**. Final S-antigen concentration was 1.5 mg/mL, total IgG concentration was 10 mg/mL. **(A–D)**, mean and range of four replicates. **(E,F)**, mean and range of three wells of a single GIA assay, representative of data from two replicate GIA assay runs.

quantitatively in terms of their potency (**Figure 3A**) and their ability to combine with rabbit anti-RH5 IgG antibodies (7) to give a synergistic level of GIA (**Figures 5A,B**). Consistent with a previous report on these two antigens (41), the combination of anti-CyRPA (Gly KO) and anti-RH5 IgG here showed synergy in the assay of GIA across two replicate assays. Aside from the amino acid substitutions to remove potential sites of N-linked glycosylation (S147A, T324A, T340A, schematic in **Figure S6**), these constructs differed markedly. The CyRPA (GlyKO) expression plasmid was a kind gift from Gavin Wright and colleagues, who use murine Ig signal peptide, and notably include a 20.4 kDa epitope tag on CyRPA (Gly KO) derived from rat CD4 domains 3 and 4 (CD4d3+4) (**Figure S6**) (48). However, before investigating which, if any, of these differences in construct design had led to differing qualities of anti-CyRPA IgG, we sought to reproduce the synergy result with the CyRPA (Gly KO) vaccine and immunized new cohorts of mice and rabbits with a new batch of CyRPA (Gly KO) protein. The IgG antibodies elicited by the CyRPA (Gly KO) antigen formulated with AddaVax™ reproducibly showed GIA against 3D7 clones parasites in both mice (**Figure 5C**) and rabbits (**Figure 5E**). We also tested formulation with Poly(I:C), a fully aqueous molecular adjuvant system, and saw diminished GIA activity by comparison to AddaVax™ adjuvant in mice (**Figure 5D**). The rabbit anti-CyRPA antibodies also showed high-level neutralization of the FVO strain (**Figure 5F**). However, the synergy observed in our initial experiment (**Figure 5A**) was not observed in subsequent experiments using IgG purified from newly immunized mice (**Figures 5C,D**) or rabbits (**Figure 5G**); only an additive effect was observed.

Given these conflicting data, we sought to confirm the validity of the initial result showing synergy between antibodies against CyRPA (Gly KO) and RH5. It was observed in the initial experiment (**Figure 5A**) that the anti-CyRPA (Gly KO) purified IgG antibodies caused agglutination of the RBC in the GIA assay, and we sought to exclude this as a mechanism of GIA. We found that pre-depletion of the mouse IgG antibody sample with human RBC ablated the agglutination observed and had no effect on the GIA, either as a single specificity or its ability to synergize with anti-RH5 IgG (**Figure S7A**). To exclude any

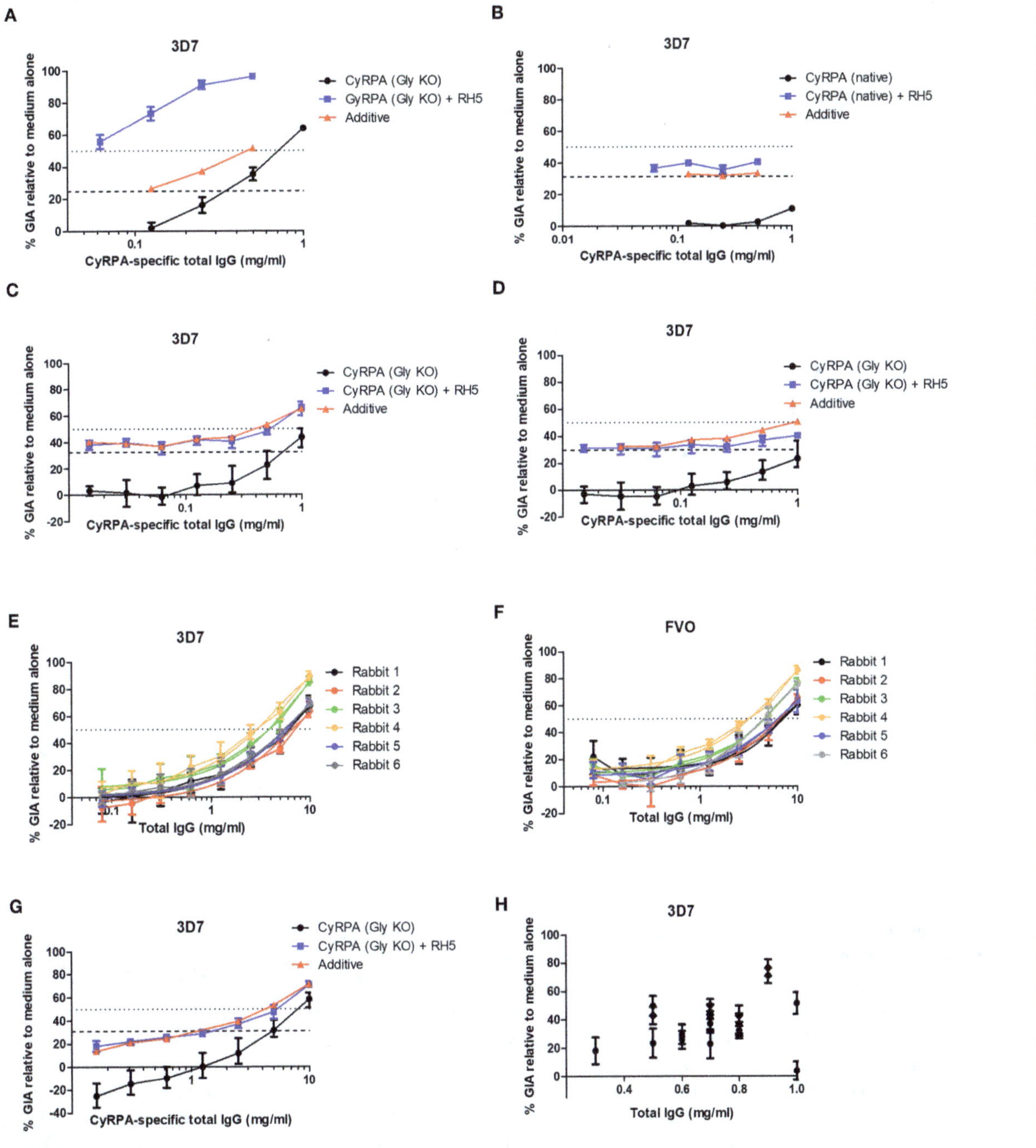

FIGURE 5 | Functional activity of anti-CyRPA antibodies in the *in vitro* assay of GIA. **(A,B)** Titration of the anti-CyRPA purified IgG samples (from **Figure 3A**) against 3D7 clone parasites, with (blue line) and without (black line) addition of a fixed concentration (1.25 mg/mL) rabbit anti-RH5 purified IgG antibodies. Dashed line shows the activity of the anti-RH5 IgG alone tested at the single fixed concentration and red line shows the calculated activity of the mixture, assuming Bliss additivity (30). Dotted line indicates 50% GIA. **(C)** A new sample of mouse anti-CyRPA (GlyKO) IgG was generated and assessed as in **(A)**. **(D)** A new sample of mouse anti-CyRPA (Gly KO) IgG was generated using an identical immunogen to **(A,C)**, but using Poly(I:C) adjuvant for formulation. **(E,F)** Six rabbits were immunized with CyRPA (Gly KO) in AddaVax^{TM} and their total IgG tested in a titration series for GIA against 3D7 clone and FVO strain parasites. **(G)** Pooled IgG antibodies from the six rabbits in panels **(E,F)** were tested for synergy against the 3D7 clone with anti-RH5 IgG antibodies as in **(A,B)**. **(H)** GIA of total IgG purified from 20 individual mice immunized with CyRPA (Gly KO) and AddaVax^{TM}, each tested at a different concentration as defined by IgG yield in the sample. All panels show representative results from two replicate GIA assays, except **(E)** which was repeated 3 times. Each point shows the mean of three replicate wells; error bars show the range of three replicates wells.

effect of possible anti-rat CD4d3+4 antibodies we also generated recombinant CyRPA with a C-terminal four amino acid C-tag (25), which contained the same CyRPA (Gly KO) sequence but lacked the CD4d3+4 domain, called CyRPA (Gly KO)-C-tag (see **Figure S6** for construct comparisons). A vaccine containing CyRPA (GlyKO)-C-tag yielded functional antibodies comparable

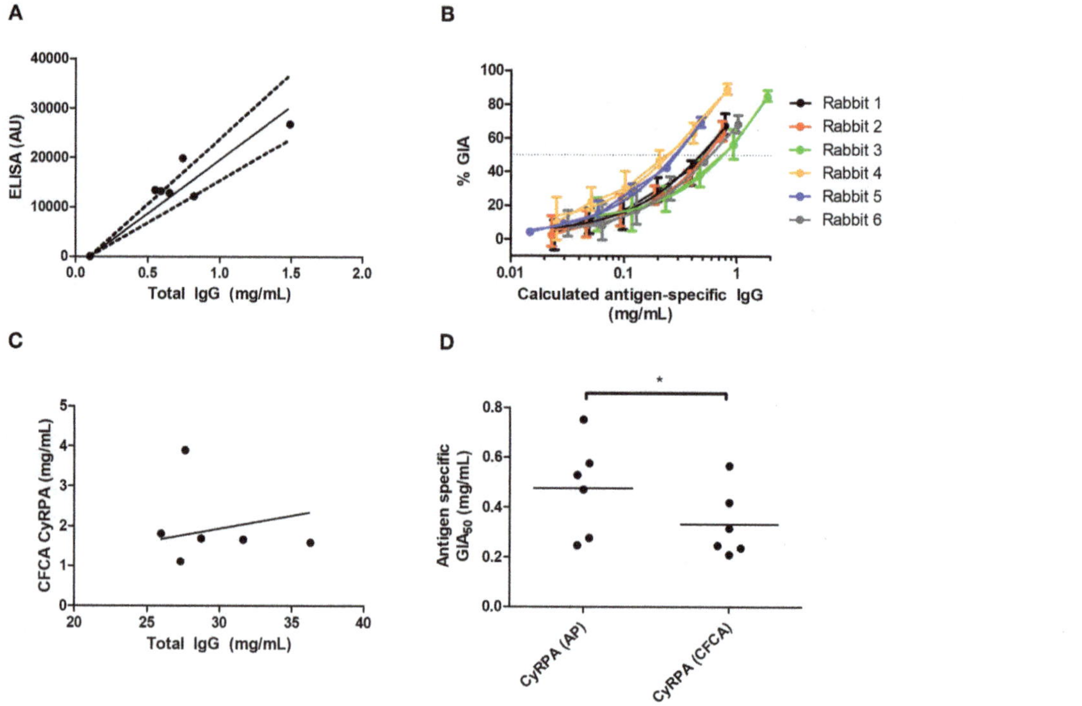

FIGURE 6 | Potency of vaccine-induced anti-CyRPA antibodies from six individual rabbits. See **Figure S8** for experimental schematic. A second batch of IgG was purified from the six rabbits shown in **Figures 5E,F**, as well as one pool of pre-immune IgG, using protein G. **(A,B)** Calculation of antigen-specific IgG concentration by affinity purification (AP) and ELISA analysis. **(A)** Total IgG from six individual rabbits was passed over a CyRPA-sepharose column and the six eluates were analyzed for total protein concentration by OD_{280}, and assayed for CyRPA binding by ELISA, to generate a conversion factor for each rabbit. Points are individual rabbits, solid line is mean conversion factor (shown for information only—not used in calculations), dashed lines 95% CI (actual calculations were performed with separate conversion factors for each individual rabbit). **(B)** GIA data from **Figure 5E** transformed using the conversion factors determined for individual rabbits in panel A, to show CyRPA antigen-specific IgG concentration. Points are means of 3 assay well replicates, error bars show range of three replicates. **(C)** Calibration-free concentration analysis (CFCA). Total IgG was analyzed for total protein concentration by OD_{280}, and anti-CyRPA antigen-specfic IgG concentration by CFCA. Pre-immune IgG gave a sub-detectable CFCA response. **(D)** Interpolated GIA EC_{50}s for the six CyRPA immunized rabbits. Points are individual rabbits, bars are means.

to the parental CyRPA (Gly KO) construct as a single specificity, however, these also showed additivity, but not synergy, with anti-RH5 IgG antibodies (**Figure S7B**), meaning that a role for anti-CD4 IgG cannot be excluded in the results from **Figure 5A**. Consequently, in a final effort to understand the mechanism of the synergy seen in **Figure 5A**, we immunized with CyRPA (Gly KO) and harvested IgG from individual mice, aiming to isolate monoclonal antibodies (mAbs) from mice whose serum polyclonal IgG showed synergy with anti-RH5 antibodies. IgG yields from individual mice were variable, necessitating GIA screening at a range of concentrations (**Figure 5H**). Although IgG from most mice showed GIA, not one of the IgG samples isolated from these 20 mice showed synergy with anti-RH5 antibodies and isolation of mAbs was not pursued (data not shown). Therefore, given the inconsistency of synergy observed in our study, we attempted to replicate as closely as possible the initial report of anti-CyRPA and anti-RH5 IgG antibody synergy, which used rat immunization with Freund's adjuvant (41). A pair of Wistar rats and a pair of Sprague Dawley rats were immunized with CyRPA (Gly KO) in Freund's adjuvant. Total IgG isolated from these rats showed 60–90% GIA at the highest concentrations tested, and some degree of additivity with anti-RH5 rabbit IgG, but no synergy was seen (**Figures S7C–F**). Thus, these data suggest that anti-CyRPA IgG raised in mice, rats and rabbits can elicit substantial GIA and that this is most consistently additive when combined with anti-RH5 rabbit IgG.

Assessment of Anti-CyRPA Specific IgG Potency

Given immunization against CyRPA could reliably elicit functional antibodies, we next aimed to better assess CyRPA's suitability as a candidate vaccine antigen by quantifying its susceptibility to vaccine-induced polyclonal antibody. We and others have previously reported similar analyses for polyclonal antigen-specific IgG against RH5, AMA1, and MSP1 in different species ranging from mice through humans (1, 4, 30). Here, for rabbit anti-CyRPA antibody, the mean total IgG concentration giving 50% GIA (EC_{50}) against the 3D7 clone parasite was 5.07 mg/mL (95% CI, 3.61–6.54, **Figure 5E**) and against the FVO strain was 5.34 mg/mL (95% CI, 3.83–6.86, **Figure 5F**). However, the antigen-specific IgG is typically only a small fraction of the total IgG; so we next determined the proportion of total IgG which is CyRPA-specific using two methods: (i) affinity purification of specific IgG using chromatography columns loaded with CyRPA antigen; and (ii) surface plasmon resonance analysis by calibration-free concentration analysis

(CFCA) using recombinant CyRPA coated onto a capture chip. The experimental schema is shown in **Figure S8**.

When using the affinity-purification method, CyRPA-specific IgG was purified from total rabbit IgG using CyRPA-immobilized sepharose columns. The total protein concentration (assumed to be all antigen-specific IgG) was then analyzed by OD_{280} measurement as well as measured for anti-CyRPA responses in arbitrary units (AU) by ELISA (**Figure 6A**). This was used to calculate a conversion factor for ELISA AU to a specific concentration of anti-CyRPA rabbit IgG antibodies in mg/mL for each individual rabbit (for information only, mean conversion factor: CyRPA-specifc IgG concentration (μg/mL) = 0.046 (ELISA AU)−0.1; slope 95% CI 0.058–0.043). We then measured the ELISA units of the IgG stocks used to perform the GIA in **Figure 5E** and replotted GIA against CyRPA-specific IgG (**Figure 6B**).

For CFCA, total IgG from individual rabbits was analyzed to assess the concentration of anti-CyRPA antibodies in samples whose total protein concentration was measured by OD_{280} (**Figure 6C**). For the pre-immune rabbit IgG pool, the anti-CyRPA CFCA response was sub-detectable. For the six immune IgG samples, the mean proportion of CyRPA-specific IgG as measured by CFCA was 6.78% of the total IgG (95% CI, 2.86–10.7%). With the proportion of total IgG that was specific for CyRPA now determined for each rabbit, GIA was replotted against CyRPA-specific IgG (not shown), and the antigen-specific GIA EC_{50} values calculated with each method were compared (**Figure 6D**). The CyRPA-specific rabbit IgG GIA EC_{50} was calculated to be 470 μg/mL by the affinity purification method (95% CI: 270–680 μg/mL) and 330 μg/mL for the CFCA method (95% CI: 190–480 μg/mL), with the figure determined by affinity purification significantly higher than by CFCA ($P = 0.031$, Wilcoxon matched-pairs signed rank test). Both figures suggest that relatively high Ag-specific antibody concentrations are required for CyRPA polyclonal IgG mediated GIA.

DISCUSSION

RH5 has emerged as a leading blood-stage vaccine candidate antigen, and vaccination with this antigen appears to elicit a potent growth-inhibitory antigen-specific antibody response (1, 12). A recombinant protein vaccine called RH5.1 based on this antigen is currently in Phase I/II clinical trials (11). The objective of this study was to shed light on whether there are other antigens that could supersede or synergize with RH5 in their ability to elicit growth-inhibitory antibodies against blood-stage *P. falciparum*. This will inform the approach taken to improve on the present RH5 vaccine and/or develop next-generation vaccine formulations targeting multiple antigens to achieve even higher levels of growth inhibitory antibodies.

To meet this objective, we tested a range of merozoite proteins in as unbiased a manner as possible, testing their ability to elicit antibodies with functional GIA. RH5 was used as a "gold-standard" antigen. Fifty-five proteins of interest were selected for study: 15 were selected from the literature as having properties desirable in a vaccine antigen; while the other 40 proteins were selected on the basis of a bioinformatically predicted role in merozoite invasion (18). These 40 proteins were selected from a shortlist of 70 on the basis of having a higher number of SNPs. Of the 55 proteins selected, 20 were successfully expressed, and for 18 we were able to raise an antibody response that showed binding to fixed schizonts. While an expression success rate of 20/55 proteins is high compared to an expression library effort using a bacterial system (49), and in line with a recent study using suspension HEK293 cells (42), this leaves 35 proteins unaddressed by this study. Alternative expression systems using insect cells (29) and protozoan cells (50) may achieve a higher success rate in future studies.

When tested for function in the *in vitro* assay of GIA, three antibody specificities showed functional activity when tested alone: S-antigen; AARP and CyRPA. While our finding that S-antigen can be a target of neutralizing antibody is novel, AARP and CyRPA have been the subject of previous publications highlighting promise for these proteins as clinical candidate vaccine antigens. We therefore scrutinized the latter two antigens particularly closely, to help inform the immediate prioritization of antigens for inclusion in the next generation of clinical vaccine candidates. For S-antigen, purified IgG samples from immunized mice and rabbits (that had also been pre-depleted with RBC) were able to inhibit growth in a reproducible manner, and this effect could be reversed by pre-incubation with S-antigen protein. S-antigen has been largely unstudied since the 1980s, and was included in this screen because of statements in review articles authored by Cowman *et al.* that S-antigen is refractory to genetic ablation (51, 52). Interestingly, while most of the 14 other proteins that were initially selected based on literature reports as showing a role in merozoite invasion would also have been identified using the bioinformatics approach used to identify the other 40 proteins (18), S-antigen was not identified bioinformatically as having a role in this process. It is therefore surprising that S-antigen appears to be the target of neutralizing antibody in the GIA assay. Given the extreme variability of S-antigen between strains [**Figure S4**, and also (53)], the ability of antibodies raised to the 3D7 clone sequence of S-antigen to neutralize the FVO strain was particularly unexpected. Although we did not follow-up this result further, our data suggest S-antigen may warrant re-visiting in future vaccine studies, with particular emphasis on defining the neutralizing epitopes and understanding the effect of polymorphism between strains.

Different antibody samples raised against AARP did not show consistent functional GIA, and further investigation suggested the function was likely mediated through off-target binding of antibodies to the RBC. Notably, previous publications ascribing a high level of neutralization activity to anti-AARP antibodies do not describe an RBC pre-incubation step in the purification and preparation of IgG from serum (9, 47), and we were unable to reproduce these results with a similar, albeit not identical, immunogen. Our negative results for AARP in rabbits are consistent with those described in a separate, recent antigen screen (54). Although we elected to not study this antigen any further, future identification of the RBC moiety bound by the neutralizing anti-AARP IgG samples could potentially yield important information about the mechanism of invasion of RBC by merozoites.

In the case of our final "hit," immunization with CyRPA-based constructs could reproducibly elicit antibodies from mice, rats and rabbits with invasion-blocking activity. The first mouse IgG sample we produced exhibited synergy when combined with anti-RH5 rabbit IgG antibodies across numerous replicate assays, in line with an earlier report on this antigen combination (41). However, the fact that multiple subsequent immunizations did not yield GIA with this synergistic property, including rats immunized using an almost identical protocol to that used by Reddy et al. (41), suggests that it is highly likely a result of rare antibody clones binding to specific epitopes. It could be that use of AddaVax^{TM} adjuvant biased the antibody response toward a non-synergistic repertoire of epitopes, although a similar result was obtained when using Freund's adjuvant in rats. Although synergy between RH5 and CyRPA IgG specificities was inconsistent, the combination did consistently result in additive GIA in our hands, in agreement with some other reports. Bustamante et al. found that the combination of RH5 and CyRPA total IgG from immunized rabbits alternated between synergy and sub-additivity in the GIA assay depending on the concentration used (54), while Favuzza *et al.* appear to observe an additive interaction between RH5 and CyRPA mAbs (55). Given CyRPA, RH5 and Ripr form a complex (56, 57), it is possible that individual antibody clones that block or stabilize different aspects of complex formation could mediate either synergistic or additive interactions with anti-RH5 antibodies. However, the relationship between antibody potency and the role of the target antigen protein in merozoite invasion is far from clear: we have previously found that antibodies to RH5 interact synergistically with antibodies to RH2, RH4, and EBA175, additively with antibodies to MSP1 and sub-additively with antibodies to AMA1 (30), none of which are known to interact directly with RH5.

Further characterization of the rabbit anti-CyRPA IgG indicated that the antigen-specific GIA EC_{50} is substantially higher than that of vaccine-induced antibodies to RH5 (30) and AMA1 (58), and more akin to the levels required when targeting MSP1 (4). These data would argue against prioritization of CyRPA over RH5 for inclusion in a single-subunit blood-stage malaria vaccine. However our results are inconsistent with recent work published by Bustamante et al., who found that anti-CyRPA rabbit antibodies are at least as potent as anti-RH5 antibodies (54). Indeed, the GIA EC_{50} reported by Bustamante *et al.* for total IgG from CyRPA-immunized rabbits against 3D7 clone parasites is 0.3834 mg/mL. This is more than 10 times lower than our total IgG GIA EC_{50} of 5.07 mg/mL, and equivalent to our calculated antigen-specific GIA EC_{50}. Both studies used very similar immunogens and also the same contractor for rabbit immunization (Cambridge Research Biochemicals). The differences in the GIA results could have arisen from other methodological factors, which could include GIA assay format and potentially differences in adjuvant selection and/or immunization regimen. We, and others, have noted quite marked differences in rabbit immunization studies with regard to overall endpoint titres raised against protein antigens, which may easily explain the discrepancy of the results for total IgG. Moreover, it is wholly possible the immunization protocols affected the quality of anti-CyRPA IgG induced in the rabbits, and this would suggest careful monitoring of the protein formulation and anti-CyRPA IgG quality is warranted in future studies. Nevertheless, the results in our present study are concordant with those published by Reddy et al. (41) and in line with the observation that the most potent anti-CyRPA mAbs yet described have a GIA EC_{50} of at least 250 μg/mL (55, 59–61); by contrast, the most potent anti-RH5 mAbs have a GIA EC_{50} of ~15 μg/mL (62). Taken together, it does appear that total IgG from RH5-based immunization tends to be more potent than IgG from CyRPA-based immunization. However, if the epitopes responsible for synergy between anti-RH5 and anti-CyRPA IgG could be identified and antibodies robustly elicited against them in combination, this could form the basis for a more effective bivalent next-generation blood-stage vaccine.

A final unexpected result from our screen was the failure of antibodies to both the glycan-ablated or the native version of SEA-1 to exhibit any GIA. Raj et al. found that SEA-1 antibodies are associated with protection from clinical malaria, and also showed that vaccination with PbSEA-1 can protect mice from *P. berghei* rodent malaria (40). Our results do not necessarily contradict these findings, because protection from malaria by anti-SEA-1 antibodies might well be mediated by Fc-dependent immune effector functions not measured in the GIA assay such as complement fixation and myeloid cell activation. However, our finding that anti-SEA-1 antibodies did not have GIA does conflict with Raj et al.'s finding that anti-SEA-1 serum antibodies, as well as mAbs, can block growth in *in vitro* cultures (40). It is possible that our protein was not folded correctly, or was insufficiently immunogenic when immunized into mice with AddaVax^{TM} as an adjuvant, leading to a negative result. Fortunately Raj *et al.* produced mAbs to SEA-1 (40), and testing these in the standardized assay of GIA as operated by the International GIA Reference Laboratory should resolve this discrepancy.

With respect to the process used to select the "bioinformatically selected panel" of 40 proteins, even in retrospect it is difficult to say whether the approach taken was optimal. Of the 15 literature-selected proteins, 8 would have been identified with the bioinformatic selection algorithm. Among the 2 robust hits from the screen, CyRPA would have been selected using the bioinformatic approach whereas S-antigen would not have (**Table S1**). This result does suggest that there may be other invasion-blocking candidate antigens which were not identified as part of the "Merozoite invasion sub-network" by Hu et al. (18). It is difficult to say whether our decision to prioritize the moderately polymorphic proteins at the expense of non-polymorphic proteins was the right one. CyRPA and S-antigens, the two robust hits from this study, both came from the literature-selected panel. CyRPA has one SNP of >10% prevalence, which would mean that had it been in the 'bioinformatically-selected' panel it would have been brought forward whether we selected the 40 most polymorphic or the 40 least prevalent genes. S-antigen is so polymorphic that with the data available at the time it was not possible to actually count SNPs, and even with data available now a full discussion of polymorphism in S-antigen is beyond the scope of this paper. Both of these antigens elicit antibodies capable of neutralizing 3D7 and FVO, which differ markedley in their S-antigen sequences, suggesting that polymorphism is not always predictive of strain-specific neutralization.

While this study has focused on the assay of GIA, as one defined mechanistic correlate that is causative of protection against blood-stage *P. falciparum* (63) it should be recognized that alternative assays of anti-merozoite antibody efficacy do exist, including phagocytosis assays (64), the assay of antibody-dependent respiratory burst (65), and the assay of antibody-dependent cellular inhibition (66). Antibody performance in each of these assays has been shown to correlate with protection from clinical malaria in the context of naturally-acquired humoral immunity. However, there are technical challenges with using these assays for antibodies derived from different species as in this study. We selected the assay of GIA because our goal was to benchmark against antibodies to RH5, which are functional in this assay.

In summary, no antibody specificity in this study outperformed anti-RH5 antibodies in the GIA assay. Neither did any polyclonal antibody specificity robustly synergize with or enhance the GIA of anti-RH5 antibodies, although additivity with anti-CyRPA IgG was generally consistent. While we attempted to make this screen as comprehensive as possible, we were not able to express every candidate antigen in HEK293 cells, and new antigens continue to be described that were not included in our original list of proteins. Bustamante *et al.* have very recently reported that SERA9, RAMA, MSRP5, and EBA181 are targets of neutralizing antibody which potentially synergize with anti-RH5 antibodies (54). The RH5-interacting protein (Ripr) is another protein with a strong rationale for testing as a vaccine antigen, but which has not been well studied due to the difficulty of expressing it in bacterial and mammalian cell systems (26, 67). It now remains a priority to test these proteins in human compatible vaccine-delivery systems to find out if their inclusion in a multi-valent vaccine offers a realistic possibility of improving on RH5 alone.

ETHICS STATEMENT

Animal experiments and procedures were performed in accordance with the UK Animals (Scientific Procedures) Act Project License (PPLs 30/2889 and PA7D20B85) and were approved by the University of Oxford Local Ethical Review Body.

AUTHOR CONTRIBUTIONS

JI: wrote the paper. JI and SD: conceived the study. JI, DA, MS, KW, AD, GL, JC, DP, and MH: produced and characterized proteins. JI, LB, DP, and SdC: performed animal immunization studies. JI, RB, JM, and DQ: performed GIA assays. SS and HB: performed affinity purification and Biacore analysis on CyRPA-specific antibodies. JI and JW: selected genes of interest.

FUNDING

This work was supported in-part by funding from the European Union's Horizon 2020 research and innovation programme under grant agreement for OptiMalVax [number 733273]. JI held a Ph.D. studentship in the Wellcome Trust Infection, Immunology and Translational Medicine Ph.D. Programme [105399/Z/14/Z]; DA held a UK MRC iCASE Ph.D. Studentship [MR/K017632/1]; AD holds a Wellcome Trust Early Postdoctoral Research Training Fellowship for Clinicians [201477/Z/16/Z]; MH is a Wellcome Trust Senior Investigator [101020/Z/13/Z]; and SD is a Jenner Investigator; a Lister Institute Research Prize Fellow and a Wellcome Trust Senior Fellow [106917/Z/15/Z].

ACKNOWLEDGMENTS

The authors are grateful for the assistance of Julie Furze, Adrian Hill, Jing Jin, and Amelia Lias (Jenner Institute, University of Oxford); Dominic Kwiatkowski (Wellcome Trust Centre for Human Genetics, University of Oxford) for useful discussions; Edmond Remarque (BPRC, Netherlands) for providing the BG98 anti-AMA1 antibodies for assay standardization; Yves Durocher for provision of HEK293E cells (CNRC-NRC, Canada); and Gavin Wright for sharing the CyRPA (Gly KO) via Addgene (plasmid number: 50823).

REFERENCES

1. Draper SJ, Sack BK, King CR, Nielsen CM, Rayner JC, Higgins MK, et al. Malaria vaccines: recent advances and new horizons. *Cell Host Microbe.* (2018) 24:43–56. doi: 10.1016/j.chom.2018.06.008
2. RTS,S Clinical Trials Partnership. Efficacy and safety of RTS,S/AS01 malaria vaccine with or without a booster dose in infants and children in Africa: final results of a phase 3, individually randomised, controlled trial. *Lancet.* (2015) 386:31–45. doi: 10.1016/S0140-6736(15)60721-8
3. Olotu A, Fegan G, Wambua J, Nyangweso G, Leach A, Lievens M, et al. Seven-year efficacy of RTS,S/AS01 malaria vaccine among young african children. *N Engl J Med.* (2016) 374:2519–29. doi: 10.1056/NEJMoa1515257
4. Miura K, Zhou H, Diouf A, Moretz SE, Fay MP, Miller LH, et al. Anti-apical-membrane-antigen-1 antibody is more effective than anti-42-kilodalton-merozoite-surface-protein-1 antibody in inhibiting *Plasmodium falciparum* growth, as determined by the *in vitro* growth inhibition assay. *Clin Vaccine Immunol.* (2009) 16:963–8. doi: 10.1128/CVI.00042-09
5. Weiss GE, Crabb BS, Gilson PR. Overlaying molecular and temporal aspects of Malaria parasite invasion. *Trends Parasitol.* (2016) 32:284–95. doi: 10.1016/j.pt.2015.12.007
6. Bustamante LY, Bartholdson SJ, Crosnier C, Campos MG, Wanaguru M, Nguon C, et al. A full-length recombinant *Plasmodium falciparum* PfRH5 protein induces inhibitory antibodies that are effective across common PfRH5 genetic variants. *Vaccine.* (2013) 31:373–9. doi: 10.1016/j.vaccine.2012.10.106

7. Douglas AD, Williams AR, Illingworth JJ, Kamuyu G, Biswas S, Goodman AL, et al. The blood-stage malaria antigen PfRH5 is susceptible to vaccine-inducible cross-strain neutralizing antibody. *Nat Commun.* (2011) 2:601. doi: 10.1038/ncomms1615
8. Douglas AD, Baldeviano GC, Lucas CM, Lugo-Roman LA, Crosnier C, Bartholdson SJ, et al. A PfRH5-based vaccine is efficacious against heterologous strain blood-stage *Plasmodium falciparum* infection in aotus monkeys. *Cell Host Microbe.* (2015) 17:130–9. doi: 10.1016/j.chom.2014.11.017
9. Pandey AK, Reddy KS, Sahar T, Gupta S, Singh H, Reddy EJ, et al. Identification of a potent combination of key *Plasmodium falciparum* merozoite antigens that elicit strain-transcending parasite-neutralizing antibodies. *Infect Immun.* (2013) 81:441–51. doi: 10.1128/IAI.01107-12
10. Crosnier C, Bustamante LY, Bartholdson SJ, Bei AK, Theron M, Uchikawa M, et al. Basigin is a receptor essential for erythrocyte invasion by *Plasmodium falciparum. Nature.* (2011) 480:534–7. doi: 10.1038/nature10606
11. Jin J, Tarrant RD, Bolam EJ, Angell-Manning P, Soegaard M, Pattinson DJ, et al. Production, quality control, stability, and potency of cGMP-produced *Plasmodium falciparum* RH5.1 protein vaccine expressed in Drosophila S2 cells. *NPJ Vaccines.* (2018) 3:32. doi: 10.1038/s41541-018-0071-7
12. Payne RO, Silk SE, Elias SC, Miura K, Diouf A, Galaway F, et al. Human vaccination against RH5 induces neutralizing antimalarial antibodies that inhibit RH5 invasion complex interactions. *JCI Insight.* (2017) 2:96381. doi: 10.1172/jci.insight.96381
13. Baum J, Chen L, Healer J, Lopaticki S, Boyle M, Triglia T, et al. Reticulocyte-binding protein homologue 5 - an essential adhesin involved in invasion of human erythrocytes by *Plasmodium falciparum. Int J Parasitol.* (2009) 39:371–80. doi: 10.1016/j.ijpara.2008.10.006
14. Rodriguez M, Lustigman S, Montero E, Oksov Y, Lobo CA. PfRH5: a novel reticulocyte-binding family homolog of *Plasmodium falciparum* that binds to the erythrocyte, and an investigation of its receptor. *PLoS ONE.* (2008) 3:e3300. doi: 10.1371/journal.pone.0003300
15. Wright KE, Hjerrild KA, Bartlett J, Douglas AD, Jin J, Brown RE, et al. Structure of malaria invasion protein RH5 with erythrocyte basigin and blocking antibodies. *Nature.* (2014) 515:427–30. doi: 10.1038/nature13715
16. Paus D, Winter G. Mapping epitopes and antigenicity by site-directed masking. *Proc Natl Acad Sci USA.* (2006) 103:9172–7. doi: 10.1073/pnas.0600263103
17. Scibienski RJ. Denaturation of lysozyme by Freund's complete adjuvant. *J Immunol.* (1973) 111:114–20.
18. Hu G, Cabrera A, Kono M, Mok S, Chaal BK, Haase S, et al. Transcriptional profiling of growth perturbations of the human malaria parasite *Plasmodium falciparum. Nat Biotechnol.* (2010) 28:91–8. doi: 10.1038/nbt.1597
19. Manske M, Miotto O, Campino S, Auburn S, Almagro-Garcia J, Maslen G, et al. Analysis of *Plasmodium falciparum* diversity in natural infections by deep sequencing. *Nature.* (2012) 487:375–9. doi: 10.1038/nature11174
20. Miotto O, Almagro-Garcia J, Manske M, Macinnis B, Campino S, Rockett KA, et al. Multiple populations of artemisinin-resistant *Plasmodium falciparum* in Cambodia. *Nat Genet.* (2013) 45:648–55. doi: 10.1038/ng.2624
21. Mu J, Awadalla P, Duan J, McGee KM, Keebler J, Seydel K, et al. Genome-wide variation and identification of vaccine targets in the *Plasmodium falciparum* genome. *Nat Genet.* (2007) 39:126–30. doi: 10.1038/ng1924
22. Volkman SK, Sabeti PC, DeCaprio D, Neafsey DE, Schaffner SF, Milner DA, et al. A genome-wide map of diversity in *Plasmodium falciparum. Nat Genet.* (2007) 39:113–9. doi: 10.1038/ng1930
23. Krogh A, Larsson B, von Heijne G, Sonnhammer EL. Predicting transmembrane protein topology with a hidden Markov model: application to complete genomes. *J Mol Biol.* (2001) 305:567–80. doi: 10.1006/jmbi.2000.4315
24. Sridhar S, Reyes-Sandoval A, Draper SJ, Moore AC, Gilbert SC, Gao GP, et al. Single-dose protection against *Plasmodium berghei* by a simian adenovirus vector using a human cytomegalovirus promoter containing intron A. *J Virol.* (2008) 82:3822–33. doi: 10.1128/JVI.02568-07
25. Jin J, Hjerrild KA, Silk SE, Brown RE, Labbé GM, Marshall JM, et al. Accelerating the clinical development of protein-based vaccines for malaria by efficient purification using a four amino acid C-terminal "C-tag". *Int J Parasitol.* (2017) 47:435–46. doi: 10.1016/j.ijpara.2016.12.001
26. Zenonos ZA, Rayner JC, Wright GJ. Towards a comprehensive *Plasmodium falciparum* merozoite cell surface and secreted recombinant protein library. *Malar J.* (2014) 13:93. doi: 10.1186/1475-2875-13-93
27. Durocher Y, Perret S, Kamen A. High-level and high-throughput recombinant protein production by transient transfection of suspension-growing human 293-EBNA1 cells. *Nucleic Acids Res.* (2002) 30:E9. doi: 10.1093/nar/30.2.e9
28. de Cassan SC, Forbes EK, Douglas AD, Milicic A, Singh B, Gupta P, et al. The requirement for potent adjuvants to enhance the immunogenicity and protective efficacy of protein vaccines can be overcome by prior immunization with a recombinant adenovirus. *J Immunol.* (2011) 187:2602–16. doi: 10.4049/jimmunol.1101004
29. Hjerrild KA, Jin J, Wright KE, Brown RE, Marshall JM, Labbé GM, et al. Production of full-length soluble *Plasmodium falciparum* RH5 protein vaccine using a *Drosophila melanogaster* Schneider 2 stable cell line system. *Sci Rep.* (2016) 6:30357. doi: 10.1038/srep30357
30. Williams AR, Douglas AD, Miura K, Illingworth JJ, Choudhary P, Murungi LM, et al. Enhancing blockade of *Plasmodium falciparum* erythrocyte invasion: assessing combinations of antibodies against PfRH5 and other merozoite antigens. *PLoS Pathog.* (2012) 8:e1002991. doi: 10.1371/journal.ppat.1002991
31. Miura K, Orcutt AC, Muratova OV, Miller LH, Saul A, Long CA. Development and characterization of a standardized ELISA including a reference serum on each plate to detect antibodies induced by experimental malaria vaccines. *Vaccine.* (2008a) 26:193–200. doi: 10.1016/j.vaccine.2007.10.064
32. Shinde V, Fries L, Wu Y, Agrawal S, Cho I, Thomas DN, et al. Improved titers against influenza drift variants with a nanoparticle vaccine. *N Engl J Med.* (2018) 378:2346–8. doi: 10.1056/NEJMc1803554
33. Podda A, Del Giudice G. MF59-adjuvanted vaccines: increased immunogenicity with an optimal safety profile. *Expert Rev Vaccines.* (2003) 2:197–204. doi: 10.1586/14760584.2.2.197
34. Wilkins AL, Kazmin D, Napolitani G, Clutterbuck EA, Pulendran B, Siegrist C-A, et al. AS03- and MF59-adjuvanted influenza vaccines in children. *Front Immunol.* (2017) 8:1760. doi: 10.3389/fimmu.2017.01760
35. Petersen TN, Brunak S, von Heijne G, Nielsen H. SignalP 4.0: discriminating signal peptides from transmembrane regions. *Nat Methods.* (2011) 8:785–6. doi: 10.1038/nmeth.1701
36. Bruder JT, Stefaniak ME, Patterson NB, Chen P, Konovalova S, Limbach K, et al. Adenovectors induce functional antibodies capable of potent inhibition of blood stage malaria parasite growth. *Vaccine.* (2010) 28:3201–10. doi: 10.1016/j.vaccine.2010.02.024
37. Draper SJ, Moore AC, Goodman AL, Long CA, Holder AA, Gilbert SC, et al. Effective induction of high-titer antibodies by viral vector vaccines. *Nat Med.* (2008) 14:819–21. doi: 10.1038/nm.1850
38. Kang Y, Calvo PA, Daly TM, Long CA. Comparison of humoral immune responses elicited by DNA and protein vaccines based on merozoite surface protein-1 from *Plasmodium yoelii*, a rodent malaria parasite. *J Immunol.* (1998) 161:4211–9.
39. Galaway F, Drought LG, Fala M, Cross N, Kemp AC, Rayner JC, et al. P113 is a merozoite surface protein that binds the N terminus of *Plasmodium falciparum* RH5. *Nat Commun.* (2017) 8:14333. doi: 10.1038/ncomms14333
40. Raj DK, Nixon CP, Nixon CE, Dvorin JD, DiPetrillo CG, Pond-Tor S, et al. Antibodies to PfSEA-1 block parasite egress from RBCs and protect against malaria infection. *Science.* (2014) 344:871–7. doi: 10.1126/science.1254417
41. Reddy KS, Amlabu E, Pandey AK, Mitra P, Chauhan VS, Gaur D. Multiprotein complex between the GPI-anchored CyRPA with PfRH5 and PfRipr is crucial for *Plasmodium falciparum* erythrocyte invasion. *Proc Natl Acad Sci USA.* (2015) 112:1179–84. doi: 10.1073/pnas.1415466112
42. Crosnier C, Wanaguru M, McDade B, Osier FH, Marsh K, Rayner JC, et al. A library of functional recombinant cell-surface and secreted *P. falciparum* merozoite proteins. *Mol Cell Proteomics.* (2013) 12:3976–86. doi: 10.1074/mcp.O113.028357
43. Srivastava A, Singh S, Dhawan S, Mahmood Alam M, Mohmmed A, Chitnis CE. Localization of apical sushi protein in *Plasmodium falciparum* merozoites. *Mol Biochem Parasitol.* (2010) 174:66–9. doi: 10.1016/j.molbiopara.2010.06.003
44. Zuccala ES, Gout AM, Dekiwadia C, Marapana DS, Angrisano F, Turnbull L, et al. Subcompartmentalisation of proteins in the rhoptries correlates with

ordered events of erythrocyte invasion by the blood stage malaria parasite. *PLoS ONE.* (2012) 7:e46160. doi: 10.1371/journal.pone.0046160

45. Sanders PR, Gilson PR, Cantin GT, Greenbaum DC, Nebl T, Carucci DJ, et al. Distinct protein classes including novel merozoite surface antigens in raft-like membranes of *Plasmodium falciparum*. *J Biol Chem.* (2005) 280:40169–76. doi: 10.1074/jbc.M509631200
46. Elsworth B, Sanders PR, Nebl T, Batinovic S, Kalanon M, Nie CQ, et al. Proteomic analysis reveals novel proteins associated with the plasmodium protein exporter PTEX and a loss of complex stability upon truncation of the core PTEX component, PTEX150. *Cell Microbiol.* (2016) 18:1551–69. doi: 10.1111/cmi.12596
47. Wickramarachchi T, Devi YS, Mohmmed A, Chauhan VS. Identification and characterization of a novel *Plasmodium falciparum* merozoite apical protein involved in erythrocyte binding and invasion. *PLoS ONE.* (2008) 3:e1732. doi: 10.1371/journal.pone.0001732
48. Bushell KM, Sollner C, Schuster-Boeckler B, Bateman A, Wright GJ. Large-scale screening for novel low-affinity extracellular protein interactions. *Genome Res.* (2008) 18:622–30. doi: 10.1101/gr.7187808
49. Mehlin C, Boni E, Buckner FS, Engel L, Feist T, Gelb MH, et al. Heterologous expression of proteins from *Plasmodium falciparum*: results from 1000 genes. *Mol Biochem Parasitol.* (2006) 148:144–60. doi: 10.1016/j.molbiopara.2006.03.011
50. Fernández-Robledo JA, Vasta GR. Production of recombinant proteins from protozoan parasites. *Trends Parasitol.* (2010) 26:244–54. doi: 10.1016/j.pt.2010.02.004
51. Cowman AF, Crabb BS. Invasion of red blood cells by malaria parasites. *Cell.* (2006) 124:755–66. doi: 10.1016/j.cell.2006.02.006
52. Cowman AF, Baldi DL, Healer J, Mills KE, O'Donnell RA, Reed MB, et al. Functional analysis of proteins involved in *Plasmodium falciparum* merozoite invasion of red blood cells. *FEBS Lett.* (2000) 476:84–8. doi: 10.1016/S0014-5793(00)01703-8
53. Saint RB, Coppel RL, Cowman AF, Brown GV, Shi PT, Barzaga N, et al. Changes in repeat number, sequence, and reading frame in S-antigen genes of *Plasmodium falciparum*. *Mol Cell Biol.* (1987) 7:2968–73. doi: 10.1128/MCB.7.8.2968
54. Bustamante LY, Powell GT, Lin Y-C, Macklin MD, Cross N, Kemp A, et al. Synergistic malaria vaccine combinations identified by systematic antigen screening. *Proc Natl Acad Sci USA.* (2017) 114:12045–50. doi: 10.1073/pnas.1702944114
55. Favuzza P, Guffart E, Tamborrini M, Scherer B, Dreyer AM, Rufer AC, et al. Structure of the malaria vaccine candidate antigen CyRPA and its complex with a parasite invasion inhibitory antibody. *Elife.* (2017) 6:e20383. doi: 10.7554/eLife.20383
56. Volz JC, Yap A, Sisquella X, Thompson JK, Lim NTY, Whitehead LW, et al. Essential role of the PfRh5/PfRipr/CyRPA complex during *Plasmodium falciparum* invasion of erythrocytes. *Cell Host Microbe.* (2016) 20:60–71. doi: 10.1016/j.chom.2016.06.004
57. Wong W, Huang R, Menant S, Hong C, Sandow JJ, Birkinshaw RW, et al. Structure of *Plasmodium falciparum* Rh5–CyRPA–Ripr invasion complex. *Nature.* (2019) 565:118–21. doi: 10.1038/s41586-018-0779-6
58. Miura K, Zhou H, Moretz SE, Diouf A, Thera MA, Dolo A, et al. Comparison of biological activity of human anti-apical membrane antigen-1 antibodies induced by natural infection and vaccination. *J Immunol.* (2008b) 181:8776–83. doi: 10.4049/jimmunol.181.12.8776
59. Chen L, Xu Y, Wong W, Thompson JK, Healer J, Goddard-Borger ED, et al. Structural basis for inhibition of erythrocyte invasion by antibodies to *Plasmodium falciparum* protein CyRPA. *Elife.* (2017) 6:e21347. doi: 10.7554/eLife.21347
60. Dreyer AM, Matile H, Papastogiannidis P, Kamber J, Favuzza P, Voss TS, et al. Passive immunoprotection of *Plasmodium falciparum*-infected mice designates the CyRPA as candidate malaria vaccine antigen. *J Immunol.* (2012) 188:6225–37. doi: 10.4049/jimmunol.1103177
61. Favuzza P, Blaser S, Dreyer AM, Riccio G, Tamborrini M, Thoma R, et al. Generation of *Plasmodium falciparum* parasite-inhibitory antibodies by immunization with recombinantly-expressed CyRPA. *Malar J.* (2016) 15:161. doi: 10.1186/s12936-016-1213-x
62. Douglas AD, Williams AR, Knuepfer E, Illingworth JJ, Furze JM, Crosnier C, et al. Neutralization of *Plasmodium falciparum* merozoites by antibodies against PfRH5. *J Immunol.* (2014) 192:245–58. doi: 10.4049/jimmunol.1302045
63. Douglas AD, Baldeviano GC, Jin J, Miura K, Diouf A, Zenonos ZA, et al. A defined mechanistic correlate of protection against *Plasmodium falciparum* malaria in non-human primates. *Nat Commun.* (2019) 10:1953. doi: 10.1038/s41467-019-09894-4
64. Osier FH, Feng G, Boyle MJ, Langer C, Zhou J, Richards JS, et al. Opsonic phagocytosis of *Plasmodium falciparum* merozoites: mechanism in human immunity and a correlate of protection against malaria. *BMC Med.* (2014) 12:108. doi: 10.1186/1741-7015-12-108
65. Joos C, Marrama L, Polson HE, Corre S, Diatta AM, Diouf B, et al. Clinical protection from falciparum malaria correlates with neutrophil respiratory bursts induced by merozoites opsonized with human serum antibodies. *PLoS ONE.* (2010) 5:e9871. doi: 10.1371/journal.pone.0009871
66. Khusmith S, Druilhe P. Cooperation between antibodies and monocytes that inhibit *in vitro* proliferation of *Plasmodium falciparum*. *Infect Immun.* (1983) 41:219–23.
67. Chen L, Lopaticki S, Riglar DT, Dekiwadia C, Uboldi AD, Tham WH, et al. An EGF-like protein forms a complex with PfRh5 and is required for invasion of human erythrocytes by *Plasmodium falciparum*. *PLoS Pathog.* (2011) 7:e1002199. doi: 10.1371/journal.ppat.1002199

Permissions

All chapters in this book were first published by Frontiers; hereby published with permission under the Creative Commons Attribution License or equivalent. Every chapter published in this book has been scrutinized by our experts. Their significance has been extensively debated. The topics covered herein carry significant findings which will fuel the growth of the discipline. They may even be implemented as practical applications or may be referred to as a beginning point for another development.

The contributors of this book come from diverse backgrounds, making this book a truly international effort. This book will bring forth new frontiers with its revolutionizing research information and detailed analysis of the nascent developments around the world.

We would like to thank all the contributing authors for lending their expertise to make the book truly unique. They have played a crucial role in the development of this book. Without their invaluable contributions this book wouldn't have been possible. They have made vital efforts to compile up to date information on the varied aspects of this subject to make this book a valuable addition to the collection of many professionals and students.

This book was conceptualized with the vision of imparting up-to-date information and advanced data in this field. To ensure the same, a matchless editorial board was set up. Every individual on the board went through rigorous rounds of assessment to prove their worth. After which they invested a large part of their time researching and compiling the most relevant data for our readers.

The editorial board has been involved in producing this book since its inception. They have spent rigorous hours researching and exploring the diverse topics which have resulted in the successful publishing of this book. They have passed on their knowledge of decades through this book. To expedite this challenging task, the publisher supported the team at every step. A small team of assistant editors was also appointed to further simplify the editing procedure and attain best results for the readers.

Apart from the editorial board, the designing team has also invested a significant amount of their time in understanding the subject and creating the most relevant covers. They scrutinized every image to scout for the most suitable representation of the subject and create an appropriate cover for the book.

The publishing team has been an ardent support to the editorial, designing and production team. Their endless efforts to recruit the best for this project, has resulted in the accomplishment of this book. They are a veteran in the field of academics and their pool of knowledge is as vast as their experience in printing. Their expertise and guidance has proved useful at every step. Their uncompromising quality standards have made this book an exceptional effort. Their encouragement from time to time has been an inspiration for everyone.

The publisher and the editorial board hope that this book will prove to be a valuable piece of knowledge for researchers, students, practitioners and scholars across the globe.

List of Contributors

Jennifer Hanley and Sue D. Xiang
Department of Immunology and Pathology, Faculty of Medicine, Nursing and Health Sciences, Central Clinical School, Monash University, Melbourne, VIC, Australia

Dodie Pouniotis
School of Health and Biomedical Sciences, RMIT University, Bundoora, VIC, Australia

Kirsty L. Wilson and Magdalena Plebanski
Department of Immunology and Pathology, Faculty of Medicine, Nursing and Health Sciences, Central Clinical School, Monash University, Melbourne, VIC, Australia
School of Health and Biomedical Sciences, RMIT University, Bundoora, VIC, Australia

Charles Ma and Ross L. Coppel
Department of Microbiology, Monash University, Clayton, VIC, Australia

Rinter Kimathi, James Mburu, Kennedy Mwai, Nelson Kibinge, Reuben Yaa, Emily Chepsat, James M. Njunge, Timothy Chege, Linda M. Murungi and Philip Bejon
KEMRI-Welcome Trust Research Programme, Centre for Geographic Medicine Research—Coast, Kilifi, Kenya

Micha Rosenkranz and Roland Frank
Centre for Infectious Diseases, Parasitology, Heidelberg University Hospital, Heidelberg, Germany

Gathoni Kamuyu
KEMRI-Welcome Trust Research Programme, Centre for Geographic Medicine Research—Coast, Kilifi, Kenya
Centre for Infectious Diseases, Parasitology, Heidelberg University Hospital, Heidelberg, Germany

James Tuju
Department of Biochemistry, Pwani University, Kilifi, Kenya

Marisa Chong Kwan and Sam Hawkings
Arrayjet, Innovative Microarray Solutions, Edinburgh, United Kingdom

Fatuma Guleid
Department of Pathology, University of Cape Town, Cape Town, South Africa

Christopher K. Kariuki
Department of Tropical and Infectious Diseases, Institute of Primate Research, Nairobi, Kenya
Cellular and Molecular Immunology, Vrije Universiteit Brussels, Brussels, Belgium

Samson M. Kinyanjui
KEMRI-Wellcome Trust Research Programme, Centre for Geographic Medicine Research—Coast, Kilifi, Kenya
Department of Biochemistry, Pwani University, Kilifi, Kenya
Centre for Tropical Medicine and Global Health, Nuffield Department of Clinical Medicine, University of Oxford, Oxford, United Kingdom

Faith H. A. Osier
KEMRI-Wellcome Trust Research Programme, Centre for Geographic Medicine Research—Coast, Kilifi, Kenya
Centre for Infectious Diseases, Parasitology, Heidelberg University Hospital, Heidelberg, Germany
Department of Biochemistry, Pwani university, Kilifi, Kenya
Centre for Tropical Medicine and Global Health, Nuffield Department of Clinical Medicine, University of Oxford, Oxford, United Kingdom

Anna Färnert
Division of Infectious Diseases, Department of Medicine Solna, Karolinska Institutet, Stockholm, Sweden
Department of Infectious Diseases, Karolinska University Hospital, Stockholm, Sweden

Kevin K. A. Tetteh
Immunology and Infection Department, London School of Hygiene and Tropical Medicine, London, United Kingdom

James G. Beeson
Burnet Institute, Melbourne, VIC, Australia
Central Clinical School, Monash University, Melbourne, VIC, Australia
Department of Medicine, University of Melbourne, Melbourne, VIC, Australia

David J. Conway
Pathogen Molecular Biology Department, London School of Hygiene and Tropical Medicine, London, United Kingdom

Kevin Marsh
KEMRI-Wellcome Trust Research Programme, Centre for Geographic Medicine Research—Coast, Kilifi, Kenya
Centre for Tropical Medicine and Global Health, Nuffield Department of Clinical Medicine, University of Oxford, Oxford, United Kingdom
African Academy of Sciences, Nairobi, Kenya

Julian C. Rayner
Wellcome Sanger Institute, Hinxton, Cambridge, United Kingdom

Leslie S. Itsara, Yaxian Zhou, Julie Do, Alexis M. Grieser and Anil K. Ghosh
MalarVx, Inc., Seattle, WA, United States

Ashley M. Vaughan
Seattle Children's Research Institute, Seattle, WA, United States

Florian Brod, Iona Taylor, Yuanyuan Li, Arianna Marini, Ahmed M. Salman, Alexandra J. Spencer and Sumi Biswas
Jenner Institute, University of Oxford, Oxford, United Kingdom

Kazutoyo Miura and Carole A. Long
Laboratory of Malaria and Vector Research, National Institute of Allergy and Infectious Disease, National Institutes of Health, Rockville, MD, United States

Yun Shan Goh
Singapore Immunology Network (SIgN), Agency for Science, Technology and Research (A_STAR), Biopolis, Singapore, Singapore

Daniel McGuire
Singapore Immunology Network (SIgN), Agency for Science, Technology and Research (A_STAR), Biopolis, Singapore, Singapore
School of Biological Sciences, Nanyang Technological University, Singapore, Singapore

Laurent Rénia
Singapore Immunology Network (SIgN), Agency for Science, Technology and Research (A_STAR), Biopolis, Singapore, Singapore
School of Biological Sciences, Nanyang Technological University, Singapore, Singapore
Department of Microbiology and Immunology, Yong Loo Lin School of Medicine, National University of Singapore, Singapore, Singapore

Aloysious Ssemaganda, Ashwini Kumar Giddam, Mehfuz Zaman, Danielle I. Stanisic and Michael F. Good
Institute for Glycomics, Griffith University, Southport, QLD, Australia

Mariusz Skwarczynski
School of Chemistry and Molecular Biosciences, the University of Queensland, Brisbane, QLD, Australia

Istvan Toth
School of Chemistry and Molecular Biosciences, the University of Queensland, Brisbane, QLD, Australia
School of Pharmacy, the University of Queensland, Brisbane, QLD, Australia
Institute for Molecular Bioscience, the University of Queensland, Brisbane, QLD, Australia

Rajiv Kumar
Department of Biochemistry, Institute of Science, Banaras Hindu University, Varanasi India
Centre of Experimental Medicine and Surgery, Institute of Medical Sciences, Banaras Hindu University, Varanasi, India

Susanna Ng and Christian Engwerda
Immunology and Infection Lab, QIMR Berghofer Medical Research Institute, Brisbane, QLD, Australia

Kwadwo Asamoah Kusi and Michael Fokuo Ofori
Department of Biochemistry, Cell and Molecular Biology, West African Centre for Cell Biology of Infectious Pathogens, College of Basic and Applied Sciences, University of Ghana, Accra, Ghana
Immunology Department, College of Health Sciences, Noguchi Memorial Institute for Medical Research, University of Ghana, Accra, Ghana

Augustina Frimpong
African Institute for Mathematical Sciences, Cape Coast, Ghana

Wilfred Ndifon
African Institute for Mathematical Sciences, University of Stellenbosch, Cape Town, South Africa

Georgina Bowyer, Amy Grobbelaa, Tommy Rampling, Navin Venkatraman, Adrian V. S. Hill and Katie J. Ewer
The Jenner Institute, University of Oxford, Oxford, United Kingdom

Danielle Morelle and Ripley W. Ballou
GSK Vaccines, Rixensart, Belgium

Xi Zen Yap and Gaoqian Feng
Burnet Institute, Melbourne, VIC, Australia
Department of Medicine, The University of Melbourne, Parkville, VIC, Australia

Joanne Pooley
Department of Biochemistry and Molecular Biology and Biomedicine Discovery Institute, Monash University, Clayton, VIC, Australia

Meredith O'Keeffe
Burnet Institute, Melbourne, VIC, Australia
Department of Biochemistry and Molecular Biology and Biomedicine Discovery Institute, Monash University, Clayton, VIC, Australia

James G. Beeson
Burnet Institute, Melbourne, VIC, Australia
Department of Medicine, The University of Melbourne, Parkville, VIC, Australia
Department of Microbiology, Monash University, Clayton, VIC, Australia
Central Clinical School, Monash University, Melbourne, VIC, Australia
Department of Medicine, Dentistry, and Health Sciences, The University of Melbourne, Parkville, VIC, Australia
Department of Microbiology and Central Clinical School, Monash University, Clayton, VIC, Australia

Rajeev K. Tyagi
Division of Gastroenterology, Hepatology and Nutrition, Department of Medicine, Vanderbilt University Medical Center, Nashville, TN, United States
Biomedical parasitology Unit, Institute Pasteur, Paris, France
Department of Global Health, College of Public Health, University of South Florida, Tampa, FL, United States

Nikunj Tandel and Richa Deshpande
Institute of Science, Nirma University, Ahmedabad, India

Robert W. Engelman
Department of Pediatrics, Pathology and Cell Biology, University of South Florida, Tampa, FL, United States

Satish D. Patel
Zydus Research Centre, Ahmedabad, India

Priyanka Tyagi
Department of Basic and Applied Sciences, School of Engineering, GD Goenka University, Gurgaon, India

Rachel J. Lundie
Burnet Institute, Melbourne, VIC, Australia
Department of Biochemistry and Molecular Biology, Biomedicine Discovery Institute, Monash University, Clayton, VIC, Australia

D. Channe Gowda and Xianzhu Wu
Department of Biochemistry and Molecular Biology, The Pennsylvania State University College of Medicine, Hershey, PA, United States

Colin J. Sutherland
Department of Immunology and Infection, Faculty of Infectious and Tropical Diseases, London School of Hygiene and Tropical Medicine, London, United Kingdom

Joseph J. Illingworth, Daniel G. Alanine, Rebecca Brown, Jennifer M. Marshall, Helen E. Bartlett, Sarah E. Silk, Geneviève M. Labbé, Doris Quinkert, Jee Sun Cho, David J. Pattinson Lea Barfod, Alexander D. Douglas, Michael W. Shea, Simone C. de Cassan and Simon J. Draper
Jenner Institute, University of Oxford, Oxford, United Kingdom

Susheel K. Singh and Michael Theisen
Department for Congenital Disorders, Statens Serum Institut, Copenhagen, Denmark
Centre for Medical Parasitology at Department of International Health, Immunology and Microbiology, University of Copenhagen and Department of Infectious Diseases, Copenhagen University Hospital, Rigshospitalet, Copenhagen, Denmark

Jonas A. Kengne-Ouafo and Gordon A. Awandare
West African Centre for Cell Biology of Infectious Pathogens, University of Ghana, Accra, Ghana

Susan Thrane, Bishwanath K. Chourasia, Morten A. Nielsen, Ali Salanti and Adam F. Sander
Centre for Medical Parasitology at Department of International Health, Immunology and Microbiology, University of Copenhagen and Department of Infectious Diseases, Copenhagen University Hospital, Rigshospitalet, Copenhagen, Denmark

Karina Teelen, Wouter Graumans, Rianne Stoter, Geert-Jan van Gemert, Marga G. van de Vegte-Bolmer, Robert W. Sauerwein and Matthijs M. Jore
Department of Medical Microbiology, Radboud University Medical Center, Nijmegen, Netherlands

Xi Zen Yap
Burnet Institute, Melbourne, VIC, Australia
Department of Medicine, Dentistry, and Health Sciences, The University of Melbourne, Parkville, VIC, Australia

Britta C. Urban
Faculty of Biological Sciences, Liverpool School of Tropical Medicine, Liverpool, United Kingdom

Bismarck Dinko
Department of Biomedical Sciences, School of Basic and Biomedical Sciences, University of Health and Allied Sciences, Ho, Ghana

Jason P. Wendler
Wellcome Trust Centre for Human Genetics, University of Oxford, Oxford, United Kingdom

Katherine E. Wright and Matthew K. Higgins
Department of Biochemistry, University of Oxford, Oxford, United Kingdom

Index

www.ingramcontent.com/pod-product-compliance
Lightning Source LLC
LaVergne TN
LVHW081029210926
848485LV00004B/978